The Evolution of Social Behaviour

How can the stunning diversity of social systems and behaviours seen in nature be explained? Drawing on social evolution theory, experimental evidence and studies conducted in the field, this book outlines the fundamental principles of social evolution underlying this phenomenal richness. To succeed in the competition for resources, organisms may either 'race' to be quicker than others, 'fight' for privileged access, or 'share' their efforts and gains. The authors show how the ecology and intrinsic attributes of organisms select for each of these strategies, and how a handful of straightforward concepts explain the evolution of successful decision rules in behavioural interactions, whether among members of the same or different species. With a broad focus ranging from microorganisms to humans, this is the first book to provide students and researchers with a comprehensive account of the evolution of sociality by natural selection.

Michael Taborsky is Professor of Behavioural Ecology at the University of Bern, Switzerland. His research focuses on evolutionary principles underlying social behaviour, combining empirical research on insects, spiders, fish, birds and mammals with theoretical and conceptual approaches.

Michael A. Cant is Professor of Evolutionary Biology at the University of Exeter, UK. His research focuses on the evolution of animal societies. His work combines theoretical modelling with empirical tests in social insects and cooperatively breeding mammals.

Jan Komdeur is Professor of Evolutionary Ecology at the University of Groningen, The Netherlands. His research focuses on the evolution of social and cooperative behaviour. He tests theoretical concepts using experimental approaches combined with long-term studies in a variety of insects and birds.

The Evolution of Social Behaviour

MICHAEL TABORSKY
University of Bern

MICHAEL A. CANT
University of Exeter, Cornwall Campus

JAN KOMDEUR
University of Groningen

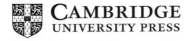
CAMBRIDGE
UNIVERSITY PRESS

CAMBRIDGE
UNIVERSITY PRESS

University Printing House, Cambridge CB2 8BS, United Kingdom

One Liberty Plaza, 20th Floor, New York, NY 10006, USA

477 Williamstown Road, Port Melbourne, VIC 3207, Australia

314–321, 3rd Floor, Plot 3, Splendor Forum, Jasola District Centre, New Delhi – 110025, India

103 Penang Road, #05–06/07, Visioncrest Commercial, Singapore 238467

Cambridge University Press is part of the University of Cambridge.

It furthers the University's mission by disseminating knowledge in the pursuit of
education, learning, and research at the highest international levels of excellence.

www.cambridge.org
Information on this title: www.cambridge.org/9781107011182
DOI: 10.1017/9780511894794

© Michael Taborsky, Michael A. Cant and Jan Komdeur 2021

First published 2021

Printed in the United Kingdom by TJ Books Limited, Padstow Cornwall

A catalogue record for this publication is available from the British Library.

ISBN 978-1-107-01118-2 Hardback
ISBN 978-1-108-74616-8 Paperback

To our students, present, past and future

Contents

Foreword by Nick Davies   *page* xiii
Preface   xv

1   Introduction   1
  1.1   A Historical Perspective   3
  1.2   Dealing with Competition   6
    1.2.1   Competition for Food   8
    1.2.2   Competition for Shelter   8
    1.2.3   Competition for Mates and Social Partners   10
    1.2.4   Competition for Multiple Resources   12
  1.3   The Tension between Conflict and Cooperation   13
  1.4   Conceptual and Semantic Confusions   13
  Box 1.1   The Meaning of Terms and a Glossary for the Concepts
    of Social Behaviour, Conflict and Cooperation   15
  1.5   The Focus of this Book   20
  CASE STUDY A: SEYCHELLES WARBLER   25

2   Non-interference Rivalry   35
  2.1   Competition: The Engine of Natural Selection   35
  2.2   Ecological Influences on the Nature of Competition   36
    2.2.1   Resource Availability and Renewal   37
    2.2.2   Clumping in Space and Time   38
    2.2.3   Predictability in Space and Time   39
    2.2.4   Divisibility   41
    2.2.5   Predation and Other Ecological Features   41
  2.3   Scramble Strategies and Animal Distributions   42
    2.3.1   Evolving Scramble Effort   44
  2.4   Competition and Collective Movement   46
  2.5   Competition for Information   48
    2.5.1   Social Learning and Recruitment of Others   48
    2.5.2   Producers, Scroungers and Deception   50
  2.6   Social Influences on Competition   52
    2.6.1   Population Density and Competition   53
    2.6.2   Sexual Conflict   55

2.6.3	Alternative Reproductive Tactics	55
2.6.4	Conditional Strategies	58
2.7	Conclusions	59
	CASE STUDY B: BANDED MONGOOSE	61

3 **Conflict** 67

3.1	Conflict and Cooperation	67
3.2	Sources of Conflict in Social Groups	72
	3.2.1 Conflict over Group Membership	72
	3.2.2 Conflict over Rank	77
	3.2.2.1 Dominance–Submission	80
	3.2.3 Conflict over Reproduction	82
	3.2.3.1 Reproductive Skew	82
	3.2.3.2 Mating Skew	87
	3.2.3.3 Parental Care	88
	3.2.3.4 Conflict over Helping	90
3.3	Social Conflict: Theoretical Approaches	92
	3.3.1 Structured Population Models	92
	3.3.2 Sealed Bid Models: Battleground and Resolution	97
	3.3.2.1 Battleground Models	97
	3.3.2.2 Resolution Models	99
	Box 3.1 Contest Success Functions	101
	3.3.2.3 Evolving Peace	105
	3.3.3 Behavioural Conflict: Threats, Negotiation and Assessment	106
	3.3.3.1 Threats and Coercion: Sequential Models	107
	3.3.3.2 Negotiation Models	112
	3.3.3.3 Assessment Models	113
3.4	Evolutionary Routes to Conflict Reduction	117
	3.4.1 Kin Selection	117
	3.4.2 Repression of Competition	118
	3.4.2.1 Reproductive Dictatorship	118
	3.4.2.2 Reproductive Levelling	118
	3.4.2.3 Life History Segregation	119
	3.4.2.4 Outgroup Threat	120
3.5	Intergroup Conflict and Cooperation	121
	3.5.1 Consequences of Intergroup Conflict: Empirical Patterns	124
	3.5.2 Intergroup Cooperation and the Major Transitions	126
3.6	Conclusions	128
	CASE STUDY C: PAPER WASP	130

4 **Cooperation** 136

4.1	Cooperation for Fitness Benefits	137
	4.1.1 By-product Benefits or Mutualism	139
	Box 4.1 Mutual Fitness Benefits by Group Augmentation	140

Box 4.2 Mutualism, By-product Mutualism and 'Pseudoreciprocity':
    What is the Difference? 142
    4.1.2   Correlated Pay-offs 144
        4.1.2.1   Reciprocity 145
            4.1.2.1.1   Three Types of Information; Three Types of
                Reciprocity 145
            4.1.2.1.2   Generalized Reciprocity 146
Box 4.3 Conditions and Mechanisms for the Evolution of
    Generalized Reciprocity 146
            4.1.2.1.3   Direct Reciprocity 149
            4.1.2.1.4   Indirect Reciprocity 149
            4.1.2.1.5   The Importance of Information 149
            4.1.2.1.6   Cooperation on Networks and Graphs 151
            4.1.2.1.7   When Should We Expect Reciprocity? 160
            4.1.2.1.8   Which Type of Reciprocity Should We
                Expect? 166
Box 4.4 Reciprocal Cooperation in Norway Rats 167
Box 4.5 Biological Markets and Cooperation 175
            4.1.2.1.9   Negotiations and Trading 177
        4.1.2.2   Kin Selection 180
            4.1.2.2.1   Evidence for Kin-directed Care in Social
                Systems 184
            4.1.2.2.2   Mechanisms to Promote Kin-directed
                Helping 186
            4.1.2.2.3   Inadvertent Kin-directed Care 187
                4.1.2.2.3.1   Longevity as a Driver for
                      Inadvertent Kin-directed
                      Cooperation 189
                4.1.2.2.3.2   Limited Natal Dispersal 192
                4.1.2.2.3.3   High Breeding Site
                      Fidelity 195
                4.1.2.2.3.4   Lekking and Mate Sharing 196
Box 4.6 Nepotistic Cooperation in Alarm-calling and Vigilance 197
                4.1.2.2.3.5   Dispersal in Kin
                      Coalitions 202
            4.1.2.2.4   Kin Discrimination Involving Kin
                Recognition 202
Box 4.7 Fitness Benefits of Dispersing in Coalitions of Relatives 203
            4.1.2.2.5   Mechanisms Underlying Active Kin
                Discrimination 209
            4.1.2.2.6   Ecological Determinants of Kin-clustering
                and Cooperation 213
            4.1.2.2.7   Kin Selection and Sexual Conflict
                Resolution 216

4.1.2.2.8 Kin Associations Do Not Always Lead to
Cooperation   221
4.1.2.2.9 Inbreeding and Kin-selected Benefits   226
Box 4.8 Selective Paternal Care and Cannibalism in Fish Males   230
4.1.2.2.10 Absence of Adjustment of Social Behaviour
to Kinship   233
4.2 Forced Cooperation   237
4.2.1 Coercion   238
4.2.1.1 Power Symmetry   238
Box 4.9 When Does Punishment Create Cooperation, and How Common is
it in Nature?   239
4.2.1.2 Power Asymmetry   243
4.2.2 Surreptitious Exploitation   246
4.3 Conclusions   247
CASE STUDY D: SOCIAL CICHLID   251

5   Interspecific Relations   263
5.1   Types of Interspecific Interactions   266
5.2   Non-interference Rivalry   266
5.2.1   Character Displacement   266
5.2.2   Specialists versus Generalists   268
5.3   Conflict   271
5.3.1   Interspecific Resource Monopolization   271
5.3.2   How to Deal with Predators: Interspecific
Associations   274
Box 5.1   Interspecific Brood Mixing in Cichlids Through Passive or
Active Processes   277
5.3.3   Host–Parasite Relations   280
5.4   Cooperation   284
5.4.1   Commensalism   285
5.4.2   Mutualism   286
5.4.3   Reciprocity   288
5.4.4   Manipulation   294
5.5   Conclusions   294
CASE STUDY E: AMBROSIA BEETLE   297

6   Synopsis   309
6.1   Race   309
6.2   Fight   310
6.3   Share   312
6.4   Interspecific Interactions   315
6.5   General Conclusions   317
6.5.1   Optimal Responses to Competition   317
6.5.2   Future Directions   318

6.5.3   Less Encouraged   319
6.5.4   Final Inference   320

CASE STUDY F: *HOMO SAPIENS*   321

References   327
Subject Index   398
Taxonomic Index   404

Colour plates can be found between pages 174 and 175.

Foreword

The fruitful interplay between social theory and field studies, which forms the central theme of this wonderful book, will be inspirational to new students and experienced researchers alike. Without theory, both to guide our observations and to interpret them, we 'might as well go into a gravel-pit and count the pebbles' wrote Charles Darwin in 1861 in a letter to a colleague. He was referring to geological studies, but his remarks, of course, apply with equal force to studies of social behaviour.

When I was a young student in the early 1970s, my bird watching was rescued from pebble counting by the ideas of David Lack, who had shown how an ecological stage of food resources and predation risk provides selection pressures which shape the evolution of avian social behaviour. I then remember my excitement, a few years later, when I first encountered Bill Hamilton's theory of kin selection and the ideas of Robert Trivers and Geoff Parker on sexual and family conflicts.

Suddenly, a whole new world was opened up, one in which the stage for behavioural evolution was set not only by ecological pressures but by social pressures, too. At around the same time, DNA profiling became available as a method for precise measures of maternity and paternity in wild populations. This thrilling combination of new ideas and new techniques led to a blossoming of field studies of social behaviour, and discoveries of how individual decision making influences fitness, which have continued ever since and which are celebrated in this volume.

The tensions between social cooperation and conflict are familiar themes in our own lives and for centuries they have inspired our art and literature. Why, then, did it take so long to realize that these same tensions also seethe away in animal societies? Perhaps it was wariness of anthropomorphism; yet imagining what you yourself might do in a particular social situation, if you were a dungfly or a dunnock, for example, is a powerful way of gaining insights into evolution because assessing the costs and benefits in order to choose the best course of action simulates the workings of natural selection.

The three authors here make a brilliant team. They have themselves made novel contributions to theory, but they have also all gone out into the field to test the ideas, with long-term studies of complex social systems: of cichlid fish in Lake Tanganyika (Michael Taborsky), of banded mongooses in Uganda and of paper wasps in Europe (Michael Cant) and of warblers in remote islands of the Seychelles (Jan Komdeur). Their painstaking field studies have shown the ingenuity needed to untangle how social behaviour influences fitness. All three parameters in Hamilton's famous rule –

B, C and r – are challenging to measure and detailed observations and elegant experiments are needed to tease apart complex selection pressures. The two-way interaction between theoretical insights and field studies has revealed unsuspected richness in social behaviour in the natural world.

We are often warned how a peek at the ending before you start can spoil a book, but I recommend that this is exactly what the reader should do here. Start with the final box, a case study of our own species and how a careful consideration of kinship theory, evidence and comparison with another long-lived mammal, killer whales, gives new insights into the evolution of the menopause. Then work your way back to the front of the book through all the other boxes of the authors' case studies (ambrosia beetles, social cichlids, paper wasps, banded mongooses, Seychelles warblers). You'll then have experienced just the right mix of theory and respect for the complexities and wonders of the natural world to be ready to start at the beginning and to be inspired as you read the book right through.

Nick Davies
Department of Zoology, University of Cambridge, UK

Preface

The study of social behaviour is the most relatable of scientific topics, because all humans study social behaviour. Of course we spend a great deal of our time studying each other, but our fascination extends far beyond humans. As children we delight in poking insects or tadpoles to see what happens; later many of us become avid pet-watchers or naturalists. Our media wow us with stories about the curious lives of organisms we've never heard of, or new insights into the minds of the animals that we think we know best. All of us are captivated by wildlife films full of drama, struggle, and beauty. No doubt there are deep evolutionary reasons for our fascination with the behaviour of other organisms, and what they can tell us about ourselves. And, increasingly, we desire ultimate, evolutionary explanations of behaviour. It is no longer enough to describe what other organisms do. We want to know why.

This book is our attempt to explain why, or as much about why as we currently know. Behind the breathtaking film sequence or curious news story typically lies the quiet work of researchers and students who are, like us, fascinated by the why questions. We describe the evolutionary theories that attempt to explain why different patterns of social behaviour evolve and the evidence for or against these theories. Like any scientific subject, the study of social evolution is a Petri dish of evolution itself: a fierce competition of ideas, subject to fashions and fads, dissension and debate. An example is the group selection/kin selection debate, which has generated lots of heat *and* light. We've tried to concentrate on the light that is produced when brilliant ideas collide, and avoid where possible being drawn off course by whirlpools of debate.

We have two major foci that are evident throughout the book. The first is a focus on theory. The theory of social evolution has transformed our understanding of social behaviour over the last 60 years, and applies to every taxon of life. One of the most active frontiers of research is the social evolution of microbes, where experiments can follow the evolution of social behaviour over hundreds or thousands of generations in the laboratory. In the same university department one might find researchers using cultural evolution theory to understand the spread of human traditions and innovations over the last 10,000 years. The formal theories employed, rooted in population genetics and game theory, are the same whether the study system is a virus or a cancer, a slime mould or a human society, and whether information is inherited genetically or culturally or, increasingly, digitally. The reach of social evolution theory is remarkable, and provides an overarching framework for thought and experiment on vastly different natural phenomena. This is one aspect of studying social behaviour that makes us feel fortunate in our choice of topic.

The second focus is on field research and reflects our own experience as behavioural ecologists who work primarily on wild animals. Field research is difficult to carry out and difficult to fund. It also has some powerful advantages. Studying natural populations gives us a picture of what variation is available to natural selection, and allows us to measure the fitness outcomes associated with this variation. Evolutionary models explore the evolution of adaptations, where an adaptive trait is that which has the highest fitness out of those traits that are available to natural selection. Fitness itself is a notoriously slippery concept to define, never mind measure, but field biologists have grown expert at measuring proxies of fitness such as the number of surviving offspring or, better still, lifetime reproductive success. In this way field research, particularly long-term research, can quantify the fitness consequences of alternative behaviour in animals living in the environment in which they evolved, exposed to their (coevolved) predators and pathogens, buffeted by unpredictable and uncontrolled ecological variation. The result is a line-of-sight connection between theory and the things being measured, and the chance to feed back lessons from reality, in all its messiness, into the neat and tidy models. Experiments under natural or semi-natural but controlled conditions can then nail down causal effects.

The book was motivated and organized by Michael Taborsky, who had the original concept and approached Jan and Mike to share the writing. Each section was spearheaded by one of the three authors, with lots of discussion and input from the other two. We completed much of the writing at a series of writing retreats in Switzerland, The Netherlands and the UK, where we could escape other responsibilities and talk at length in between putting pen to paper. Along the way we found many topics on which we had complementary expertise, but also different perspectives, gleaned from years spent watching and thinking about very different types of animal. Finding common ground by talking out our differences has been one of the most rewarding and interesting aspects of the work. Needless to say, we don't agree on everything, and we decided early on that the book was best served by allowing each of us to shape our parts of the text as we wished. So while we haven't tried to homogenize our voices, we've tried to find some kind of harmony between them, and to capitalize as much as possible on our varied experiences and study organisms.

This book aims to serve varied purposes. When thinking about fundamental concepts and the evidence for or against particular ideas, we had in mind our colleagues who would put our conclusions to the test. When outlining our framework and logic of thought, we tried to envisage how our information would help students to understand the evolutionary processes governing social behaviour. When indulging in our fascination for the staggering wealth of social patterns in nature, we thought of the interested amateur who might be prompted to take a closer look at behaviour and to make sense of the ecological circumstances that call forth one pattern rather than another. Above all, our hope is to transmit our enthusiasm for this topic to everyone who shares a curiosity and motivation to understand the sublime diversity of form and function in the world, and how we got here.

We are grateful to our universities for making this work possible and to Cambridge University Press for their patience and continued support, with a heartfelt thank you to our editors, Aleksandra Serocka, Jenny van der Meijden and Megan Keirnan. We acknowledge particularly our graphical designers, Michelle Gygax and Dick Visser, for their excellent illustrations, and Claudia Leiser for preparing the indices. We thank our colleagues Gerry Carter, Darren Croft, Raghavendra Gadagkar, Sjouke Kingma, Bram Kuijper, Nick Royle, Barbara Taborsky and Franjo Weissing for reading the book manuscript and helping us greatly to improve it. Last but not least, we owe thanks to our loved ones who generously condoned our occupation with this inspiring but time-draining endeavour.

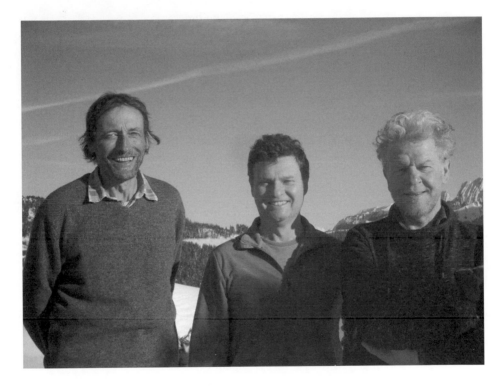

The authors arriving at one of their writing retreats at a Swiss chalet.

1　Introduction

Why is the evolution of social behaviour interesting? For one thing, if we wish to comprehend the origin, maintenance and functionality of any biological trait, we need to understand its *evolution*. At the same time, each behaviour is *social* in essence; it affects the survival, production and reproduction of others in some way or another. 'Others' encompasses social partners including mates, offspring, competitors, friends and foes regardless.

But what is it that brings animals together? Why are individuals attracted by others, interact with them or form groups? What explains the staggering diversity of animal social systems? To start to address these questions it seems useful to distinguish between ecological causes and the functions of social behaviour. For instance, it may be safer to be in a group because of high predation pressure, which represents an ecological cause for social contact, or it may be beneficial to aggregate to choose a mating partner, which is a functional reason for social attraction. Obviously, ecological causes and social functions can be intertwined. In any case, living together entails competition for resources and involves different types of interactions between conspecific contenders, which show different functional characteristics and fulfil different roles (Wilson 1975).

A conspicuous attribute of social units that immediately catches one's eye is the size of a group. Clearly, the smallest social unit is a group of two or a 'dyad', whereas there is no defined upper limit to group size, if we imagine vast fish schools, ant colonies or herds of wildebeest. But not only is the number of partners important for the evolution of adaptive responses to the challenges involved in social interactions, the relationship between partners and the dynamics of group membership are also essential. At one end of the spectrum, groups may form in which there is little or no relationship between members; for instance, aggregations may just reflect the distribution of resources. At the other end of the spectrum, groups may consist of particular individuals that are not exchangeable because they fulfil certain roles that are complementary, or are characterized by individual (personalized) relationships among group members. Hence social units can be characterized both by group size and composition and by their membership dynamics.

Dyads refer to interactions between two players, corresponding to the most basic units of sociality. Dyadic interactions may be short-term, such as when an intruder confronts a territory owner or when a male and a female mate in a promiscuous mating system. In contrast, they may last for extended periods, perhaps an entire lifetime, such as when sibling partners share resources and mates (Maynard Smith & Ridpath 1972; Foster 1977, 1981; Packer & Pusey 1982; Packer et al. 1991; Krakauer 2005; Krakauer & DuVal 2011), and in permanent monogamous pairs (Klug 2018; Kvarnemo 2018). As dyads constitute the simplest social structure, most theoretical models dealing with behavioural decisions in competitive situations have focused on this interaction unit (Kokko 2013). Well-known examples include the game-theoretical treatments of pair-wise contests (Maynard-Smith 1982a), whether in singular (e.g. one-shot games; Rand et al. 2013) or repeated interactions (e.g. iterated prisoner's dilemma games; Axelrod & Hamilton 1981). Experiments using dyads to study social decisions are also abundant due to the methodical manageability and clear predictability of behaviour (Hsu et al. 2006; Arnott & Elwood 2009; Lehner et al. 2011; Green & Patek 2018; Schweinfurth & Taborsky 2018a, 2018b).

Multi-member open groups denote assemblies of individuals characterized by dynamic membership and are often rather temporary. Examples include foraging and mating aggregations, migratory groups, schools, shoals, swarms and flocks. The functional causes of such aggregations may be the underlying distribution of used resources (Bentley et al. 2001; Bos et al. 2004; Masse & Cote 2013; Halliwell et al. 2017), reproduction (Domeier & Colin 1997; Campbell et al. 2008), the reduction of predation risk (Foster & Treherne 1981; Pitcher 1986; van der Marel et al. 2019), or the use of public information either to find resources (Coolen et al. 2003; Canonge et al. 2011; Laidre 2013; Bijleveld et al. 2015) or to increase safety (Thünken et al. 2014a; Mehlis et al. 2015).

Multi-member closed groups are characterized by more or less stable membership. Such groups may be rather unstructured, like certain aggregations that remain localized but lack specific relationships (such as dominance) among group members (e.g. long-term, localized, non-reproductive aggregations in cichlid fish; Taborsky & Limberger 1981). Alternatively, closed groups with little immigration, if any, may be characterized by individualized relations and a clear structure. In most cases, the functional background of such groups is reproduction, and their specific organization is determined by relatedness, dominance and sex of group members. The simplest and most widespread social units of this type are families with one or both parents caring for their offspring, which often coincides with resource monopolization (Clutton-Brock 1991). Sometimes, such groups persist beyond the completion of brood care, which may coincide with cooperative care of subsequent offspring by parents and young of previous broods (Skutch 1961; Taborsky 1994; Cockburn 1998; Koenig & Dickinson 2016). Alternatively, several group members may reproduce more or less independently and raise their offspring jointly (Eisenberg et al. 1972; Kappeler & van Schaik 2002; Riehl 2011, 2013). The most advanced closed multi-member groups exhibit various levels of task sharing among their members (Lacey & Sherman 1991; Bruintjes & Taborsky 2011; Holbrook et al. 2011; Pruitt & Riechert 2011; Parmentier et al. 2015), which culminates in the lifelong division between reproduction and labour by different castes (Hölldobler & Wilson 1990, 2009; Benton & Foster 1992; Crespi 1992; Thorne 1997; Bornbusch et al. 2018).

So it seems there are numerous reasons why animals get together and form groups of various sizes, compositions and membership dynamics. On the face of it, sociality seems to offer distinct advantages over solitary life, but we need to remember that organisms live in a world of competition. Behind every thicket, over and under every surface, from microbes to humans: individuals compete. And not just individuals; cultures compete, economies compete, ideas compete. Nature is red in tooth and claw in endless variations. Charles Darwin (1859) conceptualized competition for resources as the motive force in the evolution of life. Even in a land of plenty, organisms will reproduce at maximum output until they find themselves in a situation of resource limitation. The ineluctable nature of competition is one of the basic elements of ecology and a major theme in evolutionary research (Begon et al. 2006).

1.1   A Historical Perspective

How individuals of the same species compete for food, shelter, mates and other resources required for survival and reproduction is among the most obvious and enthralling observations to be made in nature. Conspecifics typically have exactly the same requirements, hence they are each other's greatest competitors. For this reason we cannot easily explain cases where individuals forgo benefits that would otherwise raise their own fitness in order to support conspecifics, that is, to accept costs for the benefit of others. This problem – explaining the evolution of cooperation and altruism – is thus one important focus of this book.

Darwin recognized that cooperative behaviour for the good of others was a critical challenge to his theory of evolution. In *On the Origin of Species*, he writes that 'Natural Selection will never produce in a being anything injurious to itself, for natural selection acts solely by and for the good of each' (Darwin 1859). Consequently, observations of apparent altruism, where individuals accept to pay a cost for the benefit of somebody else, represented a fundamental problem for Darwin's theory, as he was the first to point out: 'I will confine myself to one special difficulty, which at first appeared to me insuperable, and actually fatal to my whole theory. I allude to the neuters or sterile females in insect-communities ... this is by far the most serious special difficulty, which my theory has encountered'. This 'special difficulty' of altruistic behaviour, the sacrifice of own fitness for the sole benefit of someone else, has intrigued evolutionary biologists ever since. After all, 'altruism is the very opposite to the survival of the fittest' (Sober & Wilson 1998, p. 19), causing the progenitor of 'sociobiology', Edward O. Wilson, to call it 'the central theoretical problem of sociobiology' (Wilson 1975, p. 3). Some ethologists thought they had solved the problem by assuming that individuals act not for their own benefit but for the good of the species (Lorenz 1963). Similar ideas thrived in ecology (Wynne-Edwards 1962), when William Hamilton worked out a formal solution to the problem of altruism, which was at the same time both logically rigorous and remarkably intuitive: the idea that natural selection acts on inclusive fitness, not just personal fitness (Hamilton 1963, 1964). Hamilton's theory transformed evolutionary thinking by highlighting the importance of relatedness between the altruist and the recipient of a helpful act. This seemingly simple but essential insight revolutionized behavioural and evolutionary biology (Williams 1966; West-Eberhard 1975; Wilson 1975; Dawkins 1976; Brown 1983). Suddenly, the altruistic help of close kin was understood as an inherent component of an individual's Darwinian fitness, removing much of the mystery from the problem that had troubled Darwin more than a century before.

The advent of kin selection theory did not solve all problems encountered in the context of cooperation and altruism (see Box 1.1 for definitions). Kin selection cannot explain many aspects of cooperation occurring among relatives and, in addition, behaviour causing costs to an actor at the benefit of a recipient is not limited to social interactions between relatives. This observation led evolutionary biologists to search for alternative explanations of altruism in nature. Robert Trivers (1971) proposed that if an individual helps another one this could be paid back in the future, thereby initiating reciprocal altruism. Numerous formal models have attempted to show that the adoption of the simple decision rule 'help an individual that has helped you before' can establish evolutionarily stable levels of cooperation in a population ('direct reciprocity'; Axelrod & Hamilton 1981; Killingback & Doebeli 2002; Andre 2015). Both simpler and more sophisticated decision rules have also been proposed and formally checked for their potential to generate evolutionarily stable levels of cooperation in a population. The simplest such rule, 'help anyone if helped by someone', involves few cognitive demands ('generalized reciprocity'; Boyd & Richerson 1989; Pfeiffer et al. 2005; Rankin & Taborsky 2009; Barta et al. 2011), whereas a rule demanding higher cognitive abilities is 'help someone who has helped someone else' ('indirect reciprocity'; Alexander 1974; Nowak & Sigmund 1998; Milinski 2016). All these decision rules have been shown to create evolutionarily stable levels of cooperation by various modelling approaches, but the cognitive demands for these mechanisms are obviously very different, which may influence their prevalence in nature (Stevens et al. 2005; Schweinfurth & Call 2019a).

We should stress at this point that if actions are beneficial to an actor and at the same time benefit others, these positive by-effects do not need sophisticated evolutionary explanations. The inherent property of such mutualisms is that an action is positively selected by the direct fitness benefits to the actor, which implies that effects to other beneficiaries do not need to feed back to the actor's fitness. What may look like an act of altruistic cooperation is indeed an outcome of the pursuit of self-interests, just like Darwin had claimed (Dugatkin 1997; Taborsky et al. 2016). Such forms of mutualistic cooperation are known from both intraspecific and interspecific interactions (Frank 1994; Clutton-Brock 2009), but they are much more conspicuous – and hence better known – if different species are involved. Also, we should acknowledge that many forms of cooperation do not involve higher costs than benefits to an actor, either concerning immediate fitness effects or long-term fitness consequences. Cooperative acts may even 'produce' resources due to synergistic effects (Corning & Szathmary 2015), for instance when interacting agents benefit from division of labour. Therefore, the social dilemmas getting most attention in evolutionary theory might be less widespread and important than the impression this extraordinary focus may convey.

Last but not least, behavioural and evolutionary biologists have realized that altruism can be forced by a receiver against the fitness interests of the actor. The raiding of other ants' nests by slave-making ants to recruit workers in order to raise their broods is a vivid case in point (Brandt et al. 2005). Other extreme cases of such forced 'cooperation' or altruism, in the form of interspecific social parasitism, include the raising of broods by the hosts of brood parasites (Davies & Brooke 1989a; Davies 2000). There are many examples of exploitation of the behaviour of one party by another (Barnard 1984) and they are particularly conspicuous if different species are involved (Feeney et al. 2014; Soler 2014; Suhonen et al. 2019). Nevertheless, similar cases of brood parasitism occur within species (Andersson 1984; Petrie & Moller 1991; Field 1992; Zink 2000; Tallamy 2005). Often, individuals exploiting the effort of others against the latters' interest act surreptitiously and succeed if they remain undetected. Alternatively, animals may punish conspecifics that do not deliver the goods and services they demand (Boyd & Richerson 1992; Clutton-Brock & Parker 1995), which may simply reflect a credible threat to desert the interaction (McNamara & Houston 2002). Credible threats can induce cooperative behaviour, especially if alternative options for the social partner are poor (Cant & Johnstone 2009; Cant 2011; Hellmann & Hamilton 2018).

Despite these various alternative explanations of cooperation, the kin selection hypothesis is currently the predominant concept used to explain cooperation among conspecifics (Gadagkar 1997; West et al. 2007c; Bourke 2011; Green et al. 2016). This may be partly because many social interactions, and thus also many acts of cooperation, occur among kin, as in natural populations dispersal tends to be limited and hence interaction partners share genes by common descent (Lehmann & Rousset 2010; Koenig & Dickinson 2016). Moreover, cooperative behaviour seems to be common especially if social and mating patterns result in regular interactions between close kin (Boomsma 2007; Hughes et al. 2008; Cornwallis et al. 2010; Lukas & Clutton-Brock 2012). This does not mean, however, that altruism cannot evolve when relatedness is low (Refardt et al. 2013; Riehl 2013; Quinones et al. 2016; Taborsky et al. 2016). Furthermore, it also does not mean that direct fitness benefits are unimportant when closely related individuals interact with each other (Queller 1985; Frank 1998; Richardson et al. 2002; Griffin & West 2003; Jungwirth & Taborsky 2015). Competition between kin can outweigh the indirect fitness benefits of helping kin (Taylor 1992; Wilson et al. 1992; Queller 1994a; West et al. 2002; Platt & Bever 2009), and examples from several taxa show that kinship can even enhance aggression between group members or adversely affect cooperation propensity among social partners ('negative kin discrimination'; Zöttl et al. 2013a; Dunn et al. 2014; Thompson et al. 2017a; Schweinfurth & Taborsky 2018a). Hence, the widespread tendency to assume that kin selection explains cooperation between relatives seems detrimental to a comprehensive understanding of the evolution of cooperation. Throughout this book, we argue that there is much to learn from a genuine attempt to understand indirect *and* direct fitness effects of behaviour, irrespective of whether it is observed between related or unrelated individuals, and we extend our view across species borders also.

1.2   Dealing with Competition

What can individuals do in the struggle for resources that everyone needs? There are three principal tactics to cope with competition for resources: *race* for them (i.e. be there quicker), *fight* for them (i.e. try to monopolize), or *share* them (i.e. concede a quota to competitors). Accordingly, these alternative ways to cope with social competition are a recurring theme in this book. Clearly, there are points of intersection between these solutions. For instance, 'race' and 'fight' are not necessarily mutually exclusive tactics but may co-occur. When individuals scramble to obtain resources from patches that vary in quality, which can result in an 'ideal free distribution' (Fretwell & Lucas 1970) among the competitors, more capable individuals can gain from attempting to hold off competitors from the most profitable patches. In these circumstances, a mixture of 'race' and 'fight' can ensue, causing an 'ideal despotic distribution' (Fretwell 1972; reviewed in Tregenza 1995).

The type of resources competed for has a strong influence on social interactions, which may in turn affect social structure. Even if competition among social partners is often not confined to one type of resource, to deal with different needs separately may illustrate general principles of how to cope best with resource competition. In the following, we shall outline how different needs and functional contexts of resource competition may select for one or the other behavioural tactic; that is, whether it is best to be quick in obtaining a resource (*race*), to monopolize it (*fight*), or to concede some of it to others (*share*).

1.2.1   Competition for Food

Competition for food alone (i.e. when not competing for other resources concomitantly) may cause individuals either to *race* or to *share*, but perhaps more rarely to *fight*, as food is often a sharable resource. Hence, if individuals compete mainly for food, we would predict them either to avoid each other or to combine efforts in order to benefit from synergistic effects (e.g. by being more efficient or facing lower risk when hunting or foraging in a group; Packer & Ruttan 1988; Krause & Ruxton 2002; Corning & Szathmary 2015). Importantly, cooperation may even produce public goods and thereby reduce competition (Platt & Bever 2009). Sometimes, food may be economically defendable by individuals or groups, which then can select for monopolization (i.e. *fight*: Dill 1978; Kotrschal et al. 1993).[1]

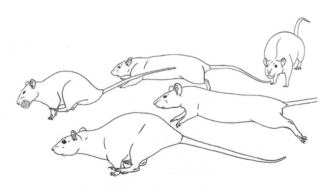

---

[1] All sketches of Norway rats were drawn by Michelle Gygax.

(a) Race

Individuals often aggregate to find food (Valone 1989; Templeton & Giraldeau 1995; Krause & Ruxton 2002). This is particularly common when food is hard to find or unpredictable. Another precondition is that food cannot be economically monopolized (Brown 1964; Maher & Lott 2000; Sorato et al. 2015). In such conditions, individuals benefit from joining others because of the increased chances to find the required resources according to the German and Dutch proverb 'four eyes see more than two'. Such aggregations of food-seeking individuals, which may also contain individuals from different species (Farine et al. 2012; Sridhar et al. 2012), create a paradoxical situation, because now the competitors for a resource do not space out, but instead connect to each other. Fighting over these desired resources does not pay, however, if they cannot be defended economically. If the food is plentiful locally or temporally, i.e. sufficient to satisfy everyone's need, there is no inter-individual conflict. Typical examples include mixed herds of grazers (Lucherini & Birochio 1997; Owen-Smith et al. 2015) and shoals/schools of fish (Baird et al. 1991; Foster et al. 2001; Hintz & Lonzarich 2018). If there is limitation, however, it is important to be quicker than others, i.e. to race (Recer et al. 1987; Shaw et al. 1995), which may come at the cost of impaired accuracy in foraging decisions. In zebra finches racing for feed, for instance, faster individuals are more likely to overlook food items (David et al. 2014). The use of a racing tactic in competitive situations has been demonstrated, for instance, in flocks of waders (Beauchamp 2012) and groups of folivorous primates (Teichroeb & Sicotte 2018), and its occurrence was experimentally shown to increase with group size in songbirds (Rieucau & Giraldeau 2009). Scramble may also lead to innovative food acquisition tactics, which can increase feeding efficiency (Morand-Ferron & Quinn 2011).

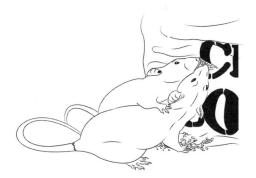

(b) Share

When several individuals obtain food that is sharable, each of them may do best by sharing with others instead of fighting over it (Elgar 1986; Caine et al. 1995), irrespective of whether the acquisition of the desired resource is incidental or resulting from shared effort. The important precondition for this type of social response is that the benefit of sharing is greater than the alternative possibility of trying to monopolize it by fighting (Dugatkin 1997). The typical food supply selecting for this type of response is ephemeral or bonanza resources (Heinrich 1988; McInnes et al. 2017), or resources that can be better obtained by group efforts (e.g. by cooperative hunting; Packer & Ruttan 1988; Herbert-Read et al. 2016; Dumke et al. 2018).

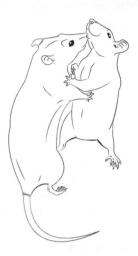

(c) Fight

When food can be economically defended (Brown 1964; Rousseu et al. 2014; Sharpe & Aviles 2016) or the renewal rate of a local food source is high enough (Waser 1981; Houston et al. 1985), it may be beneficial to defend either the food itself or an area large enough to sustain the defender. This is exemplified by feeding territories in nectar-feeding birds (Gill & Wolf 1975) and algae-feeding fish (Robertson 1984; Barlow 1993; Kotrschal & Taborsky 2010), or aquatic insects and juvenile salmonids that defend their feeding stations while feeding mainly on drift food (Dill et al. 1981; Hart 1987; Gunnarsson & Steingrimsson 2011; Nicola et al. 2016). Food may be economically defended especially at intermediate abundance, when it pays best according to the threshold model of feeding territoriality (Carpenter & Macmillen 1976; Wilcox & Ruckdeschel 1982; Carpenter 1987; Grant et al. 2002; Toobaie & Grant 2013).

1.2.2   Competition for Shelter

If individuals compete for shelter, one might expect them to either *fight* or *share*, because shelters can either be monopolized or shared, but they are typically needed for extended periods of time, so being there first (i.e. to *race*) bears little benefit. Nevertheless, there may be an element of scramble when individuals compete for resources that can be monopolized, because of the common convention 'owner wins'. Those occupying a territory first thereby may benefit from this somewhat 'uncorrel-ated asymmetry' (i.e. an asymmetry not related to their actual resource holding potential, or RHP; Maynard Smith 1974; Parker 1974; Hammerstein 1981; Hammerstein & Parker 1982).

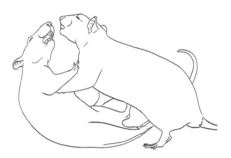

(a)   Fight

If shelters are limited but important for survival and/or reproduction, and sharing is physically impossible (e.g. due to limited den size), risky (e.g. due to increased exposure to threats), or otherwise costly (e.g. parasite transmission at close contact with conspecifics), they should be defended. This is particularly true in cases where shelters are individually produced and therefore costly, like in many plant-dwelling arthropods (Lill & Marquis 2007; LoPresti & Morse 2013; Cornelissen et al. 2016), fossorial mammals (Nevo 1979; Lacey et al. 1998) and aquatic larvae (Hershey 1987), or where shelter use is vital, such as in hermit crabs (Laidre 2011). Shelters are beneficial not only as an efficient measure to reduce predation risk, but may have additional functions such as thermoregulation, which seems to be one reason why many cave-nesting birds also use nest boxes as roosting sites outside the breeding season (Mainwaring 2011). Similarly, small lemurs on Madagascar also make use of thermoregulatory benefits when choosing tree holes as sleeping sites (Schmid 1998; Dausmann et al. 2004; Lutermann et al. 2010). Regardless of which important functions burrows or shelters serve, competitors should be kept at bay (Takahashi et al. 2001; Smyers et al. 2002; Koga & Satoshi 2010; Morgan & Fine 2020).

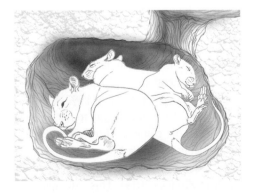

(b) Share

Often, shelters may be sharable without noteworthy costs. If the benefits of sharing outweigh the costs, monopolizing shelters seems unprofitable, which may lead to joint use of roost sites, such as typically shown in bats (Kunz 1982; Kerth 2008), or of burrow systems, such as in fossorial rodents (Santos & Lacey 2011; Lacey et al. 2019). Thermoregulatory benefits may also select for grouping in shelters (Gilbert et al. 2010), as for instance in hibernating marmots (Arnold 1988, 1990b) and socially roosting birds (Paquet et al. 2016) and primates (Eppley et al. 2017; Campbell et al. 2018).

1.2.3 Competition for Mates and Social Partners

Individuals competing for sexual or social partners, e.g. mates or collaborators, should usually either *race* to outcompete others by being there first, or *fight* to get privileged access. Sharing of mates with a same-sex partner is usually costly, particularly for males, because males often compete in a zero-sum fashion for the same total amount of obtainable paternity. If fitness interests are correlated between competitors, however, sharing partners may be beneficial (Packer 1977; Packer & Pusey 1982; Cant & Reeve 2002; Krakauer & DuVal 2011).

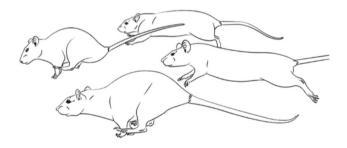

(a) Race

In the mating competition it can be uneconomic to monopolize reproduction with particular sexual partners, because due to the time involved (i.e. opportunity costs), this may prevent successful reproduction with alternative mates (Herberstein et al. 2017). This applies particularly when there is little investment involved in obtaining mates or fertilizations, such as with external fertilization observed in aquatic environments (e.g. in pelagic broadcast spawners: Shapiro et al. 1988; Levitan 1995; Domeier & Colin 1997; Crimaldi 2012), leading to promiscuous mating patterns. Here, it may pay to release gametes in large quantities at the right time, i.e. when the gametes of the other sex are available (Babcock et al. 1986, 1992; Levitan et al. 1991; Levitan 1995; Kaniewska et al. 2015). Turbulence and water flow processes greatly influence the outcome of the gametic race (Crimaldi & Zimmer 2014). This situation selects for high investment in gonads and gametes instead of in tendencies to monopolize mates or germ cells (Parker et al. 2018).

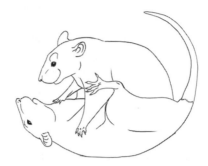

(b) Fight

If partners can be economically monopolized, this will render the highest pay-off (e.g. Crook 1972; Poethke & Kaiser 1987; Sandell & Liberg 1992; Schacht & Bell 2016). The adult sex ratio is an important factor affecting fitness pay-offs through either monopolizing partners or opportunistic promiscuity (Harts & Kokko 2013; Szekely et al. 2014; Kappeler 2017). Numerous examples exist where males monopolize partners either by direct defence against competitors or by providing resources to females (Emlen & Oring 1977; Andersson 1994; Clutton-Brock & Huchard 2013), but vice versa, females may also monopolize males (Andersson 2005). Monogamy is a special but widespread mating pattern where both partners more or less monopolize access to each other (Wickler & Seibt 1981, 1983; Klug 2018; Kvarnemo 2018), which may occur also among simultaneous hermaphrodites exchanging gametes with one another (Pressley 1981). Competition can exist for social (i.e. not *reproductive*) partners as well. For example, in some cooperatively breeding birds, brood care helpers are even kidnapped at times from other groups (white-winged chough: Heinsohn 1991; banded mongoose: Müller & Bell 2009; pied babbler: Ridley 2016).

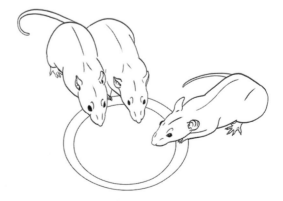

(c) Share
     If the fitness pay-offs are correlated, e.g. when potential competitors are related or
     able to reciprocate service, it may pay to share instead of fighting for privileged
     access to mates. This happens frequently in fish (Taborsky 1994, 2008; Diaz-Munoz
     et al. 2014), and also in some birds (Maynard Smith & Ridpath 1972; Burke et al.
     1989; Goldizen et al. 1998a, 1998b; DuVal 2007a) and mammals (Packer & Pusey
     1982; Feh 1999; Chakrabarti and Jhala 2017; Connor et al. 2017), including
     primates (Packer 1977; Bercovitch 1988; Watts 1998; Bissonnette et al. 2014).

1.2.4   Competition for Multiple Resources

If several resources are contested at the same time, either *fight* or *share* should be the
optimal response, because to outcompete others by being there first (*race*) is rare in
such circumstances (Foley et al. 2018), except for the influence of 'owner wins'
conventions (see Section 1.2.2). Most often, such competition is associated with
multi-purpose territories (Brown 1964), and the defended areas can be monopolized
singly (Hinsch & Komdeur 2017) or shared among a group (Port et al. 2017).

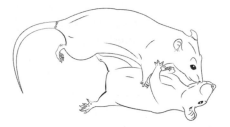

(a) Fight
     If several resources are contested at the same time, it may pay to monopolize
     an area containing these resources and/or providing access to required
     resources for potential partners and offspring, instead of competing for
     each resource separately. This is reflected in the widespread phenomenon of
     multi-purpose territories in which several activities occur, e.g. hiding,
     foraging, mating and breeding (Brown 1964; Keen & Reed 1985; Maher &
     Lott 2000).
(b) Share
     As monopolization of multiple resources by defending multi-purpose
     territories can be very costly, it may pay to share these costs by joining forces
     and dividing the benefits. This is a principle underlying the most complex
     social organizations of individuals observed in nature, including cooperative
     breeding and eusocial systems (Koenig & Dickinson 2016; Rubenstein &
     Abbott 2017).

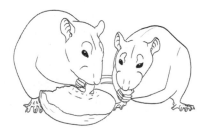

1.3   The Tension between Conflict and Cooperation

The first of our three strategies to deal with competition, outcompeting others simply by speed (i.e. *race*), provides little incentive for social interaction. Success in a race for resources is based on the ability to maximize individual consumption, not fighting or forming relationships. In this book we shall direct most of our attention to the second and third strategies of competition: fighting (in various ways) to monopolize resources, or sharing them. These are the basic strategies of conflict and cooperation in dyads and multi-member groups. Racing can, however, play a role in the formation of social groups, as we shall discuss in Chapter 2.

What is the role of conflict and cooperation in social evolution? Steven Frank argues that 'Social evolution occurs when there is a tension between conflict and cooperation' (Frank 1998, p. xi). On this basis, our aim here is to show that conflict and cooperation are not divergent phenomena, but are often intricately intertwined. if individuals cooperate, conflict may be an important part of the interaction (e.g. as is evident in negotiations; Kokko et al. 2002; Bergmüller & Taborsky 2005; Hamilton & Taborsky 2005b; Melis et al. 2009; Raihani et al. 2012; Fischer et al. 2014; Quinones et al. 2016; Thompson et al. 2017a); on the other hand, cooperation may be an efficient means to settle conflict with third parties (e.g. in coalitions; Maynard Smith & Ridpath 1972; Packer 1977; Chakrabarti & Jhala 2017). Throughout this book we shall discuss the implications of these different strategies of responding to competition. Our main focus will be on the types of interactions prevailing between individuals, and, in this context, the evolutionary mechanisms that underlie behavioural responses to environmental and social challenges, and the consequences for social structure that thereby ensue.

1.4   Conceptual and Semantic Confusions

By relieving the brain of all unnecessary work, a good notation sets it free to
concentrate on more advanced problems . . .
               A.N. Whitehead (1911) *An Introduction to Mathematics*

In science a good terminology, like a good notation in mathematics, can make it easier to think about difficult problems and work out ways to solve them. But while mathematicians get to choose their own notation, biologists frequently use everyday words in a technical way, and universal agreement over definitions is hard to find. In the study of social behaviour and cooperation, the number of definitions included in the literature has steadily increased as researchers from different scientific backgrounds have been drawn to tackle the same questions. The situation has not improved much since Jerram Brown (1983) called for caution in the use of terms when communicating about traits and concepts of sociality, almost four decades ago. Numerous attempts have been made towards a clarification of 'social semantics' (e.g. West et al. 2007a), yet there is little agreement on which terms to use for which concept. This may be due partly to the complexity of the subject and the different views on the underlying concepts of ultimate and proximate mechanisms of sociality. Evolutionary biologists tend to define terms according to the evolutionary function of traits, in essence their fitness effects. Physiologists and psychologists tend to define terms according to the physiological or psychological significance, i.e. their proximate mechanisms. Even within disciplines, opinions diverge greatly (e.g. social semantics in evolutionary biology: West-Eberhard 1975; Brown 1983; Dugatkin 1997; Bergmüller et al. 2007; Taborsky 2007; West et al. 2007a; Engelhardt & Taborsky 2020). Consensus about a particular semantic framework is not in sight, hence there is always a need to be explicit about one's own use of important terms. Divergent semantics undoubtedly complicate communication, but instead of yielding to frustration one might argue for an attitude of pluralism. Semantics are based on concepts (cf. Figure 4.2), and sometimes multiple words for related concepts can provide new perspectives, as long as terms used are consistent, transparent and sound. The terms we find useful as operational definitions (Box 1.1) may seem less suitable when working on microbes or interspecific mutualisms, for example. Clearly, we do not need to all agree on terms to make progress in the study of social behaviour.

In this book we prefer to use descriptive terms that do not imply different, narrower, or more specific meanings than their common connotations in everyday language (see the glossary in Box 1.1). For instance, we do not think it is helpful to define a familiar term such as 'cooperation' to imply specific underlying evolutionary mechanisms (e.g. Bergmüller et al. 2007; West et al. 2007a), as this may impede communication among scientists within and between disciplines, and between scientists and lay persons (Taborsky 2007). We also attempt to avoid excessive subcategorization of terms, which may hamper understanding and flow of reading. For instance, we fear that exhaustive labelling of reciprocal exchanges of goods and services between different parties (Connor 1995; Bergmüller et al. 2007) might deter rather than assist comprehension and clear exchange about underlying concepts (Clutton-Brock 2009).

In order to avoid conceptual confusion, an important distinction to make is the level of analysis, i.e. whether our aim is to identify the proximate (causal) or ultimate (functional) basis of a trait (Tinbergen 1951, 1963; Mayr 1961; Bateson & Laland 2013). Obviously, both levels need to be considered in any thorough appraisal of the foundation of a biological trait (Laland et al. 2011; MacDougall-Shackleton 2011; Hofmann et al. 2014; Taborsky & Taborsky 2015), but we should always be clear about which level we aim to address at any particular point (West et al. 2007c). In addition to separating between proximate and ultimate causes, it is also helpful to specify whether one deals with the level of genotype, which reflects the evolutionary history and dynamics of a trait, or the level of phenotype, which incorporates all the influences on the expression of traits in an individual (Taborsky 2014). A classificatory scheme that is based on 'Tinbergen's four questions' (Tinbergen 1963; Bateson & Laland 2013), but avoids some inconsistencies contained in the original formulation, addresses a trait both at the phenotype levels of 'fitness effects' and 'underlying machinery', and at the genotype levels of 'evolutionary history and dynamics' and the 'gene/environment interplay' (Table 1.1).

Box 1.1 The Meaning of Terms and a Glossary for the Concepts of Social Behaviour, Conflict and Cooperation

> Science depends upon precise, reliable communication among scientists. This is hindered by careless misuse of terms and unnecessary redefinition of widely used terms.
>
> (Jerram Lee Brown, 'Cooperation – A Biologist's Dilemma', *Adv. Stud. Behav.*, 1983)

Danger lurks when science borrows terms from everyday language. The temptation is to use terms from common language to denote concepts that are rigorously defined within a theoretical framework, despite different or much broader connotations in everyday life. For example, it has been suggested that 'a behaviour is only classed as cooperation if that behaviour is selected for because of its beneficial effect on the recipient' (West et al. 2007a, p. 419). Even if it seems plausible to define a trait so specifically in the context of natural selection, there are potential problems with this practice. First and most importantly, non-scientists will inevitably misunderstand what scientists communicate if the same terms mean different things. Second, different disciplines in science will most likely redefine the same everyday terms with divergent meanings, causing a communication barrier between different fields of science. And third, even within a discipline, scientists understand everyday terms differently, depending on their own cultural background and personal experience, hence defining them rigorously may elicit confusion. For instance, one could easily argue that the above definition implies that courtship is cooperation, whereas biparental care is not.

What is the remedy? One way out is to create new terms that have no equivalent in everyday language. For instance, the terminology of genes encoding certain functions (*lacZ*, *ABCA1*, *Insr* or *F7*) does not evoke unjustified conclusions. In the behavioural context, terms like trophallaxis, inquilinism and phototaxis do just that; compound expressions such as operant conditioning, reafference principle or filial imprinting fulfil this aim closely, even if they are combined of words with different meaning

Box 1.1 (*cont.*)

when used apart. The danger of using novel, specialist terms is that what scientists communicate with each other is largely incomprehensible for everyone else.

A second possibility is to use everyday language terms in the way most closely resembling the connotation they have in daily life. Such descriptive terminology is standard when addressing simple behaviours, such as swimming, sitting, scratching or yawning. It is undisputed also in many cases where more complex meanings are implied, for instance with terms like defence, courtship, brood care or flocking. Awkwardly, when it comes to the realm of cooperation, terms used in evolutionary biology tend to lose their everyday connotation. The meaning of 'cooperation', for instance, one of the most widespread nouns in daily language in a societal context, has been redefined in evolutionary biology in various ways, often restricting the meaning to traits with specified fitness effects. As described above, one definition requires that cooperation is selected for because of its beneficial effect on a recipient (West et al. 2007a). A slightly different definition confines the term cooperation to 'an interaction between individuals that results in net benefits for all of the individuals involved' (Bergmüller et al. 2007). This means that (1) when talking about cooperation, one needs to specify the particular definition implied by the term (e.g., *sensu* West et al. 2007a, or *sensu* Bergmüller et al. 2007); (2) scientists from other fields, e.g. neuroethology, psychology, medicine, anthropology or sociology, as well as lay persons, will not understand the connotation of the term in such text; and (3) the fitness consequences of a behaviour (Bergmüller et al. 2007) or the underlying selection (West et al. 2007a) need to be known *before* it can be named as 'cooperation'. We feel that this is impractical and hampers communication (Taborsky 2007).

Attempting to avoid such ambiguity, our aim is to use the terms with their usual, everyday connotations or as closely as possible to their original meaning. In everyday language, behaviours are usually defined by their form (e.g., quiver, peck, lick) or apparent function (threat, submission, cleaning). Transferred to biological context, this means that terms usually address the descriptive or phenotypic level. We think that this should be considered when using everyday terms in science. For instance, the term 'altruism' in everyday language refers to unselfish behaviour benefitting recipients at some cost to a donor. Typically, this does not make assumptions about lifelong consequences, e.g. implying that an altruistic act will reduce a donor's legacy or number of children. Rather, the *immediate* consequences to the donor (e.g. costs in time, energy, comfort or money) are implied (cf. Trivers 1971). Therefore, it seems too restrictive to define altruism in biology purely at the *genetic* level (i.e. meaning a reduction of *lifetime* direct or inclusive fitness), at least when not using further specification (such as '*reproductive* altruism'). By paying attention to common connotations in our use of terms we aim to diminish the risk of unfortunate misunderstandings. We are aware that we may not succeed everywhere, but stress that this is our policy.

In addition to our intention to revert terms referring to social behaviour to their common meaning, we aim to simplify the terminology in this field wherever

Box 1.1 (*cont.*)

fragmentation of terms in myriad subcategories seems superfluous. Definitions can constrain as well as clarify, and confusion can result from inadvertent exclusions and logical errors made in attempting to formulate definitions (Tregenza et al. 2006). We address this in the main text where appropriate. We think that social behaviour involves a limited number of basic principles, which need to be represented by appropriate terms. This is the reason why we do not define here a great number of social terms that in our view can be spared without losing essential means of communication.

Many terms used in everyday language in the social context imply costs and benefits of some sort. The currency differs with regard to the particular context and may involve time, energy, money, or other commodities. In evolutionary biology, the ultimate currency is Darwinian fitness, which may be subject to some specification, such as direct, indirect, or inclusive fitness. If not specified otherwise, costs and benefits refer to direct fitness in the definitions given below, without implying *lifetime* effects.

Glossary

Altruism (defined by the *immediate* consequences of an action; cf. Trivers 1971): A behaviour or trait by which an individual (actor) benefits someone else (receiver(s)) at some immediate cost to itself. This does not make assumptions about whether and how these costs may be compensated by e.g. future benefits (cf. reciprocal altruism) or fitness benefits to non-descendant relatives (indirect fitness benefits).

Altruistic punishment: Action against an individual contingent on harm received from it, involving fitness costs to the actor.

Biological market: Exchange of goods and services between individuals following the law of supply and demand (Noë et al. 1991).

By-product benefits: Benefits accrued to a social partner by a trait benefitting the bearer of the trait.

By-product mutualism: Synonymous to 'mutualism' (see below). As behaviours or other traits must have beneficial fitness effects to each actor *by themselves* to classify as mutualism, the benefits to interaction partners are of secondary importance for the trait to be selected.

Coaction: Concurrent 'acting together' of two or more individuals.

Coercion: Imposition of behaviour by one or several individuals on another individual.

Communal breeding: Different parents raise offspring jointly that were produced by >1 female.

Competition: Rivalry for resources. According to Charles Darwin (1859), competition is the principal impetus in the evolution of life.

Box 1.1 (*cont.*)

Conflict: A state of competition or rivalry between individuals, often (but not always) manifested in aggressive or agonistic behaviour. It is worth noting that conflict is not simply the opposite of cooperation (see Chapter 3).

Contest: An attempt to outcompete others, typically by direct interference.

Cooperation: By Latin origin, this term means literally 'working together'. It refers to the simultaneous or consecutive acting of two or more individuals by same or different behaviours to achieve a shared goal. Costs and benefits to either partner are not implied (i.e. net fitness benefits of cooperation may or may not result to one or all involved parties).

Cooperative breeding: Joint raising of offspring by their parent(s) and non-parents ('helpers' or temporary 'workers').

Coordination: Mutual adjustment of behaviour between two or more individuals.

Correlated pay-offs: This refers to the fitness effects of a trait on two or more individuals. Altruistic behaviour can be favoured by natural selection if its fitness effects on donor and recipient are positively correlated (Taborsky et al. 2016).

Direct fitness: Genetic fitness of an individual as affected by its own phenotype and the phenotype of its neighbours (Hamilton 1970). Direct fitness refers to a change in an actor's offspring number.

Eusociality: Cooperative breeding involving non-parents that themselves do not reproduce independently throughout life (i.e. committing complete reproductive sacrifice). 'Primitive eusociality', in contrast, is synonymous with cooperative breeding, i.e. group members are 'totipotent', which means that in principle they are able to reproduce independently.

Filial cannibalism: The consumption of part or all offspring of a brood, either eggs or young.

Genetic altruism (reproductive sacrifice): Altruistic help involving complete reproductive sacrifice (such as exhibited by workers and soldiers in eusocial animals). This addresses the same phenomenon as 'reproductive altruism', but with focus on gene level.

Group augmentation: Enhancement of group size, typically thought to cause fitness benefits to those group members inducing it.

Hamilton's rule: Generally, Hamilton's rule specifies the change in genetic fitness of an actor in relation to the change of genetic fitness in receivers of an act times the coefficient of relationship between them (Wright 1922; Hamilton 1964; see Chapter 4). Most frequently, Hamilton's rule is used to explain the conditions under which altruism can evolve, which applies when the product of positive fitness effects on receivers (benefits) times their relatedness (r) to the actor exceeds the negative fitness effects (costs) to the actor.

Help, **helping**: Action of an individual to the apparent benefit of one or several receivers. This term is devoid of assumptions about potential costs to the actor.

Box 1.1 (*cont.*)

Inclusive fitness: A combination of direct and indirect fitness. The idea behind this concept is to partition natural selection into its direct and indirect components, thereby referring to the total effect of an actor's behaviours on allele frequency change in a population.

Indirect fitness: Change in the offspring number of a recipient of an act multiplied by the relatedness between actor and recipient (cf. Hamilton's rule).

Kin discrimination: The differential treatment of conspecifics as a function of their genetic relatedness to the actor.

Kin recognition: The ability to identify or distinguish genetically related individuals (kin) from unrelated ones (nonkin).

Kin selection: Following John Maynard Smith (1964) who coined the term, kin selection refers to the evolution of characteristics which favour the survival and/ or reproduction of relatives of the affected individual. This is mathematically represented in 'Hamilton's rule'.

Mutualism: A cooperative trait or behaviour enhancing the (inclusive) fitness of each involved party. The behaviour *by itself* has beneficial fitness effects, irrespective of the behaviour of the interaction partner. Therefore, it cannot be cheated, which distinguishes it from reciprocity.

Pay-to-stay: Tolerance of subordinates by dominants contingent on the delivery of some service or commodity (such as paying 'rent'; cf. 'trading of service and commodities').

Prosocial behaviour: An act of one individual apparently benefitting others than the actor.

Public good: An amenity benefitting the whole group or population, which can be enhanced by members contributing to the common good. This can be exploited by non-cooperative individuals.

Punishment: Action against an individual contingent on actions adversely affecting the punisher.

Reciprocal altruism (*sensu* Trivers 1971): A principle by which the costs of an altruistic act are compensated in the future by some form of reciprocal return benefit.

Reciprocity (synonymous to '**reciprocal cooperation**'): This is essentially a proximate (i.e. mechanistic) concept implying decision rules evolved through certain cost/benefit relationships (Box 4.2). At the ultimate (i.e. evolutionary) level, this term refers to an apparently cooperative trait or behaviour that benefits a receiver of the act at immediate costs to the actor. At the same time, it increases the probability of receiving benefits in return, from the same or different partners. Reciprocation is hence intrinsically altruistic and prone to cheating. At the proximate level, there are three forms of reciprocity with different decision rules:

> **Box 1.1** (*cont.*)
>
>> **Generalized reciprocity**: help anyone if helped by someone
>> **Direct reciprocity**: help someone who has helped you before
>> **Indirect reciprocity**: help someone who is helpful
>
> **Relatedness**: Genetic similarity by common descent, typically expressed by Sewall Wright's (1922) coefficient of relationship (r).
>
> **Reproductive altruism**: Reproductive sacrifice of an individual over its lifetime to the benefit of someone else. The resulting total loss of the actor's direct fitness can be compensated only by respective indirect fitness benefits of related recipients (e.g. reproductives in eusocial animals). Similar to 'genetic altruism', but with focus on (lack of) participation in reproduction.
>
> **Sexual conflict**: Inevitable consequence of diverging fitness interests between the sexes.
>
> **Sociality**: Association among conspecifics. The term 'advanced sociality' refers to group living involving individual relationships between group members depending on their status, state and/or relatedness.
>
> **Strategy**: Synonymous to tactic (Taborsky et al. 2008).
>
> **Tactic**: Trait or set of traits serving a particular function. The term is typically used for, but not confined to, behavioural phenotypes.
>
> **Trading of service and commodities**: Concurrent or consecutive exchange of work or goods between individuals, either in the same or different currencies.

1.5   The Focus of this Book

Every compilation of an extensive topic needs selectivity and focus. When pondering on the scope of this book, we soon realized that evolutionary mechanisms of conflict and cooperation pervade all of biology, from meiosis to human organ donation. We had to select our conceptual and empirical bias. We decided to put our major focus in this book on 'the individual' (Bouchard & Huneman 2013). Individuals may be viewed as inherently independent units that can gain or lose by selfish or altruistic decisions, and so offer a window into the evolutionary forces that shape social traits and promote or fracture cooperation among self-interested, autonomous agents. Alternatively, one might instead focus on evolutionary mechanisms governing multi-cellularity or intragenomic conflict, for example, where genes have phenotypic effects promoting their own transmission at the expense of the transmission of other genes in the same genome. However, in that case the crucial processes underlying present-day phenotypes, i.e. multicellular organisms or the rules of gene transmission, have occurred way back in evolutionary history. This does not render them less interesting, but makes them largely inaccessible to experimental scrutiny. It is difficult to unravel the processes leading to the evolution of genomes from independent replicating

Table 1.1. Classificatory scheme of the levels of analysis inspired by Tinbergen's 'four problems of biology' (Taborsky 2014), © 2014 Blackwell Verlag GmbH. Fitness effects refer to survival value and reproduction, underlying machinery incorporates all morphological and physiological structures and processes responsible for the expression of a trait (i.e. Tinbergen's 'causation'), evolution includes both the course of evolution ('evolutionary history') and the dynamics, as outlined by Tinbergen (1963, pp. 427–429), and gene/environment interplay concerns the processes involved in the translation of genetic information, including epigenetic effects.

	Ultimate	Proximate
Phenotype	Fitness effects	Underlying machinery
Genotype	Evolution	Gene/environment interplay

molecules, for example, because this transition occurred billions of years ago under conditions about which we know little. We prefer to focus on decisions that can be studied experimentally by manipulating intrinsic and extrinsic conditions, both in the laboratory and in the wild. Individuals offer tractable and powerful opportunities for critical tests of general evolutionary hypotheses.

Our second bias is on *behavioural* decisions, instead of dealing with physiological and morphological adaptations. The reason is that behaviour is the level at which an organism interacts most directly with its environment, be it physical, animate or social. Hence, adaptive responses to environmental challenges should be best detectable at this level, even if it is the underlying mechanisms that actually evolve (McNamara & Houston 2009; Blumstein et al. 2010; Fawcett et al. 2013). Apart from this rationale, addressing this essential interface between an organism and its environment provides essential practical benefits by, again, allowing rigorous experimentation and feasible measurement of responses to specific manipulations.

These two predilections cause another bias in the conceptual and empirical treatment of our theme: we shall strongly focus on types of social organization in which there is a continuous need to make decisions about the degree of selfish or unselfish responses. We address the type of group living where individuals have the opportunity to decide whether to stay or leave, to dominate or surrender, to reproduce or abstain from reproduction, and whether to help, defect, punish or exploit others. This type of social organization, which is usually referred to as *cooperative breeding* or *primitive eusociality*, hence provides ample opportunities to unravel processes underlying natural selection. Even if this is obviously not the most widespread form of social organization, this focus allows us to discuss solutions to the permanent conflict between self-interests and the interests of social partners, because at this organizational level little has been settled yet in the previous evolutionary history. This is different, for instance, in eusocial organisms with specialized castes and more or less inflexible roles regarding the types of decisions mentioned above. In cooperative breeders, the entire scope of conflict and cooperation between independent units (individuals) is predicted to constantly influence the dynamics of social decisions.

Chapters 2–5 deal with the different manifestations of competition between organisms, from non-interference rivalry to highly organized interactions involving cooperation, negotiation and enforcement. Interspersed between these main chapters outlining the conceptual framework of the mechanisms underlying social evolution, we present six case studies, ranging from insects to humans, in order to illustrate the evolutionary mechanisms of conflict and cooperation at different levels of biological organization (Case Studies A–F).

In Chapter 2, we focus on *race* as the solution to competition for resources, which has been referred to also as 'scramble' (Parker 2000). If resources are not economically defendable, the optimal strategy to outcompete others can be to go for the resource directly, which means to seize it quickly, or to intensify search. This can apply, for example, when resources are divisible, or plentiful (temporally and/or locally), or when the renewal rate of resources is too slow to be worth local defence (territoriality). Even when individuals do not directly interfere with each other, they will need to take account of what others are doing, and in turn their own behaviour will affect others; they may also benefit from each other (e.g. by vigilance and warning cues). Therefore, in the broad sense, their behaviour is 'social' and must be considered when discussing evolutionary mechanisms of social behaviour. We shall particularly focus on the conditions (attributes of resources and competitors) under which to race for resources is the best response, and investigate the respective rules of this form of resource competition.

Chapter 3 will discuss when and how *fight* can be the optimal response to resource competition. Conflict behaviour is a way to deal with resource competition by interacting with competitors, which usually involves costs, including energy expenditure, opportunity losses and potential injury. When resource competition involves fighting, natural selection favours traits of organisms that will reduce costs and/or increase the chances of victory. The battleground of conflicting fitness interests between contestants may be defined largely by their genetic relatedness, ecological constraints, and the importance of group membership and group stability. In this chapter, we develop a general perspective of the selection mechanisms responsible for optimal decisions of individuals in all kinds of social conflicts. We discuss why the intensity and frequency of aggression varies within and between species, and which conditions can promote peaceful conflict resolution and diminish selection for selfishness within groups. We further ask how conflict and cooperation can coevolve, and how intergroup competition can select for conflict reduction and the proliferation of cooperative behaviour within groups.

The different selection mechanisms responsible for cooperation based on direct and indirect fitness benefits are the main focus of Chapter 4. Concordance of interests may prompt parties to cooperate in order to reach their goal. This can result in the most efficient use of resources, because of synergistic effects. By cooperating, social partners can 'produce' something new, thereby enhancing the fitness of all participants. But this does not necessarily apply. If an action that benefits a social partner has itself positive fitness effects on the actor, no feedback from the partner is required to select for the occurrence of cooperation (mutualism). If, however, an action benefitting a social partner has immediate negative fitness effects on the actor, such behaviour will only be positively selected if the actor increases their chances to get some fitness compensation in return, which can occur through trading and reciprocity, or though shared genes. Philopatry, limited or joint dispersal, and more generally any form of population viscosity, will lead to preferential interactions among related individuals. This may select for costly cooperation without direct fitness benefits to the actor, even if no mechanisms of actual kin discrimination exist. Alternatively, related individuals may assort deliberately to reap shared fitness benefits, if kin discrimination is effective. In this chapter we illustrate with examples of highly social taxa the apparent importance of kin directed cooperation, but we also outline the potential limitations of relatedness as the sole or major driver of cooperation. Groups of kin are not devoid of conflict, as their members compete for resources and often also for reproduction. Important modifiers of the balance between conflict and cooperation in kin groups include individual characteristics such as sex, age, dominance rank, personality traits, and variation among individuals in experience, condition and state.

Alternatively to cooperation based on direct or indirect fitness benefits, one party may force or trick another one to deliver something in their own interest, even if this involves fitness costs to the manipulated partner. If a potential recipient can force the social partner to act in their own interest, the fitness effects to this partner are primarily important to the extent to which they might select for resistance (forced altruism). In Chapter 4 we elucidate how this may lead to an arms race among conspecifics, just like in interspecific social parasitism.

Evolutionary mechanisms responsible for the form and function of social interactions among conspecifics also control relationships between individuals of different species. This will be discussed in Chapter 5, where we emphasize similarities and differences in the importance and operation of the major solutions to resource competition, i.e. *race*, *fight* or *share*, between interactions among conspecifics and members of different species. The narrow margin between conflict and cooperation can be well illustrated by comparing cases where both involved parties are in control of the interaction, with others where one party attains help from the other through deception or coercion. We shall also focus on interactions at the level of individuals in this chapter, and put this into the context of well-known paradigms of interspecific relationships such as social parasitism, facultative and obligatory mutualisms and symbioses.

In our synopsis in Chapter 6, we recapitulate the different manifestations of social responses to resource competition. We discuss evolutionarily optimized individual strategies based on conflict and cooperation, which work irrespective of whether interactions happen between related or unrelated individuals, within or between sexes, among parents and offspring, within or between groups, and among conspecifics or members of different species. We shall also outline future directions in the study of evolutionary mechanisms underlying social behaviour, and we caution against the pursuit of avenues providing poor prospect.

In between these main chapters of the book, we provide insight into case studies illustrating the general principles discussed in this book. The choice of these examples has been guided by their relevance to the concepts we wish to highlight, by the availability of information from a particular social system, and by our own insight into the respective examples. We have aimed to comprise a broad taxonomic spectrum with these case studies (Taborsky et al. 2015). The focus is on social systems characterized by a certain level of complexity, which are well suited to illustrate ecological and social causes for conflict and cooperation, as well as respective behavioural solutions. Together with the main text of this book, our hope is that these examples serve to elucidate the evolutionary mechanisms underlying social behaviour.

Understanding the Evolution of Variation in Helping Behaviour Between and Within the Sexes

Summary

The entire Seychelles warbler (*Acrocephalus sechellensis*) population on Cousin Island has been extensively documented and sampled at the individual level for more than three decades. The study system provides a rare opportunity to monitor the survival, reproduction and lifetime fitness of nearly all individuals over multiple generations. Environmental quality (food availability in each warbler territory) has been measured for all individuals and mapped in detail during every year of the study period. These long-term field data provide a fabulous wealth because they enable the clarification of general principles, beyond the influence of erratic and random environmental quirks. Not only is habitat saturation important for the occurrence of philopatry and cooperation, but variation in habitat *quality* also drives cooperation. Dominants benefit from helpers in terms of higher reproductive output. Subordinates gain survival benefits from staying on the natal territory, and both indirect fitness benefits and direct reproductive benefits from helping. Importantly, direct fitness benefits exceed those derived from kin-selection. The habitat of the Seychelles warbler population has improved in 'quality' over the course of the study due to habitat restoration, resulting in all territories becoming more equal in quality over time. Despite the increase in territory quality, variation in the degree of cooperative breeding remained. Not only habitat quality but also nest predation is crucial for the social system, including tolerating others to stay and breed, and
decisions to cooperate. The higher the local egg predation risk, the more cooperative becomes incubation attendance, which enhances egg survival. With high predation risk, dominants may allow subordinate females to lay eggs with them in return for incubation assistance; subordinate females that reproduce always help with incubation (Richardson et al. 2003a, 2003b). This might be a case of negotiated cooperation. The sociality of Seychelles warblers arises because of the specific island situation that enhances the effects of habitat saturation, and perhaps also of predation.

Introduction

The Seychelles warbler is a small passerine endemic to the Seychelles archipelago in the Indian Ocean that has been used to study the evolutionary ecology of cooperative breeding for many decades. The destruction of natural habitat for the planting of coconut trees (*Cocus nucifera*) and the introduction of mammalian predators in the early 1900s resulted in the disappearance of warblers from nearly all islands where they had previously occurred. Only on the tiny island of Cousin (29 ha), which remained free of predators, did a tiny warbler population of only 26–50 individuals persist between 1940 and 1967 (Figure A.1). They survived in a small mangrove patch (ca. 1 ha) in which the coconut trees did not thrive (Collar & Stuart 1985). The implementation of habitat restoration (removal of coconut trees and allowing the native vegetation to regrow from remnant patches) from 1968 onwards was successful and by 1982 much of Cousin was covered with native forest, and the warbler population had

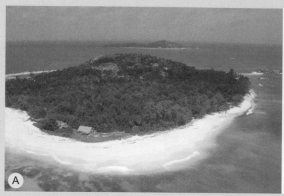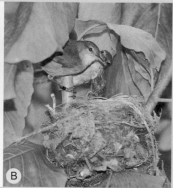

Figure A.1 (A) Cousin Island (photograph by L. Brouwer). (B) Seychelles warblers feeding nestling (photograph by D. Ellinger). (A black and white version of this figure will appear in some formats. For the colour version, please refer to the plate section.)

recovered. Since 1982, the warblers on this island have been at the maximum carrying capacity, which corresponds to about 320 birds inhabiting around 110 territories. Since that saturation point, there has been a continuous surplus of (unpaired) adult birds on the island (Komdeur 1992; Komdeur & Pels 2005). Given the low probability of any warblers moving to other islands themselves (see below) and the vulnerability of a species that is confined to a single small population, several new populations were successfully established by translocations of birds from Cousin to four other islands. The world population of Seychelles warblers is now estimated at 2750 adult birds across five islands, and the conservation status of the Seychelles warblers has been reduced from endangered to vulnerable (IUCN 2013).

The entire population on Cousin has been studied from 1981 onwards. From 1997 onwards nearly all individuals, including fledglings, have been captured, colour-ringed, blood-sampled, sexed and monitored for breeding, dispersal and social status. Molecular tools have been used to assign the sex and genetic parentage of young birds and to determine levels of relatedness between individuals. The lack of inter-island dispersal (Komdeur et al. 2004a) combined with continuous sampling of virtually the entire population, including behavioural

and annual fitness parameters, provides a rare opportunity to monitor the survival, reproduction and lifetime fitness of nearly all individuals within the population, both within and across generations. The long-term research and large-scale experiments (translocating part of the population to new islands) allow testing for how social and ecological factors influence the evolution of cooperation.

Group Living

The Seychelles warbler is a facultative cooperative breeder that lives either in pairs or small groups. Breeding groups normally consist of a dominant pair and one to three sexually mature male and/or female subordinates. Paired dominant birds often remain for life with the same partner on the same breeding territory, sometimes for up to 14 years (Komdeur 1992; Richardson et al. 2007). Subordinates are often independent offspring that have delayed dispersal and remained in their natal territory (Richardson et al. 2002). Subordinates may help the dominant pair to raise the chicks, by aiding in nest building (mainly females), incubation (females), guarding the clutch (mainly males) and/ or nestling and fledgling provisioning (males and females; Komdeur 1994a; Richardson et al. 2003a, 2003b). Cooperative breeding in this species was first observed in the early 1970s, when the population of adult birds became greater than the number of breeding positions available on territories, indicating that the lack of vacant territories could have an important influence on the emergence of cooperative breeding. This was demonstrated by the fact that vacancies created on Cousin Island through translocations of dominant birds to previously uninhabited islands were filled immediately by subordinate helpers from other territories (Komdeur 1992; Eikenaar et al. 2008b). Furthermore, subordinate birds translocated to new islands bred independently rather than becoming subordinate helpers (Komdeur 1992; Komdeur et al. 1995).

Interestingly, however, cooperative breeding on Cousin Island was observed well before the island was completely saturated with territories (which did not occur until 1982), indicating that habitat saturation was not the only parameter driving the development of cooperative breeding. The amount of insect prey present in a territory was also an important factor. There was marked variation in territory quality, with the lusher insect-rich territories being mainly found in the centre of the island and the poorer territories on the coast. For Seychelles warbler pairs without helpers, territory quality was positively correlated with breeder survival and reproductive success. As a consequence, fewer vacancies arose on high-quality territories. The options for young warblers were either to fill a vacancy in a low-quality territory, where the probability of immediate breeding was higher, or to remain as a subordinate in a higher-quality territory. For a subordinate, breeding success and survival benefits of remaining and helping in high-quality territories outweigh the benefits of independent breeding in lower-quality areas. In accordance with this observation, offspring from high-quality territories rarely disperse to breed in lower-quality areas (Komdeur 1992). This was also observed in the new populations established via translocations to other islands. At first, individuals settled only in the high-quality habitat. When the population increased in numbers such that the high-quality breeding habitat was fully occupied, individuals remained as subordinates in high-quality areas rather than dispersing

to breed independently in lower-quality areas (Komdeur et al. 1995). Also, vacancies on Cousin Island created by the translocation of breeders were filled only by subordinates from territories of equivalent or poorer quality (Komdeur 1992). These results are consistent with both the 'benefits of philopatry' hypothesis (Stacey & Ligon 1987, 1991) and the 'ecological constraints' hypothesis (Emlen 1982, 1991), which reflect two sides of the same coin, emphasizing either the benefits of staying or the costs of leaving.

Costs and Fitness Benefits of Philopatry and Helping Behaviour

In the Seychelles warbler not all subordinates present in groups help (Komdeur 1994b; Richardson et al. 2003b). Moreover, there is considerable variation in the extent to which subordinates help. Even within the sexes, the amount of helping varies substantially within and among individuals. In some cases some dominant birds are demoted and become subordinates, usually for the second time, after occupying the dominant position for an extended period (Richardson et al. 2007). What causes this variation in helping behaviour? Is the variation in helping behaviour determined by an interaction between costs and benefits of helping? The act of helping is energetically expensive (Heinsohn & Legge 1999) and the amount of help given may therefore depend on the helper's physiological condition. In the Seychelles warbler there is evidence that helping results in a decline in condition, and that only subordinates in sufficiently high condition can afford to help (van de Crommenacker et al. 2011b). Nonetheless, condition dependency cannot explain why helpers would help in the first place. Therefore it is important to understand how the costs of helping can be outweighed by adaptive benefits of such seemingly altruistic behaviour.

Indirect Fitness Benefits of Helping Behaviour

For helpers to gain indirect fitness benefits, helping must result in a net benefit in terms of relatives they help to produce (Hamilton 1964; Maynard Smith 1964). On high-quality territories, the presence of helpers increases the number of young produced. The removal of the helper from three-bird groups on high-quality territories resulted in lower reproductive success for the breeding pair (Komdeur 1994b). In a later study it was shown that fledging success and first-year survival of young were correlated with the number of birds actually helping, not with the total number of birds present in the territory, which includes non-helping subordinates (Brouwer et al. 2012). The increase in the number of fledglings produced as a result of helping and the fact that subordinates are normally helping their parents indicates that subordinates increase their indirect fitness by helping (Komdeur 1992). At the time when this conclusion was drawn, it was assumed that all helpers were non-breeding and helping their parents. However, when microsatellite-based genotyping became available a decade later, the genetic relatedness between subordinates remaining in their natal territory and nestlings they help to raise is lower than expected for first-order relatives. There are two reasons for this. (1) Males from outside the group sire about 40 per cent of offspring (Richardson et al. 2001; Hadfield et al. 2006), and only 36 per cent of subordinates and offspring present on the same territory share the same father, which in turn reduces the degree of relatedness between them. (2) Approximately 44 per cent of subordinate females also reproduce by adding their own egg in the dominant female's nest. Multiple offspring in a territory may therefore have different mothers, which further reduces relatedness between subordinate and offspring (Richardson et al. 2003a). This means that the indirect fitness benefits of helping are much smaller than assumed before the ability to assess relatedness through molecular techniques.

Despite the apparently low indirect fitness benefits of helping, subordinate females possess a mechanism for assessing their kinship to nestlings and direct help toward those to which they are most highly related. A subordinate female's provisioning is predicted by the continued presence of the dominant female, her putative mother, but not by the continued presence of the dominant male. This is because lack of intraspecific parasitism (females do not lay eggs in extra-group nests) and the presence of high rates of extra-pair paternity make maternity more certain than paternity. As such, the putative mother's continued presence reliably indicates a subordinate's relatedness to the nestling, whereas the continued presence of the dominant male does not reliably predict kinship between subordinates and nestlings due to the high frequency of extra-pair paternity (Richardson et al. 2003b). However, this cue for kin-discrimination will only work reliably for subordinates that were raised in a territory without female helpers present. If, for example, a subordinate was raised in a territory with more than one female, then the subordinate could not reliably assess kinship from the continued presence of the dominant female, because it might have been produced by a subordinate female. However, it is currently unclear if and how subordinates that were raised in groups of multiple females discriminate kin. For instance, subordinates may base their decision to help on the continued presence of the female that fed them the most. Alternatively, because both the breeding and helping females within a group are often related (Richardson et al. 2002), the subordinate may help to feed the nestling if *either* the breeding *or* helping female (potential mother) remain present, as this will still indicate an above average relatedness between the subordinate and the nestling.

Direct Fitness Benefits of Staying and Helping

Given that indirect fitness benefits gained from helping in the Seychelles warblers are relatively small (Figure A.2) and that there is still large variation in helping behaviour that cannot be explained by variation in relatedness to dominants, other proposed benefits of helping were explored. Across cooperative breeders, only a small part of variation in helping behaviour (ca. 10 per cent) can be explained by indirect benefits (Griffin & West 2003; Cornwallis et al. 2009), which suggests that additional explanations for helping behaviour should be involved. For example, subordinates may gain directly through increasing their own survival and future reproduction by helping others

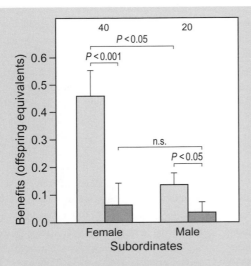

Figure A.2 Fitness benefits (± SE) of cooperative breeding gained by female and male subordinate Seychelles warblers (1997–1999). Both female and male subordinates gain significantly higher direct (pale columns) compared to indirect (dark columns) fitness benefits (female: $Z = 4.22$, male: $Z = 2.39$). Direct fitness benefits were significantly higher in females than in males ($Z = 2.29$), but there was no significant difference between the sexes in indirect benefits ($Z = 0.21$). Numbers indicate sample size (from Richardson et al. 2002) © 2002 Society for the Study of Evolution.

(Kingma et al. 2014). Alternatively, they may be forced by dominants to provide help in order to be allowed to stay in the territory and use its resources ('pay-to-stay': Gaston 1978; Taborsky 1985; Mulder & Langmore 1993). In the Seychelles warbler, female subordinates often gain parentage within their own group by laying an egg in the dominant bird's nest (44 per cent successfully produce offspring in a breeding season), whereas male subordinates rarely gain parentage within the group (15 per cent successfully produced offspring in a breeding season; Richardson et al. 2001, 2002). The direct fitness benefit gained through own parentage is three times higher for female subordinates than for male subordinates (Figure A.2).

It was also found that helping behaviour provides important breeding experience, which allows these individuals to be more productive when they obtain a breeding position themselves. This was tested by translocating similar-aged females and males with different breeding and helping experiences to a new island. On these islands, individuals with previous helping experience produced their first fledgling as fast as experienced breeders, which was significantly faster than individuals without helping experience (Komdeur 1996a). Inexperienced females took more than a year to produce their first fledgling, whereas females with helping experience produced their first fledgling within four months. This is because experienced females built stronger nests that were less prone to be blown away by wind, and they spent more time incubating, resulting in higher hatching success.

In contrast to what has been shown in several other cooperatively breeding species (Balshine-Earn et al. 1998; Leadbeater et al. 2011), helping in the Seychelles warblers does not lead to a higher chance of inheriting the territory after the death of the same-sex dominant when compared to non-helpers. Territory inheritance in the Seychelles warbler is extremely rare (only 4 per cent of subordinates inherited their natal territory), and it is not associated with helping (Eikenaar et al. 2008a, 2008b).

Subordinates may also help in order to enhance group size. It has been hypothesized that larger groups may increase the survival chances of all individuals in the group, because they are better at competing with other groups for gaining access to food resources (Kingma et al. 2014). It was found that the presence of helpers enhances group size because the number of helpers in a territory is positively associated with the chances that offspring survive to adulthood. However, larger groups are not beneficial to adults, as individuals in larger groups had lower survival probabilities than individuals in small groups due to increased competition for food (Brouwer et al. 2006). Although subordinates do disperse and occasionally settle as subordinates in other groups (23 per cent; Eikenaar et al. 2007), they generally do not join smaller groups to offset the negative effects of larger group size on survival (Groenewoud et al. 2018), as is the case in, for example, brown jays (*Cyanocorax morio*: Williams & Rabenold 2005) and stripe-backed wrens (*Campylorhynchus nuchalis*: Piper 1994). The negative effects of increasing group size on individual survival may be counterbalanced by a gain in the reproductive success of subordinates within their own group (Richardson et al. 2002). For female subordinates, and to a limited degree also for male subordinates, the direct benefits are substantially higher than the indirect benefits of helping (Figure A.2), and therefore they appear to be more important for the evolution of helping behaviour in the Seychelles warbler.

Costs and Benefits of Subordinate Helpers to Dominant Breeders

Although having more subordinates has a positive effect on the reproduction of the breeders, the survival effects described above demonstrate that there are also disadvantages to living in larger groups. If dominants are to accept subordinates, these disadvantages need to be outweighed by the benefits of the presence and help of subordinates. What are the benefits of tolerating subordinates in the first place? Dominants may benefit if the subordinates within the group actively help and improve their

reproductive success. In the Seychelles warblers, the presence of helpers on high-quality territories is associated with higher reproductive success of the breeding pair, but not for breeding pairs living on low-quality territories (Komdeur 1994b). At the time when this was known, it was also shown that most helpers are females, usually daughters from previous broods, and that males typically disperse from their natal territory. Remarkably enough, females modify the sex of their single-egg clutches according to the abundance of insect food and the number of helpers already present in the breeding territory (Komdeur et al. 1997). This seems to reflect an adaptive response to the particular ecological and social situation. Breeding pairs in high-quality territories produce mainly female offspring, i.e. the helping sex, which results in having helping subordinates in the next year. In contrast, pairs breeding in low-quality territories produce mainly male offspring, which due to their dispersal will not increase group size in the next year. Interestingly, females on high-quality territories where subordinates are already present mainly produce male offspring (the dispersing sex), which means that their group size does not increase (Komdeur et al. 1997; Kingma et al. 2017).

Over the course of our long-term study, the habitat of the Seychelles warbler population has improved in 'quality' due to habitat restoration, resulting in all territories becoming more equal in quality over time (Figure A.3). At the time of writing, all the low- and medium-quality territories had become high-quality territories, and with that the variation in habitat quality across territories has more or less disappeared (Komdeur et al. 2016). However, despite the general increase in territory quality, variation in the degree of sociality and cooperative breeding has remained. In the Seychelles warbler dispersal is energetically costly and poses a risk, which may be another reason for subordinates to stay (Kingma et al. 2016b). Subordinates engaging in prospecting trips from their resident territory in search for a breeding vacancy were attacked by other territory owners, leading to reduced food intake, lower body mass

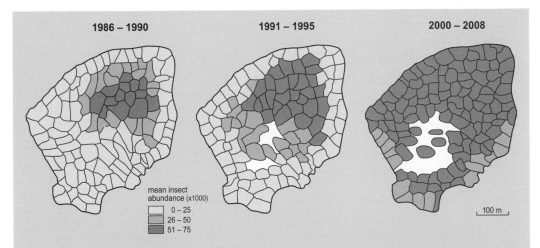

1986 – 1990   1991 – 1995   2000 – 2008

mean insect
abundance (x1000)
☐ 0 – 25
▨ 26 – 50
▨ 51 – 75

100 m

Figure A.3 Map of Cousin Island with Seychelles warbler territories and mean insect abundance present in each territory during the periods 1986–1990 (from Komdeur 1992; © 1992 Springer Nature), 1991–1995 (from J. Komdeur, unpublished data) and 2000–2008 (from Komdeur & Pels 2005; © 2005 Elsevier Ltd). White areas: absence of territories, because of rocky, barely vegetated areas; light grey: low-quality territories; medium grey: medium-quality territories; dark grey: high-quality territories.

and higher mortality compared to non-prospecting subordinates (Kingma et al. 2016a).

Also for dominants it may pay to keep some subordinates in their own group to boost up their reproductive success and survival. In addition to habitat quality, nest predation is also a crucial driver of cooperation. Seychelles warblers experience high rates of egg predation by the Seychelles fody (*Foudia sechellarum*), which is also endemic to the Seychelles archipelago. The fitness costs of egg loss are considerable, because thereby the birds lose an entire clutch, as most warblers have clutches of a single egg only (Komdeur 1994a, 1994b; Bebbington et al. 2017). Egg predation only takes a couple of seconds and occurs during incubation breaks (Komdeur & Kats 1999). The presence of a female helper significantly increases the proportion of time that the eggs are incubated (from 45 per cent without a helper to 71 per cent with a helper: Komdeur 1994a), and consequently, it reduces predation risk. Thus, helping females have a substantial effect on breeders' reproductive success.

The presence of helpers may also increase the long-term survival of dominants. Seychelles warblers that receive help with parental care reduce their effort spent with raising their offspring due to load lightening (Van Boheemen et al. 2019). These resources may then be redirected to improve their own condition, which may alleviate senescence. Indeed, the presence of helpers slows down the ageing process. Older birds without helpers have a smaller chance of survival. Received help slows down ageing, especially for female dominants (Figure A.4). Survival of female dominants that were not assisted by helpers declined strongly with age, but the survival of dominants that received help showed little age-dependence and the late-life decline was much less pronounced. There is also evidence for an association between helper presence and age-dependent survival of male dominants, but this effect is apparently smaller. The difference in the effect of helpers on female and male age-dependent survival may be due to helpers reducing the costs of incubation and investment in eggs for the dominant female (Vehrencamp 1978; Russell

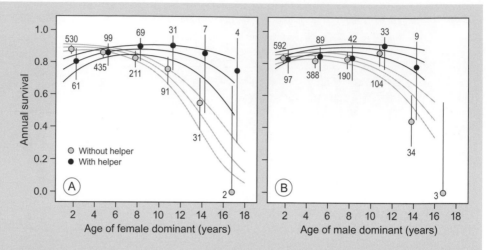

Figure A.4 Age-dependent survival of dominant Seychelles warblers in relation to helper presence. (A) Dominant females, (B) dominant males. Black lines are model-predicted slopes ± SE for dominants that were assisted by helpers during the main breeding season, and grey lines are those for dominants without helpers. Data shown are means (circles) and 95 per cent binomial confidence intervals (error bars) for 3-year age intervals (e.g. 1–3 years combined, 4–6 years combined) based on raw data (from Hammers et al. 2019). Creative Commons, open access.

et al. 2007a); in the Seychelles warbler only the female incubates. Intriguingly, older birds tend to be more social in their behaviour as they appear to recruit more helpers (Hammers et al. 2019). Together, these results suggest that helpers alleviate senescence in breeders and that older individuals may, in some way, encourage receipt of help. However, it remains to be investigated whether there are any benefits for helpers that assist older individuals.

The long-term study of the Seychelles warbler has shown that not only habitat saturation but also variation in both habitat quality and predation risk are important drivers for philopatry and cooperation.

Towards New Frontiers

In the current era of rapid and extreme climate change, organisms, populations and species are increasingly facing environments in which food availability can quickly decline or become highly unpredictable (Hoffmann & Sgrò 2011; Garcia et al.

2014; Unnemhofer & Meehl 2017; Neukom et al. 2019). The dynamics of these challenges may exceed the potential for genetic adaptation to keep pace (Bell & Collins 2008; Hof et al. 2011; Hoffmann & Sgrò 2011; Garcia et al. 2014; van de Pol et al. 2017). Sufficient flexibility and phenotypic plasticity may be required to cope with such conditions, which might be easier for animals forming groups and cooperating in important tasks that critically affect survival and reproduction.

The evolution of cooperative breeding is generally considered a two-step process in which the formation of groups precedes the possibility of cooperation (Emlen 1991; Komdeur 1992; Cockburn 1998; Hatchwell 1999; Hatchwell & Komdeur 2000; Ligon & Burt 2004; Jennions & Macdonald 2007; Griesser et al. 2017). By forming groups in which subordinates assist dominant breeders with resource defence and brood care, the reproductive output of breeders can be enhanced and the variance in productivity may be reduced (Koenig et al. 2019). Importantly, the formation of groups may buffer a decline in reproductive output caused by poor environmental conditions. Theoretical studies have suggested that reducing variance in reproductive output can contribute as much to fitness as improving the mean reproductive output (Gillespie 1977; Tuljapurkar 1990; Lehmann & Baloux 2007; Sæther & Engen 2015). But does it in natural systems? Recent comparative studies of birds and mammals revealed a higher prevalence of grouping and cooperative breeding in geographical regions with large spatial and temporal variability or uncertainty in environmental conditions (Rubenstein & Lovette 2007; Jetz & Rubenstein 2011; Rubenstein 2011; Shen et al. 2012; Sheehan et al. 2015; Koenig & Dickinson 2016; Cornwallis et al. 2017; Lukas & Clutton-Brock 2017; Kennedy et al. 2018). However, these studies did not consider the impact of those conditions on individual dispersal and group formation, which are important prerequisites for cooperative breeding in many species (Griesser et al. 2017). Also, the reproductive output of groups and their different types of members was not investigated, and the impacts of group living and cooperation on dispersal into environments with varying quality, and the associated colonization success, are still unknown.

It would hence be a worthwhile challenge to explore how ecology (e.g. food availability) and sociality may shape the adjustment of animals to rapid and extreme environmental change. Seychelles warblers live in environments where food availability can vary considerably over space and time owing to changing patterns of vegetation defoliation that result from seasonal changes in annual rainfall and prevailing wind directions (e.g. Komdeur 1992, 1993, 1994c; Dowling et al. 2001; Komdeur & Daan 2005; Komdeur & Pels 2005; Brouwer et al. 2006, 2009; van de Crommenacket et al. 2011a; Komdeur et al. 2016; Figure A.5). This species is purely insectivorous, taking insect food from leaves, and insect availability is highly variable between years and between and within warbler groups across years. Fluctuations in rainfall and insect availability within and between years affect breeding success (Komdeur 1996b), survival (Brouwer et al. 2006) and population size (Komdeur et al. 2016); nestlings regularly face mortality from starvation (Komdeur et al. 1995; Komdeur 1996b; Komdeur & Daan 2005). Our research on the Seychelles warblers over the past 35 years on Cousin Island provides accurate records of food availability, group size, conditions [weight, health (as measured by telomere attrition), group size and composition], dispersal, survival, status (dominant, subordinate helper, non-helping subordinate, floater) and breeding success (genetic data) across the whole lifespans of each member of all warbler groups (~100–120 annually).

Therefore, Seychelles warblers provide a unique opportunity to examine how behaviour and sociality shape adaptive potential by (1) identifying how changes in ecology and social factors impact on dispersal behaviour and group formation, and how within-group interactions affect immigration into existing groups; we expect that variation in food availability, group size and composition will influence individual foraging success, growth and the response to stress, reproductive output and survival, which in turn should affect social interactions among group members, dispersal behaviour, immigration success into groups, and group formation; (2) exploring the life histories of group members, and how food availability and group characteristics and dynamics directly affect the fitness of group members and potential immigrants, which should in turn influence group formation and immigration success; substantial differences between groups regarding reproductive output will contribute to variation in their persistence; we expect that with increasing size groups will persist longer, especially during years with low or unpredictable food availability; (3) investigating – at the population level – the long-term effects of variation in dispersal behaviour, group size and group dynamics on colonization, demography and population viability; why do individuals form groups and cooperate in environments with low and unpredictable food availability? When groups experience low or unpredictable food availability and they consequently decline in size,

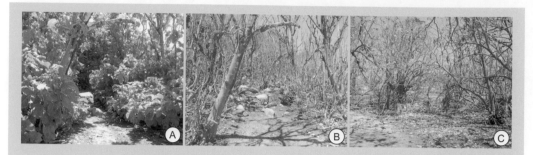

Figure A.5 The patterns of local vegetation vary greatly between breeding seasons in the same part of Cousin Island (temporal variation; A, B) and between different parts of the island (spatial variation; A, C). Warbler groups and individuals are exposed to large fluctuations in temperature, rainfall and wind exposure, which in turn are responsible for large fluctuations in vegetation growth and concurrent insect availability within and between years. These conditions generate differences in fecundity and survival between individuals and groups (Komdeur 1996b; Komdeur & Daan 2005; Komdeur & Pels 2005; Brouwer et al. 2006; Komdeur et al. 2016. Photographs: Van de Crommenacker). (A black and white version of this figure will appear in some formats. For the colour version, please refer to the plate section.)

we expect dominant breeders to show increased tolerance towards immigrants and to allow subordinates to participate in reproduction (Keller & Reeve 1994). Under these conditions, larger groups should generate benefits for survival and per capita breeding success, and hence persist longer. We are confident that future research into these topics will reveal important causes and consequences of variation in the social dynamics of this intensely studied model system.

2 Non-interference Rivalry

Competition occurs when a number of animals (of the same or of different species) utilize common resource the supply of which is short; or if the resources are not in short supply, competition occurs when the animals seeking that resource nevertheless harm one or the other in the process.

Charles L. Birch (1957)

2.1 Competition: The Engine of Natural Selection

Competition for resources is the fundamental process generating selection on social behaviour. Individuals compete with family members, with other conspecifics, and with the members of other species for food, shelter and other resources that are essential for survival and reproduction. Conspecifics also compete for access to social partners and mates, and hence selection acting on strategies of social competition is particularly intense (West-Eberhard 1979). However, competition is not simply a repellent force in the lives of organisms, driving them apart; it is often a social attractor, bringing individuals together and setting the stage for social evolution. In particular, where resources such as food and mates are clumped in the environment or predictable in time, competition has the effect of drawing individuals together into aggregation and possible social interaction, selecting for strategies that maximize fitness by exploiting, parasitizing, following, or even cooperating with other individuals of the same or different species.

The form of competition and the behavioural strategies that individuals employ to cope with competition depend to a large extent on the ecology of the environment in which competition occurs. Nicholson (1954) distinguished between two types of competition, scramble and contest, which have very different consequences for variation in fitness among members of the population and arise in different ecological conditions. Pure scramble competition is a race for resources in which individuals are selected to maximize their rate of consumption, rather than directly interfering with or hobbling their competitors. By contrast in pure contest competition individuals maximize their success by fighting for resources, or defending access to territories containing them.

Whether competition takes the form of a scramble or a contest depends on the distribution of resources in the environment. To illustrate scramble competition,

Nicholson used the analogy of sweets scattered in front of schoolchildren. Faced with such a scattered, synchronously available resource, each child does best to race to collect as many sweets as possible, rather than attempting to stake out and defend a territory. To extend this analogy, consider the case where a large bag of sweets is delivered at predictable intervals to the centre of the group. In this case competition would swiftly turn from a scramble into a contest, with one or a few larger or more aggressive children dominating the central territory.

Nicholson's (1954) emphasis was on the consequences of scramble versus contest competition for population growth: in scrambles, he argued, individuals race to obtain as much resources as they can, but because many may fail to secure enough resources to reproduce, a significant proportion of the total resources available to the population are likely to be dissipated without contributing to population growth. By contrast, in contest competition, where individuals fight over discrete parcels of resource (e.g. territories, breeding vacancies, hosts or major prey items), all of the population resources are carved up among contest winners, and no resources are dissipated (Nicholson 1954; Parker 2000). In a 'pure scramble' all competitors obtain some share of the resources proportional to their intrinsic competitive ability or quality: an example would be blow fly (Calliphoridae) larvae competing to consume a piece of flesh (Birch 1957), or a school of fish consuming plankton (Ritz et al. 2011). In 'pure contest' the resources obtained or controlled by the winners are the same as in the absence of competition; for example, when two hermit crabs (*Pagurus bernhardus*) fight over possession of a shell, the winner gains the full value of the prize (minus the costs of fighting) while the loser ends up with nothing (Arnott & Elwood 2009; Courtene-Jones & Briffa 2014).

In this chapter we examine the ecological factors that set the stage for racing versus fighting, the forms and consequences of scramble competition. Scramble competition is our focus here because it is the most basic of social interactions and generally involves the least-complicated behaviour. Animals often simply race to consume resources. Contest competition, on the other hand, leads to more varied, intimate and potentially complex social interactions to resolve conflict, such as signals and threats, assessment and negotiation. These more complex social behaviours will be considered in subsequent chapters.

2.2   Ecological Influences on the Nature of Competition

Ecological factors influence the nature of competition because they affect the 'economic defendability' of resources in the environment. Economic defendability is a measure of the degree to which attempting to defend or monopolize access to a given resource yields a net fitness benefit, compared to alternative behaviours such as scrambling or leaving to seek alternative resources (Brown 1964). Contest competition is expected to evolve where economic defendability is high, which in turn depends on how resources are distributed in the environment in time and space and the degree to which they can be shared. Brown (1964) introduced the concept of economic defendability as a way to explain variation in territorial behaviour in birds.

Since then, economic defendability has become something of a unifying principle in behavioural ecology. An explicit economic consideration of the benefits of defending a resource versus pursuing alternative strategies has been used to explain variation in animal spacing patterns (Brown & Orians 1970; Hinsch & Komdeur 2010; Parker et al. 2019), mating systems (Emlen & Oring 1977; Davies & Lundberg 1984; Sandell & Liberg 1992; Patricelli et al. 2011; Klug 2018), fighting behaviour (Parker 1974; Hinsch et al. 2013; Broom et al. 2015; Klug 2018), social organization (Lott 1991), mutualisms (Dubois & Giraldeau 2003) and reproductive skew (Vehrencamp 1983; Reeve & Ratnieks 1993; Cant & Johnstone 2009; Johnstone & Cant 2009).

Where resources are economically defendable, we expect animals to engage in contest competition, that is, to fight for possession of a resource, to drive off competitors and to defend exclusive control and access to it. A high degree of economic defendability may also set the stage for more nuanced social interactions as alternatives to fighting, such as peacefully sharing the resource, or taking it in turns to monopolize it. By contrast, there are many ecological circumstances that can render the defence of food, mates, or other resources unprofitable, leading to a scramble or race to exploit them. Below we consider four features of the ecological environment that will influence whether competitions take the form of scrambles or contests, and hence whether selection will favour strategies of fighting or sharing versus racing. Our scheme is adapted from Grant (1993), who discusses the effect of ecological variability on selection for resource defence.

2.2.1   Resource Availability and Renewal

The availability of a resource depends on its density in the environment (measured as the amount of resource per unit area) and its renewal rate (measured as the rate at which the resource is produced per unit area; Warner & Hoffman 1980; Waser 1981). When resources are scarce in time and space, defending particular resources or territories may be unprofitable, and individuals will be selected to roam widely in a race to find and consume resources. Above a certain threshold, resource defence is predicted to become more profitable, favouring more aggressive strategies and a shift towards contest competition (Parker 1984; Figure 2.1A). Finally, some theoretical models predict that resource defence will no longer pay when resources become superabundant, because in this case any resources taken by other individuals are surplus to requirements, and can be replaced at little or no cost (Carpenter & Macmillen 1976; Davies & Houston 1981; Doyle & Talbot 1986; Grant 1993). These considerations suggest that resource defence should be observed for an intermediate range of resource availability (Carpenter & Macmillen 1976; Grant 1993).

Several field and laboratory studies of foraging competition have found support for threshold effects of resource availability on resource defence, measured as food-related aggression or territoriality. For example, several studies of hummingbirds (Trochilidae) have shown evidence of an upper threshold above which aggression or territoriality declines (Gill & Wolf 1975; Carpenter & Macmillen 1976; Ewald & Carpenter 1978; Powers 1987). There is also some evidence of a lower threshold of

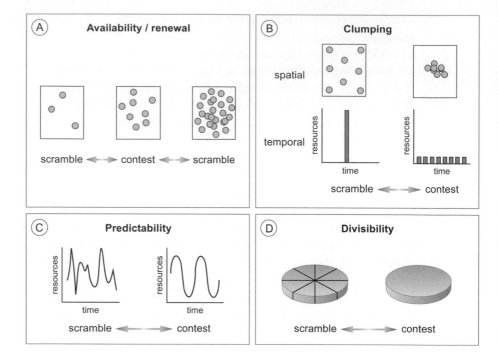

Figure 2.1 How ecological resource distributions affect the form of resource competition. The schematic depicts the hypothesized influence of (A) resource availability (or renewal), (B) clumping in space and time, (C) predictability and (D) divisibility on selection for strategies of scramble (racing to consume resources) versus contest (fighting for or defending access to resources).

flower density below which territoriality doesn't pay (Carpenter & Macmillen 1976). Several laboratory studies of fish report a dome-shaped relationship between resource input level and aggression, consistent with the prediction that contests over food occur in an intermediate range of resource availability (Grant & Noakes 1988; Grant et al. 2002). For example, convict cichlids *Archocentrus nigrofasciatum* that are fed food pellets at an intermediate rate were more aggressive than those fed at lower or higher rates (Grant et al. 2002). Similarly, water striders *Gemmis remiges* in the laboratory defend exclusive territories only at intermediate levels of resource availability (Wilcox & Ruckdeschel 1982). Overall, there is evidence of both lower and upper thresholds to resource defence. Scramble should therefore be more likely at very low and very high resource levels. However, Grant (1993) argues that upper thresholds may be difficult to detect in natural populations because resources in nature are rarely so abundant that resource defence is unprofitable.

2.2.2   Clumping in Space and Time

The patchiness or clumping of resources refers to the variance in resource availability in time or space. When resources are evenly scattered in space, individuals will search widely for resources, rather than defending them. As resources grow progressively more clumped, investment in the defence of clumped patches will become more profitable, shifting the nature of competition from scramble to contests. Clumping of resources in time can be expected to have the opposite effect: where resources are highly clumped in time, such that they appear together everywhere in a synchronous burst, they cannot be monopolized by particular individuals and we should expect a shift from contests to scramble (Blanckenhorn & Caraco 1992). Only if the availability of resources is spread out over time does investment in resource defence pay (Figure 2.1B).

Studies of foraging competition support the prediction that spatial dispersion is associated with reduced aggressive competition. In a classic early study, Monaghan and Metcalfe (1985) measured aggression of wild brown hares *Lepus americanus* foraging on highly clumped versus widely spaced pieces of apple. As predicted, aggression was much lower when food was spaced out, because individuals rarely came into direct contact. When food was clumped, aggression was much more frequent, because dominant individuals were frequently aggressive to subordinates (Figure 2.2). Similar impacts of spatial clumping have been reported in a range of other vertebrates, including pygmy sunfish *Elassoma elogladei* (Rubenstein 1981), dark-eyed juncos *Junco hyemalis* (Theimer 1987), wild ruddy turnstone *Arenaria interpres* (Vahl et al. 2007) and zenaida doves *Zenaida aurita* (Goldberg et al. 2001). In captive black-handed spider monkeys *Ateles geoffroyi*, spatial clumping of food is associated with reduced feeding rate and increased levels of physiological stress (Rangel-Negrín et al. 2015).

Grant and Kramer (1992) investigated the predicted impact of temporal clumping on aggression and resource monopilization in zebrafish *Brachydanio rario*. As predicted, when feeding events were spread out over time, dominant fish were more aggressive and better able to monopolize food. By contrast, provision of the same amount of food over a short period led to reduced aggression and more even sharing of resources, consistent with a shift to more scramble-like competition.

Temporal clumping has also been invoked as a major factor in the evolution of mating systems. Where many females in the population become sexually receptive at the same time, dominant males will be less likely to monopolize access to one female after another. Evidence in support of this hypothesis comes from a comparative analysis of 43 primate species, which shows that paternity skew declines as the synchrony of female receptivity increases (Ostner et al. 2008). Temporal clumping combined with spatial dispersion can also explain the evolution of monogamy in mammals. When females are widely dispersed and synchronously receptive, males are selected to remain monogamous rather than attempt to mate multiply (Kappeler 2013; Lukas & Clutton-Brock 2013).

2.2.3 Predictability in Space and Time

Spatial predictability is a measure of the consistency or the autocorrelation of good or poor sites over time (Warner & Hoffman 1980). Unpredictable resources favour

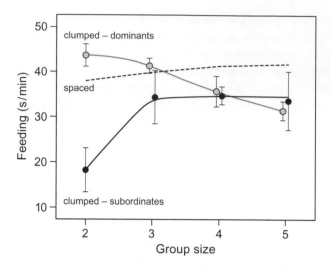

Figure 2.2 Clumping of resources leads to contest competition; spacing of resources leads to scramble. The plot shows the feeding rate (proportion of time spent feeding) of dominant and subordinate hares competing for ~60 apple pieces that were either clumped together (a pile 0.5 m in diameter) or spaced out (over ~50 m^2; Monaghan & Metcalfe 1985). When resources are clumped, a socially dominant individual could monopolize the patch against a single subordinate. Resource defence was less effective against multiple subordinates. When food was spaced out, dominant individuals could not monopolize food and hares obtained a similar pay-off (with relatively low variance) irrespective of group size. © 1985 Elsevier Ltd. Redrawn from Monaghan and Metcalfe (1983), with permission from Elsevier.

scramble competition over resource defence, because a site that is profitable now may easily become unprofitable shortly. Predictability in time is the autocorrelation of particular times in terms of whether they are resource-rich or -poor. For example, in strongly seasonal environments certain times of year are predictably much better than others. Increasing predictability of resources in time should increase the profitability of resource defence (Figure 2.1C).

Feeding experiments on Zenaida doves support the predicted effects of temporal predictability on resource defence (Goldberg et al. 2001). Increasing temporal predictability of resources led to increased aggression, but only when resources were spatially clumped. Similarly, spatial clumping increased aggression, but only when resources were temporally predictable. This study shows neatly how multiple ecological factors may interact in complex ways to determine the type of competition in which animals engage. While unpredictability should be associated with reduced contest competition, there may be substantial costs arising from physiological stress and changes in activity schedule. For example, Jones et al. (2012) subjected groups of Atlantic salmon parr (*Salmo salar*) to predictable or unpredictable feeding regimes. Predictable treatment fish tanks received food at the same time each day; unpredictable treatment tanks received food at a random time each day. Predictability of feeding was associated with elevated aggression, as theory predicts. However, unpredictable feeding was associated with reduced welfare (as measured by fin damage). Similar negative impacts of unpredictability of feeding times on welfare have been reported in pigs (Carlstead 1986) and horses (Zupan et al. 2020).

2.2.4   Divisibility

The divisibility of a resource is the degree to which it can be shared with competitors while still retaining its function or value. Where resources are indivisible, they cannot by definition be shared either through scramble competition or the granting by dominant individuals of 'concessions' or tolerated shares (Clutton-Brock et al. 2001), and the predicted outcome is contest competition (Figure 2.1D). A hermit crab, for example, cannot physically share its shell with another individual, if it is to retain the ability to move with its shelter. As we might expect, hermit crabs engage in elaborate, aggressive contests over the most valuable shells (Briffa & Sneddon 2007; Briffa & Fortescue 2017). Other examples of indivisible resources are the holes used by tree-nesting birds and dominance rank in strict hierarchies (see Section 3.2.2). Vahl and Kingma (2007) tested the impact of divisibility on foraging competition in ruddy turnstones *Arenaria interpres* using experimental food pits in which mealworms were either clustered together in a single layer (indivisible) or divided using tiles into separate layers (divisible). They found that the asymmetry in pay-offs between a dominant and a subordinate bird was reduced when food was divisible. When food was indivisible, the dominant bird completely monopolized the food pit through aggressive threat behaviour. However, dominants could not monopolize food only when pits were spaced far apart, confirming the role of spatial dispersion as a promoter of scramble competition.

Some resources are divisible, but only up to a point. For example, clownfish (Amphiprionini) live and reproduce within coral anemones, which provide protection from predators. Larger anemones can accommodate a larger number of clownfish (Ross 1978), which arrange themselves in a strict size hierarchy (Buston 2003; Buston & Cant 2006). However, when an upper group size has been reached (determined by the size of largest individual, the reproductive female) no further division of the resource is permitted. In nesting and roosting insects and vertebrates, similar constraints of divisibility will be set by the physical dimensions of a nest or roost site.

2.2.5   Predation and Other Ecological Features

In addition to these four features of resource distributions and divisibility, there are many other features of habitats that can influence the nature of competition, including the distribution of predators and pathogens, and habitat structure and complexity. Predation risk is often considered to promote scramble competition because resource defence behaviours are conspicuous to predators and costly to perform when the risk of predation is high (Martel & Dill 1993; Martel 1996). For example, juvenile coho salmon *Oncorynchus kisutch* that are exposed to the chemical stimuli of a predator show reduced aggression toward a mirror 'competitor' and reduced maximum attack distance to floating prey (Martel & Dill 1993). In natural streams, exposure to predator stimuli leads Atlantic salmon *Salmo salar* to defend smaller territories (Kim et al. 2011).

The distribution of predators in an environment contributes to a 'landscape of fear', influencing the time and energy available to prey individuals to allocate to competition with conspecifics for food versus vigilance or predator avoidance (Lima & Dill 1990; Laundré et al. 2001; Shrader et al. 2008). A landscape of fear can also bring prey into closer, more intense direct competition by forcing them to forage together on clumped patches of resources. In the forests of Poland, for example, predation by wolves forces deer to feed in small, resource-rich forest gaps (Schmidt & Kuijper 2015). These gaps are targeted by lynx *Lynx lynx* and wolves *Canis lupus*, turning them into 'death traps' for the prey species. In this system there is no easy way for prey to avoid predators, and the deer are forced to forage together, with a continuous high risk of predation.

Scramble competition may be more likely to evolve in 'complex' habitats (i.e. those that are physically, structurally, or biologically heterogeneous; Loke et al. 2015), or those within which visibility is limited, because these factors increase the cost of patrolling and defending exclusive access to a resource (Schoener 1987). In groups of zebrafish, for example, competition became more scramble-like in habitats featuring simulated vegetation (plastic strips) compared to simple habitats without added plastic (Basquill & Grant 1998). Later experiments on zebrafish suggest that this effect may not be due to habitat complexity per se, but because complex habitats were perceived by the fish as carrying a lower risk of predation (Hamilton & Dill 2002). In safer habitats (areas of a tank that were covered by plastic mesh, rather than uncovered) food was shared more evenly between fish, leading to the conclusion that reduced predation risk in this case promotes scramble-like competition. Note that this is the opposite conclusion to the studies of coho and Atlantic salmon described above (Martel & Dill 1993; Kim et al. 2011). The impact of predation risk and the landscape of fear on forms of intraspecific competition is not straightforward and merits further study.

2.3   Scramble Strategies and Animal Distributions

In this section we take a closer look at scramble competition and its consequences for individual behaviour and populations. We consider a simple model of individual effort in scramble competition, and the predicted outcome of selection acting at an individual level on animal distributions and resource utilization in heterogeneous environments.

Fretwell and Lucas' (1970) Ideal Free Distribution (IFD) model explores the consequences of scramble competition on individual patch choice decisions in a heterogeneous environment. Their original model was motivated by the problem of predicting the distribution of birds among habitats that vary in 'suitability', but the logic of the model applies generally to understanding the match between animal and resource distributions in natural populations (Tregenza 1995). The basic IFD model does not allow competitive behaviour to evolve, and there are no costs of scrambling: an individual's fitness pay-off depends only on the amount of resources arriving in a patch and the number of competitors in its patch.

Let the environment consist of a large number of patches that vary in the rate of resource input, which is assumed to be continuous. The animals compete on equal terms for each unit of resource that arrives in the patch. For example, this model might apply to fish feeding on prey that drift downstream, or swarming midges waiting to grasp an incoming female. All individuals are assumed to be identical, so an individual's fitness pay-off in patch i, W_i, depends only on the resource input rate into that patch R_i, and the number of competitors n_i, and is given by

$$W_i = \frac{R_i}{n_i}$$

If individuals have perfect information about the amount of resources and number of competitors in each patch, and can move freely to any patch of their choosing, the resulting distribution of animals will satisfy

$$W_i = \frac{R_i}{n_i} = W_j = \frac{R_j}{n_j} = C$$

for all patches i, j, k in the population, where C is a constant.

In other words, individuals will distribute themselves across patches of varying resources such that the fitness pay-offs of all individuals are equal. It follows that animals should distribute themselves according to the 'input-matching rule' $n_i = R_i/C$, that is, the number of competitors in a patch should be proportional to the input rate (or total resource input in a given period) received by that patch.

Several field and laboratory studies have found support for the input-matching rule (reviewed by Tregenza 1995). For example, fish faced with a choice between two feeding stations (Milinski 1979; Godin & Keenleyside 1984), or male dung flies (*Scatophaga stercoraria*) competing for females arriving at cowpats (Parker 1970; Reuter et al. 1998; Blanckenhorn et al. 2000), arrange themselves so that the number of individuals at each site matches the rate at which resources arrive or appear at that site. In each of these systems resources arrive at a patch one at a time, and can only be used by one individual. Hence the primary type of competition at each patch is scramble: individuals compete indirectly simply by consuming resources, which are then unavailable for use by their competitors. In a Panamanian population of algae-grazing catfish (*Ancistrus spinosus*), the density of fish in freshwater pools closely tracked the density of algae, and grazing rates were similar despite wide variation in the number of catfish per pool (Power 1983).

In many cases, however, animal distributions deviate from the predictions of the basic IFD model. A commonly observed deviation is 'undermatching', whereby richer patches are occupied by fewer individuals than predicted and poorer patches are over-occupied, so that individuals on the best patches have higher energy intake or fitness (Parker 2000). The degree of undermatching is often exacerbated at higher population densities (Shaw et al. 1995). These observations can be explained by variants of the original IFD model that incorporate biologically reasonable features of populations and allow for different forms of competition. For example, undermatching is expected if competition takes the form of contest competition (or 'interference' competition; Park 1954) rather than scramble (or 'exploitation') competition (Tregenza 1995). In many real systems, stronger individuals are able to defend access to the best patches, pushing the rest of the population into inferior habitats and resulting in an 'ideal despotic distribution' rather than the IFD (Fretwell 1972[2020]; Parker & Sutherland 1986; Tregenza 1995). Interference can also waste time and energy and hence reduce the pay-off gained at rich patches, causing dispersal of competitors onto lower quality sites (Sutherland 1983). Undermatching is also the predicted outcome if information is not 'ideal', for example where foragers face perceptual constraints and find it hard to discriminate between patch profitabilities that are less than a certain magnitude (Abrahams 1986). Tregenza (1995) discusses the effects of other important ecological and cognitive factors (such as resource dynamics and patch assessment rules) on the predicted equilibrium distribution of animals in their environment.

2.3.1   Evolving Scramble Effort

How might we expect natural selection to influence scramble strategies? In particular, how hard should individuals compete depending on resources and the number of competitors in each patch? Parker (2000) analysed a game-theoretical model of competitive effort in scramble competition and the predicted consequences for animal distributions. A key determinant of effort in this model is the assumed relationship $R(n)$, which describes how the amount of resources over which individuals compete changes with the number of competitors (or 'group size') n. Parker (2000) focused on two extreme cases. In the the first case, total resources R is independent of the number of competitors, so per-capita resources available declines with group size in proportion to R/n. This might be the case, for example, where resources are clumped in a single patch or individuals are unable to leave to seek resources elsewhere. The prediction in this case is that individuals will compete less intensely as group size increases, because the benefits of competing are lower when the fixed 'pie' of resources must be shared with a greater number of competitors (Figure 2.3A).

In the second case of Parker's (2000) model, R is assumed to increase at a constant rate with group size n, so that the per-capita amount of resources (R/n) is constant. A positive relationship between the amount of resources available and the number of individuals in a patch might arise because larger groups are more effective at finding or producing resources, or because a greater number of individuals are attracted to richer patches. The prediction in this case is that individuals should compete *more* intensely in larger groups, because the costs of competing in larger groups are offset by the benefits of winning a share of an ever-increasing 'pie' (Figure 2.3A). Parker's (2000) model also shows that undermatching is expected whenever there are additive personal fitness costs of scrambling (Figure 2.3B). The less sharply accelerating the costs of scrambling (the lower the value of a in Parker's model), the greater the

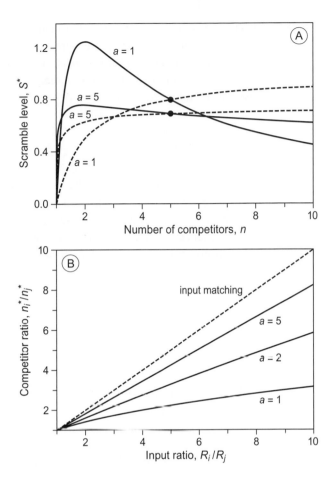

Figure 2.3 Geoff Parker's model of scramble competition. (A) Scramble level (or effort) as a function of the number of competitors, for two different levels of cost: $a = 1$ (linearly increasing costs with increasing scramble effort) and $a = 5$ (sharply accelerating costs with increasing scramble effort). Scramble level is plotted for the case when total resource input R is held constant (continuous line) or where per-capita resource input R/n is held constant (dashed line). Where total resource input is constant, scramble level declines with number of competitors (for $n > 2$); where per-capita resources are constant, scramble level increases with number of competitors. However, where costs of scramble are sharply accelerating ($a = 5$), the two cases give similar ESS scramble levels. (B) ESS ratio of competitors in patch i compared to those in an alternative patch j, in relation to the ratio of resource inputs to the two patches Ri/Rj. Redrawn with permission from Parker (2000).

deviation of the predicted evolutionarily stable strategy (ESS) distribution of competitors from the input matching rule.

To summarize, pure scramble competition leads to a predictable match between the distribution of resources in an environment and the distribution of animals. However, selection acting on scrambling effort is expected to lead to undermatching of animals to resources, with fewer individuals occupying the best patches than would be expected from the IFD model. Undermatching is also expected where there is variation in competitive ability, perceptual constraints and resources are economically defendable. As competition shifts from scramble towards contest, the result is ever-greater inequality in fitness outcomes, and ever-greater divergence between the distribution of animals and the distribution of resources.

2.4   Competition and Collective Movement

In the IFD model, it is assumed that individuals suffer the costs of competition inflicted by other individuals in their resource patch, and gain no benefit from the presence or proximity of other conspecifics. In many cases, however, competition can have more complex fitness consequences, and individuals that vie for the same resources may nevertheless gain from coordinating together. Schools of fish come together to avoid predation, but compete to avoid standing out from the crowd. Scavengers are drawn towards feeding conspecifics so that they can steal a share of their food finds. In this way, competition for resources can drive grouping, coordination and remarkable patterns of collective decision making.

The degree to which the fitness interests of aggregating individuals overlap or diverge may shape the emergent properties of groups, such as their form, movement and degree of internal structuring. Two examples help to illustrate this point. First, consider a mating swarm of chironomid midges, such as those of the European species *Chironomus plumosus*. In Europe these swarms are a common sight in early summer, typically forming in the early evening next to landmarks such as trees or the edges of buildings. Each swarm is made up of hundreds or thousands of males, each of which possesses elongated and elaborately feathered antennae that are tuned to detect the relatively slow wingbeat of gravid females who visit the swarm to find a mate. The males need to aggregate into a swarm to have any chance of attracting females, but otherwise they are in direct competition with one another for matings. When a female enters the swarm she is immediately grabbed by a male and the pair fall to the ground to mate. Any given male chironomid midge in a mating swarm probably has little information about the best position to take up to intercept the next incoming gravid female, and so it has little to gain from defending a particular location, or attempting to displace others. Time and effort spent trying to obtain or defend a particular spot would be better spent on movement and search within the swarm (Neems et al. 1992). Moreover, any particular male midge does best to move around and search the swarm independently of the others, as his goal is to 'get there first', that is, to be the first to grab hold of an incoming female (Crompton et al. 2003).

Contrast this example with a tightly packed school of mackerel. Like the midge in the swarm, an individual mackerel also probably has little or no information about where a predator will attack next. However, unlike the midge case, in a fish school each individual benefits from matching the orientation and velocity of its immediate neighbours to avoid standing out from the crowd. In addition to benefits in terms of reduced predation risk (Magurran 1990; Handegard et al. 2012; Ioannou et al. 2012), schooling brings considerable energetic and hydrodynamic benefits to swimming fish (Johansen et al. 2010; Burgerhout et al. 2013). The goal here is 'don't be last' rather than 'get there first'. Experiments using real fish predators (the bluegill sunfish *Lepomis macrochirus*) and simulated prey show that more coordinated fish are less likely to be attacked (Ioannou et al. 2012).

These differences in the fitness benefits of proximity, alignment and coordination with other members of a group can explain the incredibly rich variety of patterns of grouping and collective movement observed in nature. Simulation models suggest that many of these examples can be reproduced by assuming that each individual is a 'self-propelled particle' whose behaviour is governed by a few simple physical rules. For example, the models of Couzin and collaborators (2002; Couzin & Krause 2003) show that variation in just three parameters – the zone of attraction, repulsion and the propensity to align with others – can explain variation in group movement from the chaotic dance of insect swarms to the exquisite coordination of mackerel schools or starling flocks.

The assumptions of these simple models of collective movement fit well with experimental data in schooling fish (Huth & Wissel 1994; Hoare et al. 2004; Gautrais et al. 2009; Katz et al. 2011), but there are also important limitations in the ability of these simple models to capture the dynamics of animal groups. In particular, most models assume that aggregations consist of identical individuals which are modelled as physical 'particles', subject to social forces of attraction, repulsion and so on. In reality, groups of animals are composed of individuals of different quality, state, or capacity for movement, and the benefits and costs of aggregation may be asymmetrical for different individuals within the group. Within-group heterogeneity and sensitivity to variation in the individual movement of neighbours appear to be important influences on group movement in single-species fish schools (Katz et al. 2011) and mixed-species flocks of birds (Goodale et al. 2010; Demsar & Bajec 2013). Consistent individual differences in behaviour (or 'personality') can have a particularly strong impact on collective behaviour, and give rise to variation in leadership and group structure. For example, in shoals of sticklebacks *Gastero aculeatus*, swimming speed and foraging performance of a group depend on the composition of groups in terms of two major personality traits, 'sociability', or tendency to favour proximity to other individuals, and exploratory tendency or 'boldness' (Jolles et al. 2017). Individuals with low sociability tended to swim faster and lead the group. At a group level, groups composed of less sociable and more exploratory individuals found and depleted food patches more quickly (Figure 2.4).

Understanding the impact of within-group heterogeneity on collective behaviour is a topic of much current theoretical and empirical interest, because it is predicted to influence the transmission of information in social groups (Conradt et al. 2009; Goodale et al. 2010), the efficiency with which collective decisions are made (Petit & Bon 2010) and the spatial and social structure of groups (Conradt et al. 2009; Jolles et al. 2013, 2020). A key question is how individuals reach consensus given that each may have different physiological constraints, aptitudes, or be able to sustain different costs in group movement. In pigeons (*Columba livia*), for example, birds of different body mass and flying ability must deviate from their preferred solo flying speed in order to fly as a group (Figure 2.5). Heavier individuals slow down, lighter individuals

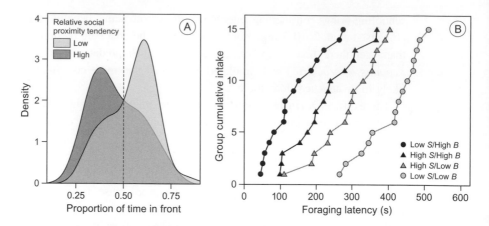

Figure 2.4 Personality traits can affect leadership and group efficiency. (A) Density plot of the proportion of time individuals spent at the front of a group, as a function of their social proximity tendency or 'sociability', a consistent behavioural tendency. Less-sociable individuals lead more often. (B) The effectiveness of groups in finding food depends on their average composition with respect to two personality traits, sociability *S* and exploratory tendency (or 'boldness' *B*). Groups that are composed of individuals with low average sociability and high average boldness are more successful at finding and consuming food. Redrawn with permission from Jolles et al. (2017). Open access.

speed up, and intermediate individuals fly at their preferred and presumably optimal speed (Sankey et al. 2019). Selection for group consensus may favour individuals that are neither too fast nor too slow, or more generally, those that possess intermediate trait values (dubbed the 'Goldilocks' principle). Alternatively, conflict over group coordination can be resolved by taking turns. For example, pairs of sticklebacks that were trained, individually, to expect delivery at different ends of a fish tank resolved conflict over where to go by taking turns to lead the pair to their preferred feeding site (Harcourt et al. 2010).

2.5   Competition for Information

The IFD model and its variants explore how information can influence the predicted distribution of animals engaged in scramble competition (Section 2.3). However, information about food, mates, predators and so on is itself a source of competition. Selection to transmit or parasitize information can lead to the formation of social groups, and to complex strategies of signalling and deception.

2.5.1   Social Learning and Recruitment of Others

A long-standing hypothesis to explain why birds and bats aggregate in giant colonies is that these colonies act as 'information centres', within which each individual

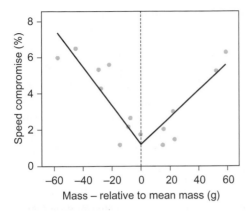

Figure 2.5 Individuals of different physical or physiological capacity must deviate from their optimal behaviour to achieve consensus. Absolute compromise in speed (per cent of preferred solo flying speed) exhibited by pigeons of different body mass versus individual body mass relative to mean body mass of the group. To reach consensus group flight speed, lighter birds speed up, heavier birds slow down and intermediate birds fly at or close to their their preferred speed. Redrawn from Sankey et al. (2019). © 2019 The Association for the Study of Animal Behaviour.

benefits reciprocally from sharing information about where to forage (Ward & Zahavi 1973; Wilkinson 1992). Evidence that foragers gain mutual information benefits from grouping has been found in evening bats *Nycticeius humeralis* (Wilkinson 1992), Bechstein's bats *Myotis bechsteinii* (Kerth & Reckardt 2003), short-tailed fruit bats *Carollia perspicillata* (Ratcliffe & ter Hofstede 2005), cliff swallows *Hirundo pyrrhonota* (Brown 1986) and ravens *Corvus corax* (Marzluff et al. 1996). In many cases, however, information transfer is a one-way street in which naive or inferior foragers learn to use the location of other individuals as means to locate resources (Krebs 1974; Weatherhead 1983, 1987; Buckley 1997; Galef Jr & Giraldeau 2001; Keynan et al. 2015). This form of social learning, known as 'local enhancement' (Thorpe 1956), is observed in a wide range of species (Galef Jr & Giraldeau 2001; Hoppitt & Laland 2013). A classic example is seen in vultures (*Coragyps atratus*), where individuals searching for carcasses are drawn to groups of already-feeding birds that are visible from afar (Buckley 1996). Local enhancement is a simple mechanism through which competition to obtain resources can promote group formation owing to the benefits of information transfer gained via eavesdropping on others. Individuals will continue to join groups until per-capita success is reduced by competition to the point that they would do better to move elsewhere (see Section 3.2.1).

In some social and cooperative species local enhancement is actively promoted because successful foragers use specialized recruitment calls to attract others to food sources (Elgar 1986; Hauser et al. 1993; Caine et al. 1995; Troisi et al. 2018). These recruitment calls can benefit the signaller where membership of a larger group increases individual foraging success (Marzluff & Heinrich 1991), deters rivals (Furrer & Manser 2009), reduces individual predation risk (Manser 2001), or where food calls attract mates (Stokes 1971; Marler et al. 1986a, 1986b). Recruitment calls may also be used strategically depending on whether the resource can be monopolized, or on the relationship of the signaller to the audience. House sparrows (*Passer domsesticus*), for example, give chirrup calls which attract conspecifics to a feeder when presented with breadcrumbs that are not economically defendable, but refrain from calling when the same quantity of bread is presented in a chunk that they can defend (Elgar 1986). Chimpanzees at a food patch are selective in their use of food calls, preferring to call to subordinate individuals or those with which they have a strong affiliative relationship (Schel et al. 2013). In pied babblers, adults give purr calls to attract young, inexperienced foragers to high-quality food patches, but chase off older individuals that utilize the same signal (Radford & Ridley 2006). Recruitment calls in pied babblers represent a form of altruism (Hamilton 1964) or local helping (Lehmann & Rousset 2010), and are predicted to evolve in stable groups where successful foragers have a genetic interest in attracting other group members to a food source, either because the receivers of signallers are genetic relatives, or because their own fitness is interdependent (i.e. positively correlated) with the fitness of other group members (Roberts 2005).

2.5.2   Producers, Scroungers and Deception

In the absence of grouping or inclusive fitness benefits, individuals that find food will suffer a cost if they are subsequently joined by conspecific or heterospecific competitors. Populations can in theory evolve to an equilibrium mixture of 'producers', i.e. individuals that attempt to find food, and 'scroungers', who focus on trying to steal the food finds of others (Barnard & Sibly 1981; Beauchamp & Giraldeau 1997; Afshar & Giraldeau 2014). Experimental tests of this hypothesis in spice finches (*Lonchura punctulata*) show that individuals employ flexibile foraging tactics according to the opportunities for exploitation, and rapidly converge on the producer–scrounger equilibria predicted by theory (Mottley & Giraldeau 2000). In house sparrows, whether individuals choose producer or scrounger tactics depends on their previous experience of pay-offs for the two tactics, suggesting that early experiences may influence the development of exploitative versus productive tendencies (Mottley & Giraldeau 2000). In five wild subpopulations of great tits (*Parus major*), individuals that were presented with a socially learnt foraging task came to adopt consistent producer or scrounger tactics, and these individual tactic specializations persisted over three years of the study (Aplin & Morand-Ferron 2017).

Those with the best information about where to find food or mates stand to lose out if this information becomes widely available, and so can gain from concealing rather than advertising the location of good food sources (Hasson 1994). Mitri et al. (2009) explored the evolutionary stability of 'information suppression' of this kind using a population of foraging 'robots' which could be evolved experimentally over 100s of generations. The robots possessed a rudimentary form of communication: each robot could randomly emit light and detect the light emitted by other individuals. When let loose in a virtual arena containing a food source, the robots rapidly evolved to cue in on areas of high light intensity, emitted by robots foraging at the food source. Because information parasitism of this kind reduced the fitness of individuals that found food, the robots soon after evolved to reduce the rate at which they emitted light, although never to switch off their light completely. The optimal rate of light emission never evolves to zero in this case because selection against signalling weakens as the information content of the signal declines (Hasson 1994; Mitri et al. 2009).

In biological systems, some degree of information parasitism may often be unavoidable if successful foragers cannot escape scroungers, or conceal all of the inadvertent cues that scroungers might use to follow their movements. Ravens, for example, frequently cache their food finds and attempt to raid the food caches of conspecifics (Bugnyar & Kotrschal 2002). In aviary studies, cachers withdrew out of sight of conspecifics to cache their food, or hid food behind structures in their environment (e.g. tree trunks and rocks). Intriguingly, raiders kept a discrete distance from individuals that were caching food, apparently so as not to alert them to the fact that they were being observed. In this case attempts by cachers to suppress information about the location of food often failed because of the surreptitious counter-tactics adopted by raiders.

Individuals in possession of advantageous information sometimes engage in active deception to avoid information parasites, rather than simply suppressing this information. In further aviary experiments on ravens, for example, subordinate individuals actively misled dominants about the location of food by leading them away from boxes that they knew to contain food to clusters of boxes they knew to be empty, while the subordinates themselves quickly returned to the profitable boxes (Bugnyar & Kotrschal 2004). Tactical deception by leading competitors away from profitable food areas has also been reported (anecdotally) in chimpanzees (Whiten & Byrne 1988; Goodall 2000). Male primates engage in a variety of deceptive tactics to obtain matings or avoid punishment, such as mating surreptitiously away from dominant males (Le Roux et al. 2013), or giving false alarm calls (Whiten & Byrne 1988). However, tactical deception is not confined to species with a large brain, as shown by the striking courtship behaviour of male mourning cuttlefish (*Sepia plangon*). In this species, males have the remarkable ability to display a pulsing striped courtship pattern to a receptive female on one side of their body, while simultaneously displaying a mottled camouflage pattern, characteristic of a female, to a watching male positioned on the other side (Figure 2.6; Brown et al. 2012). This tactical duplicity allows males to complete courtship of females while remaining undetected and unmolested by male rivals.

The theoretical difficulty raised by such examples of deceptive signalling is one of evolutionary stability: where signals are routinely false, receivers should evolve to ignore them. But signal stability can in theory be maintained if deceptive signallers occur at low frequency in the population, or if signallers produce a mixture of honest and deceptive signals. Fork-tailed drongos (*Dricrurus adsimilis*) in the Kalahari give false predator alarm calls to meerkats and pied babblers, sending them fleeing and

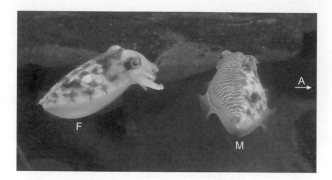

Figure 2.6 Tactical deception in male mourning cuttlefish. Male cuttlefish (M) displaying a male-specific pattern towards a female (F) while simultaneously displaying deceptive female colouration towards a rival male (A). Reproduced with permission from Brown et al. (2012). © 2012 The Royal Society. (A black and white version of this figure will appear in some formats. For the colour version, please refer to the plate section.)

allowing the drongo to steal food finds (Flower 2011). They even use a mixture of their own 'drongo alarm' calls and numerous (over 40) mimicked alarm calls, such as a 'meerkat alarm' and a 'babbler alarm', which are acoustically indistinguishable from the real alarm calls of their duped victims. In this system, the targets are quick to wise up if repeatedly exposed to playbacks of false alarms by drongos, but deceptive signalling appears to persist because individual drongos produce a mixture of honest and false signals, and 'change up' by using a different type of false alarm if their victims stop responding (Flower et al. 2014).

The deceptive behaviour of cuttlefish and drongos raises the question of whether we should expect biological signals used in competition to be honest, and what mechanisms animals might use to assess each other's competitive ability and motivation to fight. These questions are particularly important in the context of contest competition, and are considered in the next chapter (Section 3.3.3).

2.6   Social Influences on Competition

In Section 2.2 we considered how the distribution and type of resources in the environment influence the costs and benefits of racing to consume them or fighting to defend them. We now return to consider another, critical influence on the profitability of different competitive strategies: the social environment, in particular the number of competitors, and their relative strength or resource holding potential (RHP). Different individuals will experience different costs and benefits of racing versus fighting depending on their RHP and information about the environment, and so may employ different strategies in the same ecological environment. Game-theoretical models tell us that the fitness pay-offs of alternative behavioural strategies typically depend on the frequency with which different strategies are encountered in the population (Grafen 1979; Queller 1984; Houston & McNamara 1991; Kokko & Ots 2006). In many cases, strategies such as scrounging, sneaking or escalating become less profitable the more common they are, a phenomenon known as negative frequency-dependent selection, or negative frequency dependence. Where strategies are negatively frequency-dependent, populations may evolve to an equilibrium (or evolutionarily stable state; Taylor & Jonker 1978) at which the strategies have equal pay-off. Negative frequency dependence provides one explanation for why different alternative strategies can persist in populations over evolutionary time.

2.6.1   Population Density and Competition

The simplest social influence on competition is population density. Classic ecological theory predicts that populations will increase in density to the point where each individual can only produce one offspring, on average (Varley & Gradwell 1960; May et al. 1974). Variation in equilibrium population density (and, in dynamic environments, fluctuations in density) has important consequences for the frequency of social encounters and the costs and benefits of competitive behaviour. It has been hypothesized that contests will be observed at intermediate equilibrium levels of population density (Warner & Hoffman 1980; Grant 1993), similar to the predicted effect of resource availability on territoriality (Carpenter & Macmillen 1976). According to this hypothesis, where there are few competitors in the environment, social encounters will be rare, in which case there may be little to be gained from defending resources or territories containing them. Resource defence is also proposed to become unprofitable at very high population density, when defenders are swamped with intruders. In theory, therefore, aggressive resource defence should pay at intermediate population densities.

Empirical support for this prediction in laboratory cichlids was found by Noël et al. (2005; Figure 2.7). Groups of juvenile convict cichlids that were kept at intermediate competitor-to-resource ratios showed the highest rates of feeding aggression (Figure 2.7B). Moreover, this elevated aggression resulted in winners and losers and hence increased variance in body size (Figure 2.7C). In guppies (*Poecilia reticulata*), male–male courtship displays are highest at intermediate densities (Jirotkul 1999).

There is evidence that above a certain population density, aggression and contest competition is reduced. A common finding in fisheries research is that very high population density is associated with lower aggression (Wallace et al. 1988). In crickets (*Gryllus* species), males sit and call to attract females when the population density is low, but at high density they give up calling and instead start wandering, with the aim of encountering females by chance (Buzatto et al. 2014). In *Gryllus* species (French & Cade 1989; Cade & Cade 1992), damselfish *Chromis cyanea* (De Boer 1981), sticklebacks *Gasterosteus aculeatus* (Wootton 1985) and rhesus macaques *Macaca mulatta* (Wootton 1985), male–male aggression declines with increasing population density as males shift to using alternative tactics to acquire mates (reviewed by Knell 2009).

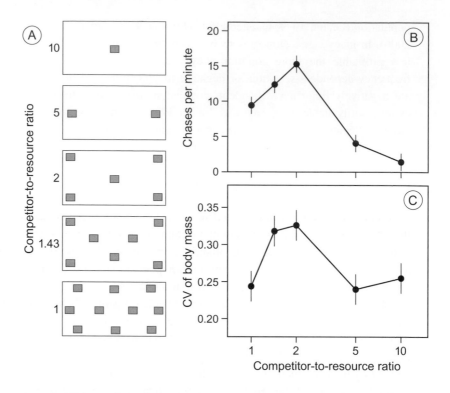

Figure 2.7 Consequences of varying resource competition for aggression and body size in convict cichlids. (A) Top view of experimental tanks showing the location of food patches (dark squares) in the five competitor-to-resource ratio treatments. (B) Aggressive behaviour associated with the five treatments. (C) Coefficient of variation in body mass at the end of the trials. Groups of fish reared at intermediate competitor-to-resource ratios showed both higher aggression and variation in final body mass (redrawn with permission from Noël et al. 2005). © 2009 The Authors. Journal compilation © 2009 The Zoological Society of London; John Wiley.

Evidence for a lower population density threshold, below which resource defence becomes unprofitable, is less common (Grant 1993). The experimental manipulations of Noël et al. (2005) on convict cichlids (Figure 2.7) and Jirotkul (1999) on guppies provide evidence of a lower threshold for resource defence. In the African striped mouse *Rhabdomis pumilio* (Schradin & Lindholm 2011), some males defend territories at high population density, but all males switch to a roamer strategy at low density (see Section 2.6.4).

Very low population density can create strong incentives to find a partner. For example, a very low density of females in the environment may promote mate-guarding and monogamy in male mammals (Schacht & Bell 2016). When females are very scarce, the best option of males may be to remain with any female they find and guard them against competitor males. In deep-sea anglerfish, very low population density and encounter rates likely explain why males fuse with females for life (Pietsch 2005). By contrast, in the Seychelles warbler, rates of 'divorce' are lower at high population density compared to low population density (Komdeur & Edelaar 2001). Increasing population density may therefore have contrasting impacts on selection for monogamy and the degree of conflict between males and females over parental investment (Chapter 3).

2.6.2   Sexual Conflict

While some resources, such as shelter, light and water, are 'passive' features of the abiotic environment, resources such as prey items and mates can be considered active 'players' in the evolution of competitive strategies. These players will distribute themselves in time and space in a way that maximizes their own fitness, which may be directly counter to the fitness interests of the individuals that compete for them as a resource. For example, dominant males may gain from monopolizing access to multiple females, but if this is not in the interest of females then they can be expected to evolve countermeasures to prevent monopolization, such as dispersal or synchronous reproduction. In these cases female behaviour has the effect of shifting the nature of male–male competition from contest towards scramble. Underlying ecological resources (such as food and water) will influence the distribution and population density of females and hence their economic defendability. However, a second major determinant of the form of male–male competition is the degree to which females can prevent males from monopolizing or controlling their mating behaviour. In banded mongooses, for example, older males closely mate-guard oestrous females in their group, following them nose-to-tail all day long, for days at a time (Cant 2000). Nevertheless, females are adept at escaping their mate guard to mate with other males in the group. When there is a high risk of inbreeding within their own group, females incite intergroup fights and use the cover of battle to escape their mate guards and mate with males from rival groups (Johnstone et al. 2020).

On the other hand, it may sometimes pay females to shift competition in the other direction, that is, to incite contest competition among males so that they are able to mate with males of the highest quality. The females of some lekking ungulates, for example, are widely dispersed with large home ranges, which should tend to reduce contest competition and lead to relatively even distribution of paternity among males (Balmford et al. 1993; Clutton-Brock et al. 1993). However, because females choose only to mate with males that cluster at particular lekking sites, they can effectively force males into a form of contest competition, allowing them to choose to mate with the highest-quality male (Bro-Jørgensen 2003; Isvaran & Ponkshe 2013). The outcome is a very strong skew in the distribution of paternity, which may be in the interests of females, but not in the interests of the majority of males, who have little or no chance of obtaining a mating.

2.6.3   Alternative Reproductive Tactics

Animal populations exhibit considerable variation in fitness-related traits such as quality, size and personality (Cam et al. 2004; Clutton-Brock & Sheldon 2010;

Wilson & Nussey 2010; Wolf & Weissing 2012). Increasing population density can generate stabilizing or directional selection on these traits, for example if smaller individuals are excluded from limited resources while larger individuals enjoy more than their fair share. Alternatively, intraspecific competition can lead to evolutionary diversification and polymorphism of behavioural strategies among individuals of different size or quality (Gross 1996; Brockmann 2001; Svanbäck & Bolnick 2005; Brockmann & Taborsky 2008; Taborsky & Brockmann 2010). For example, males of many species adopt different reproductive tactics depending on their body size or RHP (Emlen 1997; Moczek & Emlen 2000). Larger males can expect to maximize their fitness by engaging in contest competition, fighting for and defending access to females. Smaller males that would do poorly in such fights can gain from alternative 'sneaky' strategies, for example by avoiding dominant males and mating surreptitiously with females (Taborsky et al. 2008), or staying close to dominant males in the hope of intercepting incoming females.

There is a continuum in flexibility of alternative reproductive tactics, from genetically encoded, inflexible morphs to behaviours that are highly sensitive to the social and ecological context. In lek-breeding ruffs, for example, there are three genetically determined male reproductive morphs: dark-plumed, territorial 'independent' males; white-plumed, non-territorial 'satellites'; and female mimics or 'faeder' males. These morphs are inflexible to the individual's condition or environmental conditions (Lank et al. 1995). In dung beetles of the genus *Onthophagus*, males develop into two morphs: 'majors' that possess an enlarged pronotal horn used to fight other males, and 'minors' that develop rudimentary horns and sneak compulations from females that are guarded by majors (Cook 1990; Moczek & Emlen 2000; Simmons & Kotiaho 2007). The dimorphism is influenced by the paternal genotype and patterns of maternal allocation: mothers invest more in offspring that are sired to major males (Kotiaho et al. 2000). In some frogs and toads, small males or those in poor condition adopt 'satellite' tactics, remaining silent beside calling males in an attempt to sneak matings with incoming females (Zamudio & Chan 2008; Berec & Bajgar 2011). In the tropical frog *Physalaemus signifer* the first males to arrive at a breeding site become caller males, while later-arriving males become satellites (Wogel et al. 2002, cited in Zamudio & Chan 2008). In this study there was no difference in body size between callers and satellites, suggesting that each frog adjusts its tactics according to its social circumstances. Sensitivity of reproductive tactics to social conditions, particularly the density of breeding aggregations, is characteristic of mating behaviour in amphibians (Zamudio & Chan 2008).

Classic game-theoretical analyses suggest that where alternative strategies exhibit negative frequency dependence, populations may evolve to an evolutionarily stable state at which the different strategies have the same pay-off (Maynard Smith & Price 1973; Taylor & Jonker 1978; Maynard Smith 1982a). The equilibrium solution to these models may equally describe a polymorphic population consisting of an equilibrium mixture of alternative discrete strategies (e.g. p sneaker morphs and $1 - p$ territorial morphs), or monomorphic population consisting of individuals who each adopt a probabilistic continuous strategy, behaving like a sneaker with probability p, and like a territory holder with probability $1 - p$. However, the discrete and continuous cases may yield different evolutionarily stable states if competition occurs between individuals that are genetically related (Grafen 1979).

The prediction that, at equilibrium, the fitness pay-offs of alternative strategies will be equal has received surprisingly little empirical support as yet. In the marine isopod *Paracerceis sculpta*, there are three genetically discrete male morphs: alpha males who defend harems, beta males who mimic females, and tiny gamma males who sneak into large harems (Shuster & Wade 1991). Average reproductive success of the three morphs is equal. Similarly, in the side-blotched lizard *Uta stansburiana*, three male morphs coexist and experimental manipulation of morph frequencies revealed that the common phenotype lost fitness to its antagonist as predicted by negative frequency dependence (Bleay et al. 2007). In the cooperatively breeding greater ani (*Crotophaga major*), most females start the season by nesting in cooperatively breeding groups consisting of two or three mated pairs that build a communal nest. However, if their clutch is predated, some females in the population switch to a parasitic strategy of laying their eggs in another group's nest, avoiding the cost of rearing young. Other females never switch to the parasitic tactic and remain 'pure cooperators'. Pure cooperators lay larger clutches and have more surviving young than parasites, so that across years, the fitness pay-offs of the two strategies is approximatey equal (Riehl & Strong 2019).

If population density or other ecological factors change, the intersection point of frequency-dependent fitness curves can be shifted to a new, different equilibrium mixture of strategies, resulting in a different 'switchpoint' between alternative tactics or morphs. Tomkins and Brown (2004) tested this prediction by examining the relative frequency of two different morphs of the European earwig *Forficula auricularia* in island populations with varying population densities (Figure 2.8A). In this species males guard burrows and females, and use their rear forceps in both courtship and fights with other males over females. Males develop into one of two morphs, which possess small and large forceps, respectively. Small males tend to develop small forceps, and large males large ones, but the threshold body size or switch point between these two strategies varies depending on population density. Large forceps confer less of an advantage when rival males are unlikely to be encountered, which in theory should increase the threshold body size at which large forceps yield the higher pay-off. As predicted, on islands with a higher population density the switch point between the two morphs was lowered, so that a larger fraction of males developed large forceps (Figure 2.8B).

Population density has the opposite effect on the fitness of fighter males in the acarid mite *Sancassania berleisei*. Here males of a 'fighter' morphs develop a thickened third pair of legs and use these to kill other males. A second 'scrambler' morph has unmodified legs. Fighter males have higher fitness only at low densities; as population density increases fighter males suffer costs and damage as they are involved in frequent fights (Timms et al. 1982). The proportion of larvae developing into the fighter morph declines when larvae are kept at high density. In this case chemical cues of high density at the larval stage appear to be used to make a

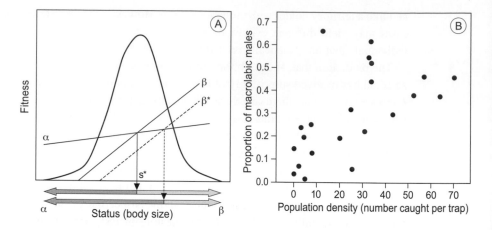

Figure 2.8 Density-dependent morph-switching threshold in the earwig *Forficula auricularia*. In this species there are two morphs, with either short forceps (brachylabic) or long forceps (macrolabic) (A). Graphical model of a status-dependent switching threshold. α and β show fitness pay-offs of two alternative tactics (for example, short and long forceps, respectively) as a function of status (here, body size). Long forceps (the macrolabic morph) are most advantageous for individuals of large body size. However, the threshold body size or switch point above which the macrolabic morph is favoured may be sensitive to population density or other environmental factors. For example, a decline in population density can be theorized to shift the fitness function of macrolabic males from β to β*, reducing the proportion of individuals that fall above the switching threshold. (B) Proportion of macrolabic males in island populations of *F. auricularia* as a function of population density. The proportion of macrolabic males varies widely with demographic factors, even over very small geographic scales. Redrawn with permission from Tomkins and Brown (2004). Copyright © 2004, Macmillan Magazines Ltd. Reprinted/adapted by permission from Springer Nature.

developmental decision about which adult morph is likely to yield the highest fitness pay-off (Tomkins et al. 2004).

2.6.4 Conditional Strategies

In many circumstances individuals adopt very different reproductive tactics, but the pay-offs of these alternatives are far from equal (Gross 1996; Schradin 2019). Low-quality individuals may be forced to make the 'best of a bad job' by avoiding contest competition, instead sneaking food or matings whenever they can, while high-quality individuals defend territories or resources (Gross 1996; Engqvist & Taborsky 2016). Variation in tactics in this case derives from environmentally or developmentally induced variation in size or quality, rather than negative frequency-dependent selection. Small males of the rove beetle *Leistotrophus versicolor* avoid being attacked by larger males by mimicking females and engaging in courtship behaviour, up to but not including copulation (Forsyth & Alcock 1990). Amphibian males that adopt satellite behaviour generally obtain reduced reproductive success compared to calling males

(Zamudia & Chan 2008). Surprisingly, these small males still manage to obtain some matings with females, even while they are in the middle of courting another male. In the African striped mouse (*Rhabdomis pumilio*), breeding males achieve approximately 10 times the reproductive success of roamers, and 100 times the reproductive success of sneakers when population density is high (Schradin & Lindholm 2011). At intermediate population density, however, the fitness pay-offs of breeding and roaming are approximately equal, and at low density all males become roamers. In many fish, birds and mammals, individuals adopt sneaker tactics when young, and compete for matings only when they are older (Oliveira et al. 2008).

Where low-quality or subordinate males are unable to defend territories or females themselves, they may use other tactics to circumvent the control that stronger, dominant individuals hold over a resource. In the striped parrotfish *Scarus croicensis*, for example, subordinate individuals that cannot obtain a territory form schools and together overcome the efforts of dominant individuals to defend exclusive access to resources (Robertson et al. 1976). In this case the school represents a form of coalition to overcome the suppression of a dominant individual, promoting a more egalitarian, scramble-like outcome of competition. This kind of 'dominance of the subordinates' has been invoked as the mechanism that stabilizes the egalitarian power structures of human hunter-gatherers (Boehm 1999). Individuals that attempt to assert power over the group are kept in check by the coordinated behaviour of other, weaker individuals, through social ostracism or verbal castigation (Section 3.4.2). Alliances of the weak against the strong to maintain egalitarian outcomes of competition can evolve when individuals experience accelerating benefits with increasing share of a contested resource (Gavrilets 2012).

The examples above of male and female banded mongooses locked in competition to achieve their preferred distribution of paternity, or parrotfish subordinates banding together to overcome dominant individuals, are far from the original conception of scramble competition as a race to exploit resources. The competition in these cases is a contest where each party is selected to fight back against the attempts by another party to control its behaviour. The outcome depends on the ability (or power) of each to enforce its own preference or optimum resolution, and the degree to which competing individuals are bound together in social interaction. The ecological and social conditions that shift competition towards contests are often associated with kin structure and repeated interactions in stable groups. In this case the parties involved can be said to be involved in social conflict, rather than scramble competition. These social conflicts and their resolution are the subject of the next chapter.

2.7   Conclusions

Competition is a fundamental force shaping social interaction. The form of competition and its consequences for evolution depend crucially on the ecological distribution of resources in time and space. We have focused on the ecological factors that push individuals towards strategies of scramble competition, or racing to consume resources, rather than fighting to defend them; and the consequences of such competition for food, space and information. Strategies of scramble evolve where resources are not economically defendable, because they are widely scattered, unpredictable in space, or because they appear synchronously everywhere.

Where competition takes the form of scramble, pay-offs from competition depend primarily on the amount of resources at stake and the number of competitors. The IFD then provides a simple, idealized account of how animal distributions will map to resource distributions in a heterogeneous environment. The model highlights that selection acting on individual decision-making can scale up to have predictable, population-level consequences. Adding in biological detail about physical or ecological constraints (such as perceptual constraints, or resource dynamics) may help to explain deviations between theory and data. These models and tests provide confirmation of the usefulness of game-theoretical approaches to understand evolution of social behaviour.

The presence and proximity of conspecifics can bring benefits as well as costs, and lead to remarkable examples of social coordination and collective movement. Individuals can be selected to follow each other closely, or to stand out from the crowd, depending on the fitness benefits of proximity, alignment and coordination. Where individuals differ in size or strength, group coordination may require the emergence of leaders and followers, or forms of compromise such as turn-taking. Consistent individual differences can lead to the emergence of coordination and influence group success. Whether and how consensus emerges depends on the intensity of competition and the degree of divergence of fitness interests among competitors.

A key resource in the life of animals is information, for example information about the location of food or mates, and about relative competitive ability. Animals exploit cues in the environment, including those produced by conspecifics. Selection in turn can favour suppression of cues and hiding of food, or flexible use of signals to recruit others to resources when this is advantageous, and hide resources that might otherwise be stolen. The remarkable cognitive abilities of some animals appear to be the result of selection to exploit and suppress information about food or to deceive rivals.

Population density exerts a fundamental social influence on the frequency and intensity of scramble competition and the form of competitive behaviour. Increasing density can amplify variation in fitness among individuals that vary in size or strength, and lead to evolutionary diversification via selection for alternative reproductive or social tactics, and polymorphism. The binding of individuals by their ecology in stable groups, engaging in repeated interactions over defendable resources, selects complex behavioural strategies of competition, such as fighting, coercing, negotiating and cooperating.

Cooperative Breeding in the Face of Intense Reproductive Competition

Summary

Banded mongooses exhibit remarkable patterns of cooperation and conflict, providing an opportunity to test how conflicts over reproduction are resolved, and the causes and consequences of helping behaviour. Unlike most cooperatively breeding mammals, there is no reproductive suppression among females. All females breed regularly from the age of one year, and usually give birth together on exactly the same day. Synchronous reproduction appears to have evolved as a means to mix up cues to maternity so that subordinate females can escape reproductive control by infanticidal dominant females. Unable to prevent subordinates reproducing, dominant females control reproductive competition in the group by violently evicting females en masse, particularly younger females who are close relatives. Helping behaviour takes the form of babysitting offspring at the den, followed by a form of one-to-one helping behaviour known as 'escorting'. Escorts are often males and pups are no more closely related to their escort than to a random group member. Escorts transmit foraging preferences and skills to the pup in their care; cultural inheritance of foraging niche lasts a lifetime. There is intense competition and extreme aggression between rival groups, during which adults and offspring are commonly injured and sometimes killed. There is growing evidence that intergroup conflict is a primary driver of helping behaviour in this system, similar to the proposed role of such conflict in the evolution of human cooperation.

Introduction

The mongoose family, the Herpestidae, consists of 34 species which vary widely in patterns of sociality, ecology and life history. Most species of mongoose are nocturnal and solitary, but nine species are known to be group-living, and three species – meerkats, banded mongooses and dwarf mongooses (*Helogale parvula*) – are obligate cooperative breeders. These three species are diurnal, territorial and live in mixed-sex groups of 5–30 individuals. Each species has been the subject of intense long-term studies that have yielded numerous insights into vertebrate social evolution and cooperative behaviour.

The Banded Mongoose Research Project is a long-term study based at Mweya peninsula in Queen Elizabeth National Park, western Uganda (Figure B.1). The study was started in 1995 by Michael Cant, then a PhD student supervised by Tim Clutton-Brock, and building on earlier work by Daniela de Luca (de Luca & Ginsberg 2001). Banded mongooses were of particular interest because reports from the 1970s suggested that groups typically contained multiple co-breeding females. By contrast, in meerkats and the dwarf mongooses, reproduction was known to be monopolized by a single dominant female and subordinate females rarely reproduced. At the time there was much interest in the idea that a single 'optimal skew' model might explain variation in reproductive skew within and between species, in animals ranging from insects to primates (Vehrencamp 1983; Reeve & Ratnieks 1993). This model assumed that dominant individuals had full control over reproduction, but could gain by offering shares of reproduction to subordinates as a 'staying incentive' to retain them as helpers in the group. Banded mongooses, in

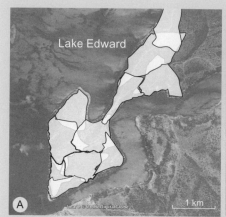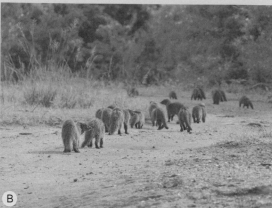

Figure B.1 (A) Map of Mweya peninsula, Queen Elizabeth National Park, Uganda, showing approximate home ranges of 11 study groups. At the study site in Uganda banded mongooses live in groups averaging 20 adults, plus offspring. Groups give birth on average four times per year, and offspring are kept underground for the first month of life. After pups emerge from the den they travel with the group and are provisioned by adults for a further 6 weeks. Females produce their first litters at around 1 year of age. Males form a dominance hierarchy in which the oldest two or three males in each group monopolize matings and paternity. For a detailed account of the study site and system, see Cant et al. (2013, 2016). (B) Banded mongooses setting out on a foraging trip. Groups sleep together each night in one of many underground dens in their territory, emerging at dawn to forage together for several hours, scouring the ground and digging for insects, arachnids and small vertebrates. (B) © Faye Thompson. (A black and white version of this figure will appear in some formats. For the colour version, please refer to the plate section.)

which reproductive skew among females appeared to be unusually low and potentially highly variable, offered an ideal opportunity to test the model. As it turned out, the findings from the study did not fit the assumption that dominant individuals controlled reproduction, stimulating the development of alternative models of reproductive skew based on incomplete control (Cant 1998; Cant & Johnstone 1999; Johnstone & Cant 1999).

Reproductive Competition

The first research of the project confirmed earlier reports that there was almost no reproductive suppression in banded mongooses (Cant 2000). All females from the age of around 9 months are potential breeders, although older females (3+ years) breed more frequently, and produce larger litters,

than younger females. Early observations showed that all breeding females in each group typically synchronize birth to the same day, or even the same morning. One day all the heavily pregnant females in the group can be observed waddling around with the rest of the group; the next morning all these females remain in the den, and only the males and juveniles in the group emerge to go foraging. In late morning breeding females typically reappear, clearly having given birth. In 63 per cent of breeding attempts, all breeding females in the group (average = 4) give birth on the same day (Hodge et al. 2011); up to 12 females have been observed to synchronize birth in this way. Extreme birth synchrony appears to be an adaptation to escape infanticide. When females give birth on different days, i.e. asynchronously, the litters of early-birthing females appear to be killed shortly after birth, whereas the litters of last-birthing females survive. This pattern and experimental suppression experiments suggest that pregnant females, particularly older, socially dominant females, are infanticidal towards other newborns in the group, until their own litter is born (Cant et al. 2014). Birth synchrony appears to remove cues to maternity, so dominant females refrain from infanticide when the communal litter contains their own offspring.

Birth synchrony and the consequent lack of reproductive suppression has cascading effects on many other aspects of the social system. Because older females appear to be unable to stop younger females from giving birth, these females start to suffer major costs of reproductive competition as the number of potential breeding females in the group grows large (Cant et al. 2010). Older females respond to this reproductive competition by violently evicting younger females from the group (Thompson et al. 2016). Pregnant females that are evicted often spontaneously abort their litter and subsequently regain admittance to the group. Older females target more closely related females for eviction, possibly because these females are less likely to put up a serious fight against a closely related dominant female (Figure B.2) (Thompson et al. 2017a). By evicting younger, closely related females, a cohort of dominant females increase their own reproductive success (Figure 3.4) and at the same time reduce the average degree of relatedness among their same sex group members.

The mass eviction of females, and sometimes males alongside them, affects the genetic structure of the population. New groups are founded when evicted groups of females meet groups of males that have also been evicted, or have left their group voluntarily. At group formation, therefore, females are related to other females, and males to other males, but inter-sex relatedness is close to zero. Because most individuals of both sexes live and die in their natal group, inbreeding leads to an increase in relatedness between breeders over time. After 10 years of breeding together, inter-sex relatedness has on average risen from around zero to around 0.25 (Nichols et al. 2012a). Inbreeding is a

serious risk, and is associated with inbreeding depression: inbred offspring are lighter at adulthood, and have lower annual reproductive success (Wells et al. 2018). In response to this rising risk of inbreeding, females in relatively old groups increasingly seek out matings with the members of neighbouring groups. These intergroup matings result in fitter, outbred offspring, but come at the cost of violent intergroup fights (see below).

Helping Behaviour

Banded mongooses exhibit two main types of communal care: babysitting and escorting pups. After the communal litter is born, two or three individuals remain behind at the den to babysit while the rest of the group goes off to forage. All individuals contribute to babysitting, but subordinate males babysit more often than older males or females, and take the longest shifts (Cant 2003). Babysitters play a crucial role in defending the litter against predators and, importantly, neighbouring groups of mongooses, which frequently attack and exterminate the offspring of rival groups. Babysitting can yield substantial inclusive fitness benefits because the mean relatedness of adults to the communal litter is quite high (around 0.25); and litters that are left undefended, or defended by only a single babysitter, are very likely to be killed (Marshall et al. 2016). There is no evidence that babysitters are coerced into helping, or gain future direct fitness from staying behind to look after the offspring (Thompson et al. 2016).

Escorting occurs after pups have emerged from the den and started to travel with the group on foraging trips. Pups aggressively compete for access to particular adult carers, or 'escorts', following them around and continuously begging for food; there is also evidence that escorts choose to help particular pups (Gilchrist 2008). Some pups receive constant care and attention from the same escort day after day, while other pups have no clearly identifiable escort and receive much less care overall, with the result that these pups grow less quickly and have lower survival. Pups observe and imitate the foraging techniques of their escort, with the consequence that pups learn their adult foraging niche

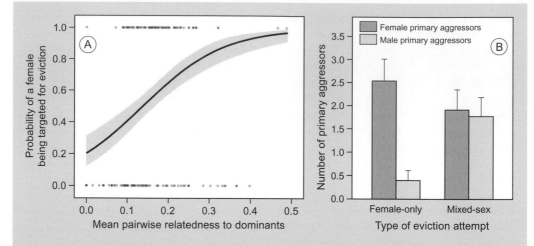

Figure B.2 Socially dominant females control reproductive competition by violently evicting groups of younger females. (A) Females target more closely related females for eviction. (B) Females are evicted as a result of aggression by other females. Occasionally groups of males are also evicted; in these cases males join in to attack evictees. (B) Redrawn with permission from Thompson et al. (2017a). © Faye Thompson.

from their escorts, rather than inheriting it from their parents (Mueller & Cant 2010). This one-to-one social transmission system helps to maintain foraging niche differentiation and reduce social competition in groups of banded mongooses (Figure B.3; Sheppard et al. 2018).

While there is strong evidence of (negative) kin discrimination during eviction events, there is no evidence of any form of kin discrimination when it comes to the care of individual young. Mothers appear to take no notice of which pups suckle from them, and pups frequently move from one mother to another in a single suckling bout (Cant 2000). Escorts do not associate with pups that are more closely related than the average for the litter. Instead, helping effort is influenced by simple rules of thumb based on the individual's own breeding status and sex. Females, for example, are more likely to babysit the communal litter if they have given birth themselves, and males are more likely to escort offspring if they are the fathers of some of the pups in the litter. There are strong sex-biases in the targeting of care within litters: females direct care at female pups and males at male pups (Vitikainen

et al. 2017). Sex-specific helping may have future fitness benefits because both male and female adults benefit from a large same-sex cohort when it comes to dispersal or defending the group.

Intergroup Conflict

Banded mongoose groups are highly territorial and frequently fight each other for access to mates and territory (Thompson et al. 2017b). These fights are violent and can lead to injury and even death. The mortality rate from intergroup fighting in banded mongooses (0.5 per cent of adults per year) is higher than in meerkats and chimpanzees, and comparable to the mortality costs of warfare in small-scale human societies. There is evidence that females lead their group into intergroup encounters to obtain benefits from outbred matings, and use the cover of battle to escape mate-guarding males (Section 3.5; Johnstone et al. 2020).

Pups are particularly vulnerable to intergroup attack, especially in their first month of life. If a neighbouring group discovers a natal den guarded by adult babysitters, they usually try to drive off the adults and, if successful, kill the entire litter. The

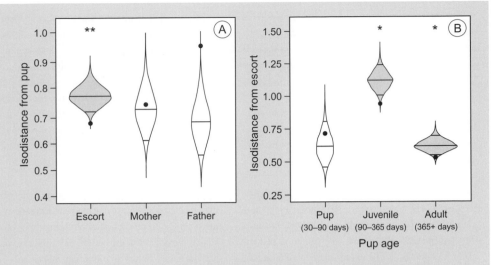

Figure B.3 (A) Pups inherit the isotopic foraging niche of their escort, not their parents. Isotopic niche distance (isodistance) of pups compared to their escort, genetic mother and genetic father. The violin plots show the null distribution based on isodistances to all group members sampled at the same time as the pup. Filled dots indicate mean observed isodistance. (B) Culturally inherited foraging niche persists across the lifespan. Redrawn with permission from Sheppard et al. (2018). $*P < 0.05$; $**P < 0.01$. Open access.

risk of intergroup attacks on the natal den explains why litter survival to emergence increases sharply with the average number of babysitters left behind to defend them (Marshall et al. 2016). Small groups are unable to leave many babysitters behind each day, and are consequently more vulnerable to lethal intergroup raids on the communal litter. The greater vulnerability of small groups to attacks on adults and offspring results in strong Allee effects in our study population: groups that dwindle to 5 or 6 individuals often go extinct within a year or so.

As discussed in Chapter 3, theoretical models suggest that severe intergroup conflict may have driven the evolution of large-scale cooperation and patterns of ethnic conflict in ancestral humans. In principle, these models should apply well to the banded mongoose system, in which intergroup conflict is severe and groups exhibit striking forms of cooperation. However, it is not yet known whether attacks from other groups cause individuals to invest more in the cooperative care of young. While there has been much research in primates and other social vertebrates on the immediate behavioural responses to intergroup attack or simulated intrusions, there are currently almost no data on the longer-term consequences of intergroup fights for group cohesion and helping effort. Banded mongooses, in which fights between groups are frequent, violent and variable, may be particularly well-suited to address this question.

Towards New Frontiers

Banded mongoose society possesses many unusual features – low female reproductive skew, synchronous birth, escorting, warfare – which make them an outlier among cooperatively breeding animals. Animals that don't fit an established pattern can be particularly powerful systems to test the generality of existing theory and suggest new hypotheses. One example is the hypothesis that warfare in banded mongooses is the result of exploitative leadership, which highlights a potential downside of social cohesion and resonates with our understanding of human conflict.

Synchronous birth by up to 12 females is a remarkable feat, but the mechanisms underlying this are still poorly understood. A working hypothesis is that older females produce pheromonal pulses close to birth that are used as a cue by younger females. The presence of multiple breeders per group allows experimental manipulation of maternal condition in litters that are raised anonymously with respect to offspring parentage. One long-running experiment suggests that maternal condition during pregnancy has lifelong impacts on the amount of help received and lifelong reproductive success. In this experiment, mothers that had been fed during pregnancy gave birth to larger offspring as expected, but then directed intense help towards the offspring of control, unfed mothers. The result was a levelling-up of the experimentally induced early-life inequalities among offspring in the communal litter. From behind a veil of ignorance over the maternity of offspring, mothers in good condition (i.e. those that were provisioned through late pregnancy) do best to provide remedial care to disadvantaged young, because there is a chance these young are their own.

The escort–pup system is a natural cross-fostering experiment to evaluate the role of genetic and cultural inheritance in behaviour. In theory, one-to-one social transmission should prevent blending cultural inheritance and increase behavioural heterogeneity within groups. Future research could test this prediction experimentally, using food puzzles, and determine whether one-to-one cultural inheritance has evolved to alleviate food competition among large cohorts of simultaneously born offspring. Multi-generational, individual-based field projects have a crucial role to play in advancing understanding of non-genetic inheritance in biological systems (Vitikainen et al. 2019).

Finally, in banded mongooses as in other social mammals, the advent of cheap drone technology has the potential to revolutionize understanding of collective movement in the natural environment, and in particular how intergroup conflict shapes collective decision making. Males and females have very different fitness incentives to seek out rival groups, and the degree of divergence within groups ebbs and flows across the phases of group females' reproductive cycle (and the cycle of neighbouring groups). How and why heterogeneous groups reach consensus over movement and how groups overcome collective action problems to remain cohesive in the face of battle are topics for future study, made tractable by innovations in tracking technology.

3   Conflict

The previous chapter examined the factors that shape the evolution of competitive behaviour, focusing primarily on forms of scramble competition or racing to consume or exploit resources. Competition also occurs between individuals that interact repeatedly – what we term social conflict – which may lead to the evolution of more complex strategies of competition. In some circumstances, individuals may be selected to put their differences aside and work together as a team to outcompete other teams. Such transitions from outright conflict to cooperation have been called 'major transitions in evolution'. The theory of major transitions tries to explain how and why many forms of life have become more complex over time, from self-replicating molecules to animal societies. Understanding how major transitions occur requires an explanation of how individual conflicts of interest can be suppressed for the good of the group. Many of the major transitions in evolution happened billions or hundreds of millions of years ago, and are difficult to study. However, a recent major transition occurred with the evolution of cooperative animal societies from solitary ancestors, and hence these societies are tractable systems to investigate how strategies of conflict and cooperation coevolve. This chapter explores the forms of conflict that arise in cooperative societies, and the social behaviours that individuals use to shift the resolution of conflict in their own favour, from aggression and escalated fighting to more subtle forms of negotiation. We show how selection can lead to the suppression of competition and peaceful resolution of conflict among social partners, uniting their fitness interests and paving the way for the final stage of a major transition, the evolution of a new, higher level of biological complexity.

3.1   Conflict and Cooperation

Given the historical perception of natural selection as a nakedly competitive process ('nature red in tooth and claw'), it is an irony that the evolution of life is now recognized as a story of cooperation. Life forms are a nested hierarchy of cooperative teams: teams of replicating molecules, genes, chromosomes, cells and individuals. Each new level of the hierarchy appears to have arisen via a major transition in which competition among lower-level units was repressed for the benefit of fitness at the level of the collective (Alexander 1987; Buss 1987; Maynard Smith 1988; Maynard Smith & Szathmary 1995; Okasha 2006; Bourke 2011; West et al. 2015).

In the process of this transition, the collective emerges as a new target or level of natural selection. The action of selection at this level favours the evolution of adaptations to maximize collective fitness, that is, the success of collectives at producing descendent collectives.

The origin of life must have involved a major transition of this kind, from some kind of simple replicating unit or molecule to interacting networks of molecules that replicated more efficiently together than alone (Vaidya et al. 2013; Szathmáry 2015). Subsequent major transitions include the evolution of chromosomes, the evolution of simple cells, the transition from prokaryotic to eukaryotic cells, and the major transition from unicellular to multicellular life forms that has occurred dozens of times over the last billion years (Bonner 1998). Over the last 50–100 million years a new tier has emerged, composed of individual partnerships (Eshel & Shaked 2001) and animal societies that exhibit group-level adaptive behaviour, as exemplified by the colonies of eusocial insects (Hölldobler & Wilson 2009).

How can self-interested agents make the transition to cooperation? Bourke (2011) divided cooperative transitions into three stages: social group formation, social group maintenance and social group transformation (Bourke 2011; Ågren 2014; Figure 3.1). Social group formation concerns the processes that result in grouping and the formation of social networks within a larger population of individuals (where 'individual' can be defined as the lowest level undergoing selection, or responding to selection; Goodnight 2013b). Social group maintenance refers to processes by which conflicts of interest between group members are resolved or repressed in the interest of group stability and efficiency. Social group transformation refers to the processes that lead to the emergence of the group as an integrated whole, a new evolutionary 'individual' (Buss 1987) or 'organism' (Queller & Strassmann 2009) with adaptations that serve primarily to maximize organismal fitness, not the fitness of its constituent units.

At each level of organization, evolutionary conflict arises whenever the fitness optima of individual subunits cannot be satisfied simultaneously (West & Ghoul 2019). The disparity between the fitness optima of constituent units gives a measure

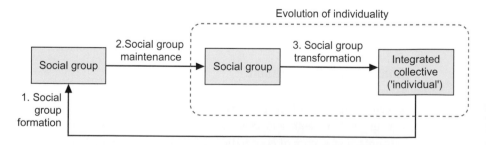

Figure 3.1 Stages involved in a major evolutionary transition (redrawn with permission from Bourke 2011). In stages 1 and 2, groups consist of individual subunits with varying fitness interests. In stage 3, conflict between subunits is suppressed or eradicated and the fitness interests of subunits aligned, setting the stage for the next transition. © Oxford University Press. Reproduced with permission.

of potential conflict within the group; actual conflict occurs when this potential conflict gives rise to costly or damaging behaviour which reduces individual and/or group fitness. In many cases the same ecological and social factors can be expected to influence levels of conflict and cooperation within groups, but conflict is not simply the opposite of cooperation. Social groups can exhibit lots of conflict and cooperation at the same time: this is the case in human societies, and in cooperatively breeding insects and vertebrates. Meerkats, for example, cooperate intensely to rear offspring and to warn each other of danger, but also engage in conspicuous acts of aggression and infanticide (Clutton-Brock & Manser 2016). Indeed, high levels of conflict may be tolerated in these systems precisely because there are large gains from cooperation (Queller & Strassmann 2009). Likewise, many social groups feature very little conflict but also little cooperation. For example, a clone of aphids living together on a plant exhibit little or no conflict behaviour, but they are also not cooperative, possibly because there is not much they can do to boost each others' fitness. Queller and Strassmann (2009) propose that these two axes, the levels of (actual) conflict and cooperation among constituent parts, define the degree to which biological entities should be considered 'organismal', that is, an adapted functional unit with high cooperation and very low conflict among its parts (Figure 3.2). Organisms are the highest tier of hierarchical organization and possess adaptations to enhance collective fitness (Queller & Strassmann 2009; Folse III & Roughgarden 2010).

In addition to the unicellular and multicellular organisms with which biologists are most familiar, certain animal societies and interspecific mutualisms could be considered a unitary organism because they occupy a similar corner of conflict–cooperation space (Figure 3.2). The fitness of an individual coral and its symbiotic zooxanthellae algae, or an individual squid and its microbiome of bioluminescent *Vibrio* bacteria, are so tightly interdependent and mutually cooperative that they can reasonably be considered a unitary organism. Similarly, a colony of the African driver ant *Dorylus wilverthi*, in which queens produce eggs at an average rate of over 1 per second, which are raised by 10 or 20 million sterile workers (Raignier & van Boven 1955, cited in Villet 1990), functions as a single organism in much the same way as the cells that make up a jellyfish or a polar bear. In many eusocial insects, conflicts over reproduction have largely been eradicated by the evolution of a sterile worker caste, but other conflicts persist, for example over the sex ratio of reared offspring (Trivers & Hare 1976), or the parentage of male offspring (Ratnieks et al. 2006). Similarly, multicellular organisms have evolved via mechanisms that suppress social conflict between individual cells, or suppress unregulated mitotic division and cancerous growth (Korolev et al. 2014). Nevertheless, potential conflicts of interest persist within the genome. For example, conflict exists between alleles at the same locus, such as when a paternally inherited allele expressed in a developing foetus favours a higher level of investment by the mother than the maternally inherited allele (Haig 2015). Conflict exists between loci within the genome when the expression of genes at one locus results in a phenotype (such as large body size) that is beneficial for one sex of offspring but not the other (Burt & Trivers 2006; Bonduriansky & Chenoweth 2009). Potential evolutionary conflict in the genome sometimes breaks

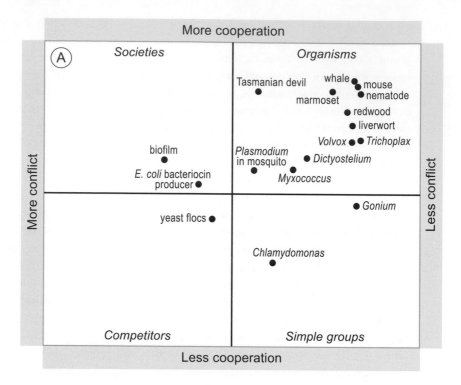

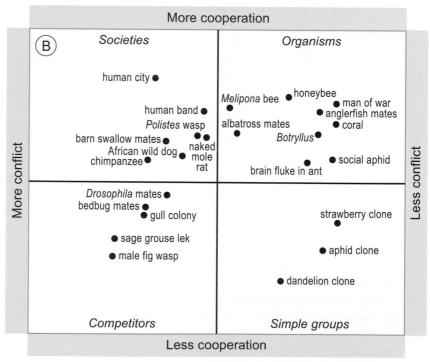

Figure 3.2 Queller and Strassmann's (2009) axes of 'organismality', as applied to (A) groups of cells and (B) groups of multicellular organisms (redrawn with permission from Queller & Strassman 2009). © The Royal Society.

out into overt conflict during phases of the life cycle, such as gametogenesis, which present opportunities for alleles to increase their own fitness at the expense of competitors.

In this chapter we address two questions: what determines the level of conflict within groups, and how is conflict suppressed in cooperative transitions? Our empirical focus to address these questions is research on cooperative animal societies, which includes eusocial, cooperatively breeding and biparental care systems. These systems are good models for the study of conflict and cooperation for several reasons. First, they possess features that are likely to have arisen in early stages in the transition to higher levels of organization (although, of course, these societies are not necessarily on an evolutionary trajectory towards ever-greater integration). Groups are formed of individuals that retain the ability to survive and reproduce as independent entities, or can break off their social interactions to seek other partners or opportunities elsewhere. The behaviour of individuals reflects the trade-off between their current versus future fitness, direct versus indirect fitness (as discussed in detail in Section 4.1.2.2), and the varying degree of overlap between their own fitness interests and those of the group. Second, animal societies offer a great deal of observable variation, the raw material to answer evolutionary questions. There is enormous variation within and between species in group size, social structure, life history, aggression, helping and self-sacrifice; and great variation in cognitive complexity, as measured by various (usually taxon-specific) cognitive tasks or batteries of tasks (Herrmann et al. 2007; Reader et al. 2011; Benson-Amram et al. 2016; Loukola et al. 2017). Patterns of cognitive variation among cooperative insects compared to among cooperative birds and mammals provide a chance to test the generality of simple models of conflict resolution, and whether behavioural mechanisms of conflict resolution (including negotiation and the use of threats) require individual recognition, assessment, or social memory.

Third, and perhaps most importantly, animal societies lack the kind of group-level adaptations that have evolved to suppress conflict among genes in genomes and cells in multicellular organisms. For diploid multicellular organisms, the single-cell bottleneck of development ensures high relatedness and low potential conflict among cooperating cells, while early sequestration of the germ line further eliminates conflict over reproduction within multicellular organisms (Buss 1987; Hochberg et al. 2008). For genomes, the machinery of meiosis and recombination is an elaborate and extremely powerful adaptation to force the interests of genes into line. A fair meiosis means that genes can only increase their own fitness by increasing the fitness of the collective. How meiosis itself evolved is controversial (Wilkins & Holliday 2009; Niklas et al. 2014; Lenormand et al. 2016; Zickler & Kleckner 2016). For animal societies (with the exception of humans) we cannot appeal to meiosis-like institutional machinery to repress competition and eliminate within-group selection. The forms and level of conflict that we see should reflect selection to maximize an individual's inclusive fitness, given the social and ecological context.

In Section 3.2 we describe some of the main sources of within-group conflict in cooperative animal societies. In Section 3.3 we discuss theoretical models of social conflict and the causes of variation in inequality and actual conflict. In Section 3.4 we discuss evolutionary and behavioural mechanisms of conflict reduction. And finally, in Section 3.5 we discuss how conflict between groups influences conflict behaviour within groups.

3.2 Sources of Conflict in Social Groups

3.2.1 Conflict over Group Membership

Social groups form when individuals have some fitness incentive to aggregate, which is sufficient to overcome the centrifugal or repellent forces of competition that drive animals apart. Clearly, competition is particularly intense between conspecifics, because they usually have similar requirements. However, despite severe competition, grouping per se can generate fitness benefits to individuals, for example through reduced risk of predation for group members or their offspring (Boland 2003), or increased efficiency in foraging (Ashton et al. 2018) or brood care (Liebl et al. 2016). Alternatively, individuals may aggregate at sites where food or mates are particularly concentrated because the benefits of doing so in terms of foraging or mating success outweigh the costs of intensified competition (Sridhar et al. 2009). In these cases groups form because the mean fitness within groups is higher than outside groups.

As pointed out by Sibly (1983), however, unless there are some barriers to group entry, joiners will continue to join groups until the benefits of grouping are dissipated in competition, and the fitness of 'insiders' is depressed to the level of 'outsiders' or solitary individuals. Paradoxically, therefore, under free entry, groups are predicted to stabilize at a larger-than-optimal size that brings no benefit from grouping (the 'group size paradox'; Giraldeau 1988; Beauchamp & Fernández-Juricic 2004). As a consequence, whenever there are benefits of grouping there is the potential for 'insider–outsider conflict' over group membership. In animal groups, this conflict is manifested in aggressive group defence and group territoriality (Brown 1987), and in some cases violent or even lethal intergroup competition (Durrant 2011; Radford et al. 2016).

An example of insider–outsider conflict is seen in the paper wasp *Polistes dominula*, where co-foundress associations form in early spring and cooperate for two months to rear the first batch of workers (Reeve 1991). Some foundresses, however, sit out this period and instead attempt to force their way into groups at a late stage, just before workers emerge (Zanette & Field 2011). Resident group members engage in fierce fights to repel these intruders, but the latter are often successful at inserting themselves into the group at rank 2 or 3 in the queue to inherit the rank 1 breeding position. They are almost never successful at usurping the rank 1 position directly, most likely because the rank 1 wasp will fight to the death to hang on to her position. A similar conflict over group membership is played out at an interspecific level in this population of wasps: females of the socially parasitic species *P. semenowi* wait until workers are about to emerge and then take over the rank 1 position in the nest. In this case the intruder is larger, stronger and more massively armoured and there is little the rank 1 host wasp can do to hold on to her position (Green et al. 2014).

Higashi and Yamamura (1993) developed a model of insider–outsider conflict to explore how relatedness and power asymmetries influence the outcome of this conflict, and the resulting stable group size. This model defines both the zone of potential conflict between competing parties (the *battleground*) and also the evolutionary process by which conflict is resolved (the *conflict resolution mechanism*). In Higashi and Yamamura's model, an outsider engages in a game of escalating costs with insiders to force access to the group, up to the point where one or the other party does best (in terms of inclusive fitness) to give up and admit defeat. The model predicts that whenever insiders have any control over group membership, groups will stabilize at a size where insiders do better than solitary individuals, thus providing an escape from Sibly's argument which applies to free-entry groups. The model predicts that insiders should prefer to accept relatives over unrelated individuals as joiners, so stable group size should increase with relatedness (Higashi & Yamamura 1993).

Shen et al. (2017) extended Higashi & Yamamura's model to consider two distinct types of grouping benefits: resource defence benefits, which derive from the presence of other group members, and collective action benefits, which require the active cooperation or coordination of group members. Figure 3.3 shows how per-capita fitness varies with group size under these two benefits, and the predicted effect of relatedness on stable group size. According to this model, the type of grouping benefit determines the pattern of group formation and the characteristics of groups. For example, groups that form because of resource defence benefits are predicted to consist predominantly or exclusively of close genetic relatives, whereas groups that form through collective action benefits may often include nonkin. The importance of resource defence as a benefit of grouping is supported by experiments that increase or decrease the (relative) quality of resources controlled by groups, leading to increased or decreased stable group size. In carrion crows, experiments to increase group resources (through provisioning) led to increased group size because offspring delayed dispersal (Baglione et al. 2006), while in superb fairy-wrens (*Malurus cyaneus*) and red-cockaded woodpeckers (*Picoides borealis*), creation of resources outside the group (through experimental creation of breeding vacancies) led to reduced group size because individuals left their group to breed independently (Pruett-Jones & Lewis 1990; Walters et al. 1992). By contrast, in sociable weavers (*Philetairus socius*), supplemental provision of food to breeding groups led to decreased group size (Covas et al. 2004), consistent with the pattern expected if individuals remain or join groups where they can be most helpful through collective action benefits.

The model of Higashi and Yamamura (1993) assumes that groups form by individuals joining each other – as birds join a flock, for example. But many if not most cooperative animal societies form by recruiting from within, via the retention of offspring. In this case, conflict often arises not over whom to permit to enter the group, but whom to allow to stay in the group, and whom to evict from it. Eviction often involves measureable costs to evictees, and sometimes also to evictors, at least in the short term (Bell et al. 2012; Thompson et al. 2016), in which case groups may

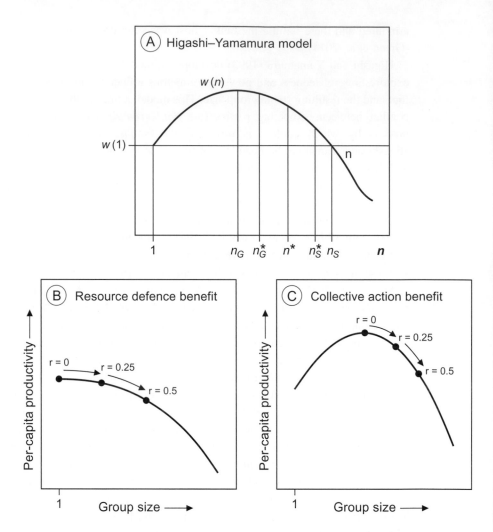

Figure 3.3 Higashi and Yamamura's (1993) model of insider–outsider conflict over group size. (A) Direct fitness of an insider, *w*, for groups of different sizes. The most productive group size is n_G, but given free entry by unrelated outsiders the stable group size is n_S. Where joiners are genetic relatives, an insider's inclusive fitness is maximized at n^*_G, while an outsider's inclusive fitness is maximized at n^*_S. Where both parties exercise partial control over the outcome the 'compromise' group size is n^*. Shen et al. (2017) adapted this model to predict stable group size for two different types of grouping benefits: (B) resource defence benefits, which accrue passively through the presence of other group members; and (C) collective action benefits, which require coordinated action or active cooperation on the part of group members. In both cases, groups of relatives are predicted to stabilize at larger size. Where grouping yields only resource defence benefits, per-capita productivity is maximized for solitary individuals and declines monotonically with increasing group size. By contrast, under collective action benefits, per-capita productivity is maximized at some intermediate group size larger than 1 (redrawn with permission from Higashi & Yamamura 1993 and Shen et al. 2017). (A) The American Naturalist © 1993 The University of Chicago Press; (B,C) © 2017 John Wiley & Sons Ltd/ CNRS.

grow larger than the size that is optimal for insiders (and greater than the stable group sizes in Shen et al.'s 2017 model, because their model assumes that insiders can evict intruders at no cost).

Forcible eviction is common in many social and cooperative species. It has been observed in fish (e.g. orange clownfish *Amphiprion percula*: Buston 2003a; emerald coral goby *Paragobiodon xanthosomus*: Wong et al. 2007; cooperative cichlid *Neolamprologus pulcher*: Taborsky 1985; Balshine-Earn et al. 1998; Dierkes et al. 1999; Fischer et al. 2014), birds (e.g. Tasmanian native hen *Tribonyx mortierii*: Maynard Smith & Ridpath 1972; pied kingfisher *Ceryle rudis*: Reyer 1986; superb fairy-wren *Malurus cyaneus*: Mulder & Langmore 1993; Arabian babbler *Argya squamiceps*: Zahavi 1990; dunnock *Prunella modularis*: Davies 1992; *Montezuma oropendola*: Webster 1994) and mammals (e.g. redfronted lemur *Eulemur rufifrons*: Vick & Pereira 1989; Kappeler & Fichtel 2012; meerkat: Young et al. 2006; banded mongoose: Thompson et al. 2016). Where the causes of eviction have been studied, eviction appears to be a response to intensified local competition for resources or reproduction, while at the same time depending on the need for cooperation. In meerkats, for example, dominant females evict subordinate females during the later stages of their own pregnancy. Subordinate evictees that are pregnant at the time of eviction suffer elevated levels of hormonal stress and abort their litter before being allowed to return to the group, reducing competition for the dominant female's own offspring in the current breeding attempt (Young et al. 2006). In the cooperative cichlid *N. pulcher*, breeders evict helpers after sexual maturation if they compete for reproduction (Dierkes et al. 1999) and if no help is needed. They are often reaccepted if help is required, e.g. to defend the territory against predators or competitors (Taborsky 1985), and in such situations even foreign subordinates may be accepted in order to join forces in warding off dangerous intruders (Zöttl et al. 2013b).

Eviction can also be used to reduce reproductive competition more permanently. In redfronted lemurs and banded mongooses, reproductive competition arises because there are multiple female breeders in each group. Socially dominant females evict other females when group size (in the case of lemurs) or the number of breeding females (in banded mongooses) grows large. Around 90 per cent of evicted redfronted lemur females (Kappeler & Fichtel 2012), and just less than half of evicted banded mongoose females (Thompson et al. 2016) permanently disperse following eviction. In banded mongooses, eviction leads to increased reproductive success for the remaining females (Thompson et al. 2017b; Figure 3.4). Voluntary dispersal by females has never been observed in either banded mongooses or redfronted lemurs, suggesting that forcible eviction is a major determinant of social and genetic structure in both systems. In banded mongooses, eviction has been shown to involve substantial costs to both evictees, in terms of subsequent fertility (Thompson et al. 2016), and evictors, in terms of survival of their current offspring (Bell et al. 2012). This cost of eviction is crucial to understanding the observed size and composition of groups in nature. For example, high costs of eviction may result in supra-optimal groups composed of unrelated, strong individuals, while weaker, related individuals are forced out (Thompson et al. 2017b).

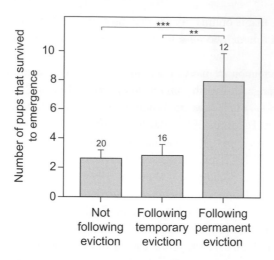

Figure 3.4 The effect of eviction on subsequent reproductive success in evicting groups of banded mongooses. Number of pups surviving to emergence from the den is shown for litters in breeding attempts where no eviction occurred ($N = 20$), following temporary eviction (where females returned to the group within 1 week; $N = 16$) and where some or all evicted females permanently dispersed ($N = 12$). $**P < 0.01$, $***P < 0.001$. (Reproduced with permission from Thompson et al. 2017b.) © 2017 Published by Elsevier Ltd on behalf of The Association for the Study of Animal Behaviour.

Eviction has been suggested to play an important role in the resolution of conflict over reproduction and investment in animal societies. For example, dominant individuals can use the threat of eviction to force helpers to exercise reproductive restraint (Johnstone & Cant 1999; Cant & Johnstone 2009), or to induce them to work harder (Gaston 1978; Bergmüller et al. 2005a; Fischer et al. 2014). Similarly, if helpers can readily disperse, they could in principle use the threat of departure to extract reproductive concessions from dominant individuals (Vehrencamp 1983; Reeve 1991). In Section 3.4.1 we discuss in more detail how threats might be used to resolve within-group conflict and to promote cooperation.

In many types of aggregation, defending or policing access to the group may be physically unfeasible or uneconomical. Examples include foraging avian flocks, insect swarms (Svensson & Petersson 1994), fish schools (Landa 1998) and ungulate herds (Creel et al. 2014). In these circumstances, Hamilton's (1971) selfish herd model suggests the theoretical outcome may sometimes be even more paradoxical than Sibly (1983) envisaged, because conflict over grouping benefits can lead to a stable outcome in which members of a group have *lower* fitness, on average, than solitary individuals. In Hamilton's (1971) model individuals compete to minimize their risk of predation. In a randomly dispersed population subject to random predation, each individual gains from moving towards other individuals to reduce their 'domain of danger', that is, the area for which they are the nearest prey item should a predator appear. He illustrated the model by imagining a snake in a lily pond, preying on frogs that are randomly distributed around its perimeter. Every now and then the snake pops up and snatches the nearest frog. If each frog is permitted to move to minimize its domain of danger, it will hop into the space between two others. The end result of the to-ing and fro-ing will be the formation of a 'selfish herd' (or, in this case, a selfish clump of frogs), but there is no guarantee that each individual will be better off at the end of this process than they were at the start. For example, aggregation can make it easier or less time-consuming for predators to catch their prey, so average fitness in the herd may turn out to be lower than it was in the original, scattered population:

The hypothesis suggests that the evolution of the gregarious tendency may go on even though the result is a considerable lowering of the overall mean fitness. At the end of our one-dimensional fairy tale, it will be remembered, only the snake lives happily, taking his meal at leisure from the scrambling heaps of frogs which the mere thought of his existence has brought into being. The cases of predators feeding on apparently helpless balls of fish seem parallel to this phantasy: here gregariousness seems much more to the advantage of the species of the predator than to that of the prey. Hamilton (1971)

The selfish herd example shows how rational decision-making that generates a short-term individual benefit (by reducing the immediate domain of danger) can lead to an evolutionarily stable outcome that is worse for all. The individuals in the population would be better off if they could all agree not to aggregate in the first place, but a population of non-aggregating, contractual 'cooperators' of this kind could be invaded by selfish mutants which at each time step acted to reduce their immediate risk. The selfish herd is thus a specific case of the well-known 'tragedy of the commons', whereby short-term self-interested behaviour can lead to catastrophic over-exploitation of a resource (Hardin 1968).

3.2.2 Conflict over Rank

Membership of a 'closed' group, in which there is a clear distinction between insiders and outsiders, brings the potential for substantial fitness benefits through coordination or cooperation, but also intensified competition for resources. How animals respond to this within-group conflict depends on the spatial and temporal distribution of resources in the environment (see Chapter 1). Group members may compete through non-interference rivalry in cases where resources are not economically defendable (Chapter 2). In many other situations, however, individuals can gain by trying to monopolize access to contested resources, and interfering with or suppressing the behaviour of rivals. In these circumstances conflict over resources leads to social aggression, fighting and, frequently, the emergence of dominance hierarchies.

The establishment of a dominance hierarchy shifts the nature of competition within stable groups from a continuous scramble over divisible resources to one or more contests over an indivisible resource, dominance status or social rank. Contests that occur during hierarchy formation and after its disturbance (e.g. the death of a dominant) may involve substantial costs of time, energy and injury, and maintaining social rank in undisturbed hierarchies can also be costly, because of the costs of threat signalling or dominance testing. However, once formed, dominance hierarchies can generate both individual and group-level fitness benefits because they ensure that individuals avoid repeatedly entering into costly fights that they are unlikely to win (Maynard Smith 1974). High social rank brings with it priority of access to resources and reproductive opportunities, but accepting low rank can be better than constantly engaging in costly competitive encounters with little chance of success (Maynard Smith & Harper 2003; Számadó 2008), and accepting a loser role can reduce contest costs (Lehner et al. 2011). Competition for rank can result in diversification of roles and a division of labour, as individuals that are unable to compete for high rank or breeding status are forced into helping roles (the 'social niche hypothesis'; Bermüller et al. 2010). For example, in both the hover wasp *Liostenogaster flavolineata* and the paper wasp *Polistes dominula*, lower-ranked individuals invest more in foraging to provision the larvae of dominant females and reduce their foraging effort when they are promoted to higher rank (Field et al. 2006). Where dominant individuals have access to better food or shelters, or suffer lower stress, small asymmetries in strength or quality between ranks can become amplified over time, with profound consequences for lifetime fitness (Clutton-Brock & Huchard 2013). Consequently, much of the social life of many cooperative animals is spent vying for social rank: fighting to establish rank, deterring challengers, engaging in submissive displays or probing others for weakness.

Social rank is often correlated with individual attributes such as size or strength, which determine absolute fighting ability or resource holding potential (RHP; Parker 1974). In many mammals, size is a good index of RHP. Where fights involve charging, shoving, striking with blows or weapons, large size is likely to increase the damage suffered by opponents while simultaneously reducing the energy required to match and exceed the competitive effort of rivals. In animals with indeterminate growth such as fish, where size variation is typically great even among adults, size and rank are usually perfectly correlated, and larger individuals evict smaller ones before they get large enough to beat them in an escalated fight (Buston 2003b; Wong et al. 2007). In other systems, where individuals do not continue to grow after maturation and size variance of adults is hence rather small, size is often not a good predictor of fighting ability. In cooperative insects, for example, asymmetry in RHP can be swamped by larger asymmetries in the value placed on resources where a challenger must invest considerable time or energy in the resource to realize its benefits (Parker 1974). In the paper wasp *Polistes dominula*, for example, around 20 per cent of dominant females (rank 1) are smaller than the rank 2 individual (Cant et al. 2006a). However, in experimentally induced fights rank 1s almost always win, most likely because a rank 1 is fighting for a nest full of her own offspring, whereas a rank 2 wasp is fighting merely for the opportunity to start reproduction almost from scratch. In other words, the value of the resource may be asymmetric for ranks 1 and 2. It is also possible that this is an example of a convention or 'uncorrelated asymmetry' (such as 'owner always wins') used to settle disputes quickly (Maynard Smith & Parker 1976; Kokko 2013). The same social rank can have different fitness values for individuals of equal strength depending on their age, experience and physiological condition; and on the time of year or season. For example, where there is a finite limit on lifespan or the length of the breeding season, as in many annually breeding social insects, a subordinate should be more likely to fight an incumbent dominant as the season progresses and hence the time available to inherit the breeding position runs out (Cant et al. 2006b).

In cooperatively breeding insects, rank is often determined by some convention such as age or order of arrival at a site. In polistine wasps (Reeve 1991) and primitively social bees (e.g. *Bombus*; van Honk & Hogeweg 1981), for example, older individuals are typically dominant to younger ones. In the hover wasp *Liostenogaster favolineata*, there is a strict age based queue (Field et al. 2006). Newly enclosed wasps join the end of a social queue to inherit dominant status. Only on rare occasions (13 per cent) do individuals attempt to jump their assigned place in the age-based queue. These rare queue-jumpers are not larger than other individuals. However, these are typically low-ranking females that previously contributed relatively little to foraging, compared to non-queue-jumpers, and so may represent a relatively rare cheater phenotype (Bridge & Field 2007). In other tropical wasps (West-Eberhard 1978; Yamane 1986) there is a reverse age-based hierarchy, whereby upon the death of the dominant female, the youngest female in the group inherits dominant status. The evolutionary causes of these two distinct conventions are currently unclear. Tsuji and Tsuji (2005) suggested that variation in the relative longevity of individuals compared to groups can explain these different patterns of age-based social rank. Specifically, Tsuji and Tsuji (2005) developed an inclusive fitness model which predicts that in systems where there is a limited breeding season, late-born, newly emerged females should accept low rank because even if they supplanted the dominant breeder they would have little time left in which to reproduce; whereas in perennial systems late-born, younger females should challenge for dominant status because by supplanting their mother they can expect a long reproductive life themselves. Thus their model can explain observed differences between some temperate and tropical wasps in age-based queueing systems. However, it does not explain the rarity of queue jumping in the tropical hover wasp *L. flavolineata* studied by Bridge and Field (2007), in which colonies are perennial and group longevity is far greater than individual lifespan.

Conflict over rank explains many of the patterns of social aggression observed in animal societies. High-ranked individuals often spend considerable time and energy being aggressive towards their subordinates – chasing, shoving, nipping, mounting and harassing them (Cant et al. 2006b). Dominant individuals typically direct the majority of their aggression toward their closest rivals, that is, the individuals that are next in line to inherit their social rank (e.g. Premnath et al. 1996; Monnin & Peeters 1999; Cant et al. 2006b; Young et al. 2006a; Ang & Manica 2010). In paper wasps (Chandrashekara & Gadagkar 1992; Cant et al. 2006b; Lamba et al. 2007), ponerine ants (Monnin & Peeters 1999) and cooperative cichlids (Wong & Balshine 2010), newly inherited dominants are hyperaggressive for the first few days, suggesting that aggression is used to cement or advertise dominant status. Subordinate individuals are also sometimes aggressive to dominants, a behaviour termed dominance testing (Reeve & Ratnieks 1993). When dominants are experimentally removed from groups of cooperative cichlids, remaining subordinates attempt to take over the dominant role

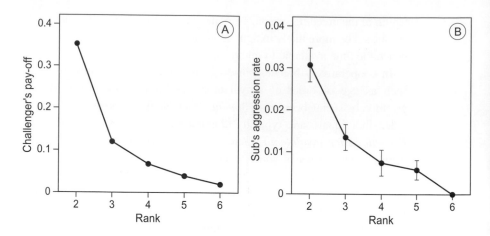

Figure 3.5 (A) Theoretical pay-offs to a subordinate challenger of fighting for the position of a dominant (rank 1) breeder, as a function of the subordinate's inheritance rank. In this model (model 1 of Cant et al. 2006b), a successful challenge leads to a reversal in dominance roles but incurs a cost to group productivity. (B) Observed aggression rate (acts per min) of subordinate foundresses of varying inheritance rank toward the dominant foundress in nests of *Polistes dominula* in Spain. The inheritance rank of subordinates was determined by repeatedly removing the rank 1 foundress and allowing the next-ranking individual to inherit the position of the dominant (rank 1) breeder (redrawn with permission from Cant et al. 2006b).

in the territory. Such attempts are typically challenged, however, by slightly larger immigrants. This leads to escalated contests usually causing one of the contenders to have to leave (Balshine-Earn et al. 1998). In social queues of the paper wasp *P. dominula*, rates of both 'upward' aggression (towards individuals one rank above) and 'downward' aggression (towards individuals one rank below) decline down the queue to inherit; and experiments show that rank causally influences aggression (Cant et al. 2006b). These results meet with prediction if the function of 'top-down' aggression by higher-ranked individuals is used to deter challenges by their subordinates and the function of 'bottom-up' aggression is to test the strength of higher-ranked individuals (Section 3.2.3; Figure 3.5).

3.2.2.1   Dominance–Submission

The presence of a dominance hierarchy is often associated with conspicuous ritualized dominance and submission behaviours. Dominance displays are often energetically costly and can be readily understood as honest signals of RHP which function to deter them from starting fights that they are unlikely to win (Maynard Smith & Harper 2003; Számadó 2011). It can therefore be in the interest of both parties, a dominant and a subordinate, for the dominant to engage in costly signalling and for the subordinate to attend to that signal (Thompson et al. 2014).

The evolution of submissive behaviour is more challenging to understand. Submissive animals crouch, roll over, freeze their position, drop their ears or antennae,

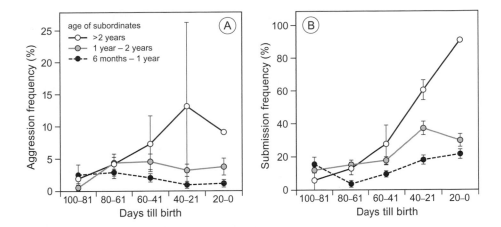

Figure 3.6 Aggression and submission in meerkats. (A) Aggression frequency of dominant females and (B) submission frequency of subordinate females as a function of the days until the dominant female gave birth. The rate of dominant aggression toward older subordinates, and the rate at which they engaged in submissive behaviour, increased rapidly as the birth date of dominant females drew near. Submission frequency did not predict whether females were evicted or not, but subordinate females that submitted *more* frequently were evicted earlier. (Redrawn with permission from Kutsukake & Clutton-Brock 2006a.) Copyright © 2005 Springer-Verlag. Reprinted/adapted by permission.

urinate, quiver, or behave like infants. These behaviours appear to signal to dominants a lack of motivation or ability to challenge the status quo. But what keeps such signals honest? Why shouldn't a subordinate signal a complete lack of motivation to challenge, or exaggerate their weakness, but then attack the dominant anyway? In rare cases, dominant individuals appear to force subordinates into a form of submission that is energetically costly and honest. In the cichlid fish *N. pulcher*, for example, subordinates engage in energetically costly submissive tail-quivering displays, which appease members of the breeding pair and obviate dominant aggression (Grantner & Taborsky 1998; Taborsky & Grantner 1998). In meerkats, subordinate females that are at risk of eviction sometimes follow the dominant female around for hours on end, crouching and engaging in what looks like begging behaviour before her (Kutsukake & Clutton-Brock 2006a; N. Kutsukake, unpublished observations; Figure 3.6).

Many examples of submissive behaviour, however, are not energetically costly per se: a paper wasp subordinate that freezes her position and allows the dominant to walk on her body and head is not expending energy; nor is a subordinate dog that rolls over and allows a dominant dog proximity to its throat. These behaviours may nevertheless be kept honest by physiological constraints on the neuroendocrinological pathways that control the expression of aggressive and non-aggressive behaviour. A subordinate that is neuroendocrinologically primed for aggression, for example through high circulating levels of testosterone, may find it difficult to fake signals of submissiveness, or allow a dominant into extremely close proximity to areas of the body (e.g. genitalia, throat, abdomen) that are vulnerable to injury. This idea is supported by studies of cooperative cichlids, where mature male subordinates showing much submissive behaviour towards territory owners have low androgen levels, implying little reproductive potential and hence competition for fertilizations (Bender et al. 2006).

Alternatively, rather than functioning as a signal of non-aggressiveness which benefits the dominant by providing information on relative strength, submissive behaviour might confound the attempts of a dominant to acquire such information. A simple conflict model (Cant 2012) predicts that where an individual knows that it is stronger on average than the pool of opponents that it will face, it pays to advertise strength; where the reverse is true it pays to conceal strength. Thus, where there is uncertainty about relative strength, but subordinates are on average weaker than dominants, subordinate individuals will be selected to engage in behaviour that conceals their underlying RHP (see also Section 3.3.2). Dominant individuals may find it hard to estimate the true strength or motivation of a potential challenger who freezes or crouches in response to a dominance display, and this may provide the selection pressure that explains the evolution of these forms of submission. Formal theoretical models would help to evaluate these hypotheses, and could shed light on the variety of submissive displays and how dominance and submission are likely to coevolve.

3.2.3   Conflict over Reproduction

3.2.3.1   **Reproductive Skew**

While dominance hierarchies are common in cooperative animal societies, there is great variation both within and between species in *reproductive skew* – the evenness with which reproduction is distributed among the members of a cooperative group. Reproductive skew is high in many cooperatively breeding insects and vertebrates, where breeding is restricted to a single queen or dominant pair and other group members are present as non-breeders. In other species (e.g. lions *Panthera leo*, banded mongooses, groove-billed anis *Crotophaga sulcirostris*, pukeko *Porphyrio porphyrio*), by contrast, skew is much lower, and multiple females and males regularly breed together and successfully raise young (reviewed by Riehl 2013). Low-skew societies are sometimes referred to as 'communal breeders', and treated as evolutionarily distinct from other cooperative breeding species (Lukas & Clutton-Brock 2012a, 2013; Koenig et al. 2016). However, this categorization obscures the striking similarities in helping behaviour in high- and low-skew societies (Cant et al. 2013), and the fact that skew is a continuous rather than a categorical measure, and varies widely within species and even within groups over time (Field et al. 1998). Across 20 species of cooperatively breeding vertebrates there is a great deal of variation in the frequency of subordinate reproduction, and often substantial differences between males and females of the same species (Figure 3.7).

Some degree of reproductive skew is expected because of individual heterogeneity in quality or fecundity. For example, older or larger females may produce larger or more competitive offspring because they benefit from greater experience or are in better

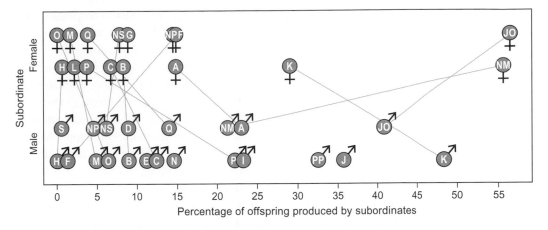

Figure 3.7 Variation in reproductive skew among males and females in cooperatively breeding vertebrates. The figure shows the percentage of group offspring that are sired by male and female subordinates in wild populations. Lines connect values for males and females from the same population. Most of the offspring produced by subordinates are sired within the group, but sometimes subordinates, usually males, gain parentage outside their own group. Although in some species subordinates refrain (almost) completely from direct reproduction, in other species they produce nearly as many offspring as the dominants in the group (e.g. pukeko, *Porphyrio porphyrio melanotus*). Furthermore, in some species, subordinates of one sex produce a considerably larger part of group offspring than the other sex (note that in some species, e.g. superb fairy-wrens and write-browed scrubwrens, no values were given for females because subordinates in these species are exclusively males). In mammals and birds, male helpers often exceed female helpers in the proportion of offspring they produce, whereas in cichlid fishes and Seychelles warblers this seems to be reversed. In all cases, parentage was assigned using molecular analyses. Species and sources: A, dwarf mongoose (*Helogale parvula*, Keane et al. 1994); B, wild dog (*Lycaon pictus*, Girman et al. 1997); C, meerkat (*Suricata suricatta*, Griffin & West 2003); F, Seychelles warbler (*Acrocephalus sechellensis*, Richardson et al. 2001); G, moorhen (*Gallinula chloropus*, McRae 1996); H, Florida scrub-jay (*Aphelocoma coerulescens*, Quinn et al. 1999); I, white-browed scrubwren (*Sericornis frontalis*, Whittingham et al., 1997); J, alpine accentor (*Prunella collaris*, Hartley et al., 1995); K, pukeko (Lambert et al. 1994); L, white-throated magpie-jay (*Calocitta formosa*, Berg, 2005); M, long-tailed tit (*Aegithalos caudatus*, Hatchwell et al., 2002); N, superb fairy-wren (*Malurus cyaneus*, Double & Cockburn, 2003); O, American crow (*Corvus brachyrhynchos*, Townsend et al. 2009); P, ground tit (*Parus humilis*, Wang & Lu, 2011); Q, red-winged fairy-wren (*Malurus elegans*, Brouwer et al. 2011); NP, *Neolamprologus pulcher* (Taborsky 2016; data combined from several studies in the field and laboratory); JO, *Julidochromis ornatus* (Awata et al. 2005); NM, *Neolamprologus multifasciatus* (Taborsky 2009; the female estimate is based on the number of broods in which >1 female participated in egg production); NS, *Neolamprologus savoryi* (Heg et al. submitted); PP, *Pelvicachromis pulcher* (Taborsky 2009); S, *Symphodus ocellatus* (Taborsky 2009).

condition, have better foraging skills, or because they are better able to choose higher-quality or genetically more compatible mates (Wasser & Barash 1983; Pusey & Wolf 1996; Koenig & Haydock 2004; Hodge et al. 2009). Alternatively, females may gain from suppressing their own fertility in times of resource scarcity or stress, if this allows them to reserve reproductive investment for future breeding attempts – the 'reproductive suppression' hypothesis (Wasser & Barash 1983). In many cases, however, differences in reproductive output among breeders are the outcome of intense competition over reproduction, in which breeders attempt to reduce the reproductive success of same-sex rivals. For example, adults may attack one another directly, which can impede growth and hence competitive potential (Buston 2003b; Heg et al. 2004b), inhibit fertility (Young et al. 2006a; Walter et al. 2011), interfere with mating or nesting attempts (Emlen & Wrege 1991; Mumme et al. 1983), or kill each other's offspring (Mumme et al. 1983; Young & Clutton-Brock 2006b; Hodge et al. 2011; Stockley & Bro-Jørgensen 2011; Clutton-Brock & Huchard 2013). Selection on males to suppress rivals often selects for large body size or weaponry, particularly where one or a few males are able to monopolize access to fertile females (Clutton-Brock 1985). Among female cooperative breeders, competition for reproduction is also intense, and results in costly and sometimes aggressive forms of overt conflict (meerkats, yuhinas *Yuhina brunnei-ceps*, smooth billed anis *Crotophaga ani*). However, because the cost of producing and rearing young is higher for females compared to males, and males often have more to gain through intrasexual competition, theory suggests that females will often resolve conflict without recourse to overt violence, for example through the use of signals or threats (Cant & Young 2013).

Female breeders may also compete via maternal effects on offspring growth, for example by priming their offspring to face competitive social environments through hormone signalling (via androgens or glucocorticoids; Dloniak et al. 2006; Sanderson et al. 2015b; Meise et al. 2016). In banded mongooses, for instance, females invest more prenatally when competing with a greater number of other breeders, and the response to competition is particularly strong when food abundance is low (Inzani et al. 2016). These effects can be interpreted as a form of 'predictive adaptive response' (PAR; Rickard & Lummaa 2007; Bateson et al. 2014), whereby mothers (or, potentially, offspring themselves) are hypothesized to adjust the developmental trajectory to ensure a match between offspring phenotype and the environment experienced postnatally or in later life (Taborsky 2006; Taborsky et al. 2007). In splendid fairy-wrens (*Malurus splendens*; Russell et al. 2007a), carrion crows (*Corvus corone*; Canestrari et al. 2011) and cooperative cichlids (*N. pulcher*; Taborsky et al. 2007), mothers reduce their investment in eggs when helpers are present (Figure 3.8), which has been interpreted as load-lightening by helpers. By contrast, in acorn woodpeckers (*Melanerpes formicivorus*) mothers produce eggs of the same size but in greater quantity (Koenig et al. 2009). These contrasting patterns may reflect between-species differences in the costs of increasing clutch size (Savage et al. 2015).

Infanticide as a means to reduce reproductive competition is found in both insect and vertebrate societies (see also Section 4.1.2). In many Hymenoptera, for example, relatedness asymmetries arising from haplodiploidy mean that workers can gain from identifying and killing unfertilized eggs laid by other workers, which would develop into male reproductives. In the honeybee *Apis mellifera*, for example, queens mate with 10–40 haploid males and produce a workforce of females who are mostly half-sisters to each other. While all workers are related to males produced by the queen by 1/4, they are related to their own sons by 1/2 and the sons of half-sisters by 1/8 (Ratnieks 1988; van Zweden et al. 2012). Consequently, workers can gain fitness

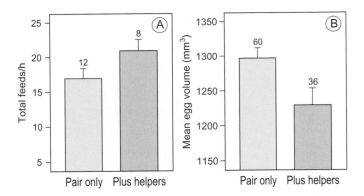

Figure 3.8 Splendid fairy-wren mothers reduce egg investment when helpers are present. (A) The presence of helpers increases the amount of food delivered to chicks. (B) This extra food compensates for the reduced investment in eggs by mothers that have helpers. Numbers above columns denote number of independent breeding units. Redrawn with permission from Russell et al. (2007a). Copyright © 2007, American Association for the Advancement of Science. Reprinted with permission from AAAS.

benefits by producing their own sons, but both queens and workers should attempt to suppress or reduce male production in other workers. In line with this theoretical prediction, workers are observed to identify and kill the male offspring produced by other workers, while letting the sons of the queen develop – which has been termed 'worker policing'. Since its discovery in the honeybee (Ratnieks & Visscher 1989), worker policing has been reported in numerous other species, including the Asian honeybee *Apis florea* (Halling et al. 2001), *Apis cerana* (Oldroyd et al. 2001), the bumblebee *Bombus terrestris* (Zanette et al. 2012), nine species of wasps and several ants (Wenseleers & Ratnieks 2006b; Figure 3.9).

Policing in honeybees is very accurate: the eggs of workers are almost 70 times more likely to be killed than are queen-laid eggs (a 'policing effectiveness' of 98.5 per cent; Wenseleers & Ratnieks 2006b). In other hymenoptera, however, policing is much less accurate. In the paper wasp *Polistes chinensis*, for example, worker-laid eggs are only 1.7 times more likely to be killed than queen-laid eggs (a policing effectiveness of 41.4 per cent). Across nine hymenopteran species (eight wasp species plus the honeybee), high policing accuracy is associated with low relatedness among workers and a low percentage of workers becoming reproductive (i.e. developing ovaries; Wenseleers & Ratnieks 2006b). Thus, policing is most accurate where workers have most incentive to cheat (i.e. where relatedness is low), and it is in these circumstances that policing is successful at suppressing worker reproduction.

Analogous examples of policing of offspring have been observed in several cooperatively breeding birds and mammals. In several joint nesting bird species, females cooperate to establish a territory and share a nest, but compete for reproduction by throwing or rolling the eggs of their co-breeders out of the nest (Riehl 2013). In smooth-billed anis (*Crotophaga ani*) and greater anis (*Crotophaga major*), females continue

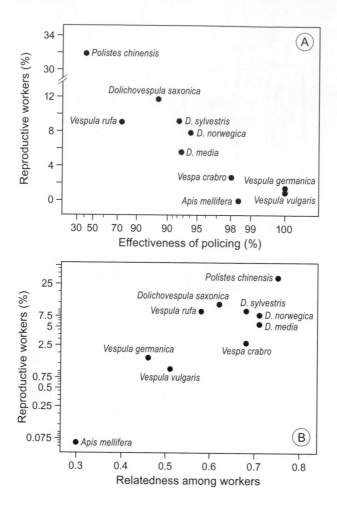

Figure 3.9 Policing as a means of reproductive suppression in social insects. (A) Across species, the proportion of workers that are reproductive declines with the effectiveness of policing, measured as $1 - W$, where W is the relative survival of worker-laid versus queen-laid eggs. (B) Policing is more effective at suppressing worker reproduction where relatedness is low. Reproduced with permission from Wenseleers & Ratnieks 2006b. Copyright © 2006, Nature Publishing Group.

with egg destruction until they lay an egg of their own (Vehrencamp & Quinn 2004; Riehl 2016). Similarly, in communally breeding house mice (*Mus domestica*) and banded mongooses, there is evidence that females kill offspring produced before, but not after, they give birth themselves (König 1994; Hodge et al. 2011; Cant et al. 2014). These observations suggest that females use infanticide as a means to increase their share of reproduction only when they can be certain not to kill their own young. A similar principle explains patterns of infanticide in polygynandrous fish (e.g. the Mediterranean ocellated wrasse *Symphodus ocellatus*), where females consume eggs in a male's nest before depositing their own (Taborsky 1994).

3.2.3.2   Mating Skew

In addition to intra-sexual conflict over shares of reproduction, there is also often intense conflict between males and females over the distribution of paternity within groups. Males typically invest less in parental care than females, and have a higher potential rate of reproduction, leading to a male-biased operational sex ratio and intense male–male competition for matings. In animal societies males reduce the individual costs of competition by forming dominance hierarchies, in which dominant males try to monopolize access to breeding females by mate-guarding. Males may also try to force copulations, or to harass females to increase the cost of their resistance to mating (Clutton-Brock & Parker 1995). In long-tailed macaques, for example, males are more aggressive to females when another male is present (Michael & Zumpe 1993). In chimpanzees *Pan troglodytes*, high-ranking males who are more aggressive to females during non-receptive (non-swollen) periods gain a greater share of paternity (Feldblum et al. 2014). This can explain why severe male attacks on females often occur for no obvious reason and outside of the receptive period (Goodall 1986). Interestingly, aggression during swollen periods results in more copulations but not more paternity. Thus, it appears that males can increase their reproductive success through long-term aggression and intimidation towards females, even outside of breeding periods. Males can also inflict physiological costs on their mating partners through the production of seminal toxins. Inflicting physiological damage during mating may make females less likely to risk remating with a different male, protecting a damaging male's paternitiy. Males can be selected to damage their mating partners, even though by doing so they reduce the fitness of their shared brood (Clutton-Brock & Parker 1995; Johnstone & Keller 2000).

Females are not passive in the face of attempts to control paternity (Carbone & Taborsky 1996). Selection on females to wrest the resolution of conflict over paternity towards their own optimum has resulted in a range of behavioural and physiological adaptations in females. Females engage in evasive behaviour and intense resistance to forced copulation (Griffith et al. 2002; Andersson & Simmons 2006; Neff & Svensson 2013). Females in many socially monogamous species regularly escape from their pair bond male to engage in extra-pair copulations (EPCs) with other males in the population (Davies 1986; Kempenaers & Dhondt 1993; Mulder et al. 1994; Forstmeier et al. 2014). Females also exercise cryptic choice after copulation to influence the probability of fertilization by particular males (Eberhard 1996; Birkhead 1998; Firman et al. 2017). For example, female feral fowl *Gallus domesticus* differentially eject sperm to avoid fertilization from socially subordinate males (Pizzari & Birkhead 2000). Other mechanisms of female choice include differential sperm storage (Ward 2000; Higginson et al. 2012) and differential mediation of sperm performance via female reproductive fluids (Gasparini & Pilastro 2011; Rosengrave et al. 2016).

Females invest in these strategies, despite the potential costs, to gain economic benefits for their offspring, or genetic benefits, for example to increase the level of heterozygosity or major histocompatability complex (MHC) variability among their offspring (Arnqvist & Rowe 2005; Løvlie et al. 2013). Sometimes multiple mating can yield both types of benefit. In the cooperatively breeding superb starling, for example, females with few helpers are more likely to share paternity with males within the group, most likely because this increases the help received by their offspring (Rubenstein 2007). In dunnocks *Prunella modularis*, a female which copulates with two males can secure paternal provisioning from both, enabling her to raise more surviving offspring (Davies 1986). In addition, females paired with relatively homozygous males copulate with males from outside their social group, resulting in increased offspring heterozygosity. In banded mongooses, relatedness within groups increases with the number of years since group founding. Females in older groups are more likely to engage in extra-group copulations, resulting in heavier, more heterozygous offspring, despite the fact that these intergroup encounters result in violent fights leading to the death and injury of fellow group members (Nichols et al. 2015). Similarly, in the Seychelles warbler females seek extra-pair copulations when paired with males that have low diversity of MHC genes, and these extra-pair copulations result in offspring that are more diverse at MHC loci compared to within-pair offspring (Richardson et al. 2005).

3.2.3.3   Parental Care

In over 80 per cent of bird species both male and female parents contribute to the rearing of offspring (Cockburn 2006). Biparental care is also observed in mammals, fish, various amphibians and many insects (Royle et al. 2012; Suzuki 2013). Conflict over investment arises because each parent stands to benefit if their partner does most of the work, or takes most of the risks, associated with parental care. The degree of conflict depends on the probability that the same two parents will remain together to reproduce in the future (Trivers 1972; Maynard Smith 1977). At one extreme, little or no conflict over parental investment is expected in long-term or lifelong monogamous species, because each parent is dependent on the health and survival of the other for its lifetime reproductive success. At the other extreme, high levels of conflict are expected in species where cooperation is limited to the production of a single brood, after which parents split up. In these circumstances, each parent would prefer the other to work themselves to death for the current brood, as long as that death occurred after the joint offspring have reached independence (Lessells 2012).

In theory, stable cooperation between two parents can be maintained if each partner partially compensates for a reduction in the effort of the other (Chase 1980; Houston & Davies 1985; McNamara et al. 1999; see also Section 3.3.3). Experimental tests of this prediction have been carried out numerous times in biparental birds, either by removing one parent or manipulating the effort of one parent while leaving the partnership intact (Wright & Cuthill 1989). A meta-analysis of 54 studies found support for the prediction of partial compensation in both cases (Harrison et al. 2009). The effect size was particularly high in studies in which one mate was removed. In studies that manipulated the effort of one parent in situ, the overall pattern supported partial compensation, particularly in the case of provisioning effort. However, there is considerable variation between individual studies in the response to manipulation, ranging from partial compensation to no response, and even effort-matching – a result not predicted by most theoretical models (Hinde & Kilner 2007).

These varied responses may reflect biological constraints on the information each individual has about the effort level of their partner, or the need for help (Manica et al. 2013). For example, effort-matching is predicted to occur if parents use the effort level of their partner to estimate the level of offspring need (Johnstone & Hinde 2006). By contrast, individuals are predicted to be unresponsive to changes in the effort of their partner in systems such as those of paper wasps where helpers cannot observe the helping effort of other group members directly (Donaldson et al. 2013).

In addition to conflict between parents over the allocation of care, conflicts arise between offspring and parents, parents and helpers, and between siblings within litters, over the amount of food provided and how it is shared out among offspring (reviewed by Kilner & Hinde 2012; Royle et al. 2016). Offspring typically prefer parents to provide more food and care for them than is optimal for the parent (Trivers 1974; Kilner & Hinde 2012). Conflict also arises within litters and between litters over the level of investment provided by parents (Kölliker et al. 2015; Kuijper & Johnstone 2018). This conflict is manifested in conspicuous begging displays, parental aggression towards offspring and sibling violence (reviewed by Mock & Parker 1997; Kilner & Hinde 2008, 2012; Mock et al. 2011). The balance of power between parents and offspring depends to some extent on the life history of parents and offspring. Where parents have little interaction with offspring (for example, where they merely prepare a nest or burrow for their offspring, before depositing eggs; Balshine 2012), parents may 'win' in the sense that offspring may have little opportunity (behaviourally at least) to shift the level of parental provisioning towards the offspring optimum. At the other end of the scale, mammalian offspring spend a large proportion of their lives in intimate contact with their mothers, and sometimes with their fathers too. Haig (1993, 2015) provided suggestive evidence that some of the features of foetal development (e.g. invasive plancentae, secretion of human placental lactogen to raise maternal blood sugar) result from selection on developing young to extract resources from mothers, sometimes to the detriment of maternal fitness.

Theoretical research on parent–offspring conflict suggests that in many cases, conflicts between parents and offspring may lead to evolutionarily unstable outcomes, rather than the evolutionarily stable resolutions typically considered in game theoretical models (Lessells 2006).

A challenge for empirical work on this and other forms of within-group conflict is to understand when the outcome of conflict is likely to be evolutionarily stable and when it is not (Lessells 2006; Kilner & Hinde 2012). Moreover, theory suggests there may often be zones of parent-offspring agreement, rather than conflict, depending on the shape of the genetic trade-offs underlying life-history traits. Kölliker et al. (2015) used selection experiments on the earwig *Forficula auricularia* to reveal the shape of these trade-off curves. Their results suggest that parents and offspring disagree about investment in pre-hatching traits such as the rate of egg development, but are in full agreement about post-hatching traits such as offspring growth rate and survival offspring. This research implies that some offspring traits represent a partnership-level adaptation between parent and offspring, which simultaneously maximizes the inclusive fitness of both parties.

3.2.3.4   Conflict over Helping

In cooperative groups, individuals often face a trade-off between investing in a group-beneficial behaviour or 'public good' and their own personal fitness interests (Archetti & Scheuring 2012). In sociable weavers, for example, numerous group members nest together and build a massive communal thatch which provides thermoregulatory benefits to all the nests in the colony (Dijk et al. 2014; Figure 3.10). Individuals could maximize personal fitness by enjoying the benefits of the thatch without paying the energetic costs involved in working to build or maintain it. In pied babblers, one group member acts as a sentinel to look out for predators while the other group members forage, emitting a regular train of peeps to signal to the others that it is on guard. Sentinels pay a personal cost because they are targeted by predators and take longer to reach cover following experimental playbacks of predator calls (Ridley et al. 2013). Again, there is a potential to free-ride because individuals could benefit from the sentinel behaviour of others without engaging in it themselves. Similar conflicts over helping effort arise within cooperative animal societies. Where helpers have some

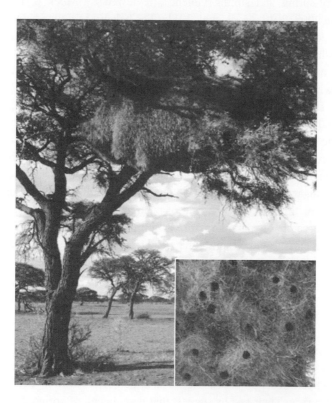

Figure 3.10 Communal thatch in sociable weavers. Inset: the downward-pointing nest chambers. Individuals (particularly males) contribute to provision of the public good (building the thatch). However, males preferentially build thatch near to their own nest chamber, and nest near to their genetic relatives. Reproduced with permission from Dijk et al. (2014). © 2014 The Authors. *Ecology Letters* published by John Wiley & Sons Ltd and CNRS. Open access.

chance of breeding themselves either currently or in the future, they should prefer to work at a lower rate than is optimal from the perspective of a dominant breeder (Cant & Field 2001).

Given an incentive to free-ride, how can stable cooperative investment be maintained? One possibility is that there is subtle kin structuring within groups, so that actions appearing to be for the public good are actually selfish and directed towards relatives (Dijk et al. 2014). In the sociable weaver example, relatedness between colony members is low overall, but individuals who build the thatch do so next to their own nest chamber and the nest chambers of relatives. The presence of defectors or free-riders at a high frequency can shift the optimum form of cooperative investment from the production of purely public good to the production of private goods which benefit the producer or their relatives (O'Brien et al. 2017).

A second possibility is that investment is maintained by punishment or coercion. In the sociable weavers, cooperative individuals were shown to target aggression towards selfish individuals, and the individuals suffering aggression perform cooperative behaviors subsequent to receiving aggression. This may suggest a pay-to-stay mechanism involving punishment of free riders (Leighton & Vander Meiden 2016), which here might act in concert with relatedness to maintain cooperation (Dijk et al. 2014). In cooperative cichlids, helpers that are prevented from helping (by denying them information about the need for help, or by physically confining them when their help is needed) are subject to increased aggression from dominant breeders (Fischer et al. 2014; Naef & Taborsky 2020b). These helpers subsequently also show elevated rates either of helping or of submissive behaviour to dominants, suggesting that cooperation and submission are used as alternative means to appease aggressive dominants (Bergmüller & Taborsky 2005; Schreier 2013; Kasper et al. 2018). Coercion of subordinates into helping probably works more effectively if dominants and subordinates are unrelated. In cichlids, for example, coercion results in higher cooperative investment by unrelated helpers than by related helpers (Zöttl et al. 2013a; Quiñones et al. 2016). In paper wasps, superb fairy-wrens, naked mole-rats and meerkats, lazy individuals or those which are temporarily removed from the group are subjected to elevated aggression by dominant individuals (Reeve 1992; Mulder & Langmore 1993; Reeve & Nonacs 1997; see Section 4.2.2).

By contrast, several other studies of birds and mammals have failed to find evidence for coercion of cooperation (McDonald et al. 2008a, 2008b; Nomano et al. 2015; Thompson et al. 2016). It is perhaps surprising that evidence for punishment is not more widespread, given that punishment is likely to be cheap for high-quality, dominant individuals (Raihani et al. 2012). It is much easier to reduce a recipient's fitness by 50 per cent (for example, by injuring it) than to boost her fitness by the same amount. However, coercion may be widespread but often remain undetected. Specifically, coercion may be difficult to detect if it is based on threats rather than actions, because acts of punishment are necessary only when the threat of punishment fails (see Section 3.4.1). Punishment might also be expected to be rare in groups of close relatives compared to groups of non-relatives for two reasons. First, in groups of close relatives helping brings inclusive fitness benefits without the need for coercion

(Quiñones et al. 2016). Second, the coercion by threats of punishment is less credible when wielded against genetic relatives, because it is not in the coercer's own interest to harm their close kin (Cant & Johnstone 2009; Thompson et al. 2017a). It is probably no coincidence that some of the clearest evidence of coercion is found in associations of unrelated individuals, for example those of cleaner fish (e.g. *Laborides dimidiatus*) and their client hosts (Raihani et al. 2010), and in anemone fish [e.g. clownfish *Amphiprion percula* (Buston 2003a; Rueger et al. 2018), coral-dwelling goby *Paragobiodon xanthosomus* (Wong et al. 2007, 2008)].

3.3   Social Conflict: Theoretical Approaches

Conflicts of interest are ubiquitous in animal societies, but there is great variation in the degree to which these conflicts are manifested as aggression, destruction or laziness. A large body of theory tries to explain this variation in overt conflict. In this section we pick out three types of modelling approach which differ in their approach and objectives: structured population models of kin selection, 'sealed bid' conflict models and behavioural models of conflict resolution.

The statistician George Box observed that 'all models are wrong, but some are useful' (Box and Draper 1987, p. 424). In the case of evolutionary models of conflict, each type of model is 'wrong' in the sense that it is based on a set of restrictive and unrealistic assumptions, but each type is useful because it provides insight into distinct questions. How do population structure and demography affect selection for harmful behaviour? How is within-group conflict resolved over evolutionary time? What determines whether underlying conflicts of interest break out into observable behavioural conflict and escalated contests? Below we describe alternative attempts to answer these questions.

3.3.1   Structured Population Models

Models of kin selection in structured or 'viscous' populations examine how patterns of life history and ecology influence selection for helping and harming traits, that is, traits that increase or decrease the fecundity and/or survival of other local group members. These models were motivated by the question of whether increased population 'viscosity', or constraints on dispersal, favour the evolution of altruism. The 'canonical' version of Hamilton's rule (Hamilton 1963, 1964), $r B > C$, gives the condition for the spread of a social trait conferring benefit B fitness units on a recipient at a cost C fitness units to an actor, where r is relatedness between them, i.e. genetic similarity relative to the population average [see Chapter 4, and Akçay & Van Cleve (2016) for a discussion of fitness in Hamilton's rule]. This inequality can be satisfied if the recipients of altruism are more closely related to the actor than the population average. This can be ensured if actors can somehow recognize individuals with which they share genes [through mechanisms of kin discrimination or 'green-beards'; Dawkins 1976 (2016)]. Alternatively, limitations on dispersal, or population viscosity, ensure that interactions occur among individuals that are genetically more similar than the population as a whole (Hamilton 1964). Viscosity is a general promoter of altruism because almost all natural populations are subject to constraints on dispersal, and hence exhibit population structure and non-random interactions between individuals (Lehmann & Rousset 2010).

The difficulty with this mechanism is that increasing viscosity leads to both high relatedness and high levels of competition among kin (see Section 4.1.2.2). To determine the direction of selection on a social trait we need to consider not just relatedness of an actor to the recipient, but also to the individuals with whom that recipient competes (Queller 1994a). This may be illustrated by developing a 'three-party' version of Hamilton's rule, which includes both the immediate consequences of a social trait for fecundity (or survival) and the knock-on effects that result from changes in the level of local competition. Consider a social trait which influences fecundity only (for simplicity). The trait results in b extra offspring for members of the local group, at a cost of c fewer offspring for the actor (Taylor 1992a; Queller 1994a). The net change in the number of offspring produced is $b - c$, and so we can expect $b - c$ offspring to be displaced somewhere in the population as a result of competition. West and Gardner (2010) call these displaced offspring 'secondary recipients', to contrast with the 'primary recipients' on whom the change of b offspring is originally conferred. Assuming population size is fixed and inelastic, selection will favour the trait if the following inequality is satisfied (equation 1 from Queller 1994a, following equation 1 in Taylor 1992a)

$$r_{xy}b - c - r_{xe}(b - c) > 0 \qquad (1)$$

where r_{xy} is the actor's relatedness to local group members (the primary recipients), and r_{xe} is the actor's relatedness to the offspring displaced by competition (the secondary recipients). If the $b - c$ additional offspring disperse away from the local patch and compete with offspring to whom the actor is unrelated, r_{xe} is zero and hence competition has no effect on the direction of selection. However, if a fraction of the $b - c$ offspring remains in the group to compete locally, r_{xe} to the offspring displaced by competition will be positive and inequality (1) is harder to satisfy. In the simplest infinite island model of Taylor (1992b) the contrasting effects of increasing viscosity on $r_{xy}b$ (promoting helping) and on $r_{xe}(b - c)$ (inhibiting helping) exactly cancel each other out, so that varying the rate of dispersal and consequently relatedness has no effect on selection for either helping or harming. Inequality (1) can be adapted to apply to heterogeneous groups consisting of classes of individuals that vary in reproductive value (Rodrigues & Gardner 2013). In this case the inhibiting force of local competition increases in proportion to the reproductive value of the secondary recipients.

Inequality (1) can be used to illustrate conditions for which selection favours harming traits, that is, behaviour which involves some fecundity cost to the actor, while at the same time reducing the fecundity of a recipient [note that if these reductions in fecundity translate into reduced lifetime fitness for actor and recipient, harm is the same as spite in Hamilton's (1964) terminology]. Overt acts of aggression, fighting, infanticide and egg destruction offer candidate examples of harming behaviour. Harming may also take more subtle forms, for example the production of larger, more competitive young when faced with reproductive competition (at a cost to the ability to invest in future offspring), or the production of costly signals which deter challenges to dominant status, or cause other local group members to exercise reproductive restraint. More broadly, basic life-history decisions such as when to breed and how many offspring to produce are likely to affect the fitness of other local group members, and may thus constitute forms of indiscriminate harming or helping (Johnstone & Cant 2008).

For the simple case where all individuals have equal reproductive value, harming can be favoured where relatedness to those offspring displaced by competition (secondary recipients) is greater than relatedness to primary recipients (because in this case $r_{xe} - r_{xy} > 0$). This can arise, for example, if a primary recipient's offspring compete directly with the actor's own offspring. In addition, if recipients vary in their reproductive value, harming can be favoured even where relatedness is higher to primary than secondary recipients, provided that secondary recipients have relatively high reproductive value (Rodrigues & Gardner 2013). Note that harming behaviour (which we observe as actual conflict) might be either selfish or spiteful at the level of an individual's lifetime fitness, depending on how the immediate impacts of a social trait on fecundity and survival convert into lifetime fitness impacts (Lehmann et al. 2006). For instance, paying an immediate fecundity cost to reduce the fecundity of a rival breeder may ultimately be selfish with regard to lifetime effects if it results in increased direct fitness in the long run, for example because it alleviates the intensity of local competition. For empirical biologists interested in understanding the causes of observed conflict, the question of whether harm is 'selfish' or 'spiteful' with regard to its lifetime fitness consequences will often be of theoretical rather than practical interest, and in any case difficult to unveil.

The key advance of structured population models over classic kin-selection models is that rather than externally assigning values of relatedness to different recipients, relatedness values and recipient kin structure are allowed to emerge endogenously from the assumed demographic features of the population, such as dispersal and mortality rates and patterns of mating. Most of these structured population models (reviewed by Lehmann & Rousset 2010; Cooper et al. 2018) are based on the 'infinite island' modelling framework of Wright (1931), which introduces population structure while retaining analytical tractability. In this framework, populations are assumed to consist of a very large number of patches or groups in which there is competition for limited resources or breeding positions (Taylor 1992a, 1992b; Irwin & Taylor 2000; Taylor et al. 2007a provide a comprehensive analysis of other dispersal assumptions). Individuals either remain in their natal patch or disperse individually to a far-flung patch which contains no relatives. Individuals proceed through discrete phases of a specified life history, for example (i) social interaction among adults (conferring bs and incurring cs); (ii) reproduction; (iii) dispersal of offspring; (iv) death of adults; (v) competition among offspring for breeding vacancies; (vi) population regulation (death of remaining offspring). The precise order of the phases can be varied according to the focus of the model. For example, helping and harming might occur among adults and offspring prior to dispersal, or among offspring themselves (Taylor 1992b; Gardner 2010). Population regulation could occur before or after dispersal, or some combination of the two (Lehmann & Rousset 2010). In addition, the models can be used to explore variation in ecology and social structure. For example, groups might vary in size (Rodrigues & Gardner 2013), resource richness (Rodrigues & Gardner 2013), reproductive skew (Johnstone 2008) or age-structure (Johnstone & Cant 2010). Dispersal might also occur in groups ('budding' dispersal) rather than individually (Gardner & West 2006; Koykka & Wild 2015). The output of the models is the equilibrium level of relatedness among different classes of individual, given the specified demography and life history. Selection for helping and harming can then be explored by deriving and comparing equivalent versions of inequality (1), each of which take into account differences between individuals in reproductive value and different ecologies (Taylor 1992a; Johnstone et al. 2012).

How does dispersal influence selection for harming behaviour? In the simplest models assuming a haploid, asexual population with non-overlapping generations and unconditional helping and harming, dispersal rate does not influence selection on social traits (Taylor 1992a). However, this conclusion no longer holds if an individual can adjust its behaviour according to whether it has dispersed or not (El Mouden & Gardner 2008). Non-dispersers experience higher than average relatedness to other local group members, whereas dispersers experience lower than average local relatedness. This asymmetry favours harming behaviour by individuals that have dispersed and, to a lesser extent, helping behaviour by individuals that remain philopatric (El Mouden & Gardner 2008). In terms of overt conflict, the model predicts that dispersers will be more aggressive than philopatric individuals, and that aggression will be most intense where ecological constraints on dispersal are most intense.

El Mouden and Gardner's (2008) model may explain the strong link between dispersal propensity and aggression in western bluebirds (*Sialia mexicana*). Over the last 30 years, western bluebirds have gradually displaced less-aggressive mountain bluebirds (*Sialia currucoides*) in the north-western USA. The invasion front of western bluebirds consisted of dispersing males that were particularly aggressive, while western bluebird males that remained in their natal population were non-aggressive. Levels of aggression declined rapidly after sites had been colonized for a few generations. This decline can be attributed to selection against aggression in established groups, given that aggression is heritable (heritability $h^2 = 0.45$) and negatively related to male reproductive success (Duckworth & Badyaev 2007).

In bacteria, these structured population models predict the degree to which bacteria inflict harm on their competitors through the secretion of lethal chemical weapons known as bacteriocins (Inglis et al. 2011); and the level of damage that viruses of bacteria inflict on their host organism (i.e. their virulence; Gardner et al. 2004; Lion & Boots 2010; Leggett et al. 2017). In fig wasps, males never disperse from their natal fig before engaging in injurious competition. In this case, structured population models predict that the intensity of local competition, not the degree of relatedness, should predict levels of harming. As predicted, the level of male injury in fights over females declines with female density but not relatedness between males (West et al. 2001). Finally, in the social aphid *Pemphigus obesinymphase*, individuals that move out of their home gall and invade the gall of a different clone change their behaviour as their social environment changes (Abbot et al. 2001). When surrounded by members of another clone, these individuals refrain from self-sacrificial defence behaviour and instead invest more in selfish reproduction. Altruistic gall defence in aphids is conditional on whether they are immigrants or natives, as predicted by formal structured population models (El Mouden & Gardner 2008).

Sex differences in dispersal also have a strong influence on selection for helping and harming. Where sex-specific dispersal rates diverge, selection almost always favours helping by the less dispersing sex and harming behaviour by the sex that disperses at a higher rate (Johnstone & Cant 2008; see also Gardner 2010). In most cooperative and social mammals, females are philopatric while males disperse; in cooperatively breeding birds, by contrast, it is typically females that disperse between groups. The model predicts that the philopatric sex is under strong selection to help, which is consistent with observed patterns of female-biased helping in mammals and male-biased helping in birds (Cockburn 1998; Russell 2004). In a meta-analysis of 20 species of cooperatively breeding birds, helping effort was biased towards males in species where males are philopatric (and stand to gain future fitness through inheritance), and biased towards females in species where females are philopatric (Downing et al. 2018). Patterns of local relatedness and the probability of inheritance may both contribute to observed sex differences in helping effort. In addition, the model predicts that selfish or aggressive harming should be more frequent in males in social mammals, and females in cooperative birds. The intensity of male (or female) aggression within groups should increase with the level of male (or female) bias in dispersal, but these predictions concerning harming behaviour remain untested.

Unusual patterns of dispersal have been proposed to explain the evolution of menopause and late-life helping in humans, resident killer whales and short-finned pilot whales (Johnstone & Cant 2010). Under male-biased dispersal and local mating (characteristic of most social mammals), the relatedness of breeding females to other local breeders present in the group declines with age, and hence selection for helping by females declines as they get older. However, two distinct demographic patterns select for strategies of reproductive competition early in life and helping later in life. Specifically, female-biased dispersal coupled with local mating (the demographic pattern characteristic not only of birds, but also of many extant apes and, potentially, ancestral humans) and low dispersal of both sexes coupled with non-local mating (characteristic of menopausal cetaceans) both select for harming early in life and helping later (Johnstone & Cant 2010; Croft et al. 2017). In both cases females have very low relatedness to group males early in life, but female–male relatedness increases as females get older and produce philopatric sons. A study of resident killer whales shows a close match between the predictions of this model and patterns of genetic relatedness within pods (Croft et al. 2017). Similarly, a recent genealogical study using a cross-cultural sample of 19 human societies showed that members of the dispersing sex become more closely related to local group members as they get older, as predicted by Johnstone & Cant's (2010) model (Koster et al. 2019). These studies support the idea that patterns of dispersal and mating determine patterns of genetic relatedness within and between animal groups and hence the potential for kin selection to shape social traits in viscous animal societies.

3.3.2 Sealed Bid Models: Battleground and Resolution

The models in the preceding section show how demography can influence the costs that individuals should be prepared to pay to inflict harm on others. But what if the costs of a harming act depend on the strength of opponents and their potential to inflict harm in return? These questions have been addressed by a number of game-theoretical models of within-group conflict. The models were originally developed to study conflict over reproductive skew in cooperative animal societies. However, because the models examine conflict over any shared resources, they can be applied with little or no modification to conflict over services or products in cooperative mutualisms, conflict over parental investment in family groups and also to conflict among cells and genes. Formal models of ecological 'scramble' competition (Parker 2000), the tragedy of the commons (Rankin et al. 2007) and intragenomic conflict between paternally and maternally imprinted alleles (Haig & Wilkins 2000) are almost identical to 'tug-of-war' models of reproductive skew (Cant 2012).

Models of reproductive conflict (like other models of evolutionary conflict, e.g. parent–offspring conflict; Godfray 1995) typically fall into one of two broad categories: battleground models and resolution models. Battleground models focus on the factors that influence the zone of conflict between the fitness interests of competitors. Resolution models focus on the coevolution of conflict strategies within the battleground and the consequences for resource sharing.

3.3.2.1 Battleground Models

Two types of constraint can determine the battleground of conflict: (1) optimization constraints and (2) outside options. Optimization constraints arise when the fitness pay-offs of social partners are positively correlated, and there are diminishing returns on conflict investment (Field & Cant 2009). For example, if they are genetic relatives and there are diminishing returns on increasing reproductive share, both players can gain from allowing their partner a share of reproduction (Figure 3.11). A second layer of constraint on the battleground is determined by the outside options available to each competitor, that is, the alternative pay-offs each could expect if the cooperative interaction were terminated. For example, where one or both players can leave or evict their social partner, the battleground is defined by the fraction of reproduction that one individual needs to concede to the other to deter it from taking up its outside option, i.e. to leave and thereby end cooperation (Reeve 2000; Cant & Johnstone 2009; Figure 3.11). This latter layer of constraint arises because of a behavioural threat: the battleground is constrained only if one or both parties are aware that their

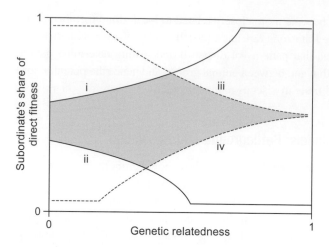

Figure 3.11 The battleground of conflict over direct fitness in animal societies. Two pairs of constraints demarcate the battleground of reproductive conflict between a dominant and a subordinate member of a cooperative group: group stability constraints (pair i and ii) and internal optima (pair iii and iv). Together these constraints define the zone for which stable groups can form (shaded area): this is the battleground within which group members compete over shares of direct fitness. In reproductive skew theory, the constraints are labelled as follows: (i) eviction threshold; (ii) staying incentive; (iii) subordinate optimum sharing; (iv) dominant optimum sharing. Lines (i) and (iii) together define the share of direct fitness obtained by the subordinate when it can choose its own optimum share, at no cost. Lines (ii) and (iv) together give the share obtained by the subordinate when the dominant can choose its own optimum share, at no cost.

partner possesses a credible threat to exercise the outside option and terminate the interaction. Behavioural threats are discussed in detail in Section 3.4.1.

The disparity between the fitness interests of social partners, as measured by the width of the battleground, gives a measure of *potential* conflict between them. In some cases, the level of potential conflict is a reasonable predictor of levels of actual conflict. In social queuing models, for example, aggression is predicted to be most intense toward the front of a queue to inherit breeding status, because the fitness pay-off associated with moving up from rank 2 to rank 1 is much greater than the fitness pay-off of moving from rank 5 to rank 4. Experimental and observational evidence of aggression in the hierarchies of cichlids and paper wasps supports this prediction (Cant et al. 2006b; Wong & Balshine 2010). In other cases, however, *potential* conflict is a poor predictor of *actual* conflict. In the sea anemone *Actinia equina*, for example, aggression increases with the degree of genetic relatedness between competitors (Foster & Briffa 2014). In this system unrelated individuals have greater potential conflict, but closer relatives appear to be more evenly matched in terms of resource holding potential, leading to a positive relationship between aggression and relatedness. In banded mongooses, dominant females preferentially target more closely related subordinate females for violent eviction, consistent with the predicted pattern if dominant females avoid attacking those victims that are most likely to fight back (Thompson et al. 2017b).

The take-home message from these studies is that the relationship between potential and actual conflict is not straightforward, and that it depends strongly on the behavioural mechanisms involved in the expression of conflict behaviour. It is not necessarily the disparity between fitness optima that is the prime determinant of observed levels of actual conflict, but the costs and benefits of effort invested in conflict to 'win' a resource, or to shift the distribution of shares of the resource in one's own favour. Two individuals may have widely different interests, but if overt conflict involves a high chance of death or injury, competitors may do better to resolve differences through less-costly forms of negotiation or signalling. Peaceful co-breeding and low reproductive skew among female lions has been attributed to the lethal weaponry and high costs of reproductive competition in this species (Packer et al. 2001). Conversely, if aggression is conspicuous but does little damage, overt conflict may be common even when there is little to fight over. If the fitness of two individuals w_1 and w_2 is a function of their own conflict effort level a_1 and that of their partner a_2, the ESS levels of effort will be determined by the partial derivatives $\partial w_1/\partial a_1$ and $\partial w_2/\partial a_2$, not the width of their zone of conflict (Cant 2006). In the next section we describe resolution models which adopt this 'marginal fitness' approach to predict actual conflict, rather than potential conflict.

3.3.2.2   Resolution Models

Resolution models focus on how competitors can shift the division of a contested resource in their favour, or win control of it outright (Reeve et al. 1998a; Johnstone 2000). The models typically examine the coevolution of blind 'sealed-bid' genetic strategies, that is, fixed genetic strategies which specify a given level of effort or investment, irrespective of the individual attributes of an opponent, or the opponent's effort. The assumption rules out the adjustment of behaviour to the specific attributes or effort level of opponents, which limits the usefulness of the models in explaining observed variation in behavioural conflict in many systems. However, sealed-bid models have much heuristic value from their advantages of mathematical tractability and generality, and can be applied to study conflict resolution at different levels of biological organization and at more than one level simultaneously (e.g. individuals and groups; Reeve & Hölldobler 2007).

Resolution models of conflict need to make some assumption about how effort invested in conflict converts to 'success' in conflict: for a non-divisible resource, success can be measured as the probability of winning; for a divisible resource, success can be measured as the fraction of the resource obtained. The function linking effort to success is known as the *contest success function*, *F*. Most models of conflict assume that the contest success function takes the form of a ratio, with a focal individual's effort as the numerator, and the mean or sum of individual efforts as the denominator. These 'ratio form' models have been developed to study evolutionary conflict in different social contexts and at different levels of organization, for example among genes, individuals and societies (Parker 1974, 1985; Frank 1995,

2003; Cant 1998; Reeve et al. 1998a; Haig & Wilkins 2000; Kondoh & Higashi 2000; Cant & Shen 2006; Reeve & Hölldobler 2007; Gavrilets 2012; Gavrilets & Fortunato 2014; Rusch & Gavrilets 2017). A second type of contest success function is the 'difference form', which assumes that contest success depends on the difference in efforts between a focal individual and its competitors (Hirshleifer 1989; Cant 2012). This contest success function is less commonly used but applies well to many biologically relevant scenarios. Contest success functions are considered in more detail in Box 3.1.

Two influential resolution models that use a ratio form contest success function are Reeve et al.'s (1998a) tug-of-war model and Frank's (1995) policing model. In the tug-of-war model, each player can invest effort to increase their share of a resource, but at a cost to the amount of resource to be shared. Thus, conflict effort gives each player a larger slice of a smaller pie. The model predicts that individual and total effort expended on conflict will decline with (1) increasing relatedness between competitors, and (2) increasing strength asymmetry between the dominant and the subordinate. Prediction (1) is a standard prediction from classic kin selection models (Section 3.2.1). Prediction (2) is similar to those derived from behavioural 'assessment' models of conflict. Thus, while there is empirical support for both predictions (e.g. Reeve & Keller 1995; Langer et al. 2004), testing the tug-of-war model is difficult because of the non-discriminating nature of its predictions.

A result not emphasized by Reeve et al. (1998a) is that at the evolutionarily stable equilibrium, the dominant's inclusive fitness declines with subordinate strength b, whereas the subordinate's inclusive fitness increases with b. This may have interesting implications for partner selection and group dynamics. In a heterogeneous population where individuals can choose to pair up with others, strong dominants should attempt to pair with weak subordinates, whereas weak subordinates should do their best to avoid strong dominants. This conflict over choice of partners might select for strategies by dominants to limit the outside options of subordinates, particularly if these are recruited from within the group, for example through retention of offspring. This suggestion is similar to the suggestion of Crespi and Ragsdale (2000) that parents could gain by reducing their offspring's dispersal options to force them into a helping role.

Whereas the tug-of-war model considers a single evolvable trait, conflict effort, Frank's (1995) policing model examines the coevolution of two traits, selfish effort x to gain a greater share of group productivity (equivalent to conflict effort in the tug-of-war); and policing effort a to eliminate selfishness. An individual that invests in policing effort a keeps a proportion a of its social interactions equitable (equal sharing). The model predicts that the evolution of policing is all or nothing: below a critical relatedness value (which is equal to the cost of policing c) all group members pay the cost of policing and all social interactions are policed (i.e. $a^* = 1$). Above the threshold value of relatedness no social interactions are policed ($a^* = 0$) and the game reduces to a simple N-player tug-of-war.

A curious feature of Frank's model is that ESS values of selfishness x^* are higher in the presence of policing than in the basic model. In the presence of policing, equilibrium selfishness is $x^* = (1 - r)/r(1 - c)$, compared to $x^* = (1 - r)$ in the absence

Box 3.1 Contest Success Functions

Economic and evolutionary models of conflict need to make some assumption about how effort converts into contest success. Contest success functions are mathematical functions that give each player's probability of winning, or each player's share of a divisible resource, as a function of all players' efforts (Skaperdas 1996). There are two canonical forms, the ratio form and the difference form (Hirshleifer 1989, 2001). These two functional forms have distinct properties and implications for the resolution of evolutionary conflict (Skaperdas 1996). Here we sketch examples of evolutionary conflict models that use these different forms of contest success function.

Ratio Form Models

Reeve et al.'s (1998a) tug-of-war considers groups composed of a dominant (player 1) and a subordinate (player 2) who can invest efforts x_1 and x_2, respectively, to increase their share of reproduction of value V. In their model, the contest success function for the dominant is

$$F_1 = x_1/(x_1 + bx_2)$$

and for the subordinate it is

$$F_2 = bx_2/(x_1 + bx_2).$$

The parameter b is a discounting factor (≤ 1) applied to the subordinate's effort to allow for asymmetry in strength between the players.

Effort invested in conflict could otherwise have been invested in cooperation, so V is a declining function of conflict efforts x and y. Specifically, Reeve et al. (1998a) assume that productivity V declines with the sum of conflict efforts: $V = 1 - x_1 - x_2$. Thus, by investing effort in the conflict, each player gains a larger slice of a smaller pie.

The direct fitness of the dominant is

$$W_1 = x_1/(x_1 + bx_2)(1 - x_1 - x_2)$$

To solve the model, Reeve et al. (1998a) use an 'inclusive fitness' approach (Hamilton 1964; Taylor et al. 2007b). The dominant's inclusive fitness can be written $I_1 = W_1 + rW_2$, where r is the relatedness (assumed symmetrical) of each individual to its partner. Likewise, the subordinate's inclusive fitness is $I_2 = W_2 + rW_1$. The ESS solutions to the model are obtained by simultaneously maximizing I_1 and I_2 with respect to x and y, respectively, to yield the equilibrium fitness maximizing effort levels ($x_1{}^*, x_2{}^*$). The main predictions of this tug-of-war model are that stronger dominants will obtain the larger share of reproduction, and that relatedness has little effect on the partitioning of shares.

By comparison, Frank's (1995, 2003) policing model uses a ratio form contest success function of the form

Box 3.1 (*cont.*)

$$F = x/\bar{x}$$

i.e. an individual's success is its own selfish effort x relative to the average selfish effort in the group $\bar{x}$. Group productivity V declines linearly with average selfishness, so that $V = 1 - \bar{x}$. The fitness of individual i is

$$W_i = x/\bar{x}(1 - \bar{x}) \qquad 3.1$$

Frank solves the model using the 'direct fitness' or 'neighbour-modulated' approach, an alternative way to formulate the process of kin selection. Maximizing W_i with respect to x (Taylor 1990; Franks 1995; Taylor & Frank 1996; Foster 2004; Taylor et al. 2007b) yields the solution $x^* = 1 - r$, where r is whole-group relatedness (mean relatedness among group members, allowing for relatedness to self). Groups of close kin should be less selfish than groups of non-relatives, but substantial levels of selfishness are expected even when relatedness is high (e.g. $x^* = 0.5$ for $r = 0.5$).

What if group members can invest in policing to suppress selfishness? Frank (1995) envisages a situation where a focal individual can invest policing effort a at a cost of ca fitness units to eradicate selfishness in any social interactions over which it has influence. If the average policing effort in the group is $\bar{a}$, a fraction $\bar{a}$ of social interactions is kept fair, in which case a focal individual's relative success is set equal to 1, and there is no damage to group productivity. The remaining fraction $(1 - \bar{a})$ of social interactions remains unpoliced: in these social interactions the focal individual's share of productivity is, as before, $x/\bar{x}$, and group productivity is $(1 - \bar{x})$. Thus, in the extended model, direct fitness is proportional to

$$W_i = [\bar{a} - ca + x/\bar{x}(1 - \bar{a})][1 - (1 - \bar{a})\bar{x}]$$

This model features two stable outcomes: full policing ($a^* = 1$) or no policing at all ($a^* = 0$). Full policing evolves where whole-group relatedness r is less than a critical threshold $1 - c$. Above this threshold r, policing does not evolve and the model results are identical to those of the basic model 3.1.

A Difference Form Model

Difference form models can be used to investigate contests in which players can gain a share of a resource even though they invest zero effort, for example when conflict takes the form of suppression, policing, or infanticide (Cant 2012). Consider the following contest success function, adapted from the economic models of Hirshleifer (1989, 2001).

$$F_1 = \frac{1}{1 + e^{d(bx_2 - x_1)}}$$

Here, x_1 and x_2 are the conflict efforts of the focal individual (player 1) and its opponent (player 2), respectively, and b measures the relative strength of player 2

Box 3.1 (cont.)

(for example, if $b < 1$, player 1 is stronger than player 2). The parameter d (for 'decisiveness') scales the advantage of superior effort invested in conflict (Figure 3.12A).

As in Reeve et al.'s (1998a) tug-of-war model, group productivity is assumed to decline with the sum of effort invested in conflict. Player 1's direct fitness is given by:

$$W_1 = \frac{1}{1 + e^{d(bx_2 - x_1)}} (1 - x_1 - x_2)$$

Cant (2012) solves the model using the inclusive fitness approach to find the evolutionarily stable values of x_1 and x_2. Unlike ratio form models, in this difference form model both mutual peace $(x_1^* = 0, x_2^* = 0)$ and one-sided peace $(x_1^* > 0, x_2^* = 0)$ can be evolutionarily stable outcomes. The stable outcome is mutual peace where $d < 2((1 + r)/(1 - r))$ (Figure 3.12B).

of policing. In other words, policing selects for greater levels of selfishness. This is difficult to reconcile with the proposed role of policing as a mechanism to enhance group productivity and repress selfishness (Frank 1995; El Mouden et al. 2010). El Mouden and collaborators (2010) highlighted this difficulty and showed that the problem lies in the assumed nature of the costs and benefits of policing. First, Frank's (1995) model assumes that the personal fitness cost of policing is a reduced share of total group productivity. This means that the absolute fitness cost of policing is lower in more selfish groups, which seems difficult to justify in many biological scenarios. Second, the model assumes that, in any given social interaction, an act of policing recovers all of the damage lost to selfishness. Selfishness inflicts damage on group productivity, but this damage is completely reversible and does not reduce selfishness in the first place. In animal societies, by contrast, policing involves steps to limit the damaging effects of selfish behaviour, for example by removing worker-laid eggs or killing subordinates' offspring to reduce the intensity of reproductive competition. In this situation, even if every interaction is policed $(a^* = 1)$, the initial damage caused by selfishness may be difficult to restore completely (El Mouden et al. 2010).

El Mouden et al. (2010) adapted Frank's (1995) model in two ways: first they assumed that the fitness costs of policing increased (rather than decreased) with the level of selfishness; second, they assumed that policing could limit damage to group productivity, but not fully restore it. The predictions of this adapted model differ from the original policing model in three important ways. First, the model predicts that a range of policing efforts can be evolutionarily stable, rather than policing at level zero or one. Second, selfishness is reduced in the presence of policing. Third, positive effort invested in policing evolves only at intermediate levels of relatedness, rather than below a critical threshold. Unlike Frank's model, therefore, El Mouden et al.'s (2010) model

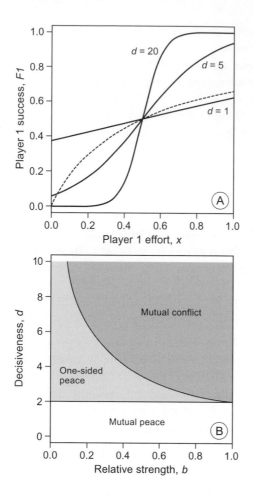

Figure 3.12 How destructive competition can lead to peaceful conflict resolution. (A) The curves plot the difference form contest success function for player 1, that is, how player 1's relative success (or relative share of a prize) increases with its conflict effort for three values of decisiveness d. For comparison, the dotted line plots the ratio form contest success function used in Reeve et al.'s (1998a) tug-of-war model. (B) Evolutionarily stable outcomes are plotted as a function of 'decisiveness' d and the relative strength of the two players b. In the mutual conflict zone, the stable solution is for both players to invest positive effort in conflict. In the one-sided peace zone, only the stronger player invests positive effort in conflict at equilibrium. In the mutual peace zone, the evolutionarily stable solution is for both players to invest zero in conflict. Other parameter $r = 0$. Redrawn with permission from Cant (2012).

predicts that selection for policing breaks down when whole-group relatedness (that is, an individual's genetic similarity to the whole group, including the effect of its own relatedness to itself) is low, for example, in very large groups. In pairs and small groups, however, whole-group relatedness is elevated by one's own relatedness to self, and so policing can readily evolve even among unrelated social partners. For this reason, El

Mouden et al. (2010) suggest that policing may be effective to reduce conflict also in interspecific mutualisms such as host–symbiont relationships.

3.3.2.3 Evolving Peace

A general feature of ratio form models is that any disparity between the fitness optima of competitors is always manifested in costly conflict. For example, in the policing model, some or all of the damage caused by selfishness can be repaired later through policing, but stable equilibria always involve some positive level of damage ($x^* > 0$). In ratio form models, zero investment in conflict always brings zero share of a resource (or zero probability of winning it, if the resource is indivisible). If other players invest zero effort, any mutant that invests an infinitesimally small level of effort wins the entire resource. Outcomes featuring 'one-sided peace' where a subset of competitors invests zero effort are evolutionarily unstable in ratio form models. In nature, however, many animal societies feature 'peaceful' outcomes, in which there is high potential for conflict, but actual conflict is absent or rare (Packer & Pusey 1982; Jamieson et al. 1994; Kardile & Gadagkar 2002; Endler et al. 2007). Other societies feature examples of 'one-sided peace', where one party (e.g. a dominant individual) engages in aggression or competitive behaviour while others do not. Indeed, far from retaliating, subordinates in many social animals respond to dominant aggression by adopting submissive postures or actively signalling their inferior quality or status, as discussed above. During sexual reproduction unrelated haploid genomes, which have great potential for evolutionary conflict, fuse with little actual conflict (Queller & Strassman 2009). How can this discrepancy between theory and data be reconciled?

Examples of peace and one-sided peace can be explained by 'difference form' models of conflict, in which contest success depends on the difference between competitor efforts, rather than their ratio. Unlike in ratio form models, in difference form models, individuals that invest zero in conflict effort can still gain some share of the resource (or, in the case of an indivisible resource, have some probability of winning it all). Whether a ratio or a difference form model best captures the gains of conflict effort depends on the mechanism by which individuals compete. To illustrate this, consider two birds laying eggs in a shared nest (as occurs in several cooperative joint-nesting species; Riehl 2013). If competition takes the form of a scramble for resources after hatching, each female's success will depend on their proportional representation in the number of eggs laid, and hence a ratio form contest success function would apply well. This is an example of 'productive' competition, where success depends on maximizing the production of competitive units (in this case, eggs), or competitive acts. If, however, competition takes the form of egg destruction or infanticide after the clutch is laid, a female that invested nothing in competition could still achieve some reproductive success (particularly if discrimination is not perfect). This is an example of 'destructive' competition, where success depends on suppressing or eliminating the competitive units produced by others, or nullifying their competitive acts. Or to use a human example, imagine an economic competition between two rival fishing firms: productive competition occurs when the firms build new ships or make their existing vessels more efficient. Destructive competition occurs when the firms invest in trying to sabotage or sink each other's ships.

Cant (2012) analysed a difference form version of Reeve et al.'s tug-of-war model, in which a focal individual's success in conflict depends on the difference between its own conflict effort x_1 and that of its opponent x_2 (Box 3.1). The model includes two other parameters: a relative strength parameter b, which gives the strength of player 2 compared to player 1; and a decisiveness parameter d, which measures the marginal benefits of superior conflict effort. When decisiveness is low, a given difference in conflict effort does not make too much difference to the difference in relative success of the two players. When decisiveness is high, a small advantage in conflict effort translates into a large advantage in relative success. Figure 3.12A illustrates the shape of the difference form contest success function for different values of the decisiveness parameter. Decisiveness can be interpreted biologically in a number of ways. Decisiveness will be high where success depends on outlasting or wearing down the resistance of one's opponent in a war of attrition. In these circumstances an individual that puts in slightly more effort than its opponent may stand to win all of the resource. By contrast, decisiveness will be low where conflicts are risky or stochastic in nature, or where individuals have little information about the likely outcome of the conflict or the strength or effort of their opponent.

This model predicts that when individuals engage in destructive competition, the same degree of potential conflict results in very different levels of actual conflict, depending on asymmetry in strength and decisiveness. Increasing strength asymmetry can shift the stable outcome from mutual conflict to one-sided peace in which only the stronger individual invests in conflict (Figure 3.12B). In this model, therefore, it can pay a subordinate individual to submit completely in the face of an aggressive dominant (see also Section 3.2.2). Mutual peace is only possible where decisiveness is low. Because mutual peace is a more efficient outcome than those involving conflict, individuals can gain by acting to reduce decisiveness below the threshold for mutual peace, for example by withholding information about their own expected conflict effort, or increasing the stochasticity of contests. This argument is similar to the idea that meiosis reduces conflict within the genome because it draws a 'veil of ignorance' over the outcome of interlocus conflict (Haig & Grafen 1991; Okasha 2012). In a fair meiosis, each allele has only a 50 per cent chance of being transmitted to any particular gamete, so a given allele is ignorant of whether other alleles at different loci are future gametic partners or future gametic rivals. The machinery of meiosis reduces information about the outcome of conflict, and hence the level of decisiveness, in any conflict between loci, which according to the destructive competition model will promote intragenomic peace.

3.3.3 Behavioural Conflict: Threats, Negotiation and Assessment

The assumption of sealed-bid models that competitors do not respond in real time to each other's behaviour is at odds with our observations of animal behaviour, particularly in the context of aggression and fighting. Combatants or competitors appear

Table 3.1 Behavioural and evolutionary mechanisms of conflict reduction. Behavioural mechanisms involve real-time assessments of and responses to changes in the behaviour of an opponent. Evolutionary mechanisms are those that shape the evolution of fixed genetic strategies over many generations. Evolutionary and behavioural mechanisms are not exclusive and may coevolve; for example, kin selection influences negotiation and threats (e.g. Savage et al. 2013; Thompson et al. 2017a).

Behavioural mechanisms of conflict reduction		Evolutionary mechanisms of conflict reduction	
Mechanism	**How is conflict reduced?**	**Mechanism**	**How is conflict reduced?**
(i) Threats	Credible threats resolve conflict without recourse to violence	(i) Kin selection	High genetic relatedness reduces the width of the battleground and the profitability of conflict effort
(ii) Negotiation	Negotiation allows fine-tuning of conflict effort and conveys information about strength or need	*Destructive competition*	Low contest decisiveness and high relatedness reduce the profitability of conflict effort
(iii) Assessment	Assessment and displays reduce uncertainty about relative strength or need	(ii) Repression of competition	
		Dictatorship	Complete suppression of subordinates aligns their fitness interests with those of the dominant
		Levelling	Enforced equality aligns the fitness interests of group members
		Life history segregation	Temporal separation of fertility schedules reduces reproductive conflict
		Outgroup threat	Existential outgroup threat aligns the fitness interests of group members

continuously to adjust their behaviour to aggression or resistance of their opponent. Behavioural models of conflict attempt to incorporate a degree of real-time responsiveness in various ways, for example by assuming that one player 'moves' first so that their behaviour can be observed by a second player before choosing their response; or by assuming that individuals interact repeatedly and can 'bargain' towards a peaceful resolution of conflict. These models are a step towards understanding the dynamics and form of fighting, policing and other forms of overt conflict, and why the form, frequency and intensity of conflict behaviour vary between groups, populations and species (see Table 3.1).

3.3.3.1   Threats and Coercion: Sequential Models

The simplest step toward a behavioural theory of evolutionary conflict is to assume that interactions involve a sequence of 'moves' rather than simultaneous sealed bids. These sequential models grew out of early models of reproductive skew, which explored how threats of departure or eviction might influence the resolution of conflict over reproductive shares. The distinction between a simultaneous and sequential game is one of information: in a sequential game, player B has information about player A's action before choosing its own response. This simple adjustment of the information structure of the game opens the door to a much wider range of strategies to influence the behaviour of partners, and a wider range of potential outcomes of evolutionary conflict. In particular, when individuals anticipate each other's responses, individuals may use threats to coerce the behaviour of opponents, rather than brute force (Cant 2011; Cant & Young 2013). The economist Schelling (1967) painted a vivid contrast between the use of brute force and coercive threats:

There is a difference between taking what you want and making someone give it to you, between fending off assault and making someone afraid to assault you, between holding what people are trying to take and making them afraid to take it, between losing what someone can forcibly take and giving it up to avoid risk or damage. It is the difference between defense and deterrence, between brute force and intimidation, between conquest and blackmail, between action and threats. (Schelling 1967, *Arms and Influence*, p. 2)

Coercion by threat is difficult to study because threats work by deterrence. If a threat of infanticide by individual A is effective at deterring individual B from breeding, no offspring need to be killed, and hence it will not be at all obvious to an observer that B's behaviour is the result of coercion. To be effective as a means for A to coerce the behaviour of B, A's threat must be both *credible* and *clear*. The threat is credible only if B believes, or is made to believe, that A would carry through with the threatened action, should B choose to defect or to resist coercion. The threat is clear if B has information about what it needs to do to avoid triggering the threatened action. To coerce B successfully, A needs to convince B that it would be better to cooperate than to defect and suffer the consequences of the threatened action. To be coercive, violence has to be anticipated, and to be avoidable by accommodation. Finally, threats need to be targeted accurately, and hence are most effective in dyadic relationships and strict hierarchies, where each individual's threat is targeted towards a single other. Threats of, say, eviction or infanticide are not credible where targeting is inaccurate, and hence restraint is not an evolutionarily stable outcome in these circumstances (Figure 3.13).

To test whether an animal's behaviour is coerced by threat, we need to perform experiments to break the rules that we suspect threats are used to enforce. Three examples illustrate how experimental manipulations can reveal hidden threats. First, in the cooperatively breeding banded mongoose, almost all females reproduce in each breeding attempt and in 64 per cent of cases synchronize birth to the same morning. In the 36 per cent of breeding attempts in which females give birth asynchronously (i.e. over several days), litters that are produced first almost always die in the first few days after birth, whereas litters that are born last almost always survive (Hodge et al. 2011). A similar pattern is seen in smooth-billed anis and communally breeding mice (Vehrencamp 1977; König 1994). Hodge and collaborators (2011) hypothesized that dominant female banded mongooses kill litters that are certain not to contain their own young and hence subordinates can escape the threat of infanticide by synchronizing birth to the same day as dominants. To test this hypothesis, Cant and collaborators (2014) used contraceptive injections to suppress reproduction in dominant or

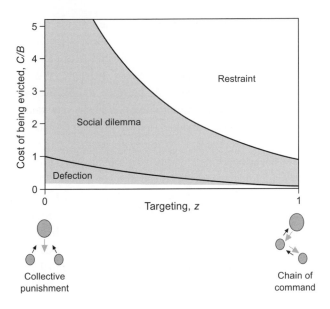

Figure 3.13 Effectiveness of threats to enforce restraint or cooperation in multi-member groups. The figure shows the results of a three-player model in which a dominant player can evict one of two subordinates if either of them defects and claims a share of reproduction. Zones for which the evolutionarily stable outcome is mutual subordinate restraint (unshaded) or defection and consequent eviction of one of the subordinates (shaded) are plotted as a function of the cost of being evicted (C, relative to the benefits of defecting and escaping punishment B) and the degree to which the dominant singles out transgressors for punishment (targeting z). The zones marked 'restraint' and 'defection' indicate areas where strategies of restraint and defection yield the highest pay-off irrespective of the strategy of the other subordinate. In the 'social dilemma' zone, defection is the evolutionarily stable strategy even though both subordinates would do better if they could agree to exercise restraint. The case where $z = 1$ applies to groups that exhibit a linear hierarchical structure, such that each individual monitors and targets its immediate subordinate for punishment (labelled 'chain of command' in the figure). In this case, restraint is stable if the cost of being evicted outweighs the benefits of claiming additional reproduction (i.e. $C/B > 1$). Reproduced with permission from Cant et al. (2010). © 2010 The Royal Society. Open access.

subordinate females, respectively. Suppression of dominants, but not subordinates, resulted in whole-litter failure immediately after birth, consistent with the hypothesis that dominant females kill litters that do not contain their own young. The results suggest that selection to avoid triggering a threat of infanticide has driven the evolution of the remarkable birth synchrony observed in this species.

A second example of effective threats in nature relates to the strict size hierarchies exhibited by several species of fish (Heg et al. 2004b; Wong et al. 2007, 2008; Ang & Manica 2010). Buston (2003b) hypothesized that discrete size intervals such as those observed in clownfish hierarchies are maintained by a hidden threat of eviction: lower-ranked individuals stop growing to avoid triggering eviction by the ⁓ individual immediately above them in rank. However, evictions are almost never observed in nature – precisely as expected if the threat of eviction is effective.

To test Buston's (2003b) hypothesis requires experiments to test what happens when lower-ranked individuals grow larger than they would in nature. Wong et al. (2007) carried out this experiment on the coral-dwelling goby *Paragobiodon xanthosomus*. In this species, smaller individuals (termed subordinates) typically maintain a size ratio of 0.9–0.95 times that of the next larger individual (termed dominants) and cease feeding to avoid growing larger than this relative size (Wong et al. 2008). Wong et al. (2007) used staged contests to show that a subordinate was usually tolerated by a dominant if she was smaller than the most common size ratio observed in natural groups (0.93) and usually evicted if she was larger than this threshold size. It was also clear from this experiment why dominants evict above a threshold of around 0.9–0.95: if the subordinate is allowed to grow larger than this, then the dominant is at risk of being evicted herself (Figure 3.14). Experimental evidence for strategic growth to maintain a certain size differential has also been demonstrated in cooperative cichlids (Heg et al. 2004b). Finally, a recent field experiment on clownfish showed that reproductively active subordinates that were introduced to groups are more likely to be evicted compared to size-matched, non-reproductive subordinates (Rueger et al. 2018). Clownfish also show competitive growth in the laboratory, growing faster when paired with a size-matched reproductive rival (Reed et al. 2019). Remarkably, the elevated growth rates of clownfish in competitive treatments were achieved despite the fish receiving no extra food.

A third, general example of the importance of threats in nature is the formation of dominance hierarchies. A stable dominance hierarchy is based on establishing credible deterrent threats of violence. To deter subordinate challenges, subordinate individuals must believe that fighting a dominant would be unprofitable. Thus, if there is any uncertainty about relative strength, it will benefit dominant individuals to advertise their superior strength (for example, through costly or aggressive displays) in order to reduce or remove this uncertainty. How frequently should a dominant display its strength? If the strength of dominants and subordinates did not vary over time, a strong dominant would have to signal once and once only in order to deter a subordinate forever. However, if strength is subject to stochastic influences (e.g. because of fluctuations in food, exposure to disease, or senescence) it would be maladaptive of a subordinate to believe a dominant's signal forever. A subordinate behaving optimally should allow its estimate of the dominant's strength to spread (i.e. increase in uncertainty) over time since the signal was last given. Dominant individuals may therefore need to repeatedly update their signal in order to effectively deter a subordinate. Thompson et al. (2014) tested this idea in foundress associations of the paper wasp *P. dominula* by manipulating the opportunity for rank 1 and rank 2 females to interact, prior to staging a contest for control of the nest. Rank 1 females that were allowed the opportunity to engage in a dominance interaction a few days before the induced contest typically retained control of the nest without a challenge from the rank 2. Denying the females this opportunity to interact frequently led to escalated and violent fights. Some of these fights lasted over 20 minutes and involved attempts to sting each other – a potentially lethal move (Reeve 1991).

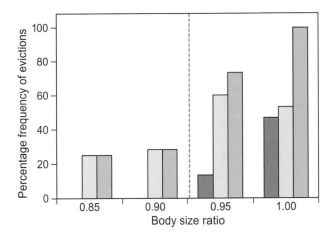

Figure 3.14 Evictions and body size in the goby *Paragobiodon xanthosomus*. Bars show percentage of experimental trials in which subordinate fish were evicted (light grey) or dominant fish were evicted (dark grey bars). The combined percentage of evictions is given by the grey bars. The vertical dashed line is the modal body size ratio observed in natural groups of clown anemonefish (0.93). (Reproduced with permission from Wong et al. 2007.) © 2007 The Royal Society.

It is important to note that punishment as a mechanism to suppress selfishness or induce cooperation largely relies on the coercive rather than the brute force effects of violence. Inflicting a cost on another individual to induce it to be more cooperative or less selfish in future works by establishing the credibility of a threat to attack again, in the event of non-compliance or defection. It follows that the most effective punishment will often rarely be observed – once credibility is established, the latent threat of punishment works silently behind the scenes to deter repeat offences.

The coercive nature of punishment is implicit in reputational models of punishment, where a reputation for punishing can induce cooperation in future interactions with the same individual or with third party by-standers (Raihani et al. 2010). However, many theoretical models assume that individuals have a single-step memory, and thereby inadvertently rule out the power of punishment to condition the longer-term behaviour of recipients. This has led some authors to argue that punishment should be more common when there are large asymmetries in strength, because strong players can punish weak ones at lower cost (e.g. Raihani et al. 2012). By contrast, if coercion takes the form of threats of punishment, punishment itself may be *less* common where there are large asymmetries in strength, because weaker recipients may be more easily deterred, and for longer. Models of aggression as a deterrent signal predict that dominant individuals will need to display less often to weaker challengers (Thompson et al. 2014a). In the dominance hierarchies of some primates, the most powerful dominants may sometimes use small signals (e.g. an eyebrow flash) to displace low-ranked group members, having already established the credibility of threats of violence.

The dynamics of punishment and recidivism, for example how much punishment should be dealt out, and how long a given punishment should function as a deterrent, remain little explored theoretically and empirically. In economics, there is a long-standing interest in whether more frequent or severe punishment is more effective in deterring crime (e.g. Becker 1968) and what are the optimal policies of punishment for deterrence (Rubinstein 1979, 1980; Burnovski & Safra 1994). The intuitive prediction of Becker (1968) that increasing the probability of punishment, or its severity, should reduce crime is challenged by data that show the opposite pattern (Tittle & Rowe 1974; Katz et al. 2003; Fagan & Meares 2008), spurring the development of new theory which incorporates factors such as social memory and self-reputation (e.g. Bernheim & Thomadsen 2005; Bénabou & Tirole 2009; Chiba & Leong 2015). These economic analyses suggest there is potential for much future development in evolutionary theory to understand variation in the effectiveness and frequency of punishment.

3.3.3.2   Negotiation Models

Models of behavioural negotiation assume that individuals engage in repeated bouts of interaction in which they can make repeated offers or bids to resolve the division of a contested resource (McNamara et al. 1999; Johnstone & Hinde 2006). Unlike traditional evolutionary game-theory models which are concerned with evolutionarily stable strategies (such as the level of effort invested in conflict), these models solve for evolutionarily stable 'response rules' that specify how individuals should react on a behavioural timescale to changes in the effort level of their social partner (McNamara et al. 1999). The models take into account the fact that social partners are bound to vary in quality or state, and so the effort that different social partners invest in the game will also vary. Individuals will know their own quality or state, but not necessarily the quality or state of their partners. Hence, each player needs a behavioural rule to follow which gives the best effort for them to invest, for any effort invested by the other player.

McNamara et al. (1999, 2003) illustrated the consequences of allowing individuals to engage in behavioural negotiation on the predicted outcome of conflict using Houston and Davies' (1985) classic game model of parental care (see also Section 3.2.3). They assume that a male and a female can engage in an unspecified period of behavioural negotiation, involving a repeated exchange of effort and counter-effort, until these efforts settle down to some equilibrium (the 'negotiated outcome') which specifies how hard they subsequently work to rear the offspring. The pay-off to each parent depends only on the final negotiated levels of investment – the period of negotiation itself is entirely cost-free. McNamara et al. showed that allowing behavioural negotiation in this way leads to some surprising outcomes. For example, in the parental care game, negotiation leads to lower levels of investment in cooperative care. Negotiation is so detrimental to cooperation in the parental care game that in some cases offspring may even be better off with a single parent than with two negotiating ones (McNamara et al. 2003).

An important question is how negotiation will affect stable levels of conflict investment. In general, negotiation is expected to help resolve conflicts at lower cost, because it can provide information about the need or state of opponents which can be used to fine-tune competitive effort. For example, Johnstone and Roulin (2003) show that in the context of siblings competing for food in a nest, offspring can gain from negotiating about the division of resources prior to the arrival of a parent with food because the negotiation process conveys information about each offspring's need. Negotiation is a particularly effective means of reducing conflict effort where resources are indivisible and where competitors are close genetic relatives.

The modelling framework of McNamara et al. is just one way of investigating the outcome of repeated behaviour negotiation. Some of the assumptions of the model, such as cost-free negotiation, are obviously unrealistic, and analytical solutions for ESS response rules are obtainable only where fitness functions take a particularly simple, quadratic form (which is not the case, for example, for classic conflict models such as the tug-of-war of Reeve et al. 1998a). Nevertheless, the main point that natural selection will lead to the evolution of stable response rules is an important one. The economist Ken Binmore (2010) suggested other approaches to modelling the evolution of negotiation strategies based on the theory of bargaining which could be adapted to a biological context. Further theoretical development in this area would help to predict and explain behavioural dynamics during conflict in a way that current sealed-bid game-theoretical approaches cannot.

3.3.3.3 Assessment Models

Because individuals with greater resource holding potential (RHP) usually win fights, selection should favour mechanisms that allow animals to assess the RHP of their opponent and themselves and so avoid fights that they are unlikely to win. Several models have been proposed to understand the process by which animals might gather and use information during a fight or agonistic interaction. These assessment models have been described as 'open box' models, because the process by which conflict effort translates into success is made explicit, rather than being encapsulated in the 'closed box' of a particular mathematical form of the contest success function (Kokko 2013).

An influential model of this kind is the sequential assessment (SA) model of Enquist and Leimar (1983, 1987). In this model (sometimes also referred to as a 'mutual assessment' model; Arnott & Elwood 2009) conflict is settled via repeated rounds of costly interactions, in which each round is an opportunity to reduce uncertainty about relative strength. This model involves mutual assessment – individuals use information about their own strength compared to that of their opponent to decide whether to continue with the contest. Such a model might be relevant to contests that involve ritualized displays, pushing or shoving contests. Fights continue until one player reaches a switching point or 'giving up threshold', that is, a threshold level of uncertainty about relative strength below which the expected pay-offs of continuing to fight are lower than the pay-off of giving up and fleeing the scene (Figure 3.15). The main predictions of this model are (i) sometimes stronger individuals will lose due to the stochastic nature of the sampling process; (ii) increased uncertainty at the start of the contest will in general lead to longer fights; (iii)

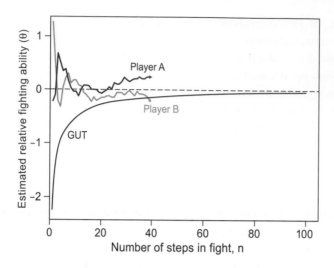

Figure 3.15 The sequential assessment game. Fights consist of a sequence of steps in which two players (A and B) exchange blows, which yields to each a sample from which to estimate relative fighting ability (θ_{AB}). Relative fighting ability is a measure of the players' ability to inflict costs upon each other ($\theta_{AB} = \ln(c_B/c_A)$, where c_A and c_B are the ability of A and B to inflict costs on each other at each step, respectively). The fight continues until one player's sampling average of θ_{AB} crosses its giving up threshold (GUT), at which point it does better to concede. In this example, player B concedes the fight at step 39 of the fight (redrawn with permission from Enquist & Leimar 1983). Copyright © 1983 Published by Elsevier Ltd.

fight duration will be longest for opponents of similar RHP; and (iv) fights will last longer where resources are more valuable.

In many cases individuals might simply persist in a contest according to an assessment of their own RHP, rather than engage in assessment of their opponents (Taylor & Elwood 2003; Arnott & Elwood 2009). This process has been referred to as 'own RHP-dependent persistence' (Taylor & Elwood 2003). An example is the energetic war-of-attrition (EWOA) model (Payne & Pagel 1997), which assumes that contestants persist until they have depleted their own energy reserves to a threshold level. In this model there is no assessment of the opponent's strength, and the costs paid by an individual depend only on its own attributes, not on the attributes of its opponent. By contrast, the cumulative assessment (CA) model (Payne 1998) assumes that the costs suffered for persistence include both internal energetic costs and costs inflicted by an opponent, as appropriate for injurious contests that involve butting, rutting, boxing or biting. A key difference between the CA and the SA models is that the CA model assumes that the rate of escalation is an evolving trait, rather than a constant or fixed feature of the interaction as assumed by the SA model (Kokko 2013). The CA model again predicts longer fights over more valuable resources and between equally matched opponents, but in addition predicts that fights will typically escalate in intensity, up to the point where the loser concedes. In some cases (particularly when contest duration is long) poorer-quality individuals are predicted to start with a low conflict intensity but escalate rapidly before giving up (Payne 1998). Importantly, CA models can predict both escalation and de-escalation over the course of the contest, whereas SA models predict only escalation (Arnott & Elwood 2009).

Determining which type of assessment model best captures contest behaviour in nature has proved difficult because different models make similar predictions, and because in reality fights can involve a mixture of self- and mutual assessment, or a mixture of personal and opponent inflicted costs. A common finding is that contest duration is negatively related to the size difference between contestants, which would appear to support the process of mutual assessment in the SA and CA models (Dowds & Elwood 1985; Dugatkin & Biederman 1991; Leimar et al. 1991; Faber & Baylis 1993; Hack 1997; Stokkebo & Hardy 2000). However, Taylor and Elwood (2003) show that this relationship does not necessarily mean that individuals assess the RHP of their opponent. A negative relationship between contest duration and size or RHP asymmetry can arise spuriously even if individuals base their persistence in a contest on their own body size only, because of correlations between own body size and absolute or relative size difference. Given that data on contest duration are inconclusive alone as a means of differentiating between assessment models, several authors have advocated a combined approach that uses information on contest dynamics and correlations between RHP (or a proxy such as body size) and costs to differentiate between assessment models (Briffa & Elwood 2009; Briffa & Hardy 2013; Briffa et al. 2013). For example, Green and Patek (2018) staged fights over burrows in the mantis shrimp *Neogonodactylus bredini* (Figure 3.16). They analysed correlations of RHP and contest intensity, and patterns of contest escalation, to disentangle between SA and CA models. Their analysis showed that the relationship between RHP and conflict intensity, and the unidirectional pattern of escalation, was consistent with a process of sequential assessment, but not cumulative assessment. The SA model provides the best model of the informational and biological factors affecting conflict dynamics and outcome of fights in mantis shrimp.

These assessment models are potentially relevant to understanding the stability of social hierarchies. Conflict over rank is often settled by bouts of escalated fighting which continue until one party 'gives up' and accepts subordinate status (Cant et al. 2006a). In both the paper wasp *P. dominula* and the cooperative cichlid *N. pulcher*, fights over dominance rank can be induced experimentally by removing a dominant individual, allowing a subordinate or usurper to inherit his or her position and then replacing the original dominant (Cant et al. 2006a; Leadbeater et al. 2010; Thompson et al. 2014; O'Connor et al. 2015). In *P. dominula*, contest duration increases with the time that the dominant is away (Cant et al. 2006a), and fights are shorter if the two contestants are allowed to interact socially midway through the removal period (Thompson et al. 2014). These results are consistent with the assumption of the SA and CA models that fight duration depends on the level of uncertainty about relative strength, and that dominance interactions can function to reduce this uncertainty. A similar pattern is observed in *N. pulcher*, where contest duration among males is also positively related to the time that a territory holder is kept away (O'Connor et al. 2015). The aggression rate of dominant males appears positively related to the

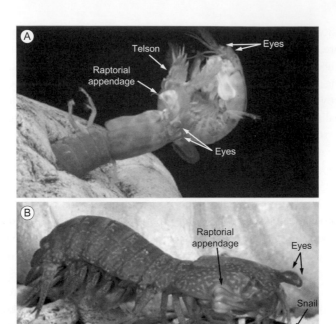

Figure 3.16 Contests with a deadly weapon in mantis shrimp. (A) Mantis shrimp of the genus *Neogonodactylus* deliver powerful strikes to opponents using a raptorial appendage. In this top image there are two shrimps: the shrimp on the right is defending against a strike by coiling its telson (terminal segment) in front of its body. (B) The shrimp use the raptorial appendage to kill prey. Here the raptorial appendage is in a raised, pre-strike position, about to deliver a blow to a snail. (Photo © Roy Caldwell. From Green et al. 2019.) (A black and white version of this figure will appear in some formats. For the colour version, please refer to the plate section.)

subjective value they place on the contested territory: males are more aggressive when trying to regain control of a sole-ownership territory compared to a polygynous set of territories in which they are likely to share paternity.

A limitation of open box models of assessment is that they typically consider one-off contests between unrelated individuals, rather than repeated interaction of the kind that occur between family members (Kokko 2013). Where contests over rank and resources occur between competitors that interact repeatedly, previous social interactions will be a major determinant of fighting intensity and contest duration (Hardy et al. 2013). As described in Section 3.4.1, selection acting on subordinate memory will favour a faster rate of 'forgetting' (i.e. disregarding) of cues or signals of an opponent's strength where strength is more variable over time (Thompson et al. 2014). Thus, we might expect the intensity or frequency of dominant aggression to be inversely related to the durability of subordinate social memory. The development of open-box models that incorporate social factors such as relatedness and social memory is a rich area for research on behavioural conflict.

3.4   Evolutionary Routes to Conflict Reduction

The models in the preceding section help to identify factors that influence the level of potential and actual conflict within groups (Table 3.1). During the latter stages of a cooperative transition, the group transformation stage, these conflicts are reduced to a very low or negligible level and groups emerge as a new tier of organization. From the perspective of multilevel selection models, reducing within-group conflict means reducing the potential for selection within groups, that is, the level of within-group variance for social traits. When within-group variance is minimized, between-group variance can select for traits which benefit group fitness at the expense of individual fitness. Okasha and Paternotte (2012), extending work by Gardner and Grafen (2009), suggest that the eradication of within-group competition is both a necessary and sufficient condition for groups to function as 'fitness maximizing agents', with adaptations to maximize mean group fitness. These models suggest that the key to group transformation is the eradication of potential conflict, as measured by within-group variance in fitness. Haig (2014), in a commentary on Grafen's (2007, 2009, 2014) 'Formal Darwinism' project, argues that the complete eradication of conflict is often unachievable, because individual alleles will almost always have differing optimal phenotypes. For Haig, successful organisms (or 'organismal lineages') are those that can effectively manage and reduce internal conflicts, rather than eliminate them entirely: other things being equal, the more effective the management of conflicts, the more successful the lineage (Haig 2014).

How can conflict over direct fitness be reduced on an evolutionary timescale? Current theory suggests that there are two main pathways to conflict reduction: kin selection (Hamilton 1964, 1970; Frank 2003) and repression of competition (Alexander 1987; Buss 1987; Frank 2003; Bowles & Gintis 2013).

3.4.1   Kin Selection

High relatedness has a dual impact on levels of within-group competition. First, it draws together the fitness optima of individual units of selection, reducing the potential for conflict. However, as discussed in Section 3.3.2, the width of the battleground does not necessarily predict the level of actual conflict, and high relatedness is often associated with intense local competition among kin, which can inhibit selection for altruism (Section 4.1.2.2). Relatedness has a second effect, however: it serves to reduce the inclusive fitness pay-offs of investing in competition over reproductive shares within groups. Genetic relatedness interacts with contest decisiveness to determine whether peaceful resolution of evolutionary conflict is evolutionarily stable. In difference form models of conflict, high relatedness and low decisiveness can favour peaceful outcomes, even among individuals with divergent fitness interests. Comparative analyses have highlighted the importance of high kinship for evolutionary transitions to cooperation in animal societies. In insects (Hughes et al. 2008), birds (Cornwallis et al. 2010) and mammals (Lukas & Clutton-Brock 2012b), monogamy (and consequent high relatedness between offspring) may have set the stage for the evolution of cooperation (see Section 4.1.2.2).

3.4.2   Repression of Competition

Repression of within-group competition can be defined as any evolved process, mechanism or convention that acts to reduce within-group variance in fitness. There are four distinct methods of reducing variance in direct fitness between members of the group.

3.4.2.1   Reproductive Dictatorship

In groups of relatives, within-group conflict over reproduction can be eradicated if reproduction is restricted to a single breeder or breeding pair and other group members are permanently sterile, as exemplified by colonies of ants and many termites. Absolute reproductive suppression via permanent worker sterility ensures that the reproductive interests of workers and the reproductives are aligned, minimizing within-group selection and facilitating the evolution of functional colony-level adaptation. In many eusocial insects and in all cooperatively breeding insects and vertebrates, however, workers retain the capacity to produce offspring. In these cases, enforcing a reproductive dictatorship requires active policing behaviour. The model of El Mouden and collaborators (2010) shows that policing can be effective at enforcing dictatorship, but not entirely: for example, policing breaks down at larger group sizes. Thus, even in the most rigid dictatorships these policing models suggest that within-group selection and conflict cannot be eradicated entirely and reproductive dissidents can persist at a low level.

3.4.2.2   Reproductive Levelling

In groups of non-relatives, fitness interests can be aligned if reproductive shares are distributed evenly among group members. In these circumstances an individual can gain in fitness (relative to the population mean) only by raising the fitness of the entire group. Within genomes and human societies, levelling can be institutionally or socially imposed. In diploid organisms, for example, meiosis ensures a rigidly fair chance that any given allele has an equal chance of representation among gametes, although some genes and selfish genetic elements have evolved to subvert this fair raffle. The term 'fair raffle' highlights the fact that levelling can work by equalizing expected or anticipated pay-offs, even if realized pay-offs vary between subunits. Meiosis equalizes anticipated pay-offs of genes in a genome by drawing a veil of ignorance over the precise fate of different meiotic products, so that each allele has the same chance of ending up in a successful gamete (Okasha 2012).

Reproductive levelling can also be enforced directly on realized shares of reproduction, through collective suppression of upstarts. In humans, hunter-gatherers are typically egalitarian in the sense that attempts by individuals (usually males) to control resources or political decision-making are immediately put down through peer criticism, ridicule, ostracism or even death (Boehm 1999; Wrangham 2018). Among the Hadza of Tanzania, for example, men that attempt to dominate others by ordering them around or taking their wives run the risk of being ambushed at night, or killed in their sleep (Woodburn 1982). Reports of the execution of men that attempt to bully or dominate are widespread in the ethnographic literature (Boehm 1999). Mild social sanctions such as peer criticism and ridicule are effective at deterring would-be tyrants because they carry the behavioural threat of escalation to more severe punishments, such as ostracism or, in the extreme, execution (Wrangham 2018).

How might collective action preventing domination by strong individuals evolve? A model by Gavrilets (2012) suggests that egalitarian social control can readily evolve where weak individuals have an incentive to intervene on each other's behalf in conflicts with stronger individuals. For example, where there are accelerating fitness returns on increasing share of a resource, weak individuals do best to form coalitions to prevent monopolization of resources by strong individuals (see also Noë's veto game played by baboons; Noë 1990). Gavrilets (2012) refers to this situation as 'egalitarian drive'. However, it is not clear why, for humans, an accelerating returns on resource share should apply, rather than the typical assumption of diminishing returns on resources that we might expect to apply to social species. For example, where the cost of offspring production increases with litter or clutch size, we expect the marginal fitness returns of increasing resource share to decline with the amount provided (Cant & Johnstone 1999). In Gavrilets' (2012) model, this diminishing returns pattern favours strong individuals monopolizing and trying to suppress any competitors, not sharing with them. There is scope for further theoretical research to understand the circumstances that promote solidarity of the weak against the strong.

3.4.2.3 Life History Segregation

A third mechanism to reduce within-group variance in fitness is life history segregation, the temporal segregation of life-history functions in groups with overlapping generations (Figure 3.17). In many cooperatively breeding mammals, for example, subordinate females suppress their ovarian function and form a queue to inherit dominant status (e.g. naked mole rats *Heterocephalus glaber*: Clarke & Faulkes 1997; Oosthuizen et al. 2008; Damaraland mole rats *Fukomys damarensis*: Cooney & Bennett 2000; Clarke et al. 2001; Young et al. 2010; meerkats: Young et al. 2006; Clutton-Brock et al. 2010). Conflict over reproduction is particularly extreme when a reproductive vacancy appears, at which point the latent conflicts of interest within the group break out into fights to inherit. At the other end of the fertility schedule, menopause in humans and killer whales helps to reduce intergenerational conflict over reproduction (Lahdenperä et al. 2012; Croft et al. 2017). In these two species (and, potentially, also in short-finned pilot whales) menopause occurs at a proximate level because the reproductive system undergoes rapid senescence midway through life, with the timing of the onset of reproductive senescence coinciding with

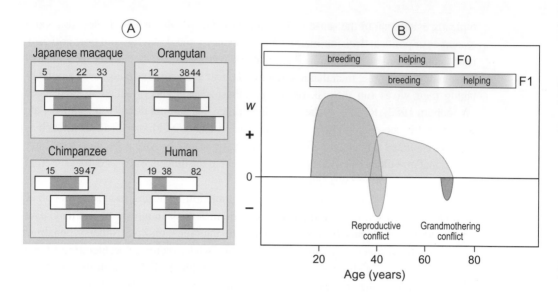

Figure 3.17 Reduction of within-group competition via life history segregation. (A) Average reproductive overlap in human hunter-gatherers and non-human primates, based on mean age at first birth (MAFB), mean age at last birth, and maximum lifespan in the wild (MLS). For each species, horizontal bars represent the maximum lifespans of three successive generations, scaled to a standard length and offset in accordance with the value of the MAFB relative to the MLS, with mean reproductive spans shaded. Human data are averaged values for two particularly well-studied hunter-gatherer populations (the Ache and !Kung). The mean reproductive overlap values for Japanese macaques, orangutans and chimpanzees are 0.71, 0.52 and 0.39, respectively. For humans, the mean reproductive overlap is 0.00 (reproduced with permission from Cant & Johnstone 2008). (B) Schematic schedule of inclusive fitness costs (negative values of W) and benefits (positive values of W) for a focal female (F0) across two generations, based loosely on findings from a longitudinal study of a historical Finnish population living in natural fertility conditions (Lahdenperä et al. 2004, 2012; Chapman et al. 2019). Bars depict overlapping life histories of F0 and F1 females (reproduced with permission from Cant & Croft 2019). © 2019 Elsevier Ltd.

the age at which the offspring of older females start to compete with the offspring of the next generation (Cant & Johnstone 2008). Reproductive suppression among younger individuals (common in cooperatively breeding birds and mammals) and reproductive suppression among older individuals (as occurs in humans, killer whales and, potentially, short-finned pilot whales) both serve to reduce within-group competition via temporal segregation of fertility. Whether selection favours suppression in older or younger generations may depend crucially on patterns of demography (Johnstone & Cant 2010; Croft et al. 2017; Section 3.3.1).

3.4.2.4   Outgroup Threat

Fourth, the shared risk of group extinction by a common enemy, such as a predator, pathogen or a rival group, can align the interest of group members, just as internal reproductive levelling mechanisms do. Where individuals live and die as a group, and/or individual survival depends on coordination or cooperative behaviour, fighting over within-group resources places all individuals at risk. Individuals will be selected to minimize within-group competitive behaviour for the good of their group (as well as themselves; Reeve & Hölldobler 2007). In animal societies, predators lead to the conspicuous suppression of internal conflicts over vigilance (Bednekoff & Naguib 2015) or movement (Ioannou et al. 2012; Herbert-Read et al. 2017). Social insects, like humans, engage in wide-ranging acts of coordination and self-sacrifice to defend members of their society against infection by pathogens and parasites (Shorter & Ruepell 2012; Cremer et al. 2007). Finally, in many animals rival groups of conspecifics pose a potentially lethal threat via intergroup aggression and warfare. This latter form of threat may have played a central role in the evolution of our own social behaviour. Theory and data suggest that warfare among ancestral bands may have promoted the evolution of intense cooperation and teamwork, even among non-relatives (Darwin 1871; Bowles 2009; Bowles & Gintis 2013), and to patterns of antipathy and hostility towards outgroups. These potential impacts of intergroup conflict on behaviour and social evolution are considered in more detail below.

3.5   Intergroup Conflict and Cooperation

In many social animals individuals compete with the members of other groups via ecological exploitation competition for limited resources, such as food or territory. However, in a few social species, including humans, individuals compete as a group through coordinated, collective attacks on rival groups, behaviour which is termed 'collective violence' (Durrant 2011) or simple 'warfare' (Thayer 2004). In ants, for example, colonies may engage in prolonged lethal fights with rival colonies of the same or different species (Wilson 1971; Hölldobler & Wilson 2009). In some cases, these ant wars continue for weeks, and involve the death of thousands of individuals. In single-piece nesting termites such as the dampwood termite *Zootermopsis nevadensis*, intergroup conflict occurs as a normal part of the life cycle, when multiple pairs found nests in the same log and grow into competing colonies. Colonies that meet each other engage in lethal aggression directed at the reproductive pairs, but after fighting groups commonly fuse into a single functional group (Thorne et al. 2003; Johns et al. 2009).

In the vast majority of social mammals, lethal intergroup conflict is absent or, where it does occur, extremely rare (Boydston et al. 2001; Lazaro-Perea 2001; Rosenbaum et al. 2016; Jordan et al. 2017). Frequent, lethal coalitionary violence, accounting for 10 per cent more of adult deaths, is probably limited to 10 or fewer mammalian species (Wrangham 1999). Social mammals that fall into this category include banded mongooses, in which intergroup interactions account for 10 per cent of total adult mortality where the cause of death is known; for juveniles this figure is 20 per cent (Nichols et al. 2015). In wolves (*Canis lupus*), relations between packs are highly aggressive and intraspecific (intergroup) killing accounts for over 40 per cent of adult deaths (Mech 2003; Cubaynes et al. 2014). In lions, almost all adult deaths are a consequence, directly or indirectly, of intergroup aggression (C. Packer, pers. comm.). In chimpanzees, rates of intergroup (or intercommunity) killing vary widely across populations (Boesch et al. 2008; Wilson et al. 2014), accounting for 17 per cent of adult deaths in one long-term study (Williams et al. 2008). Intergroup warfare by chimpanzees involves patrols and raids which exhibit elements of planning and stealth. In chimps, intergroup killing appears to be an adaptation to outcompete rival groups. By contributing to intergroup attacks an individual can increase its own group's access to territory and resources, particularly mates, increasing the individual's absolute fitness and fitness relative to neighbours (Wrangham 1999; Mitani et al. 2010; Wrangham & Glowacki 2012). In humans, the percentage of adult mortality that is attributable to war is 14 per cent for 14 Late Pleistocene and Early Holocene hunter-gatherers (Bowles 2009) and 18 per cent in 14 contemporary small-scale human societies (Gurven & Kaplan 2007; Bowles 2009).

The last decade has seen revived interest in the idea that intergroup conflict and warfare can exert a strong influence on patterns of cooperation and conflict within groups. In theory, warfare can favour altruism, despite the costs that altruists suffer compared to selfish individuals. This is an idea with a long intellectual pedigree. Darwin (1871) raised the possibility that intergroup competition could generate the selective forces necessary for the spread of self-sacrificing war-like behaviour within groups. He argued that selection at the level of the group would favour groups with a large number of war-like, aggressive individuals, while selection within groups would favour 'selfish, treacherous' individuals over brave, self-sacrificing ones. Hamilton (1975) developed a multilevel selection model of this problem and showed that limited dispersal, by increasing the mean level of relatedness within groups, can promote the spread of an altruistic war-like trait through populations, despite the personal fitness costs. This kind of altruism can spread more easily than helping behaviour because it serves to increase the level of resources or territory to which the group has access, and hence reduces rather than intensifies local competition among relatives. In a sense, this form of altruism 'produces' resources for common use. Choi and Bowles (2007) investigated the potential for warfare to select for altruism using a simulation model of the coevolution of two traits, ingroup helping (or 'altruism') and outgroup aggression (parochialism). Their model suggests a mortality rate of around 4 per cent of the population per generation is sufficient to favour the coevolution of the two traits that make up the syndrome of 'parochial altruism'. This mortality rate is substantially less than estimated mortality rate through warfare calculated from archaeological and ethnographic evidence.

Choi and Bowles (2007) suggest that relatedness plays only a minor role in the evolution of parochial altruism. However, this conclusion was contested by Lehmann and Feldman (2008), who used the infinite island modelling framework to investigate the coevolution of 'bravery' and 'belligerence' (traits which are similar to altruism and parochialism in the Choi & Bowles 2007 model). In this model, intergroup conflict can select for bravery (which increases a group's success in intergroup conflict) and belligerence (which increases the likelihood of attacking other groups) even when relatedness is zero. Nonetheless, selection for both traits is much stronger when there are constraints on dispersal and, consequently, increased relatedness between group members. They conclude that Hamilton (1975) was thus correct in his conjecture that increasing relatedness within groups promotes the development of within-group coalitions and between-group hostility.

How will intergroup conflict affect patterns of within-group conflict? Reeve and Hölldobler (2007) developed a tug-of-war model which includes allocation to both within-group and between-group conflict as a single decision. Thus, this model considers groups of n identical individuals, in a pool of N groups competing for R resources. A single trait t determines what fraction f of an individual's resources should be invested in a selfish within-group tug-of-war over group fitness, with the remaining fraction $(1 - t)$ being used to increase group competitiveness. Unlike Lehmann and Feldman's (2008) model, relatedness within groups is assigned as an external parameter, rather than emerging from the demographic assumptions of the model. In this sense the model is not well suited to disentangle the effects of local relatedness and local competition. However, the Reeve and Hölldobler (2007) model does allow for variation in relatedness between groups; in the infinite island model relatedness between groups is assumed zero by definition. In this model high within-group relatedness (relative to between-group relatedness) reduces internal conflict. Another factor is population structure: internal conflict is reduced when populations consist of large numbers of small competing groups.

Reeve and Hölldobler (2007) predict that intense between-group competition (relative to within-group competition) and high within-group relatedness (relative to between-group relatedness) both act to reduce effort expended on within-group conflict, setting the stage for transitions to 'superorganismality'. In addition, they predict that superorganisms are most likely to evolve in populations which consist of large numbers of small competing groups (large N, small n). It is notable that this prediction runs counter to observations in social insects that the most extreme cooperation occurs in the largest colonies (Bourke 1999, 2011). Reeve and Hölldobler (2007) suggest that this discrepancy can be explained if one assumes that both the number of competiting groups and number of individuals per group increase with patch richness (i.e. amount of resource per group). It would be useful to have more data on the relationship between colony size and number of competing groups in social insect populations to test this assumption.

The models of intergroup conflict described above assume that the n individuals in each group are identical. In reality there may be considerable within-group heterogeneity in strength, quality and the cost of fighting. How does this variation affect the evolution of cooperation? Gavrilets and Fortunato (2014) used economic contest theory to compare contributions to intergroup conflict in egalitarian groups, in which resources are shared equally among all group members, versus hierarchical groups, in which the share of resource obtained depends on social rank. The surprising result is that while hierarchies invest more overall in intergroup conflict than do egalitarian groups, this effort is invested almost exclusively by the strongest individual, which ends up with the smallest share of group direct fitness.

While there are considerable data to support the idea that high-ranked, stronger individuals invest disproportionately in intergroup conflict, these individuals typically gain the highest, not the lowest, share of group fitness as predicted by Gavrilets and Fortunato (2014). An economic conflict model by Garfinkel and Skaperdas (2007) provides a possible explanation for this mismatch between theory and data. In their 'guns and butter' model, individual group members choose between investing in forceful appropriation of group resources ('guns') versus activity that produces group resources ('butter'). In animal and human societies, selfish behaviour aimed at monopolizing reproduction within groups will often trade off against productive, group-beneficial activity, such as hunting for food, keeping watch for predators, or caring for young. Taking this internal trade-off into account, Garfinkel and Skaperdas (2007) find that weaker individuals should specialize in raising group fitness, while stronger individuals should specialize in appropriating it – and end up with a greater share of overall group fitness as a result. Incorporating a trade-off of this kind into Gavrilets and Fortunato's (2014) model may shed new light on the evolution of dominance hierarchies and individual task specialization within animal societies.

One long-standing explanation for why human wars are so destructive is that wars are often waged at the behest of 'exploitative' leaders that do not pay the costs of fighting, or reap a disproportionate share of the benefits. Recently, Johnstone et al. (2020) showed that this type of asymmetry can also explain the evolution of damaging intergroup conflict in animal societies. They extended the classic Maynard Smith's Hawk–Dove model (Maynard Smith 1982a) to consider conflict between groups, in which the decision about whether to fight as a collective is made by a single leader, who enjoys greater benefits or suffers lower costs of fighting. This model demonstrates that leadership of this kind can lead to much more damaging levels of intergroup conflict than would otherwise be possible, to the point where mean population fitness is negative. They then tested the model using long-term data from banded mongooses and showed that females initiate conflicts to obtain outgroup matings, but once fights start it is males that do most of the fighting and suffer almost all of the mortality and injury costs (Figure 3.18). Females lead their group into collective fights and then use the cover of battle to escape their mate guard and mate with extra-group males. The outcome is exceptionally high rates of intergroup aggression, involving mortality costs that are comparable to those seen in the most warlike mammals. Johnstone et al. (2020) suggest that the decoupling of leaders from the costs of warfare can contribute to the evolution of extremely damaging intergroup aggression in both human and non-human animal societies.

3.5.1   Consequences of Intergroup Conflict: Empirical Patterns

Empirical studies of intergroup conflict in non-human animal societies have revealed intriguing variation in the consequences of attack for within-group behaviour. A general hypothesis, linked to but distinct from the evolutionary models described above, is that groups that are exposed to intergroup conflict should become more cohesive or coordinated to increase their resilience to future attack (the 'conflict–

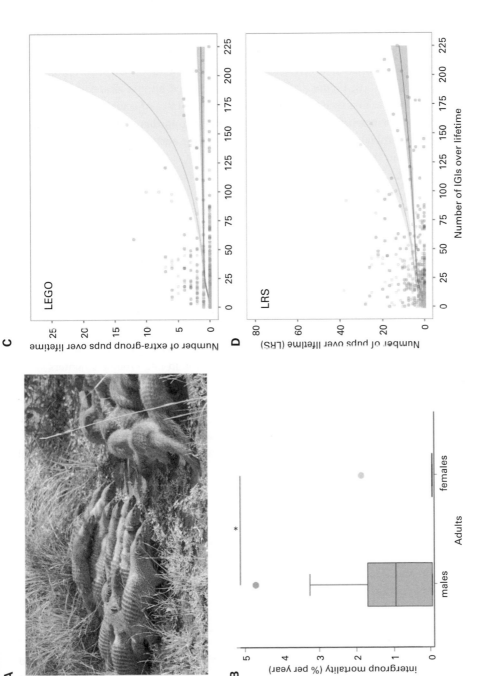

Figure 3.18 Exploitative leadership by females leads to hyperviolent intergroup conflict in banded mongooses. (A) Banded mongoose battle lines during an intergroup interaction or IGI (photo: Dave Seager). (B) Costs of intergroup aggression in male and female banded mongooses. Mortality rate of adult males and females resulting from intergroup aggression. (C) Lifetime reproductive success and intergroup conflict. Lifetime number of extra-group offspring (LEGO; top panel) and lifetime reproductive success (LRS; bottom panel) of males (blue) and females (orange) are plotted against the number of IGIs in which individuals were involved across their lifespan. $N = 499$ males and 367 female adults monitored from birth to death over 20 years. (A black and white version of this figure will appear in some formats. For the colour version, please refer to the plate section.)

cohesion' hypothesis; Radford 2008b; Thompson et al. 2020). In some species, intergroup encounters are followed by increased within-group affiliative behaviour. For example, blue monkeys (*Cercopithecus mitis*) studied in Kenya engage in frequent (every 2–3 days) agonistic territorial encounters with neighbouring groups (Cords 2002). Intergroup fights are often followed by a 'frenzy' of grooming among adult females (who are the main protagonists in intergroup conflicts; Cords 2002). Simulated intrusions by rival groups in green woodhoopoes (Radford 2008a) and cooperative cichlids *N. pulcher* (Bruintjes et al. 2016) result in an immediate increase in within-group affiliative behaviour (preening in the woodhoopoes, or soft 'bumping' behaviour in cichlids; Figure 3.19A). In the dampwood termite *Zootermopsis angusticollis*, exposure to a rival group results in increased rates of social contacts, but not allogrooming or trophallaxis (Thompson et al. 2020). In this system social contacts may serve a 'social surveillance' function, checking identity and helping to assess relative RHP in the face of attack.

In other species, by contrast, intergroup conflict results in increased within-group aggression. In a population of bonnet macaques (*Macaca radiata*) in India, for example, intergroup encounters are followed by increased aggression by males towards female members of their own group (Cooper et al. 2004; Figure 3.19B). This behaviour has been interpreted as 'herding' by males to prevent females leaving the group (Cooper et al. 2004), or as a by-product of elevated stress or anxiety following intergroup fights (Radford et al. 2016). In vervet monkeys studied in South Africa, intergroup encounters result in increased aggression by females towards certain male group members and increased grooming towards other male group members. Males that are aggressed or groomed are more likely to participate in the subsequent bouts of fighting, suggesting that females may use grooming and aggression as social incentives to increase male participation in intergroup encounters (with grooming acting as a 'carrot' and aggression as a 'stick'; Arseneau-Robar et al. 2016).

In a recent human behavioural economic experiment based on the iterated prisoner's dilemma, intergroup conflict increased within-group cooperation where other groups were perceived as an existential threat to the entire group, but it increased within-group selfishness where costs of conflict were perceived to threaten individual pay-offs (Weisel 2016). These empirical patterns suggest that, rather than increasing internal solidarity, intergroup conflict may sometimes exacerbate internal conflicts and provoke coercive behaviour. As reviewed above in the case of dyadic models of conflict between individuals (Section 3.3.2), simple sealed-bid models may underestimate the complexity of outcomes of behavioural conflict between groups. A challenge for future research is to develop models of intergroup conflict that incorporate behavioural responses and are capable of explaining this variety of empirical patterns observed in nature (Thompson & Cant 2018).

3.5.2 Intergroup Cooperation and the Major Transitions

Although much recent research on intergroup conflict in animal societies has focused on conflict between groups, there are circumstances in which the members of distinct

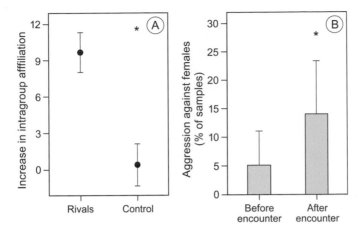

Figure 3.19 Contrasting consequences of intergroup encounters on within-group behaviour. (A) In the cooperative cichlid *N. pulcher*, simulated intrusions by individuals from a rival group were followed by increased affiliative behaviour in the 10 minutes following the intrusion (as measured by soft 'bumping' behaviour; reproduced with permission from Bruintjes et al. 2016). (B) In bonnet macaques, natural encounters between groups were followed by an immediate increase in aggression by males towards females (redrawn with permission from Cooper et al. 2004). *$P < 0.05$. Copyright © 2004, Springer-Verlag.

groups may be selected to tolerate or cooperate with one another rather than to compete. For example, tolerance between groups is expected where intergroup aggression is very costly, or where the intensity of intergroup competition is low (Robinson & Barker 2017). In small-scale human societies, for example, groups regularly engage in trade to exchange goods and services for mutual benefit; archaeological evidence confirms that trade has been a feature of human evolution for thousands of years (Oka & Kusimba 2008). Trade is especially profitable when different groups have access to different resources that each requires, or specialize on different resources or technologies. A second example of intergroup cooperation is observed in polydomous ants, in which a single 'colony' consists of several socially interacting but spatially separated nests, each of which is home to a group of ants (Robinson 2014). Polydomous nesting can confer foraging advantages and allow colonies to exploit widely dispersed resources (Thomas et al. 2006). It can also allow colonies to break out of the ergonomic, physical and group size constraints associated with a single nest (Robinson 2014). The defining feature of polydomy is lack of aggression between nests that are socially connected within the larger polydomous colony. This breakdown of inter-nest conflict is taken to its extreme in unicolonial ants (e.g. invasive populations of the Argentine ant *Linepithema humile*), which form supercolonies of thousands of nests, among which aggression is completely absent (Moffett 2012). Nevertheless, even in the Argentine ant, lethal aggression between supercolonies does occur along contact zones, which correlates with abrupt genetic differentiation between supercolonies (Thomas et al. 2006).

The evolution of intergroup cooperation requires that individuals not only discriminate ingroup from outgroup members, but also make finer distinctions of identity between cooperative and non-cooperative groups. In particular, in both the human and the ant case, individuals behave favourably towards groups that are familiar, but retain hostility or antipathy towards unfamiliar individuals and groups in the wider population. The transition from intergroup conflict to intergroup cooperation can be viewed as an expansion of the perceived ingroup to include a broader range of entities and a broader range of phenotypic identifiers. There are similarities here with the long-standing idea that a biological individual is defined by the presence of some form of immune system, which rejects some entities and accepts others (Medawar 1957; Pradeu 2010), and polices the individual to prevent selfish proliferation by lower-level units (Burnet 1970; Michod 2000; Pradeu 2013). Colonies of social insects can similarly exhibit a social immune system, where individuals act to prevent the spread of pathogens within the colony, for example by rejecting infected individuals, or allogrooming to remove parasites (Cremer et al. 2007; Meunier 2015). The immune system of the social insect colony thus has a hierarchical organization, consisting of own body–other body tissue discrimination within an individual worker or soldier, and own group–other group individual discrimination between colony-mates. It seems likely that the evolution of a hierarchy of discrimination systems may be a key component of the process of group transformation, the final stage of the transition to new levels of biological organization (Figure 3.1).

Research on the evolution of intergroup conflict and cooperation is at an early stage. The problem of cooperation between groups is to some extent a repeat of the problem of cooperation between individuals, which is the focus of the rest of this book. However, it remains to be seen which theoretical mechanisms can be scaled up and applied to explain peace and cooperation between groups. Group interactions differ in critical respects from those between individuals. For example, groups face the problem of identifying members of the ingroup from the outgroup, and groups are by definition heterogeneous compared to individuals. Some group members may refuse to participate in conflict, or may experience different costs and benefits from a fight, whereas this is clearly not the case for the cells of a multicellular individual engaging in a fight with a rival for control of a territory. Understanding how the disunity and heterogeneity of groups is overcome to permit coordinated action, whether collective aggression or collective cooperation, is a particularly promising area for future research (Radford et al. 2016; Christensen & Radford 2018; Thompson & Cant 2018).

3.6   Conclusions

The evolution of animal societies provides an opportunity to explore and test some of the general mechanisms that may underlie major transitions in evolution, and hence the evolution of biological complexity. Evolutionary conflicts arise in these societies whenever the fitness of interacting social partners cannot be maximized simultaneously. Such conflicts of interest arise during the process of group formation. For example, conflict exists over the membership of groups and over the division of the reproductive gains of cooperation. Conflict arises between insiders and outsiders as insiders attempt to preserve the benefits of grouping, leading to aggressive group defence and eviction.

A fundamental source of conflict within animal societies is reproduction. Groups can collectively control and defend disproportionate resources, resulting in strong selection for individuals to monopolize those resources for reproduction. Conflict over reproduction can be reduced via the formation of stable dominance hierarchies, in which higher-ranked individuals attempt to monopolize reproduction. Conflict over social rank explains much of the patterns of low-level social aggression within animal groups. Both males and females compete directly for shares of reproduction using aggression directed at rival breeders or their offspring. Females may also employ subtle means of reproductive competition, for example deterring rival breeders through the threat of infanticide, or upregulating prenatal offspring growth. In cooperatively breeding animal societies, conflict also arises over helping effort, that is, how hard individuals work to rear offspring. There is evidence that this conflict is resolved peacefully through a process of negotiation, and also sometimes through punishment or threats of eviction.

There are diverse theoretical approaches to study the evolution of conflict in cooperative societies; these approaches are reviewed and compared here. A new wave of kin selection models has revealed how population demography and life history can shape social behaviour and life-history strategies. Game-theoretical models examine how conflict strategies of rival parties coevolve and are resolved on evolutionary and behavioural timescales. For example, sealed-bid models provide insight into conflict resolution on an evolutionary timescale, and the conditions that can favour peaceful outcomes despite the potential for conflict. Behavioural models of conflict incorporate the ability to respond in real time to the observed behaviour of a rival. For example, many social interactions occur in sequence, with one player acting or 'moving' first and a second player choosing its optimum response. These sequential models open the door to the use of threats and commitment strategies in competition. Alternative behavioural models examine back-and-forth negotiation, or how animals use social information to resolve conflicts. These varying theoretical approaches offer complementary perspectives to examine and explain observed variation in conflict behaviour.

Synthesizing these theoretical approaches suggests two main pathways by which conflict can be reduced over evolutionary time to facilitate cooperative transitions: kin selection and the repression of competition. Several mechanisms may be involved in the repression of competition. Fitness variance among group members can be minimized through absolute reproductive dictatorship, or absolute reproductive levelling. Competition can also be minimized by evolving non-overlapping reproductive life histories, a life-history equivalent of turn-taking. Finally, intergroup conflict aligns the fitness interests of group members, reducing infighting. Intergroup conflict is emerging as an important research frontier in social evolution. A better understanding of the causes and consequences of intergroup conflict may be particularly important to understanding the final stage of major cooperative transitions, group transformation, during which group-level adaptations and new levels of biological complexity emerge.

Cooperation in the Context of Power, Submission and Subversion

Summary

The European paper wasp *Polistes dominula* has long served as a model social insect system to study the evolution of cooperation and conflict in animal societies. In the early stages of nest founding, groups are composed of females of varying genetic relatedness, all of whom are capable of founding a nest and raising a brood of workers on their own. Yet many females join cooperative groups as subordinate foragers, helping to raise the offspring of a dominant female. Here we describe research on a Spanish population of *Polistes dominula* that helps understanding of how social hiearchies form and why there is so much individual variation in helping behaviour and aggression within groups. Foundresses that join a group as a subordinate helper have a good chance of inheriting the position of breeder if the dominant dies or disappears. They may also gain a share of reproduction before they inherit. The current and future direct fitness benefits of group members explain why unrelated females gain from joining groups as subordinate helpers rather than starting a nest on their own. Foundresses form a strict dominance hierarchy or social queue to inherit breeding status, meaning that the expected future fitness of females varies system- atically with their inheritance rank. Helpers of lower inheritance rank invest the most in costly helping behaviour and reduce their helping effort as they move up through the queue. Helpers higher up the queue engage in frequent social aggression, which may serve to challenge or test the social rank of others. A combination of direct and indirect fitness can explain why individuals join cooperative teams in this species. Individual variation in cooperative and aggressive behaviour within groups is explained by variation in future direct fitness benefits, not variation in genetic relatedness. Future research to understand how individuals perceive their rank and remember their interactions with groupmates may offer general insights into the evolution of hierarchical societies.

Introduction

Wasps of the genus *Polistes* are a type of paper wasp (subfamily Polistinae) that is widely distributed and common in both temperate and tropic regions. Most of the approximately 200 species of *Polistes* live and reproduce in paper nests built from wood pulp and plant fibre, suspended from the underside of leaves, stems, crevices or other substrates in the environ- ment. In temperate regions, overwintered found- resses of the European paper wasp *Polistes dominula* start building new nests in early spring, either singly or in small groups of 2–8 foundresses. The first batch of female workers emerges two months after nest founding and helps to expand the nest and provision offspring. Across summer the next generation of reproductive males and females are produced, and existing workers and the original foundresses die off. Males die shortly after mating, while inseminated females overwinter in hiberna- cula before starting a new nesting cycle the following spring.

The species *P. dominula* has a long history as a focus for research on the evolution of social behaviour. In the early 1940s Leo Pardi from the University of Pisa published a series of papers describing the presence of a dominance hiearchy among foundresses of *P. dominula* (*née P. dominulus*, *P. gallicus*). The idea that insects could exhibit social hierarchies similar to those reported in vertebrates was criticised as an anthropomorphic fallacy (by fellow entomologist Deleurance 1950; quoted in Caniglia 2015). For Pardi, however, his findings served to highlight the underlying similarity between vertebrate and insect social systems. He saw no intrinsic difference between the dominance hierarchies observed in paper wasps and those observed in birds (Schjelderup-Ebbe 1935) or primates (Maslow 1936). Nevertheless, Pardi was so discouraged by the attacks on his work that he gave up working on wasps for 20 years.

Since these first studies, *Polistes* wasps have become a model system to investigate both social conflict and cooperation in animal societies (Turillazzi & West-Eberhard 1996; Jandt et al. 2014). *Polistes dominula* has been the subject of long-running research at several sites, including Tuscany, Italy (Beani & Turillazi 1988; Branconi et al. 2018), north-eastern USA (Ithaca, NY and Ann Arbor, MI; Reeve et al. 1998b; Sheehan & Tibbetts 2011; Tibbets et al. 2019) and southern Spain (Cant & Field 2001; Grinsted & Field 2018). Like many vertebrate cooperative breeders, foundress associations of paper wasps are composed of individuals of varying relatedness (typically full sisters, cousins, and unrelated individuals; Queller et al. 2000; Zanette & Field 2008), all of which are mated and capable of nesting independently. They show conspicuous forms of aggression, with dominant individuals chasing, mounting and occasionally biting their subordinates (Cant et al. 2006a). There are also more escalated fights that last for several minutes and can involve the use of lethal stings (Reeve 1991). However, there is also very clear helping behaviour: subordinate foundresses hunt for caterpillars and other insect food to provision the offspring of the dominant female. Foraging foundresses expose themselves to predation by invertebrate and vertebrate predators, so the question arises as to why foundresses risk their lives to help another female to breed when they are perfectly capable of breeding themselves. On a practical level, a major attraction of paper wasps for students of social evolution is their tractability. *Polistes* species build open 'carton' nests in which the behaviour of adults and their offspring is clearly visible and can be readily videoed. Group members can be easily captured, individually marked with enamel paint, temporarily removed and then replaced, and even hand-fed with tweezers (Donaldson et al. 2013).

In southern Spain, *P. dominula* was very common until recently. Foundresses frequently built their nests on *Opuntia* cactus, which was planted in dense hedges around pastures and meadows (Figure C.1). Ten years ago it was common to find 100 or even 200 nests on a single stretch of *Opuntia*. In recent years, however, *Opuntia* hedgerows at the site have been obliterated by mealybugs (*Dactylopus ceylonicus*), a biocontrol agent. Nevertheless, *Opuntia* sites dense with *P. dominula* nests are still found further inland.

Nest Founding and Cooperation

In these Spanish populations around 20 per cent of nests are initiated by single foundresses who work alone until the first batch of workers emerges, two months later. These 'solitary' foundresses nest side by side with 'cooperative' foundresses, who build their nest as a team in groups ranging from 2 to 20 foundresses (median 6; Zanette & Field 2011). Nests founded and tended by a single foundress are more likely to fail in the founding period than those tended by multiple foundresses (failure rate within first 10 days of discovery = 63 per cent and 50 per cent for single versus multiple foundress nests, respectively; Zanette & Field 2011). Solitary foundresses must leave the nest unattended to forage, and predation of the foundress results in failure of the nest. In cooperative associations, by contrast, a single dominant foundress remains on the nest while other foundresses leave to forage. Among cooperative associations, nest failure rates do not differ for groups of two to five foundresses, suggesting that a division of labour in foraging roles explains the elevated nest survival of multiple foundress groups. Why some foundresses choose to nest alone is still unclear: one possibility is that females initiate a nest in the expectation of joiners that never appear (Seppä et al. 2012).

Around 20 per cent of subordinate foundresses are unrelated to the dominant female or to any other

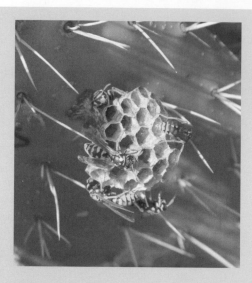

Figure C.1 A founding phase *P. dominula* nest suspended from an *Opuntia* cactus leaf at Conil de la Frontera, Spain. Six foundresses are visible on the nest. The first offspring have reached the pupal stage, visible toward the top of the nest, and will soon emerge as workers to help raise a younger brood. © Michael Cant. (A black and white version of this figure will appear in some formats. For the colour version, please refer to the plate section.)

foundress in the group. What do these females have to gain from joining unrelated individuals, and helping to rear their young? Leadbeater et al. (2011) showed that unrelated subordinate found-resses actually gain considerable direct fitness benefits from group membership and can expect to produce more direct offspring than lone breeders. Most of a subordinate's direct fitness arises because she stands to inherit the position of breeder if the dominant dies or disappears. Direct fitness benefits can explain why these females join groups and work to ensure the nest survives and has a large and productive complement of workers (Leadbeater et al. 2011). Similar future direct fitness benefits of helping explain patterns of helping across species of cooperatively breeding birds (Kingma 2017).

Individual Variation in Helping and Aggression

In most cooperatively breeding animal societies, there is considerable individual variation in patterns of helping and aggressive behaviour. In *P. dominula*

there is a single 'dominant' female on each nest, who rarely leaves the nest and is more aggressive than the other foundresses. Nearly all the foraging for food to feed larvae is done by subordinate found-resses. However, there is much individual variation in individual work rate: some subordinate found-resses spend nearly all the day foraging, returning to the nest only briefly to deliver food, whereas other members of the same group do little foraging and spend a large part of their time sitting on the nest. What could cause this great variation in helping effort among individuals of the same sex and age?

The answer lies in the fact that dominant females quite frequently die during the founding phase, and their position is inherited by one of her subordinates. Subordinate foundresses form a strict hierarchy to inherit the breeding position, which means that the expected future fitness of subordinates varies sys-tematically with social rank. A simple game-theoretical model predicts how this variation in future fitness should affect the optimal helping effort for a subordinate. The model predicts that

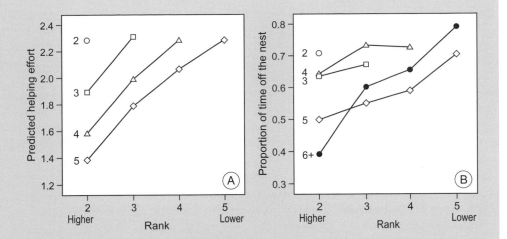

Figure C.2 Individual variation in helping effort and inheritance rank. (A) Predictions of a game-theoretical model of helping effort for individuals at different positions in a social queue, assuming that effort invested in helping reduces survival and hence the probability of surviving to reach the rank 1 position. Numbers along the left of lines indicate group size. Helping effort is predicted to increase down the queue and decline with increasing group size. Results shown assume that subordinate helping effort is controlled by the dominant foundress; a model assuming subordinates control their own helping effort produces qualitatively identical results. (B) Observed proportion of time spent off the nest (presumed foraging) for individuals of different inheritance rank in groups of different sizes. After measuring helping effort, individual inheritance rank was revealed by successively removing wasps to allow the next in line to inherit. Redrawn with permission from Cant and Field (2001). © The Royal Society.

individuals with little chance of inheriting breeding status should work harder than those individuals next in line to inherit; and that helping effort should be lower in larger groups (because inheriting a large group represents a more valuable future 'prize'). These predictions hold whether one assumes that helping effort is under the control of the subordinate themselves, or is controlled by the dominant (Cant & Field 2001).

To test these predictions, Cant and Field (2001) measured helping effort of all wasps in each group and then removed group members, starting with the dominant, to reveal the order in which they inherited dominant status. The results of this experiment are shown in Figure C.2B. As the model predicts, wasps that were higher up in the queue to inherit dominant status, and those in larger, more valuable groups, worked less hard to rear the dominant's offspring. A few years later, Field et al. (2006) tested the predicted effect of rank and group size experimentally using the Malaysian hover wasp *Liostenogaster flaveolina*. In this species groups reproduce year-round, and within groups there is a strict, age-based queue (Field et al. 2006). Experimental manipulation of rank and group size suggests that both have causal effects on helping effort in hover wasps, in the manner predicted by the model.

Given that future fitness (in the form of inheritance rank) has such a strong impact on helping effort, how might it affect patterns of conflict? Should individuals that are high up in the queue to inherit be more or less aggressive to their immediate dominant than individuals lower down the queue? How aggressive should individuals of different rank be towards their subordinates? To address these questions, Cant et al. (2006a) developed simple models to examine how the pay-off of challenging for superior rank, or defending one's own rank against a challenger, varies down a social queue. They tested the predictions of these models by videoing aggressive behaviour and then sequentially removing wasps to reveal their inheritance rank. As predicted, both 'upward' aggression (directed at the wasp one rank above) and 'downward' aggression (directed at the wasp one rank below) declined down the social queue (Cant et al. 2006a; Figure 3.5).

Aggression as a Deterrent Signal

These studies suggest that wasps 'know' their inheritance rank, before any vacancy appears, and adjust their helping effort and aggression level to maximize their inclusive fitness. Helpers at the bottom of the queue to inherit work harder and are docile; high-ranking helpers are both lazy and aggressive. Research by Thompson et al. (2014) suggests that a dominant must repeatedly aggress the rank 2 female on her nest to deter that female from challenging her position. Thompson et al. induced contests of social rank by removing the rank 1 individual, keeping her in a refrigerator for a few days, and then releasing her back to the nest. In around half of cases the result was an escalated fight between the original dominant and the rank 2, who had newly inherited the rank 1 position. Thompson et al. (2014) showed that letting rank 1s and rank 2s interact midway through the removal period greatly reduced the probability of escalated fighting when the rank 1 was finally released back to the nest, as expected if social interaction serves to refresh memories about each other's strength or motivation to fight (Thompson et al. 2014). Somewhat counter-intuitively, therefore, repeated acts of social aggression appear to stabilize the hierarchy and keep the peace in groups of paper wasps. In the language of threats (Section 3.3), social aggression serves to establish the credibility of a dominant female's threat to escalate to a full-blown (and potentially lethal) fight to defend her position.

In the *P. dominula* system, variation in genetic relatedness does not explain individual variation in social behaviour. Unrelated foundresses do not work less hard, nor are they more aggressive than full sisters of the dominant (Leadbeater et al. 2010, 2011). While the closely related *P. fuscatus* is

renowned for its ability to recognize individuals on the basis of facial patterns (Sheehan & Tibbetts 2010; Tibbetts & Sheehan 2013), in *P. dominula* there is little evidence that foundresses recognize individuals, at least of non-nestmates (Sheehan & Tibbets 2011; see below), or to discriminate degrees of relatedness among nestmates (Leadbeater et al. 2010). They do, however, discriminate inheritance ranks well and target individuals of adjacent rank for aggression. Variation among individuals in future direct fitness, not variation in genetic relatedness, explains why social behaviour varies so much between group members in this system.

Towards New Frontiers

Social behaviour in the *Polistes* system appears to be determined in large part by each individual's perception of its future fitness opportunities, which is determined by its social rank. The stability of social hierarchies depends on cognitive processes such as memory of previous interactions, recognition of individual identity or social rank, and even logical inference of the social rank of others (Tibbetts et al. 2019). There are intriguing differences in these attributes between *Polistes* species that are otherwise similar in social behaviour. Research by Elizabeth Tibbets, Michael Sheehan and colleagues has shown that foundresses of *P. fuscatus* exhibit strong individual recognition compared to *P. dominula*, despite both species exhibiting very similar social systems (Sheehan & Tibbetts 2011). *P. fuscatus* also exhibits much more variation in facial colour patterns, suggesting that facial recognition has coevolved with facial variation in this species. In these experiments, *P. dominula* foundresses showed no individual recognition in trials conducted using unfamiliar foundresses over two subsequent days. However, the observation that, within natural foundress associations, social rank has such a strong impact on social behaviour suggests that there may nevertheless be clear individual recognition of familiar nestmates in *P. dominula*. The finding that subordinate foundresses spend most of their time being aggressive to those individuals that are above and below themselves in the inheritance queue suggests that *P. dominula* may recognize individual nestmates with whom they interact repeatedly, or at least discriminate their social rank. Further research might help to test the capacity and limits of individual recognition among nestmates of *P. dominula*.

Unlike *P. fuscatus*, *P. dominula* foundresses have conspicuous and highly variable clypeal marks on the face. In a USA population there is experimental evidence that these marks function as an honest badge of status or fighting ability which helps to resolve conflict without recourse to escalated aggression (Tibbetts & Dale 2004). However, two studies on the Italian population (Cervo et al. 2008; Branconi et al. 2018) failed to find any evidence that clypeal patterning functions as a badge of status. One explanation for this discrepancy is that the USA populations are invasive, while the Italian population is native. The honesty and meaning of a badge-of-status signal may vary over time and with ecological conditions that affect the expression and frequency of the signal. In the USA around 85 per cent of wasps possess a clypeal mark, whereas the equivalent figure in Italy is 40 per cent, and only 20 per cent in the Spanish population. Moreover, there is evidence that temperature during development and exposure to parasites affect the amount and patterning of black pigmentation on the clypeus (Tibbetts et al. 2011). To add further intrigue to this story, preliminary results from the Spanish population suggest that dominant foundresses with a clear clypeal mark may be less aggressive to their subordinates, as expected if the mark does function as a non-cryptic indicator of fighting ability.

Where an opponent's strength varies over time, it may pay to update any memory of fighting ability derived from a previous encounter by testing them

or provoking them into a display. Patterns of aggression within stable groups of animals may therefore be intimately linked to the durability of memories of individual strength or identity (Thompson et al. 2014). While dyadic animal contest theory has illuminated the ways in which animals assess each other's strength and avoid damaging conflict (Section 3.3), these models often focus on single encounters between rivals rather than the repeated sequences of affiliative and competitive interactions that characterize the relationships of social animals. In *P. fuscatus*, social memories of individual identity appear to last up to a week (Sheehan & Tibbets 2008). In *P. dominula*, there is evidence that a subordinate's memories of her dominant appear to deteriorate over time (Thompson et al. 2014), but it is not clear what aspects or attributes of identity are being remembered or forgotten. The tractability of *Polistes* to new experimental approaches and manipulations may make them a future model system for exploration of the coevolution of cognition and sociality. For example, the potential for micro-CT scanning of wasp brains opens up the possibility to explore the coevolution and development of brain architecture and social behaviour. Recent experiments using classic methods from psychology have revealed transitive inference in *P. dominula*, which may help individuals to navigate the hierarchical society in which these animals live (Tibbets et al. 2019). Seventy years after Pardi's work on social dominance was attacked as an anthropomorphic fallacy (Caniglia 2015), research on *Polistes* continues to offer insights that transcend taxonomic boundaries to reveal general rules about the evolution of life in hierarchical societies.

4   Cooperation

In the previous chapters we have discussed how to succeed in obtaining resources by attempting to be quicker (*race*) or stronger (*fight*) than competitors. The third principle tactic to cope with competition for resources is to *share* them, which involves conceding a quota to competitors. This may prove to be a better choice than either *racing* or *fighting*, particularly if these tactics are too costly or unprofitable because of limited competitiveness, or due to concordance of fitness interests (Frank 2003; Taborsky et al. 2016). Sharing can also be favoured if coordinating or cooperating with other individuals increases the value of a resource, or helps to produce resources (Clark & Mangel 1986; Garfinkel & Skaperdas 2007; e.g. in cooperative hunting: Packer & Ruttan 1988; Dumke et al. 2018). Cooperation often guarantees the most efficient use of resources, because of synergistic effects (Maynard Smith 1982b; Queller 1985; Hauert et al. 2006; Gore et al. 2009; Cornforth et al. 2012; Van Cleve & Akcay 2014; Corning & Szathmary 2015). For instance, if several individuals coordinate to capture a prey that is normally difficult or risky to hunt on their own, each individual predator may gain more food at lower cost. Similarly, raising offspring in a group may allow individuals to specialize in different tasks, such as tending young, warding off predators and supplying resources, which enhances the efficiency of offspring care. Nevertheless, it is important to note that evolutionarily stable cooperative relationships generally can develop only when one of two conditions applies:

- **Cooperation for fitness benefits**. Evolutionarily stable cooperation can arise if unilateral exploitation can be avoided and either in the short or long term *all* involved partners obtain a net fitness benefit from their cooperation. In other words, the fitness benefit of a participant's action (B) outweighs its cost (C) (B/C > 1). There is a concordance of interests between the involved parties, such as in parent–offspring relationships, although there may still be conflict over the net pay-off obtained by each (Frank 1998; Taborsky et al. 2016).
- **Forced cooperation.** In this case one partner can exploit the other, surreptitiously or by coercion. What may look like 'cooperation' is, evolutionarily speaking, exploitation of one by the other, i.e. social parasitism. In that case there is no concordance of interests between the involved parties (Barnard 1984).

In this chapter we discuss the mechanisms underlying the evolution of cooperation (see Box 1.1 for definition). Based on the classification of Lehmann and Keller

(2006a) we demonstrate how these mechanisms fall into one of four distinct categories (Figure 4.2). Cooperation may provide immediate or delayed fitness benefits to the actor because the action itself is beneficial to the agent ((i) by-product mutualism), or the pay-offs are correlated either by conditional returns ((ii) reciprocity) or shared genes ((iii) relatedness, genetic correlations); finally, cooperative behaviour may be a product of manipulation of the actor by the receiver ((iv) coercion, trickery). Many attempts have been made to subcategorize these four inherently simple mechanisms (e.g. Connor 1986, 1995a; Bergmüller et al. 2007; West et al. 2007a), which in our view has caused confusion rather than clarification. Therefore, our strategy is to elucidate the underlying principles without differentiating all possible variants and categorizing them with idiosyncratic terms. We feel that this will throw light upon the jungle of social semantics (Taborsky 2007).

4.1   Cooperation for Fitness Benefits

Let's assume that helpful behaviour raises the indirect fitness of the donor, which is possible if receiver and donor are genetically related. Parental behaviour is a classic example where some individuals (parents) help others (offspring) to obtain resources such as food and shelter. Despite an apparent immediate negative cost/benefit balance of the behaviour to parents, the propensity for parents to care for their offspring can spread through the population because it benefits the latter and, as long as it has a genetic basis, it will be inherited by them. This possibility was first modelled in detail by William D. Hamilton (1963, 1964), a pre-eminent evolutionary biologist who was particularly interested in the fitness consequences of social interactions. In principle, interactions among two players can produce four different outcomes (Figure 4.1): benefits may accrue to both, one or the other, or neither of them. Subsequent research has focused mainly on the lower left square of Hamilton's scheme, where one individual pays a cost by helping another one to the latter's benefit. Such 'altruism' (see Box 1.1 for definition) can evolve if donor and receiver are related, or in other words, share genes by common descent. This mechanism for the evolution of altruism, termed 'kin selection' (i.e. the evolution of characteristics which favour the survival and/or reproduction of relatives of the affected individual; Maynard Smith 1964) has subsequently received most interest; however, Hamilton himself expressed some doubts that kin selection was the primary explanation for variation in altruism in natural populations. In the *Narrow Roads of Gene Land* (1996) he wrote:

I do believe in the existence of considerable genetical differences in altruism, in selfishness, and in many other social attributes in most social animals, and this includes in humans, but this belief is certainly not predicated directly from kin-selection theory. Rather, it is underpinned more by a belief in a complexity of life sufficient to generate genetical variability in almost everything – the variability we actually see – and also ... by modern theoretical expectations connected with reciprocation and with disease selection. It certainly does not come from kin selection *per se*. (pp. 19–20)

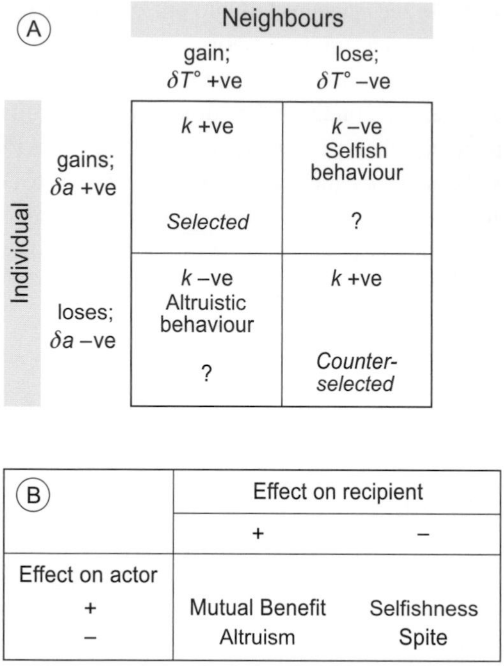

Figure 4.1 (A) Hamilton's 1964 classification of social interactions and their potential fitness consequences. Symbols: δa +ve = action beneficial to individual fitness; δa −ve = action detrimental to individual fitness; $\delta T°$ +ve = total (positive) effect on neighbours' genes; $\delta T°$ −ve = total (negative) effect on neighbours' genes; k = ratio scaling the fitness gains and losses for individuals versus neighbours. (B) Simplified version of Hamilton's (1964) classification scheme as proposed in West et al. (2007a). Drawn by the authors.

Kin selection has caused intense and often heated debate about the most appropriate way to calculate fitness or imagine its maximization (Nowak et al. 2010a; Abbot et al. 2011; Bourke 2011; Allen et al. 2013; Birch & Okasha 2015; Liao et al. 2015). An unfortunate consequence is that other selection mechanisms that can generate and stabilize cooperation in natural populations, such as mutualism, reciprocity and enforcement, have taken a back seat. We shall attempt in this chapter to balance this out by dealing with each of them in sufficient detail.

The evolution of cooperation in situations lacking unilateral exploitation can be explained in two principal ways: by-product benefits and correlated pay-offs (Figure 4.2; see Box 1.1 for definitions). Either the behaviour itself benefits each actor, implying that it is not selected because of benefits accrued to the partner (see Section 4.1.1 By-product benefits or mutualism), or each partner's behaviour is selected to benefit the other (see Section 4.1.2 Correlated pay-offs). We will discuss these two possibilities in the subsequent sections of this chapter (Section 4.1.1 and Section 4.1.2). In addition, cooperative behaviour may be favoured by group selection (Wade 1977; Craig 1982), where natural selection favours individuals in groups with a

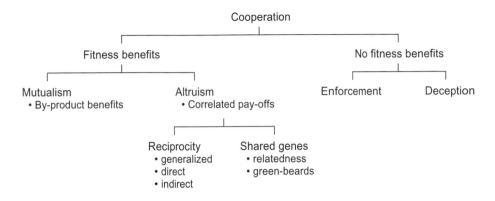

Figure 4.2 Conceptual scheme of the selection mechanisms underlying cooperation.

higher frequency of cooperators (D.S. Wilson 1975; Wade 1976; Mesterton-Gibbons & Dugatkin 1992; Sober & Wilson 1998; Okasha 2005). A prerequisite for this mechanism to work is differential productivity of trait groups (i.e. a collection of individuals sharing common properties; D.S. Wilson 1975) independent of differences in fitness-relevant traits of their members, such as the degree of cooperativeness. Because theory suggests that the evolution of cooperation via group selection occurs only in certain, restricted conditions (for example, where within-group competition is less important than between-group competition, and dispersal between groups occurs within narrow bounds; Kümmerli et al. 2009a; Gardner & Grafen 2009; Böttcher & Nagler 2016), the evolution of altruism and cooperation by trait group selection is probably rare (Williams 1966; Gadgil 1975) and its importance in nature is unclear (Goodnight & Stevens 1997). If relatedness, i.e. the sharing of genes by common descent, correlates well with the structuring of populations into groups, which is usually the case, group selection may become virtually indistinguishable from kin selection (Lehmann et al. 2007; Marshall 2011; Lehtonen 2016; see Okasha 2006, 2016 and Goodnight 2013b for discussions of the complementarity of multilevel selection and kin selection approaches to the study of social behaviour). The latter will be dealt with in Section 4.1.2.2.

4.1.1   By-product Benefits or Mutualism

In evolutionary biology, a mutualistic interaction based on by-product benefits classifies a behaviour or trait that increases the inclusive fitness of each party. By definition, the behaviour or trait *by itself* has beneficial fitness effects to the provider, irrespective of the behaviour or trait of the interaction partner. This distinguishes by-product mutualism from the concept of altruism, where an individual benefitting an interaction partner bears fitness costs by its behaviour or trait. A mutualistic behaviour selected through by-product benefits yields beneficial effects to the direct fitness of the actor. Because of such 'selfish benefits', it cannot be cheated. For this reason, this type of cooperation has been referred to also as 'by-product mutualism', 'by-product effects', 'by-product beneficence' or 'pseudoreciprocity' (Brown 1983; Connor 1986, 1995a; Mesterton-Gibbons & Dugatkin 1992; Dugatkin 1997, 2002; Bergmüller et al. 2007; Leimar & Hammerstein 2010). Mutual fitness benefits can depend on social conditions such as group size, which may select for cooperative behaviour of group members serving to enhance group size (group augmentation generating mutual or 'passive' benefits, i.e. survival benefits resulting merely from the presence of additional group members and not from their behaviour; Kokko et al. 2001; Kingma et al. 2014; see Box 4.1).

Box 4.1 Mutual Fitness Benefits by Group Augmentation

Group members may gain inclusive fitness benefits by helping to augment their group. For instance, a larger number of individuals may result in greater safety from predators, or enhance each individual's competitive advantage against (members of) other groups (Kokko et al. 2001; Garay 2009). These individual benefits can compensate for or outweigh the costs of raising the offspring of others. The benefits of group augmentation may accrue in the short or long term (Kingma et al. 2014).

Immediate benefits of group augmentation: Helpers raising the offspring of others may benefit from a greater chance of survival during their coexistence with these additional recruits in the group. Such benefits may result merely from increased group size (e.g. dilution effects or safety-in-numbers), which can also reduce the risk of group extinction (Courchamp et al. 1999). For example, in cooperatively breeding cichlids (*Neolamprologus pulcher*), where 34 per cent of groups went extinct between subsequent years, large groups survived better and reproduced more successfully than small groups (Heg et al. 2005a), suggesting positive density dependence or Allee effects (Allee 1951). Group augmentation benefits can also ensue from the performance of mutually beneficial behaviours such as shared vigilance, joint territory defence, or social thermoregulation. In dwarf mongoose (*Helogale parvula*) family groups, for instance, subordinate males are the primary sentinels guarding the group (Rasa 1989). The vigilance efficiency against ground predators is 100 per cent when guards are present, but the vigilance system becomes inefficient when too few subordinate guards are present. Mortality by predation is the major cause of reduced reproductive success in this species, and the number of young surviving is positively correlated with group size. In cooperatively breeding green woodhoopoe (*Phoeniculus purpureus*) night-time energy expenditure of individuals can be reduced by 30 per cent or more, dependent on ambient temperature, through communal roosting among group members (Du Plessis & Williams 1994). Group augmentation benefits may be associated also with reciprocal cooperation between helpers and recruits (e.g. allogrooming, sharing of food). In cooperatively breeding African wild dogs, hunting success increases with the number of group members, and per capita food intake per spent hunting effort peaks at the modal group size in nature (Creel & Creel 1995).

Delayed benefits of group augmentation: Former helpers that raised the offspring of others may benefit from the presence or action of their recruits if the latter help the previous helpers in reproduction, or enhance their survival chances

Box 4.1 (*cont.*)

(Ligon & Ligon 1978, 1983; Ligon 1983; Wiley & Rabenold 1984). This can occur when a former helper has ascended to breeder status either in its resident territory or after dispersing together with its recruits to breed somewhere else. As with short-term group augmentation gains, these beneficial effects may result merely from the presence of additional group members, or from beneficial behaviours of recruits towards the former helper (delayed reciprocity). Cooperatively breeding meerkats (*Suricata suricatta*), for example, rely heavily on communal vigilance and auditory warning against danger (le Roux et al. 2009). Reproducing

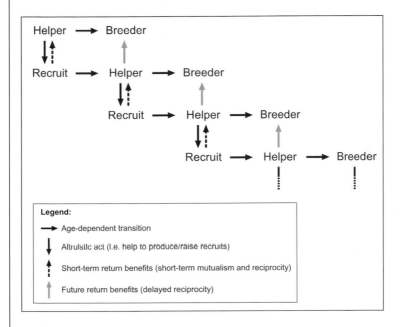

Figure 4.3 The cascading effect of immediate (or 'short-term') and delayed (or 'long-term') reciprocity between helpers and their recruits, where helpers enhance the production of recruits, which in turn become helpers after transition of their former helpers to breeder status (from Kingma et al. 2014). Copyright © 2014 Elsevier Ltd. All rights reserved.

subordinate females that have previously helped to raise offspring of the dominant can hence benefit from the enhanced group size by improved survival prospects for themselves and their offspring (Clutton-Brock et al. 1999). In stripe-backed wrens (*Campylorhynchus nuchalis*), dominants' offspring raised by former helpers become their helpers in turn when the latter take over the dominant breeding role (Wiley & Rabenold 1984), and subordinate group members in white-winged choughs kidnap and raise young from neighbouring groups apparently to receive subsequent help from them when raising own offspring (Heinsohn 1991). A comparative analysis including 20 cooperatively breeding bird species revealed that the sex that is more likely to later breed in its natal group invests more in

Box 4.1 (*cont.*)

helping, suggesting that helping in family groups may be partly shaped by future expectations of delayed reciprocity (Downing et al. 2018). This was corroborated also by Kingma (2017), who showed that in cooperatively breeding bird species where the prospects of territory inheritance are larger, subordinates provide more help, which is not preferentially directed toward relatives.

The potential immediate and delayed effects of group augmentation to helpers are depicted schematically in Figure 4.3.

A familiar example of mutualistic interaction is group hunting, where individuals join forces to detect, overcome, seize or defend prey against competitors to their mutual benefit (Packer & Ruttan 1988). Cooperative hunting is shown by many animals ranging from ants (Franks 1986; Duncan & Crewe 1994; Witte et al. 2010) and spiders (Ward & Enders 1985; Whitehouse & Lubin 2005) to fish (Partridge et al. 1983; Handegard et al. 2012; Herbert-Read et al. 2016), birds (Hector 1986; Bednarz 1988; McMahon & Evans 1992) and mammals (e.g. bats: Barak & Yomtov 1989; Dechmann et al. 2010; lions: Scheel & Packer 1991; Stander 1992; hyenas: Kruuk 1972; Drea & Carter 2009; wild dogs: Creel & Creel 1995; Rasmussen et al. 2008; dolphins: Gazda et al. 2005; Benoit-Bird & Whitlow 2009; chimpanzees: Boesch 1994, 2002; humans: Alvard & Nolin 2002; Bird et al. 2012). It is important to note, however, that an observation of cooperative hunting does not imply a mutualistic relationship per se (Bird et al. 2012).

The crucial characteristic of mutualistic interactions is that the (behavioural) trait produced by an actor has itself positive fitness effects. These are usually enhanced by the partner(s) in the mutualistic interaction, but these positive fitness returns are not required for the trait to evolve due to its inherent positive benefit–cost balance. American white pelicans, for instance, often forage in groups and synchronize their bill dipping, which serves to herd prey (McMahon & Evans 1992). Capture rates and prey size are highest for individuals hunting in a coordinated fashion in a group, thereby benefitting each participant. This means that cooperation based on mutualism cannot be cheated – the trait itself is positively selected, even without return from others. This is in sharp contrast to interactions based on reciprocity, which will be outlined in detail below. The key difference between these two concepts is that one is not cheatable (mutualism) whereas the other one is (reciprocity) (Clutton-Brock 2009). Traditionally, this important distinction has not always been made (e.g. West-Eberhard 1975; Connor 1995a), possibly causing some confusion (Box 4.2).

Box 4.2 Mutualism, By-product Mutualism and 'Pseudoreciprocity': What is the Difference?

In this book we prefer to use the term 'by-product mutualism' (Brown 1983) instead of the simpler term 'mutualism', because it stresses the fact that the behaviour or trait by itself has positive fitness effects to the actor (Connor 1995a; Dugatkin 2002; Bergmüller et al. 2007). The original definition (Brown 1983) states: 'In *by-product*

Box 4.2 (*cont.*)

mutualism, each animal must perform a necessary minimum for itself that may benefit another individual as a by-product. These are typically behaviors that a solitary animal must do regardless of the presence or behavior of others, such as hunting for food.' This describes the basic concept of mutualistic behaviours in evolutionary terms, as outlined above; therefore, strictly speaking the addendum 'by-product' is redundant (i.e. a pleonasm). Nevertheless, as the term 'mutualism' (lacking the attribute 'by-product') often causes misunderstanding due to its slightly different and generally broader meaning in ecology, we add 'by-product' to 'mutualism' in order to underline that we here deal with the evolutionary denotation of the term instead of the ecological one.

It has been proposed that a distinction should be made between 'by-product mutualism' and 'pseudoreciprocity' on the assumption that the latter involves investment of an actor generating a benefit to a recipient, which in turn benefits the actor as a by-product [e.g. birds calling in conspecifics to feed with them on swarming insects, which benefits both the responders (as they are guided to a food patch) and actors (as they may benefit from safety in numbers and more easily track the insect swarm when conspecifics participate in the hunt); Brown et al. 1991; cf. Connor 1986, 1995a; Bergmüller et al. 2007]. In this case, the behaviour (e.g. calling) might appear to be costly without immediate benefit to the actor. We think this type of interaction can be easily subsumed in the general category (by-product) 'mutualism' on the following grounds:

(1) Most importantly, the behaviour or trait by itself has beneficial fitness effects to the actor as outlined above, hence it is uncheatable; in our bird example, calling in conspecifics directly generates the benefit of group hunting. If it is not successful, i.e. no conspecifics will join the hunt, the behaviour (calling) does entail net costs, i.e. energy expenditure and potential risk due to eavesdropping predators, but this is also the case with other unsuccessful selfish behaviours (e.g. a failed prey-catching attempt, which would still fall under 'foraging'). Any investment in augmenting group size may fall in this category (Kingma et al. 2014).

(2) The term pseudoreciprocity has been coined for a form of by-product mutualism induced by a selfish act of the beneficiary of the by-product (Connor 1986). This is a central characteristic of mutualism, not an aberration. *A* creates a benefit for *B*, which consequently and *inevitably* produces something benefitting *A*. Similar relationships hold, for instance, for classical examples of mutualism, such as mycorrhiza, lichens, pollination, ungulate digestive symbiosis and coral–zooxanthellae endosymbiosis (Boucher 1985; Bronstein 1994; Bronstein et al. 2006). Flowering plants produce pollen for the purpose of fertilization, which is collected and used for food by animal pollinators. The latter benefit themselves from visiting different flowers as thereby they are collecting food, but at the same time, as a by-product they provide benefits to the plant by implementing fertilization for them. This is functionally similar to the bird/food-calling example above. Other renowned examples of interspecific mutualism include, for instance, insects tending fungi in order to benefit from the harvest thereby produced (Mueller et al.

Box 4.2 (*cont.*)

1998; Biedermann & Taborsky 2011), which bear net costs from the fungus care, but thereby generate a beneficial resource (Mueller et al. 2005), just like a territorial algae feeder does by defending its algal mat (Ferreira et al. 1998; Iguchi & Abe 2002; Peyton et al. 2014), or a squirrel by hoarding food (Winterrowd & Weigl 2006; Delgado et al. 2014). The defence of algae or the caching of food is costly, but the benefits thereby created (sustained food availability for the fish and the squirrel, respectively) are an integral part of the act, just like in fungus agriculture. At the same time, the algae benefit from the exploitation protection by the territorial fish and the nut tree from the distribution of its seeds by the squirrel. We discourage the use of different terms for the same phenomenon, or for phenomena with similar underlying functionality, by different disciplines (i.e. in ecology: 'mutualism'; in ethology: 'pseudoreciprocity').

(3) Lastly, in reality it will often be difficult to identify the immediacy of the benefit of an action or trait, and whether a mutualism is based on 'by-product benefits' from both sides or a 'pseudoreciprocal' action involving investment from partner A that benefits partner B, with the latter generating a benefit to A in return but without paying a cost (Connor 1986). We generally propose to use operational terms to describe a phenomenon that otherwise could only be addressed by its name after scrupulous clarification of immediate and long-term fitness effects on a detailed scale (Taborsky 2007).

4.1.2   Correlated Pay-offs

If a helpful behaviour causes net fitness costs, i.e. the immediate costs of acting are exceeded by its immediate benefits, such behaviour is termed altruistic (see Glossary Box 1.1). It can only be favoured by natural selection if the fitness effects of the behaviour on actor and receiver are somehow positively correlated (Frank 1998). This correlation can come about in three principal ways (Lehmann & Keller 2006a; Taborsky et al. 2016). (i) Genes shared by interaction partners through common descent, enabling kin selection to take effect (Hamilton 1963, 1964; Maynard Smith 1964; Frank 1998, 2013; Gardner et al. 2011; Bourke 2014). (ii) A genetic correlation between genes coding for cooperation and for traits enabling assortment of the bearers of such genes, e.g. traits that can be used to differentiate carriers of altruism genes allowing them to exercise selective cooperation ('green-beard effect'; Dawkins 1976; Keller & Ross 1998; Queller et al. 2003; Sinervo & Clobert 2003; Gardner & West 2010; Madgwick et al. 2019). (iii) An above-random chance that a helpful act of an individual will increase the likelihood that the costs of this act will be outweighed by future benefits accrued from receiving help in return (reciprocity; Trivers 1971; Axelrod & Hamilton 1981; Nowak 2006; Taborsky et al. 2016). We shall describe these mechanisms responsible for correlated pay-offs in detail below, starting with the most contentious.

4.1.2.1 Reciprocity

The concept of 'reciprocal altruism' (Trivers 1971) addresses an evolutionary enigma: it aims to explain how helpful behaviour can be selected despite immediate costs to the helper exceeding its immediate benefits. This might be explained by genes shared between donor and recipient, but what if donor and recipient are unrelated? According to Darwinian principles, an altruistic act will then be counterselected because it reduces the genetic fitness of the donor. Unless – and this is the principal solution suggested by Robert Trivers (1971) – the help is returned in the future: the execution of help increases the likelihood that help will be received in return (Lehmann & Keller 2006a). In a sense, 'shared genes' between social partners are replaced here by a 'shared future', likewise resulting in aligned fitness interests (Taborsky et al. 2016). If reciprocal altruism is to generate evolutionarily stable cooperation in a population, investment in a trait that does not generate immediate 'selfish' fitness benefits should increase the likelihood of obtaining fitness benefits in the future, which compensate for the costs of initial investment. Evolution of such exchange of services is hampered by the inherent temptation to cheat (Clutton-Brock 2009): individuals may simply enjoy the help of others without paying back anything in the future. This temptation can be reduced or removed, however, if the pay-offs of social partners are correlated, for example because they are likely to interact again repeatedly in the future ('shadow of the future'; Axelrod 1984).

In contrast to the term 'reciprocal altruism', which implies an evolutionary (i.e. 'ultimate') mechanism, the term 'reciprocity' or 'reciprocal cooperation' denotes a proximate mechanism. It describes the application of a decision rule, such as 'help someone if the likelihood that this individual will return the favour is sufficiently large to compensate for the immediate negative cost–benefit balance'. It is important to note that the probability that contingent return of help will fail to happen increases with the turnover rate of interaction partners and with the time interval between successive interactions among social partners (van Doorn et al. 2014). Reciprocity involves the consideration of information about the *likelihood* of obtaining fitness benefits in return for a helpful act. Therefore, a concurrent exchange of reciprocal help ('coaction') will much more easily establish stable cooperation between social partners than if a time lag is involved between actions (van Doorn et al. 2014). All else being equal, future gains are less predictable than immediate return benefits; therefore, fitness benefits expected from prospective actions should be discounted. As Robert May (1981) put it, 'One offspring in the hand can literally be worth two in the future'. Temporal discounting is a general principle of animal decision-making (Kagel et al. 1986; Hayden 2016; Vanderveldt et al. 2016) and may be one reason why reciprocity is less likely to occur with extended delays between subsequent interactions (Stephens et al. 2002).

4.1.2.1.1 Three Types of Information; Three Types of Reciprocity

In the case of uncertainty about the helpfulness of a social partner, for instance because of a time delay between successive interactions, the information individuals need for a prudent decision about whether to help a partner can primarily derive from their previous experiences or interactions. Depending on the type of information about interactions that individuals use in helping decisions –

anonymous, partner-specific, or public – reciprocal cooperation may take one of three forms: generalized, direct or indirect reciprocity (Rutte & Taborsky 2008; Herne et al. 2013; for examples see Table 4.1).

4.1.2.1.2 *Generalized Reciprocity*

Individuals interact with others in the population that may be helpful (to varying degrees) or not. If they experience help from one individual, this may influence their cooperativeness towards other individuals, resulting in *generalized* reciprocity (Hamilton & Taborsky 2005a; Pfeiffer et al. 2005; Bartlett & DeSteno 2006; Rutte & Taborsky 2007; Rankin & Taborsky 2009; Barta et al. 2011; van Doorn & Taborsky 2012). This possibility has been referred to as 'upstream tit-for-tat' (Boyd & Richerson 1989), 'upstream indirect reciprocity' (Nowak & Roch 2007), 'serial reciprocity' (Moody 2008), 'upstream reciprocity' (Iwagami & Masuda 2010), or 'pay-it-forward reciprocity' (Fowler & Christakis 2010).

The decision rule underlying generalized reciprocity is simply 'help anyone if helped by someone' (Barta et al. 2011; Box 4.3). The only information required to implement this decision rule is the actor's own social experience. Therefore, the behavioural decision mechanism involved resembles the rule that results in 'winner/loser effects' in an agonistic context, whereby individuals vary their aggressive behaviour depending on whether they have won or lost a previous encounter with some member of the population (Hsu et al. 2006; Rutte et al. 2006). As in generalized reciprocity, winner/loser effects occur because experience of an interaction made with one individual affects the behaviour shown towards another individual in a subsequent encounter, even if both these social partners are unknown or 'anonymous'. Male rats, for instance, are more likely to immediately attack an unknown competitor for food when they have previously won a contest with a different social partner, whereas they behave more submissively towards an unfamiliar conspecific after losing a contest with another individual. This contingent behaviour benefits former winners, because the subsequent encounter is settled more quickly and hence more cheaply; but it also benefits former losers, because it reduces their injury risk (Lehner et al. 2011). Hence, both sociopositive and socionegative experiences with unfamiliar individuals may change the propensity to treat others, even in a completely anonymous setting (Rutte et al. 2006; Rutte & Taborsky 2007; Gray et al. 2014; Tsvetkova & Macy 2015).

Box 4.3 Conditions and Mechanisms for the Evolution of Generalized Reciprocity

At first glance, generalized reciprocity seems unlikely to evolve because of the striking risk that cooperativeness can be exploited by cheaters, or simply, by individuals abstaining from cooperation (Boyd & Richerson 1988). Why should I help others just because someone has helped me? We have seen above that reciprocity can establish stable levels of cooperation in a population only if a cooperative act increases the chances that a helper will receive help in return. The prime reason why such enhanced probability of return benefits may also accrue when interactions involve different, even anonymous social partners lies in the fact that interactions among individuals in a population are not random. Members of

Box 4.3 (*cont.*)

natural populations are always assorted in some way or another, and so are their interactions. Panmictic populations, where all individuals interact among one another with similar likelihood, are an important tool in population genetics, but the assumption of unbiased interactions between individuals is a mathematically convenient abstraction with little correspondence in nature. Theoretical models have revealed that under the more realistic assumption that interactions of individuals are assorted in some way, for instance by population viscosity (Rankin & Taborsky 2009; Schonmann et al. 2013) or consistent interaction networks (Iwagami & Masuda 2010; Chiang & Takahashi 2011; van Doorn & Taborsky 2012), cooperation based on the decision rules of generalized reciprocity can be evolutionarily stable. The effect of population assortment is comparable to the effect of limited group size, which has been shown to favour generalized reciprocity to evolve (Boyd & Richerson 1989; Pfeiffer et al. 2005). It is important to note that these models assume the simplest possible decision rule for generalized reciprocity: 'help anyone if helped by someone'. A similarly simple decision rule would correspond to social contagion, i.e. the rule to copy what others are doing, which seems common in humans. However, experimental results with human subjects suggest that this copying rule does not seem to enhance helpfulness as much as generalized reciprocity does (Tsvetkova & Macy 2014).

Theory suggests that generalized reciprocity can still evolve under plausible conditions for a range of other decision rules and when relaxing assumptions about assortment and interaction biases (Barta et al. 2011; Chiong & Kirley 2015; Ohtsuki 2018). Depending on their experience of help or defection, an individual may decide not only whether to cooperate in a subsequent interaction, but also whether to stay or leave the group. If both these decisions can be made in response to experienced interactions, a win-stay, lose-shift rule may evolve that can establish variance between groups in a population regarding their average degree of cooperativeness (Hamilton & Taborsky 2005a). If individuals base their decision to cooperate on an internal state variable ('actual cooperativeness') that can be updated by the outcome of each interaction, generalized reciprocity may emerge and establish evolutionarily stable levels of cooperation in a population under a wide range of conditions (Barta et al. 2011). Importantly, this model is not based on a priori assumptions about assortment, interaction probabilities, group or population sizes, i.e. interactions between group members occur at random. A related theoretical approach revealed that generalized reciprocity can evolve even if social interactions happen only once ('one-shot games' as opposed to the iterated prisoner's dilemma), if social information is used in a form of indirect reinforcement learning (Chiong & Kirley 2015).

Generalized reciprocity can also evolve in connection with other mechanisms such as direct reciprocity and network reciprocity, which enhance the level of cooperation in a population (Nowak & Roch 2007) but may be sensitive to costs involved in the participation of interactions (Pena et al. 2011). Low levels of relatedness in a population can also be conducive to the emergence of generalized

Box 4.3 (*cont.*)

reciprocity (Schonmann & Boyd 2016). It is worth pointing out that all these models are based on an anonymous prisoner's dilemma situation, whereby an individual that has to decide whether to cooperate altruistically or not has no information about their future interaction partners, or reassurance that they will ever receive favours in return. This is generally regarded as the most difficult situation for reciprocal altruism to evolve. In this case the evolution of reciprocity is facilitated if cooperation is implemented as a continuous rather than a discrete decision, i.e. where individuals can choose the amount of help they provide, not merely *whether* they help. The ability to choose from a continuous helping strategy can enhance the establishment of efficient cooperation in a population (Takezawa & Price 2010). The structure of an interaction network characterized by a measure of local centrality can also influence the emergence of generalized reciprocity in a population (van Doorn & Taborsky 2012), regardless of the type of social dilemma (Stojkoski et al. 2018).

Given the varied and plausible conditions under which generalized reciprocity can evolve and establish cooperation in a population, one does wonder how frequently this mechanism occurs in nature. At present we are not able to properly answer this question because the decision rules employed in the anonymous prisoner's dilemma paradigm have been explored by rigorous experiments only for a handful of species. Nevertheless, in the cases where this was done, experimental subjects usually did apply generalized reciprocity (rats: Rutte & Taborsky 2007; Schneeberger et al. 2012; dogs: Gfrerer & Taborsky 2017; capuchin monkeys: Leimgruber et al. 2014; chimpanzees: Claidiere et al. 2015; humans, including small children: Bartlett & DeSteno 2006; Stanca 2009; Herne et al. 2013; Leimgruber et al. 2014). Due to its notable simplicity and, consequently, low cognitive demands, we assume that the simple decision rule to help others if helped oneself may actually be very widespread. In humans, for instance, generalized reciprocity appears to have stronger and more lasting effects than reputation-based indirect reciprocity in an organizational setting (Baker & Bulkley 2014). It would be intriguing to know how many of the impressive number of cases of apparent reciprocal cooperation in animals (see Table 4.1) can be explained by individuals applying this extremely simple decision rule instead of more complex ones; this will be an exciting challenge for future research. Previous studies have revealed two possibilities: individuals may apply only this simple decision rule when reciprocating received help, like in dogs (Gfrerer & Taborsky 2017), or they may apply both generalized *and* direct reciprocity rules, thus leading to different levels of cooperation, like in Norway rats (Rutte & Taborsky 2008; Schneeberger et al. 2012), chimpanzees (Claidiere et al. 2015; Engelmann et al. 2015; Schmelz et al. 2017, 2020), humans (Bartlett & DeSteno 2006; Stanca 2009; Herne et al. 2013) and possibly guppies (Edenbrow et al. 2017). The research on humans suggests that direct reciprocity may emerge from generalized reciprocity during child development (Leimgruber 2018).

4.1.2.1.3　Direct Reciprocity

If an individual has received help from a social partner, this may increase its propensity to help this partner at a subsequent occasion, thereby generating *direct* reciprocity (Trivers 1971; Axelrod & Hamilton 1981; Nowak & Sigmund 1992, 1993; Hauser et al. 2003; Krams et al. 2008; Rutte & Taborsky 2008; St.-Pierre et al. 2009; Majolo et al. 2012; Carter & Wilkinson 2013; Voelkl et al. 2015; Taborsky & Riebli 2020). The decision rule underlying direct reciprocity is basically 'help someone who has helped you before' (tit-for-tat or variations thereof; Axelrod & Hamilton 1981; Killingback & Doebeli 2002; Schweinfurth & Taborsky 2020). The information required to implement this rule is whether the individual previously received help from the same partner. This decision mechanism may resemble rules employed in the agonistic context in a conflict between social partners or neighbours that know each other from previous interactions, and which therefore have information about each other's competitive (fighting) ability. This may stabilize rank orders, the relationship between territorial neighbours and social networks (Huntingford & Turner 1987; McGregor 2005; Müller & Manser 2007; Christensen & Radford 2018).

4.1.2.1.4　Indirect Reciprocity

'Public information' is a form of indirect social information that can be used by animals in different contexts (Valone 2007). If individuals have information about the cooperativeness of social partners, for instance, they may decide to help (generally) cooperative social partners, even if they have not interacted with them before, thereby employing indirect reciprocity (Alexander 1987; Nowak & Sigmund 1998a, 1998b, 2005; Wedekind & Milinski 2000; Leimar & Hammerstein 2001; Ohtsuki & Iwasa 2004, 2006; Brandt et al. 2007). The rule underlying this decision may be based on the 'reputation' of the social partner, which reflects its (general) cooperativeness. The behavioural mechanism entailing the rule 'help someone who is helpful' depends on public information obtained, for instance, by eavesdropping (Johnstone 2001; Peake 2005), which has been shown to affect behavioural decisions in the agonistic context (Oliveira et al. 1998; Peake et al. 2001; Earley & Dugatkin 2002). Male fighting fish, for example, monitor aggressive interactions between neighbours and use the information on their relative fighting ability thereby obtained in subsequent aggressive interactions with them (Oliveira et al. 1998).

4.1.2.1.5　The Importance of Information

Our consideration shows that the three types of information that individuals may use – anonymous, partner-specific, or public – determine which form of reciprocity they can apply. The use of information may be constrained by the limited capacity of potential receivers to perceive, process, memorize and retrieve information, and by the costs of information acquisition and processing. Individuals deciding about reciprocal help should base their decision on 'economically' available information according to the 'hierarchical information hypothesis' of reciprocal cooperation (Rutte & Taborsky 2008). This concept implies that the decision to help others contingent on previously received help should take into account as much information about prospective receivers as possible, in order to maximize the probability of being helped in the future; that is, in order of complexity, animals should apply indirect, direct or generalized reciprocity according to capability.

If individuals possess pertinent information about the general cooperativeness of a social partner, they can decide to help 'cooperators' and refrain from helping 'non-cooperators' (or 'defectors'), as has been demonstrated in experiments with human subjects (*indirect* reciprocity: Wedekind & Milinski 2000; Milinski et al. 2002; Wedekind & Braithwaite 2002; Semmann et al. 2005; Seinen & Schram 2006; see Milinski 2016 for review). In these studies, subjects naïve with regard to the logic of the experiment typically receive information about the fellow players' previous generosity to others, which allows them to decide about their own generosity towards more or less helpful individuals. It has been suggested that other animals may lack the ability to employ indirect reciprocity, due to its high cognitive demands (Milinski & Wedekind 1998; Stevens & Hauser 2004; Stevens et al. 2005; Larose & Dubois 2011; Emonds et al. 2012). Advanced cognitive mechanisms required for the reputation-building process underlying indirect reciprocity may be too costly to favour the evolution of cooperation based on this mechanism alone (Suzuki & Kimura 2013). However, preconditions of this mechanism, such as information gathering by eavesdropping and contingent 'image scoring' expressed by preferential association with obliging social partners, have been demonstrated in an interspecific context in cleaner fish–host interactions (Bshary 2002; Bshary & Grutter 2006), which will be discussed in Chapter 5. Furthermore, Norway rats (*Rattus norvegicus*) and domestic dogs (*Canis lupus familiaris*) apply indirect reciprocity decision rules in controlled experimental conditions after witnessing a conspecific helping another one (Spahni 2005; Gfrerer 2017). Hence, non-human animals are obviously capable of applying indirect reciprocity, but due to the substantial cognitive costs involved in this mechanism its significance in natural conditions is dubious (Stevens et al. 2005).

If animals can remember the cooperative propensity of a particular social partner from their previous interaction(s) among each other, they may decide to be helpful contingent on the previous helpfulness of this partner – which, according to the concept of *direct* reciprocity, only pays if there is a chance that the same two partners will again interact in the future (Trivers 1971; Axelrod & Hamilton 1981; Sigmund 2010). The memory capacity required for this type of reciprocity is not as demanding as in indirect reciprocity, but it may constrain the number of interacting group members for the functioning of this mechanism (Moreira et al. 2013). Careful experimentation revealed that representatives from different taxa, including fish, songbirds, rodents, bats, primates and even polychaete worms, are capable of applying direct reciprocity (de Waal & Berger 2000; Hauser et al. 2003; Krams et al. 2008; Rutte & Taborsky 2008; Schino et al. 2009; St.-Pierre et al. 2009; Viana et al. 2010; Cheney 2011; Majolo et al. 2012; Carter & Wilkinson 2013; Dolivo & Taborsky 2015a, 2015b; Molesti & Majolo 2017; Schweinfurth & Taborsky 2017, 2018a, 2018b, 2018c; Schweinfurth et al. 2017a; Stieger et al. 2017; Gfrerer & Taborsky 2018; Picchi et al. 2018; Taborsky & Riebli 2020), and it seems to be widespread in nature in the context of allogrooming in birds and mammals in general (Hart & Hart 1992; Stopka & Graciasova 2001; Radford & Du Plessis 2006; Schino & Aureli 2008a, 2008b; Gomes et al. 2009; Cheney et al. 2010).

If individuals cooperate by direct reciprocity, theory predicts that they should consider the costs of their helpful behaviour and the benefits to the receivers of their help (Trivers 1971). In Norway rats, these predictions have been confirmed. Experimental manipulation of the costs of producing food for a social partner triggered the helping propensity of experimental subjects: the higher the energetic costs of pulling food towards a partner, the better they distinguished between partners that had provided them with food before versus those that had not (Schneeberger et al. 2012). In addition, experimental subjects provided hungry partners in bad body condition with more food than hungry partners in good condition, suggesting that the relative benefits to the receiver were considered when deciding to reciprocate previously received help. Other experiments revealed that the quality of received help influences the propensity to give help back. Social partners providing focal subjects with attractive banana induced the latter to return this favour more readily than if they only provided carrot, which is less fancied (Dolivo & Taborsky 2015a). These results reveal that animals are indeed capable of adjusting reciprocal cooperation to the costs and benefits involved in such behaviour.

If an individual remembers only whether it was previously helped, regardless of by whom, it can decide whether to cooperate simply based on this experience, thereby using the decision rule denoting *generalized* reciprocity. The use of non-specific information such as 'I received help' (irrespective of the identity of the helper) may be better than using no information, if more specific information (e.g. on individual identity) is not available. The very simple decision rule 'help anyone if helped by someone' has been found to generate evolutionarily stable levels of cooperation in a population under a wide range of conditions (Box 4.3). Humans, chimpanzees, capuchin monkeys, dogs and female Norway rats have been demonstrated to act upon this decision rule when they were permitted to help an anonymous social partner (see Box 4.3 for references). Longtailed and Barbary macaques were found to exhibit direct but not generalized reciprocity (Majolo et al. 2012; Molesti & Majolo 2017). However, in these two studies the monkeys could apply both direct and generalized reciprocity in a correlative, i.e. non-experimental, study where spatial proximity was not controlled for. Therefore, the monkeys might in fact have applied the simple decision rule of generalized reciprocity 'help anyone if helped by someone' instead of the ostensible direct reciprocity rule, as has been demonstrated in dogs (Gfrerer & Taborsky 2017). Nevertheless, in Norway rats the same experimental paradigm revealing generalized reciprocity in females failed to show it in males; instead, they did employ direct reciprocity (Schweinfurth et al. 2019).

4.1.2.1.6 Cooperation on Networks and Graphs

Theoretical models have investigated the importance of spatial relationships and interaction networks for the origin of cooperation, assuming that relationships between individuals are based on (interaction) networks or non-random connections

Table 4.1. Examples of reciprocal cooperation in vertebrates.

This table reports evidence for reciprocal cooperation among conspecifics from 180 studies (four of which were meta-analyses) of 95 vertebrate species (20 of which comprised primate meta-analyses, including humans) observed under natural, semi-natural and laboratory conditions. The evidence provided in these studies ranges from correlation analyses of reciprocal exchanges to results from stringently controlled experiments testing for the application of specific decision rules. In a large proportion of these studies, relatedness between interaction partners has been excluded as a major explanatory variable for reciprocal cooperation, either by the nature of group structure, experimental design, or statistical analysis. 'Allogrooming' or 'allopreening' refers to *reciprocal* grooming or preening between two or more individuals in a group. E = experimental; O = observational; C = captivity; W = in the wild.

Species	Common name	Order, Family	Form of reciprocity	Obs/ Exp	Capt./ Wild	References
Fishes						
Neolamprologus pulcher	Princess of Lake Tanganyika	Cichliformes Cichlidae	Commodity trading based on pay-to-stay negotiations among breeders and helpers; reciprocal shelter digging	O/E	W/C	M. Taborsky 1985; B. Taborsky 2006; Balshine-Earn et al. 1998; Bergmüller & et al. 2005a; Stiver et al. 2005; Heg & Taborsky 2010; Bruintjes & Taborsky 2008, 2011; Zöttl et al. 2013a, 2013b, 2013c; Fischer et al. 2014; Naef & Taborsky 2020a, 2020b; Taborsky & Riebli 2020
Pelvicachromis pulcher	Kribensis cichlid	Cichliformes Cichlidae	Satellite males trading fertilization access against help in brood care and defence	O	C	Martin & Taborsky 1997
Poecilia reticulata	Guppy	Cyprinodontiformes Poeciliidae	Cooperative predator inspection	E/O	C/W	Dugatkin & Alfieri 1991; Croft et al. 2006
Symphodus ocellatus	Ocellated wrasse	Labriformes Labridae	Satellite males trading fertilization access against help in territory defence and female attraction	O/E	W	Taborsky et al. 1987; Taborsky 1994, 2009; Stiver & Alonzo 2013
Siganus corallinus S. *doliatus* S. *puellus* S. *vulpinus*	Rabbitfish	Perciformes Siganidae	Reciprocal vigilance among long-term dyads	O	W	Brandl & Bellwood 2015

152

Hypoplectrus nigricans	Black hamlet	Perciformes	Serranidae	Egg trading	O	W	Fischer 1980
Serranus tigrinus	Harlequin bass	Perciformes	Serranidae	Egg trading	O	W	Pressley 1981
Serranus tortugarum	Chalk bass	Perciformes	Serranidae	Egg trading	O	W	Fischer 1984; Hart et al. 2016
Serranus tabacarius	Tobaccofish	Perciformes	Serranidae	Egg trading	O	W	Petersen 1995
Serranus subligarius	Belted sandfish	Perciformes	Serranidae	Egg trading	O	W	Oliver 1997
Gasterosteus aculeatus	Three-spined stickleback	Gasterosteiformes	Gasterosteidae	Cooperative predator inspection	E	C	Milinski et al. 1990; Huntingford et al. 1994
Birds							
Geronticus eremita	Northern bald ibis	Ciconiiformes	Threskiornithidae	Turn-taking in leading flight position	O	W	Voelkl et al. 2015
Uria aalge	Common guillemot	Charadriiformes	Alcidae	Allopreening	O	W	Lewis et al. 2007
Phoeniculus purpureus	Green woodhoopoe	Bucerotiformes	Phoeniculidae	Alloparental brood care *vs.* help in territory acquisition and alloparental care; allopreening	O	W	Ligon & Ligon 1978, 1983; Radford & Du Plessis 2006
Tyto alba	Barn owl	Strigiformes	Tytonidae	Allopreening and food donations for preening among nestlings	E	W/C	Roulin et al. 2016
Psittacus erithacus	African grey parrot	Psittaciformes	Psittacidae	Reciprocal token transfer	E	C	Krasheninnikova et al. 2019; Brucks & von Bayern 2020
Nymphicus hollandicus	Cockatiel	Psittaciformes	Cacatuidae	Exchange of co-feeding and allopreening in juveniles	E	C	Lievin-Bazin et al. 2019
Ficedula hypoleuca	Pied flycatcher	Passeriformes	Muscicapidae	Reciprocal defence of neighbours against predators	E	W	Krams et al. 2008, 2010, 2013; Krama et al. 2012
Parus major	Great tit	Passeriformes	Paridae	Parental turn-taking in chick provisioning	O	W	Johnstone et al. 2014
Sitta pusilla	Brown-headed nuthatch	Passeriformes	Sittidae	Allopreening	O	W	Cox 2012

Table 4.1. (cont.)

Species	Common name	Order, Family	Form of reciprocity	Obs/ Exp	Capt./ Wild	References
Campylorhynchus nuchalis	Stripe-backed wren	Passeriformes Troglodytidae	Alloparental care *vs.* alloparental care (delayed reciprocity)	O	W	Wiley & Rabenold 1984
Cantorchilus leucotis	Buff-breasted wren	Passeriformes Troglodytidae	Allopreening	O	W	Gill 2012
Taeniopygia guttata	Zebra finch	Passeriformes Estrildidae	Reciprocal food provisioning	E	C	St-Pierre et al. 2009
Malurus cyaneus	Superb fairy wren	Passeriformes Maluridae	Pay-to-stay interactions among male breeders and male helpers	E	W	Mulder & Langmore 1993
Corcorax melanorhamphos	White-winged chough	Passeriformes Corcoracidae	Alloparental care *vs.* alloparental care (delayed reciprocity)	O	W	Heinsohn 1991
Cyanocitta cristata	Blue jay	Passeriformes Corvidae	Reciprocal food exchange under reduced discounting effects	E	C	Stephens et al. 2002
Corvus monedula	Jackdaw	Passeriformes Corvidae	Reciprocal food exchange	E	C	De Kort et al. 2006; Von Bayern 2007
Corvus frugilegus	Rook	Passeriformes Corvidae	Reciprocal co-feeding	O	C	Scheid et al. 2008
Corvus macrorhynchos	Large-billed crow	Passeriformes Corvidae	Allopreening	O	C	Miyazawa et al. 2020
Corvus corax	Raven	Passeriformes Corvidae	Agonistic support for allopreening; Cooperation in loose-string pulling task	E	C	Fraser & Bugnyar 2012; Massen et al. 2015
Agelaius phoeniceus	Red-winged blackbird	Passeriformes Icteridae	Reciprocal nest defence among neighbours	O/E	W	Olendorf et al. 2004
Mammals						
Eulemur fulvus	Red-fronted lemur	Primates Lemuridae	Allogrooming	O	W	Port et al. 2009
Saguinus oedipus	Cotton-top tamarin	Primates Callitrichidae	Direct reciprocity in food exchange task; trading of grooming against alloparental infant carrying	E/O	C	Hauser et al. 2003; Chen & Hauser 2005; Ginther & Snowdon 2009; Cronin et al. 2010

154

Species	Common name	Order / Family	Behavior			References
Callithrix jacchus	Common marmoset	Primates Callitrichidae	Allogrooming	O	C	Campenni et al. 2015
Cebus apella	Tufted capuchin	Primates Cebidae	Reciprocal food exchange by direct and generalized reciprocity; allogrooming; grooming for infant handling opportunities; trading tools for food; trading grooming for food sharing	E/O	W/C	Izawa 1980; de Waal 1997a, 2000; DiBitetti 1997; Westergaard & Suomi 1997; Mendres & de Waal 2000; Hattori et al. 2005; Schino et al. 2009; Tiddi et al. 2010, 2011; Sabbatini et al. 2012; Suchak & de Waal 2012; Leimgruber et al. 2014; Parrish et al. 2015
Cebus capucinus	White-faced capuchin	Primates Cebidae	Allogrooming	O	W	Manson et al. 2004
Cercocebus atys	Sooty mangabey	Primates Cercopithecidae	Trading grooming for infant handling opportunities	O	W	Fruteau et al. 2011a, 2011b
Lophocebus albigena	Grey-cheeked mangabey	Primates Cercopithecidae	Allogrooming	O	W	Chancellor & Isbell 2009
Chlorocebus pygerythrus (C. aethiops)	Vervet monkey	Primates Cercopithecidae	Trading grooming for social support, food provisioning, and infant handling opportunities	E/O	W	Seyfarth & Cheney 1984; Fruteau et al. 2009, 2011a, 2011b; Borgeaud & Bshary 2015
Cercopithecus mitis	Blue monkey	Primates Cercopithecidae	Allogrooming	O	W	Rowell et al. 1991
Macaca fascicularis	Long-tailed macaque	Primates Cercopithecidae	Trading grooming for social support; allogrooming	E/O	C	Hemelrijk 1994; Gumert 2007; Gumert & Ho 2008; Majolo et al. 2012
Macaca sylvanus	Barbary macaque	Primates Cercopithecidae	Allogrooming and trading grooming for agonistic support	O	W	Carne et al. 2011; Molesti & Majolo 2017
Macaca arctoides	Stump-tailed macaque	Primates Cercopithecidae	Reciprocal agonistic support	O	C	De Waal & Luttrell 1988
Macaca mulatta	Rhesus macaque	Primates Cercopithecidae	Reciprocal agonistic support	O	C	De Waal & Luttrell 1988
Macaca fuscata	Japanese macaque	Primates Cercopithecidae	Allogrooming; covariation of allogrooming and social support	O	C	Schino et al. 2003, 2007; Ventura et al. 2006

Table 4.1. (cont.)

Species	Common name	Order, Family	Form of reciprocity	Obs/ Exp	Capt./ Wild	References
Macaca radiata	Bonnet macaque	Primates Cercopithecidae	Allogrooming; Exchange of social support and allogrooming	O	C	Sugiyama 1971; Koyama 1973; Silk 1992; Manson et al. 2004
Macaca assamensis	Assamese macaque	Primates Cercopithecidae	Allogrooming	O	W	Haunhorst et al. 2016
Macaca thibetana	Tibetan macaque	Primates Cercopithecidae	Allogrooming	O	W	Balasubramaniam et al. 2011; Xia et al. 2012
Papio cynocephalus	Yellow baboon	Primates Cercopithecidae	Allogrooming	O	W	Seyfarth 1976; Hemelrijk & Luteijn 1998
Papio ursinus	Chacma baboon	Primates Cercopithecidae	Allogrooming	O	W	Henzi et al. 1997; Barrett et al. 1999; Silk et al. 1999
Papio hamadryas	Hamadryas baboon	Primates Cercopithecidae	Allogrooming; trading grooming for social support	O/E	C/W	Leinfelder et al. 2001; Cheney et al. 2010
Papio anubis	Olive baboon	Primates Cercopithecidae	Role exchange in male coalitions against opponents; females trading grooming for infant handling opportunities	O	W	Packer 1977; Smuts 1985; Frank & Silk 2009a, 2009b
Mandrillus sphinx	Mandrill	Primates Cercopithecidae	Allogrooming; agonistic support for allogrooming	O	C	Schino & Pellegrini 2009, 2011
Hylobates lar	White-handed gibbon	Primates Hylobatidae	Mutual allogrooming; grooming for mating access	O	W	Barelli et al. 2011
Pongo pygmaeus	Orangutan	Primates Hominidae	Reciprocal token exchange	E	C	Dufour et al. 2009
Pan troglodytes	Chimpanzee	Primates Hominidae	Reciprocal agonistic support; trading grooming for social support and food; allogrooming; reciprocal exchange of food; trading of food for social support; trading social support and food for mating; direct and generalized reciprocity in food exchange tasks	O/E	C/W	De Waal & Luttrell 1988; de Waal 1989, 1997b; Hemelrijk & Ek 1991; Mitani & Watts 1999, 2001; Watts 2002; Koyama et al. 2006; Mitani 2006; Melis et al. 2008; Gomes & Boesch 2009, 2011; Gomes et al. 2009; Jaeggi et al. 2010; Newton-Fisher & Lee 2011; Crick et al. 2013;

Species	Common name	Order	Family			Behaviour	References
Pan paniscus	Bonobo	Primates	Hominidae	E/O	C/W	Allogrooming; exchange of allogrooming and food sharing	Silk et al. 2013; Wittig et al. 2014; Claidiere et al. 2015; Engelmann et al. 2015; Kaburu & Newton-Fisher 2015; Schmelz et al. 2017, 2020
14 species		Primates		O	C/W	Allogrooming	Jaeggi et al. 2013; Surbeck & Hohmann 2015
14 species		Primates		O	C/W	Trading grooming for social support	Schino & Aureli 2008a, 2010a
6 species (incl. *Homo sapiens*)		Primates		O	C/W	Reciprocal food sharing and trading other commodities	Schino 2007 Jaeggi & Gurven 2013
Apodemus microps	Herb-field mouse	Rodentia	Muridae	O	C	Allogrooming	Stopka & Graciasova 2001
Rattus norvegicus	Norway rat	Rodentia	Muridae	E/O	C	Reciprocal allonursing; generalized and direct reciprocity in food exchange task; allogrocming; trading of different commodities	Menella et al. 1990; Rutte & Taborsky 2007, 2008; Schneeberger et al. 2012, 2020; Dolivo & Taborsky 2015a, 2015b; Wood et al. 2016; Schweinfurth & Taborsky 2017, 2018a, 2018b, 2018c, 2020; Schweinfurth et al. 2017a, 2019; Stieger et al. 2017; Delmas et al. 2019; Kettler et al. 2021
Desmodus rotundus	Common vampire bat	Chiroptera	Phyllostomidae	O/E	W/C	Reciprocal food provisioning and allogrooming	Wilkinson 1984, 1986; DeNault & McFarlane 1995; Carter & Wilkinson 2013, 2015; Wilkinson et al. 2016; Carter et al. 2017
Artibeus jamaicensis	Jamaican fruit-eating bat	Chiroptera	Phyllostomidae	O/E	W	Subordinate males trade territory defence against reproduction and territory inheritance	Ortega & Arita 2000, 2002
Rousettus aegyptiacus	Egyptian fruit bat	Chiroptera	Pteropodidae	O	C	Trading food for mating	Harten et al. 2019
Suricata suricatta	Meerkat	Carnivora	Herpestidae	O	W	Reciprocal allogrooming; grooming and allonursing in exchange for social benefits	Kutsukake & Clutton-Brock 2006b, 2010; MacLeod et al. 2013; MacLeod & Clutton-Brock 2015

Table 4.1. (cont.)

Species	Common name	Order, Family	Form of reciprocity	Obs/ Exp	Capt./ Wild	References
Helogale parvula	Dwarf mongoose	Carnivora Herpestidae	Trading sentinel behaviour for allogrooming	O/E	W	Kern & Radford 2018
Canis familiaris	Dog	Carnivora Canidae	Generalized reciprocity in food exchange task	E	C	Gfrerer & Taborsky 2017, 2018
Nasua nasua	Coati	Carnivora Procyonidae	Social support	O	C	Romero & Aureli 2008
Equus caballus	Horse	Perissodactyla Equidae	Coalitionary support among males for mating access	O	W	Feh 1999
Rangifer tarandus	Reindeer	Artiodactyla Cervidae	Reciprocal allonursing	O	W	Engelhardt et al. 2015
Dama dama	Fallow deer	Artiodactyla Cervidae	Reciprocal allonursing	O	W	Ekvall 1998
Giraffa camelopardalis	Giraffe	Artiodactyla Giraffidae	Reciprocal allonursing	O	C	Gloneková et al. 2016
Aepyceros melampus	Impala	Artiodactyla Bovidae	Allogrooming	O	W	Hart & Hart 1992; Mooring & Hart 1997
Tursiops aduncus	Indo-Pacific bottlenose dolphin	Artiodactyla Delphinidae	Reciprocal flipper rubbing	O	W	Sakai et al. 2006

between neighbours on a spatial or social lattice or 'graph' (e.g. Nowak & May 1992; Nakamuru et al. 1997; Santos & Pacheco 2005, 2006; Ohtsuki et al. 2006; Santos et al. 2006; Masuda 2007; Gomez-Gardenes et al. 2007; Szabo & Fath 2007; Taylor et al. 2007a; Sicardi et al. 2009; Fu et al. 2010; Suzuki & Kimura 2011; Pena & Rochat 2012; Szolnoki et al. 2012; Utkovski et al. 2017; Stojkoski et al. 2018). In the simplest case, interactions are allowed only with the immediate neighbour of an individual, and the behavioural decision is either to cooperate or not, without behavioural contingency (Axelrod 1984). In this purely deterministic version of the prisoners' dilemma, cooperation and non-cooperation (i.e. 'defection') can coexist in a population, which coincides with chaotically changing spatial patterns of cooperators and defectors (Nowak & May 1992). These simple models usually assume unconditional cooperation between neighbours of the assumed networks. Sometimes the resulting patterns of cooperation between individuals of a population are referred to as 'network reciprocity', which is misleading as the behavioural rule does not involve reciprocal responses. The rule is simply 'cooperate' or 'defect' (i.e. help or do not help a social partner), irrespective of the previous experience of the actor. Therefore, these models test whether in certain interaction schemes unconditional cooperation can evolve and persist in a population (e.g. via 'spatial selection'; Nowak et al. 2010b), but they do not inform about the evolution of reciprocity rules (Perc et al. 2013). Hence, a more adequate term for this type of interactions is '*network cooperation*'. It should be noted in this context that certain spatial or interaction structures are not always assumed when testing for the evolutionary stability of unconditional cooperation (e.g. Masuda 2012).

In contrast to models based on spatial or interaction networks that assume purely unconditional behavioural strategies, other models have assumed that individuals apply decision rules characteristic of generalized reciprocity (e.g. Greiner & Levati 2005; Nowak & Roch 2007; Iwagami & Masuda 2010; Sigmund 2010; Chiang & Takahashi 2011; Masuda 2011; Pena et al. 2011; van Doorn & Taborsky 2012; Chiong & Kirley 2015). Social interactions among animals are structured according to different factors such as sex, age, kinship, familiarity, personality and sociability (McPherson et al. 2001; Croft et al. 2009; Schürch et al. 2010). As a result, both the quality and quantity of interactions among individuals differ, generating heterogeneous networks of social interactions within a population (Croft et al. 2009; Sih et al. 2009). Interaction networks are characterized by their size (i.e. the total number of interacting individuals) and degree of heterogeneity. Numerous studies have shown that group size, network heterogeneity, network connectivity and modularity (i.e. the cross-linking level between individuals and the division of a network into groups or clusters), participation costs and the occurrence of other forms of reciprocal cooperation in the population all may affect the establishment and maintenance of generalized reciprocity in a social network (van Doorn & Taborsky 2012, and references therein). Evidence for the use of generalized reciprocity decision rules depending on environmental conditions (predator pressure), population origin and sex exists for instance in guppies, *Poecilia reticulata*, where experimental subjects interacted more cooperatively with unfamiliar partners after receiving cooperative experience with others (Edenbrow et al. 2017). In the wild, guppy social networks are positively assorted by cooperative predator inspection behaviour (Croft et al. 2009).

4.1.2.1.7 When Should We Expect Reciprocity?

There are several conditions promoting cooperation by reciprocity.

The profitability of behaving reciprocally depends on the relationship between costs of helping to the actor (c), benefits of helping to the receiver (b) and the probability that the actor receives help of corresponding value in the future (w) (Axelrod & Hamilton 1981; Nowak 2006). Helping is favoured where

$$w > c/b$$

or

$$c < b\,w$$

This means that stable levels of cooperation by reciprocity are more likely to evolve if three conditions are met:

(1) First condition: the costs of helping to the actor are low. This seems to accord with the frequent occurrence of reciprocal grooming in mammals (see Table 4.1 for numerous examples). The temporary net fitness costs of allogrooming/ allopreening have been assumed to be low (Dunbar & Sharman 1984; Schino 2007; Clutton-Brock 2009). However, grooming involves time, effort, i.e. opportunity costs (the loss of opportunities to perform alternative behaviours such as feeding, courting or defending resources), energy expenditure and risk due to reduced vigilance (Hawlena et al. 2007). Time costs of grooming and preening have been suggested by correlative evidence in various mammals and birds (e.g. impala, Mooring 1995; moose, Mooring & Samuel 1999; baboons, Dunbar & Dunbar 1988; penguins, Viblanc et al. 2011), and they were experimentally demonstrated for instance in great tits (Christe et al. 1996), bats (Giorgi et al. 2001) and gerbilline rodents (Hawlena et al. 2007; Raveh et al. 2011). Significant energetic costs of grooming were shown in bats (Giorgi et al. 2001) and penguins (Viblanc et al. 2011), and vigilance costs of grooming were found in antelopes (Hart et al. 1992; Mooring & Hart 1995) and gerbils (Raveh et al. 2011). Grooming may also facilitate parasite transmission (Heitman et al. 2003) and involve various physiological costs (see Hawlena et al. 2007 for review). Even though most of these data were obtained on self-grooming, extrapolation to costs of allogrooming seems justified (cf. Hart et al. 1992). Therefore, the assumption that grooming is particularly cheap with regard to potential fitness effects may be unjustified. Concerning the causality of allogrooming and allopreening, the observed stress-reducing effect of social hygiene may indicate a proximate mechanism controlling reciprocal grooming against the background of apparent fitness costs (Terry 1970; Feh & Demazieres 1993; Shutt et al. 2007; Ueno et al. 2015; Teunissen et al. 2018).

In some primates, food may be shared reciprocally (Mitani 2006; Silk 2007; Jaeggi & van Schaik 2011; Jaeggi & Gurven 2013), but often food sharing reflects tolerated scrounging rather than reciprocal food offering (Schusterman & Berkson 1962; Blurton Jones 1984, 1987; Rose 1997; Jaeggi & Gurven 2013), implying that costs are negligible (Blurton Jones 1987; Winterhalder 1996). Some chimpanzee populations differ from most other primates in that caught prey is regularly shared (Boesch 1994; Silk et al. 2013), but the lack of reliable estimates of involved fitness correlates makes it difficult to assess costs involved in offering and sharing food (cf. Winterhalder 1996). In contrast, prey is rarely shared among adults in nature in most other species (e.g. capuchin monkeys: Rose 1997), whereas sharing of all sorts of food from adults to immatures is frequent (Jaeggi & van Schaik 2011; Jaeggi & Gurven 2013); nevertheless, this is usually unilateral rather than reciprocal. Coalitions formed to overcome opponents, which may involve reciprocation, can also be cheap if they deter an escalated encounter (Packer 1977). Similarly, reciprocal turn-taking when provisioning chicks may be cheap, at least relative to the costs of the parental/alloparental investment conflict (Johnstone et al. 2014), provided that it only requires marginal adjustments of individual food provisioning regimes (Savage et al. 2017). In mammals, allonursing of the offspring of other group members seems to occur mainly when costs are low (e.g. in lions: Pusey & Packer 1994; reviewed in Packer et al. 1992; MacLeod & Lucas 2014), and discrimination based on relatedness may be lacking (König 1989; Ebensperger et al. 2006). There is evidence in some species that allonursing is exchanged reciprocally between brood caring mothers (Ekvall 1998; Engelhardt et al. 2015).

(2) Second condition: the benefits to the receiver are high. This has been suggested to be the case in vampire bats, *Desmodus rotundus*, that need a blood meal about every other day, otherwise they are doomed to die from starvation (Wilkinson 1984). If an individual was not successful in foraging, it may attempt to obtain a blood meal donation from a colony mate. A high proportion of blood transfer of this kind occurs between relatives, but blood is also donated to unrelated individuals, apparently preferably to partners that are likely to pay back in the future (Wilkinson 1984). Reciprocal exchange is a proximate mechanism that also works among relatives, but the evolutionary causes of reciprocity are less clear if exchange happens among kin (Wilkinson 1988). Experimental evidence from a captive colony of vampire bats suggests that in fact food received in a previous interaction predicts food donations more closely than relatedness in this species (Carter & Wilkinson 2013; Figure 4.4). Nearly two-thirds of all blood-sharing dyads in the study involved unrelated social partners. Interestingly, the food-sharing network correlated well with mutual allogrooming, which indicates an interaction network based on service reciprocity, as suggested also by field observations of these bats (Wilkinson 1986). Allogrooming may be a first step towards creating social relationships that increasingly involve reciprocal service by raising the stakes from rather cheap (grooming) to more costly behaviours (food-sharing; Carter et al. 2020).

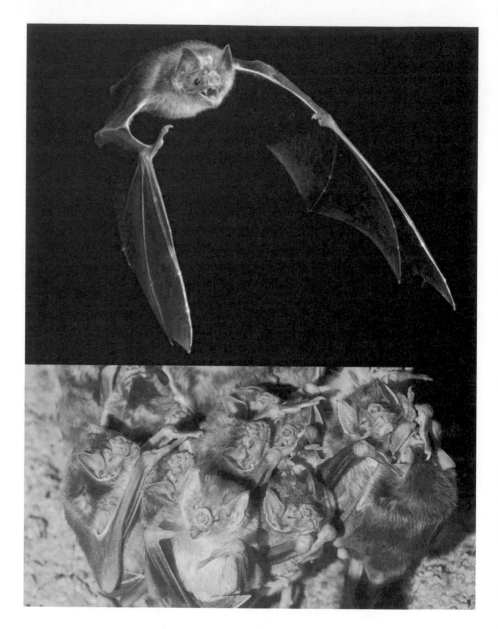

Figure 4.4A Common vampire bat in flight and resting in a social group in day roost (from Wilkinson 2019). © 2019 Elsevier Ltd. (A black and white version of this figure will appear in some formats. For the colour version, please refer to the plate section.)

Coalitions among males to obtain mating access are frequent in fish, birds and mammals (reviewed in Taborsky 1994; Olson & Blumstein 2009; Diaz-Munoz et al. 2014; see also Section 4.1.2.2.3.4, Lekking and mate sharing). They often occur among unrelated males and may enable reproductive access to individuals despite

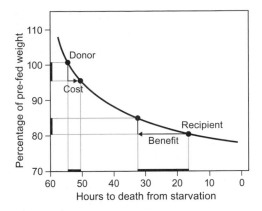 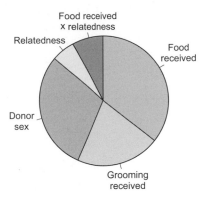

Figure 4.4B Scheme (left) of relative cost to donor and benefit to receiver of blood donation in vampire bats (after Wilkinson 1984). The nutritional value of the transferred food (measured in relative body mass; marked bold on the *y*-axis) is the same for donor and receiver, but the survival value (cost to donor and benefit to recipient; marked bold on the *x*-axis) differs between donor and receiver, due to the non-linear relationship between nutritional state (simplified: body mass) and time to starvation. Bats donate food to social partners primarily in response to received help either by previous food donations of the partner, or by previous grooming service received from the partner (right). Data from Carter and Wilkinson (2013); after Taborsky (2013).

relatively low competitive power. In fact, this may be the only chance for low-quality males to reproduce successfully (Noë 1990; Feh 1999; DuVal 2007c). Hence, even if the share of subordinate males in such coalitions is significantly smaller than that of their dominant partners, this suggests important mutual fitness benefits.

Significant fitness benefits from received help have also been shown in the context of reciprocal preening in birds (common guillemot: Lewis et al. 2007), with long-term fitness effects (increased long-term breeding success of pairs) accrued mainly by reciprocal preening of pair members, whereas allopreening of neighbours mainly provides short-term fitness returns (improved current breeding success of preening individuals). This contrasts with the assumption that mutual hygiene is a commodity of little fitness value (Clutton-Brock 2002).

(3) Third condition: the probability of receiving help or benefits in return is high. This depends on several factors, including:

(a) Group size. In small groups, (i) generalized reciprocity can be responsible for evolutionarily stable levels of cooperation (Pfeiffer et al. 2005); (ii) the surveillance of social interactions and the history of cooperation of social partners is easier and cheaper than in large groups, which can favour direct and indirect reciprocity (Nowak & Sigmund 1998b; Stevens et al. 2011); (iii) a rather fair distribution of benefits among group members in accordance with their relative power may be accomplished more easily than in large groups. This might explain why coalitions of unrelated male competitors for reproduction in order to obtain or monopolize mates are typically small (Bercovitch 1988; Packer et al. 1991; Feh 1999; for review see Taborsky 1994, 2001; Diaz-Munoz et al. 2014).

(b) Interaction frequency. The more often individuals interact with each other, the larger the probability that evolutionarily stable levels of cooperation will be established in a population, regardless of whether by generalized (Barta et al. 2011) or direct reciprocity (Nowak 2006), and perhaps less so by indirect reciprocity (Nowak 2006). Also, the time delay between subsequent interactions can be important, as outlined above; if individuals keep close contact between subsequent interactions, such as in many cooperative breeders or in primate groups, the probability that a favour will be returned is higher than in a social system where interactions happen more unpredictably (Stevens & Gilby 2004; Stevens & Hauser 2004; van Doorn et al. 2014). This might be one reason why mutual exchange based on the use of direct reciprocity rules seems particularly common in allogrooming relationships (e.g. Hart & Hart 1992; Radford & Du Plessis 2006; Schino & Aureli 2008a; Gomes et al. 2009; Schweinfurth et al. 2017a; see Table 4.1). Finally, the turnover rate of group members can affect the likelihood of interactions occurring among the same versus different individuals, which can change the balance between the occurrence of direct and generalized reciprocity (Barta et al. 2011).

(c) Relatedness. Reciprocity can generate evolutionarily stable levels of cooperation among unrelated individuals, but it can also enhance the probability of cooperation among relatives. This is due to the fact that the costs to the donor of a helpful act to a relative are devalued by the degree of relatedness (r):

$$c(1 - r) < b\,w \qquad\qquad 4.3$$

We might hence expect reciprocity to be particularly common among relatives, for the same reason that cooperation can evolve among relatives by kin selection. In other words, reciprocity can increase the fitness benefits of cooperation between relatives, thereby enhancing the occurrence of cooperation among relatives. There are several reasons why reciprocity should occur particularly often between relatives, including (i) the devaluation of fitness loss due to shared genes (Hamilton 1964), (ii) relatives interacting particularly often with each other due to spatial viscosity (Hamilton 1964, 1972; Mitteldorf & Wilson 2000; Kümmerli et al. 2009b; Lehmann & Rousset 2010), (iii) groups of relatives often being small (e.g. in cooperative breeders; Koenig & Dickinson 2016), and (iv) related recipients also having an indirect fitness incentive to return help in the future. Therefore, the danger of being exploited by free-riders is rather low if individuals perform reciprocal cooperation in groups of relatives.

On the other hand, there are compelling reasons why relatedness can in fact have the opposite effect on the probability that individuals engage in reciprocal

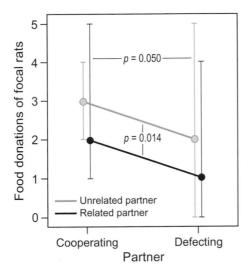

Figure 4.5 Reciprocal food donations to related and unrelated social partners in Norway rats. Focal subjects donated more food to previously cooperating than to previously defecting partners, irrespective of relatedness, but they donated overall more food to unrelated rats (grey line) than to related social partners (black line). The graph shows the median numbers of donations (+ interquartile ranges) of focal rats during the test phase (after Schweinfurth & Taborsky 2018a). © 2018 The Authors. Published by the Royal Society. All rights reserved.

exchanges. Part of the reason why applying the rules of direct or generalized reciprocity can generate evolutionarily stable levels of cooperation is that helping a social partner provides an incentive that this will be paid back, or paid forward, in the future, a process by which the pay-offs of social partners are correlated (Taborsky et al. 2016). If individuals are related, the reason for providing such incentive is less important, because one can expect helpful behaviour from a relative anyway – the fitness pay-offs of related individuals are correlated for another reason, i.e. the sharing of genes. This might be responsible for the observation that reciprocal cooperation can lead to higher levels of cooperation among unrelated than among related individuals (cf. Quinones et al. 2016). Norway rats, for instance, help each other reciprocally to obtain food in a prisoner's dilemma situation (Rutte & Taborsky 2008; Schneeberger et al. 2012; Dolivo & Taborsky 2015a, 2015b; Schweinfurth & Taborsky 2017). If social partners are related to each other, they also apply direct reciprocity rules when exchanging help to provision the partner with food, but the amount of help they provide to a related social partner is lower than the amount of help they provide to an unrelated social partner (Schweinfurth & Taborsky 2018a; Figure 4.5). In cooperatively breeding cichlids, where (subordinate) helpers pay to stay in the territory of (dominant) breeders by caring for their offspring (Taborsky 1985; Balshine-Earn et al. 1998; Bergmüller & Taborsky

2005; Bergmüller et al. 2005a; Heg & Taborsky 2010; Naef & Taborsky 2020a), helping levels are significantly lower if helpers are related to the dominant female than if they are unrelated to her (Zöttl et al. 2013a). Unrelated helpers trade their investment in alloparental care against being allowed to stay in the territory of dominants, benefitting from the protection and resources this entails. This costly effort is of less importance for related helpers, which are tolerated in the territory for other reasons, i.e. the sharing of genes with the dominants (Zöttl et al. 2013a; Quinones et al. 2016). In vampire bats, reciprocity explains a much higher proportion of the variance in altruistic blood donations between group members than relatedness (Figure 4.4B; Carter & Wilkinson 2013).

There is a surprising lack of both theoretical and empirical research on evolutionary and proximate mechanisms underlying reciprocal cooperation in groups of relatives. Often the observation of cooperative behaviour among relatives is attributed entirely to the action of kin selection, as will be outlined in Section 4.1.2.2. This assumption may mask the importance of reciprocity for decisions to cooperate with social partners. It is important to note that the concept of reciprocity refers to proximate mechanisms describing decision rules, just like the recognition of kin is required to avoid exploitation by non-related individuals when the evolution of cooperation is based on kin selection (or other mechanisms making sure that help is allocated to relatives – such as familiarity, assortment, etc.; Bourke 2011). Understanding the emergence and evolutionary stability of these decision rules is an exciting challenge for behavioural and evolutionary biologists (see Box 4.4 for an attempt to this end in Norway rats).

4.1.2.1.8   *Which Type of Reciprocity Should We Expect?*

The costs of cooperation may involve lost opportunities (e.g. to perform alternative behaviours such as feeding, courting, or defending resources) due to time constraints and trade-offs, energy expenditure and increased risk. In addition to these potential costs involved in cooperative behaviour in general, reciprocal cooperation occasions costs entailed by the acquisition, maintenance, processing and retrieval of information to allow appropriate informed decisions. As outlined above, the costs associated with information processing are very different between the three major forms of reciprocity: indirect reciprocity requires a reputation mechanism based on the performance of social partners when interacting with others (Nowak & Sigmund 1998a, 1998b, 2005; Wedekind & Milinski 2000), and hence complex social memory (Milinski & Wedekind 1998; Stevens et al. 2005; Brosnan et al. 2010). Direct reciprocity requires individual recognition and specific social memory about previous interactions with a social partner (Milinski & Wedekind 1998; Stevens & Hauser 2004; Stevens et al. 2005, 2011). Limitations in the capacity to remember a previous interaction with a social partner may affect the functionality of this mechanism. For instance, experiments in which the memory capacity of zebra finches was experimentally impaired by means of corticosterone implants occasioned reduced levels of reciprocal food donations to a partner (Larose & Dubois 2011). In humans,

---

Box 4.4 Reciprocal Cooperation in Norway Rats

Norway rats are highly social animals living in groups of variable size, ranging from just a few up to several hundred members, that exhibit a rich spectrum of social interactions, including social huddling, the sharing of food and mutual hygienic services (Barnett & Spencer 1951; Davis 1953; Barnett 1963; Telle 1966; Alberts 1978, 2007; Blanchard et al. 1984; Krafft et al. 1994; Grasmuck & Desor 2002; Schuster 2002; Schuster & Perelberg 2004; Łopuch & Popik 2011; Silberberg et al. 2014; Bartal et al. 2014; Sato et al. 2015; Tan & Hackenberg 2016). Their high degree of social flexibility and propensity to cooperate when facing environmental challenges may well be part of their ecological success. Norway rats are hence an ideal model system to study the decision processes underlying cooperative behaviour, also because they are amenable to experimental manipulation of both behaviour and social setting under rigorously controlled conditions (Wrighten & Hall 2016; Schweinfurth et al. 2019).

After humans, Norway rats were just the second species shown to apply the simple decision rule 'help anyone if helped by someone', which characterizes generalized reciprocity. After receiving help to obtain food by anonymous social partners, they are more likely to provision a novel, unfamiliar social partner with food (Rutte & Taborsky 2007). Nevertheless, if they meet the same social partner again that had been helpful before, they are even more prone to donate food; their propensity to cooperate was found to be more than twice as high if they meet a previously helpful individual than if they meet a new partner (Rutte & Taborsky 2008). In other words, altruistic cooperation can be attained by generalized reciprocity, and is amplified even further when there is an opportunity for direct reciprocity. This may reflect hierarchical information processing: when the donor has individual information about a prospective receiver it cooperates on the basis of this information, whereas without individual information cooperation is based on anonymous social experience, which is not as effective in triggering altruistic help ('hierarchical information hypothesis of reciprocal cooperation': Rutte & Taborsky 2008). This makes sense when considering the adaptive nature of such decisions, because direct reciprocity is less prone to be undermined by defection than generalized reciprocity (Pfeiffer et al. 2005; Rankin & Taborsky 2009).

Rats were shown to apply direct reciprocity rules in a range of contexts and experimental conditions (e.g. Rutte & Taborsky 2008; Schneeberger et al. 2012; Dolivo & Taborsky 2015a, 2015b; Schweinfurth & Taborsky 2016, 2017, 2018a, 2018b, 2018c; Wood et al. 2016; Schweinfurth et al. 2017a, 2019; Stieger et al. 2017; Delmas et al. 2019; Kettler et al. 2021). Typically, experiments testing the propensity of rats to apply direct reciprocity rules are based on variants of the sequential (or alternated) prisoner's dilemma, where the response of the partner to one's own altruistic help is basically unknown (Figure 4.6). However, the helpful act in itself increases the chances of receiving help back in a future interaction (Trivers 1971; Axelrod & Hamilton 1981; Killingback & Doebeli 2002; Doebeli & Hauert 2005). Importantly, the propensity to help a social partner in Norway rats is not affected

Box 4.4 (*cont.*)

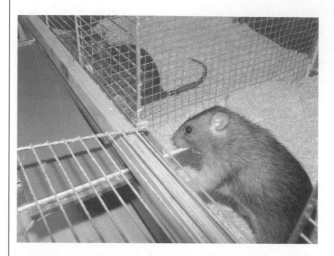

Figure 4.6 Experimental setup used to test for reciprocal cooperation between wild-type Norway rats. The individual in front pulls a tray towards the cage, an action through which the social partner in the neighbouring compartment (background) receives a treat. Subsequently, usually on the next day, that partner can return the favour by itself pulling food to the cage for the previous donor. Importantly, the donor does not get anything directly from the act of pulling, but does bear the costs of this act, implying that the behaviour is altruistic. © Res Schmid.

if the treat they receive is not provided by a conspecific (Schmid et al. 2017), meaning that they apply a decision rule of direct reciprocity while abstaining from unconditional prosociality. Nevertheless, providing help generously as a first step, i.e. without previously received help, is an important component of cooperation shown in the iterated prisoner's dilemma game (Axelrod & Hamilton 1981; Killingback & Doebeli 2002). The fact that the propensity of rats to help is raised by receiving favours does not mean that they do not help social partners at all when these partners had not been helpful before; they do so only to a lower degree. Such 'first help events' can generate series of iterated cooperation based on the decision rule of direct reciprocity (Schweinfurth et al. 2019). Moreover, rats also exhibit behaviour consistent with indirect reciprocity: they help social partners with an increased probability if they had witnessed them to be cooperative to someone else (Spahni 2005), which has not been shown in other non-human animals. Thus, there is evidence that in rats, all three forms of reciprocity can operate in parallel.

When deciding to help a social partner to obtain food, Norway rats take account of the costs involved in this effort. The more expensive the helping act gets, the more thoroughly rats discriminate whether their partner had been cooperative before or not (Schneeberger et al. 2012). They also consider the value of help they received from their social partner. Receiving high-quality food from a partner

Box 4.4 (*cont.*)

triggers higher donation levels in return than receiving less attractive fodder (Dolivo & Taborsky 2015a), and also the amount of food received predicts the size of the refund (Kettler et al. 2021). Furthermore, the hunger status of the prospective recipient determines the propensity to return received help. If a focal subject receives olfactory information revealing that the social partner is hungry, it donates food more readily and quicker to a conspecific than if the odour conveys that the partner is satiated (Schneeberger et al. 2020). In addition, hungry partners get more food from the focal subject if they are light, which implies a poor body condition, than if they are heavy (Schneeberger et al. 2012).

Norway rats do not only pay like with like. In the context of food provisioning, they may use different mechanisms to return received favours, involving, for instance, pulling a tray or pushing a lever for releasing a treat to a previously helpful partner (Schweinfurth & Taborsky 2017). Moreover, they may pay back help received to obtain food with allogrooming and vice versa, revealing that they trade different commodities with one another (Schweinfurth & Taborsky 2018b; Figure 4.7). Grooming a social partner does increase the latter's motivation to pay this hygienic service back in the same (Schweinfurth et al. 2017a) or a different currency (Schweinfurth & Taborsky 2018b), and this propensity is affected not only by received cooperation, but also by received affiliative and aggressive behaviours (Stieger et al. 2017). Interestingly, social bonds are apparently not involved in reciprocal cooperation of rats (Schweinfurth et al. 2017b), which seems to diverge from the typical situation in primates (Gomes et al. 2009; Schino & Aureli 2009; Berghänel et al. 2011).

Considering the behavioural and physiological mechanisms involved in the reciprocation of received help, it is important to know how rats obtain information about the partner: its cooperation propensity, its state and need. Do rats communicate with each other when being helpful or if in need of help? Indeed, prospective receivers in need of help to obtain a food reward address their social partner with a sequence of solicitation behaviours. First they reach out in the direction of the desired food item. If this does not release the help, they start emitting affiliative 50 kHz calls towards the partner; if the latter still does not respond appropriately, they resort to a combination of noisy behaviours directed towards the potential donor, which might be interpreted as 'attention grabbing' (Schweinfurth & Taborsky 2018c). These behaviours are effective by raising the partner's propensity to donate food to the needy signaller (Łopuch & Popik 2011; Schweinfurth & Taborsky 2018c).

In principle, received help may change one's propensity to behave cooperatively towards the benefactor in one of two ways: either consecutive experiences are integrated over some time and a number of interactions, leading to a specific attitude towards the social partner ('attitudinal reciprocity': de Waal 2000; also referred to as 'emotional bookkeeping': Schino & Aureli 2009), or only the last interaction determines one's response ('tit-for-tat'; Axelrod & Hamilton 1981). In Norway rats, a series of experiments aimed to clarify which of these two decision

Box 4.4 (*cont.*)

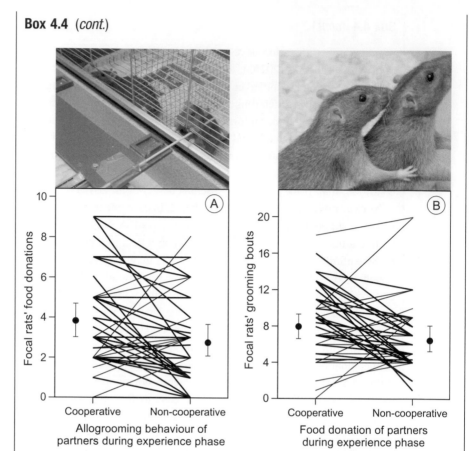

Figure 4.7 Wild-type Norway rats provided more food (A) to previously experienced cooperative grooming partners than to non-cooperative grooming partners. They also reciprocated in the reversed situation (B), where they groomed previous food providers more often than non-providers. Each line represents the raw data for a single focal rat towards its partner in two situations. The data are summarized by arithmetic means with 95 per cent confidence intervals on either side of the plots (after Schweinfurth & Taborsky 2018b). © 2018 Elsevier Ltd.

processes takes effect. Focal animals either received help from a partner on three consecutive days, or their partner refused to provide help during the same time period. On the fourth day, the treatments were switched, i.e. the partners changed either from cooperation to defection or vice versa. On the fifth day, the focal animals were tested for their propensity to help their partner to obtain food. The results were straightforward and somewhat surprising. The focal subjects clearly responded much more strongly to the behaviour of their partner shown in the last interaction, meaning that they largely disregarded the incremental experience they received beforehand. This implies that the rats are using a tit-for-tat like strategy rather than adopting attitudinal reciprocity (Schweinfurth & Taborsky 2020).

Box 4.4 (*cont.*)

Apparently, memory decay is not responsible for the application of this rather simple strategy, as has been apprehended (Stevens & Hauser 2004). When the last interaction with or without cooperation experience happened 4 days before the test, the result was very similar: the rats played tit-for-tat even if they experienced their partner in a neutral situation, without cooperation or defection, on the days in between experience and test (Schweinfurth & Taborsky 2020). When interacting with several partners consecutively, rats remember over 4 days which one was cooperative and which one was not (Kettler et al. 2021). Rats were also shown to remember individuals that had groomed them 7 days before, which significantly altered their behaviour towards these social partners even though they interacted constantly with several other individuals in between experience and test (Stieger et al. 2017).

Rats are primarily nocturnal; therefore, visual information is unlikely to be of importance when rats communicate either their need or their helpfulness. Indeed, reciprocal cooperation among Norway rats works well if they are deprived of visual cues (Dolivo & Taborsky 2015b). In contrast, both direct and generalized reciprocity only work if social partners obtain olfactory information from one another. In an experiment where the focal subjects received nothing but olfactory information from a conspecific helping another rat in a different room, this cue increased the test subject's helpfulness towards a stooge in a neighbouring cage compartment (Gerber et al. 2020). Regardless of the identity of the rat providing the olfactory information, the odour released by the helpful act triggered the cooperative response; the same individuals were used as both helpful and non-helpful experience providers in subsequent trials. This suggests there may be a characteristic 'smell of cooperation' that serves as a signal conveyed to the receivers of help, in order to reciprocate in an upcoming interaction. It is as yet unclear to what extent this cue–response relationship reflects a learned ability, but it has been shown that environmental conditions involving specific sensory modalities encountered during early adulthood have specific long-lasting effects on the learning abilities of Norway rats (Dolivo & Taborsky 2017). Furthermore, in this study environmental rather than genetic factors determined interindividual divergence, which hints at an important role of phenotypic plasticity and learning.

Nevertheless, from the aforementioned studies it is clear that basic instrumental and Pavlovian association processes cannot explain the reciprocal cooperation exhibited by Norway rats (Dolivo et al. 2016). Rather, the reciprocal cooperation of rats seems to reflect the application of more or less specific, evolved decision rules (Schweinfurth et al. 2019). How the intriguing propensity of rats to reciprocate received help plays out in nature and how it affects their Darwinian fitness is an outstanding question and an intriguing challenge for future studies. First results revealed that reciprocal allogrooming reduces health risks and raises longevity of Norway rats, at least under captive conditions (Yee et al. 2008).

experiments in which memory capacity has been challenged by demanding subjects to attend to a different task between subsequent cooperation trials, or simply by increasing the number of interaction partners, revealed an adverse impact on reciprocal cooperation (Milinski & Wedekind 1998; Stevens et al. 2011). In contrast, generalized reciprocity requires nothing but a memory of the outcome of a previous social interaction, i.e. whether one received help or not (Rutte & Taborsky 2007; Barta et al. 2011). The identity of the individual providing or withholding help is irrelevant, as is the identity of future interaction partners. This resembles the rather undemanding information processing involved in responses to escalated encounters with anonymous opponents, which cause the renowned winner and loser effects (Rutte et al. 2006). If the costs of information acquisition and management are of importance for the question of which type of reciprocity should be most common, clearly generalized reciprocity would win the game.

The capacity for the simple memory of social experience required for generalized reciprocity exists probably in all biological organisms. Bacteria, for instance, have been shown to respond to the secretion of exoproducts such as iron-sequestering siderophores by secreting these substances themselves (Darch et al. 2012; reviewed in West et al. 2007b; Williams et al. 2007) despite the potential exploitation by 'cheaters' from different clones capitalizing on their siderophore production (Diggle et al. 2007; Rumbaugh et al. 2009; Cordero et al. 2012; Dandekar et al. 2012). Therefore, if there is no mechanism selecting against public goods production contingent on others benefitting you similarly, generalized reciprocity might be expected to be a ubiquitous mechanism. Several studies have in fact suggested that the conditions for generalized reciprocity to evolve are widespread (Box 4.3). It is difficult, however, to prove that animals apply this simple rule in natural interactions, because potential alternative explanations need to be ruled out. This requires rigorous experiments involving behavioural manipulations to exclude alternative decision rules. Hitherto, only a handful of species has been studied by applying the required experimental rigor, showing that both humans and non-human animals do apply the decision rule characterizing generalized reciprocity (see Box 4.3).

The time structure of reciprocity may take two forms: simultaneous versus successive exchange of service and commodities. What might appear like a small detail can in fact make a significant difference for the functionality of reciprocal exchange.

(1) *Simultaneous exchange of services, trading of commodities and cooperative coaction*: If helping another individual is contingent on an immediate response of the receiver, it is easy to avoid being exploited (van Doorn et al. 2014). The decision to withhold effort if help is not reciprocated can be made 'in real time', i.e. the trading of commodities is transparent to all partners involved. This kind of simultaneous collaboration is apparently widespread, but has been little studied to date. Many cooperative behaviours such as predator inspection (Milinski et al. 1990; Pitcher 1991), cooperative hunting (Boesch & Boesch, 1989) or joint territory defence (Krams et al. 2008) typically rely on concurrent social information exchange. In these instances, individuals can survey the behaviour

of their partners and respond immediately to their actions (McNamara et al. 1999). Furthermore, they may actively communicate with each other while establishing or maintaining cooperation (Noë 2006). This can generate co-action and advanced forms of behavioural coordination (Boesch & Boesch, 1989; Mendres & de Waal 2000; Schuster 2002). A typical example is mutual grooming among social partners, observed for instance in male chimpanzees (Machanda et al. 2014). In humans, it has been shown experimentally that synchronous action can foster cooperation, which is a powerful mechanism as it may help to mitigate the free-rider problem (Wiltermuth & Heath 2009).

(2) *Successive exchange of services involving a time delay between reciprocal actions*: If helping others is contingent on reciprocal exchange but there is some delay between actions of involved partners, there is uncertainty whether a helpful act may be paid back (Trivers 1971). The lack of information exchange between players when time structure of reciprocal exchange is discrete facilitates exploitation of help by cheaters (Harris & Madden 2002; Clutton-Brock 2009). As a result, animals are generally unlikely to pay in advance for an uncertain future benefit (Dugatkin 1997; Stephens et al. 2002). Nevertheless, if costs to donors are low and benefits to receivers are substantial, this kind of delayed reciprocity may still generate cooperation between group members (Wilkinson 1984; Carter & Wilkinson 2013; Taborsky 2013). In vampire bats, experiments revealed that social partners exchanged blood with each other primarily depending on demand and previously received help from the same partner (Carter & Wilkinson 2013). In such interactions, a long-term relationship between social partners may be conducive to successful reciprocation, as suggested by experiments with zebra finches (*Taeniapygia guttata*). These birds maintained high levels of cooperation in an iterated prisoner's dilemma game only when interacting with a long-term social partner (St-Pierre et al. 2009). Frequent reciprocal exchange of services such as allopreening may in turn also stabilize social relationships, as suggested in family-living buff-breasted wrens, *Cantorchilus leucotis* (Gill 2012).

It is important to note that even if there is a time delay before reciprocal benefaction, the basic principles of 'trading' apply (Binmore 2010; Box 4.5). Such exchanges may happen between social partners meeting only for a certain purpose and/or for a limited period of time, such as when simultaneous hermaphrodites trade eggs with one another (Fischer 1980, 1984; Sella 1985, 1988; Petersen 1995; Sella et al. 1997; Sella & Lorenzi 2000; Hart et al. 2016; Table 4.1). Eggs are much more expensive to produce than sperm; therefore, in simultaneous hermaphrodites it is more attractive to play the male role when mating with a partner in order to produce zygotes. This is probably the reason why simultaneous hermaphrodites typically parcel their gametes in small portions, which increases the chances that an individual spawning just a few eggs will receive a number of eggs in return to be fertilized in the subsequent gamete release bout. In the polychaete worm *Ophryotrocha diadema*, for example, individuals in spawning dyads alternate sexual roles conditionally to their partner's behaviour, returning the favour of receiving eggs from their partner by quickly delivering eggs

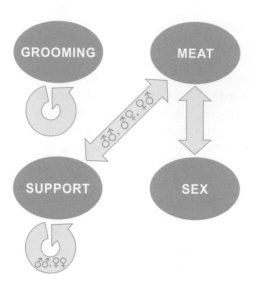

Figure 4.8 Scheme of commodity trading (also called 'interchange'; Hemelrijk 1990) in West African chimpanzees (from Gomes & Boesch 2011). Copyright © 2011, Springer-Verlag.

themselves, thereby adjusting the number of eggs they provide for fertilization to the number they have received from their partner (Picchi et al. 2018).

On the other hand, different services may commonly be traded against each other among long-term social partners or members of stable groups (Seyfarth & Cheney 1988). For instance, unrelated wild vervet monkeys, *Chlorocebus pygerythrus*, were experimentally shown to pay back (i) grooming service by social support (Seyfarth & Cheney 1984), and (ii) help they received to get food by subsequent grooming (Fruteau et al. 2009). In vampire bats, allogrooming received by a social partner caused individuals to pay back with food donations (Carter & Wilkinson 2013). In many primates, grooming is regularly exchanged against the same and other commodities, such as access to food, mating opportunities, social and agonistic support, or help in offspring care (see Table 4.1 for many examples). In chimpanzees, for example, food is traded against agonistic support and mating opportunities (Byrne 2007; Gomes & Boesch 2011; Figure 4.8), and rats were found to trade allogrooming against food donations (Schweinfurth & Taborsky 2018b; cf. Figure 4.7). A meta-analysis of the relationship between allogrooming and agonistic support including 36 studies of 14 primate species revealed an overall significant positive correlation, suggesting that allogrooming and social support might reflect a prototype of reciprocal cooperation in primates (Schino 2007). The cognitive mechanisms and decision rules underlying such type of exchanges may in fact be simple (Seyfarth 1977).

The prevalence of reciprocal cooperation in a wide range of taxa, spanning from polychaete worms to humans (Bowles & Gintis 2013; Picchi et al. 2018), supports the idea that the exchange of same or different commodities between social partners

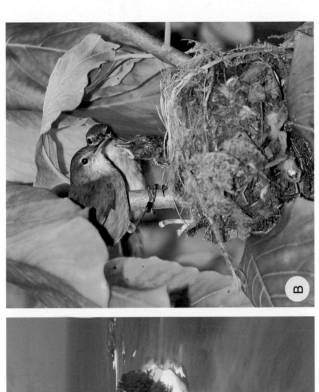

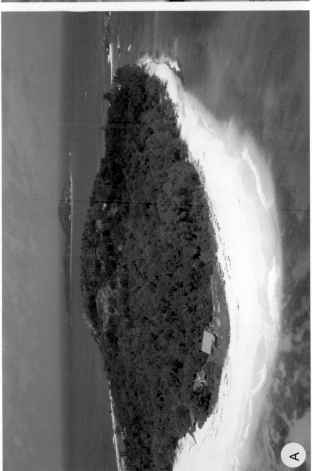

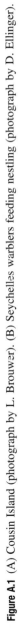

Figure A.1 (A) Cousin Island (photograph by L. Brouwer). (B) Seychelles warblers feeding nestling (photograph by D. Ellinger).

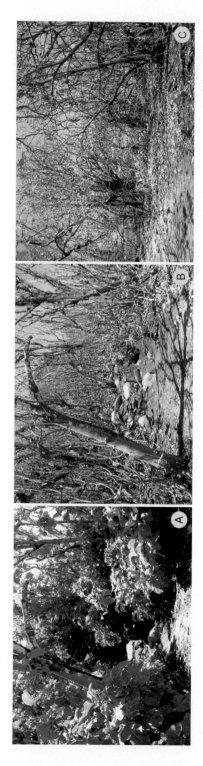

Figure A.5 The patterns of local vegetation vary greatly between breeding seasons in the same part of Cousin Island (temporal variation; A, B) and between different parts of the island (spatial variation; A, C). Warbler groups and individuals are exposed to large fluctuations in temperature, rainfall and wind exposure, which in turn are responsible for large fluctuations in vegetation growth and concurrent insect availability within and between years). These conditions generate differences in fecundity and survival between individuals and groups (Komdeur 1996b; Komdeur & Daan 2005; Komdeur & Pels 2005; Brouwer et al. 2006; Komdeur et al. 2016. Photographs: Van de Crommenacker).

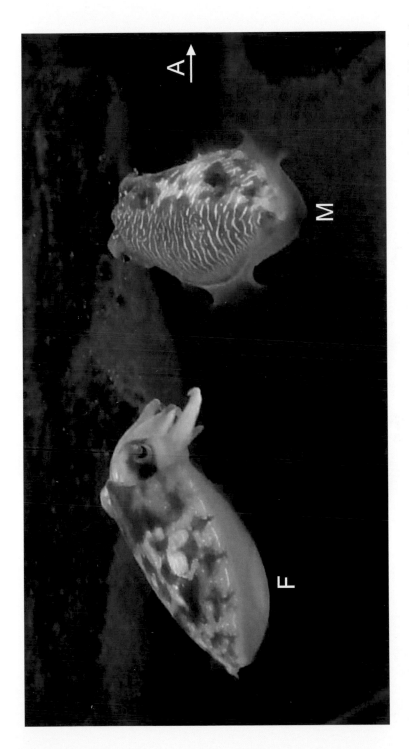

Figure 2.6 Tactical deception in male mourning cuttlefish. Male cuttlefish (M) displaying a male-specific pattern towards a female (F) while simultaneously displaying deceptive female colouration towards a rival male (A). Reproduced with permission from Brown et al. (2012). © 2012 The Royal Society.

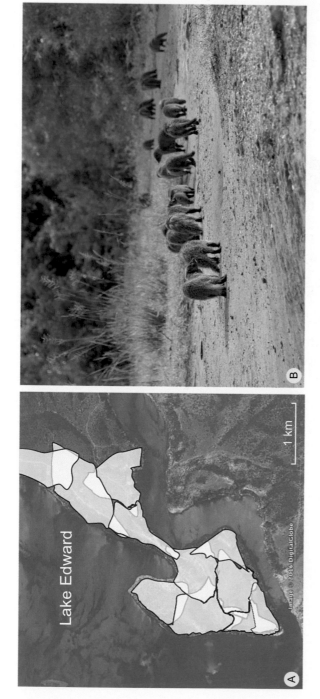

Figure B.1 (A) Map of Mweya peninsula, Queen Elizabeth National Park, Uganda, showing approximate home ranges of 11 study groups. At the study site in Uganda banded mongooses live in groups averaging 20 adults, plus offspring. Groups give birth on average four times per year, and offspring are kept underground for the first month of life. After pups emerge from the den they travel with the group and are provisioned by adults for a further 6 weeks. Females produce their first litters at around 1 year of age. Males form a dominance hierarchy in which the oldest two or three males in each group monopolize matings and paternity. For a detailed account of the study site and system, see Cant et al. (2013, 2016). (B) Banded mongooses setting out on a foraging trip. Groups sleep together each night in one of many underground dens in their territory, emerging at dawn to forage together for several hours, scouring the ground and digging for insects, arachnids and small vertebrates. (B) © Faye Thompson.

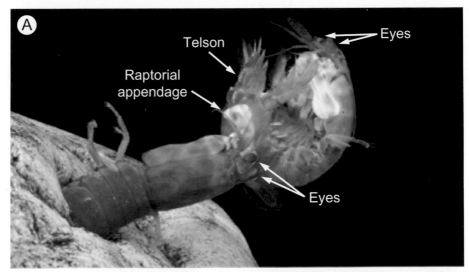

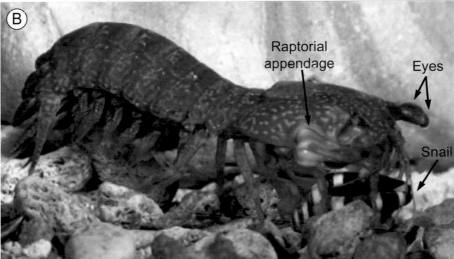

Figure 3.16 Contests with a deadly weapon in mantis shrimp. (A) Mantis shrimp of the genus *Neogonodactylus* deliver powerful strikes to opponents using a raptorial appendage. In this top image there are two shrimps: the shrimp on the right is defending against a strike by coiling its telson (terminal segment) in front of its body. (B) The shrimp use the raptorial appendage to kill prey. Here the raptorial appendage is in a raised, pre-strike position, about to deliver a blow to a snail. (Photo © Roy Caldwell. From Green et al. 2019.)

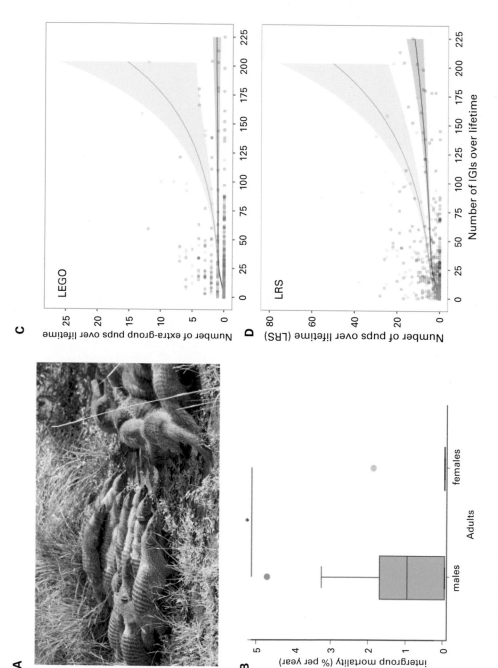

Figure 3.18 Exploitative leadership by females leads to hyperviolent intergroup conflict in banded mongooses. (A) Banded mongoose battle lines during an intergroup interaction or IGI (photo: Dave Seager). (B) Costs of intergroup aggression in male and female banded mongooses. Mortality rate of adult males and females resulting from intergroup aggression. (C) Lifetime number of extra-group offspring (LEGO; top panel) and lifetime reproductive success (LRS; bottom panel) of males (blue) and females (orange) are plotted against the number of IGIs in which individuals were involved across their lifespan. N = 499 males and 367 female adults monitored from birth to death over 20 years.

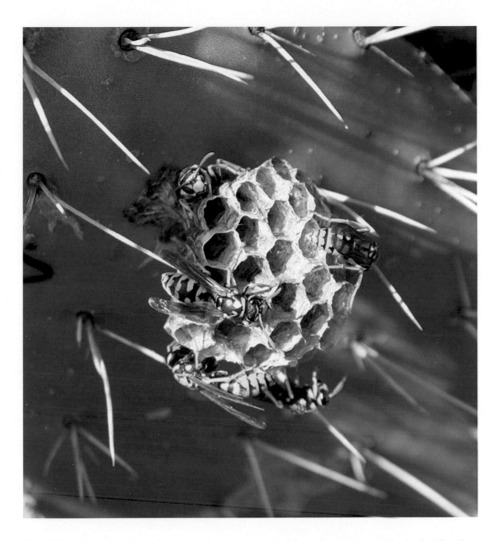

Figure C.1 A founding phase *P. dominula* nest suspended from an *Opuntia* cactus leaf at Conil de la Frontera, Spain. Six foundresses are visible on the nest. The first offspring have reached the pupal stage, visible toward the top of the nest, and will soon emerge as workers to help raise a younger brood. © Michael Cant.

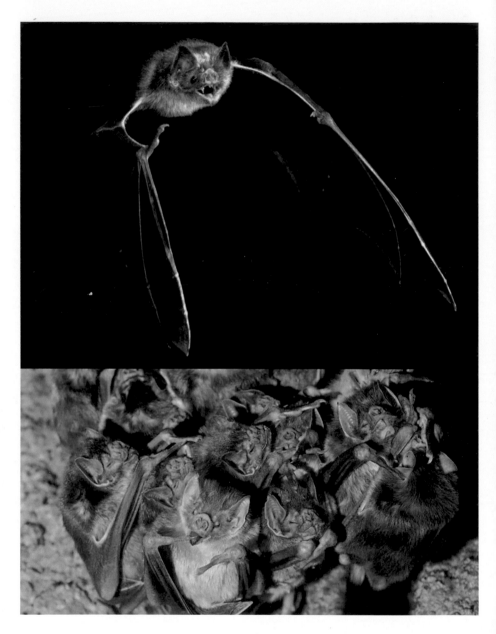

Figure 4.4A Common vampire bat in flight and resting in a social group in day roost (from Wilkinson 2019). © 2019 Elsevier Ltd.

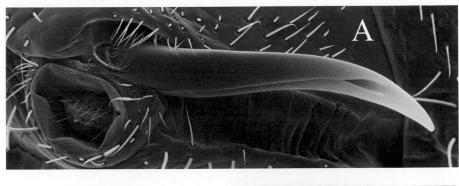

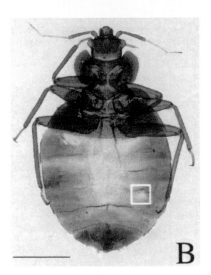

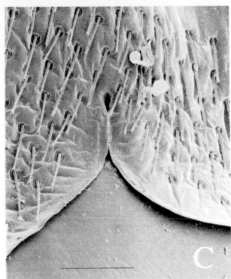

Figure 4.25 (A) The intromittent organ, specialized to deliver sperm during copulation, of the male bed bug (modified paramere). The groove in which the paramere sits when not in use is visible underneath the paramere (bar = 0.1 mm). (B) The site of copulation on the ventrum of the female's abdomen. The male always copulates at this site (bar = 1.5 mm; from Stutt & Siva-Jothy 2001). (C) Detail of the copulation site on the female's abdomen showing the incurving of the female's sternite, which acts as a guide for the male's intromittent organ (bar = 0.1 mm). (A) and (C) © Andrew Syred (Microscopix, UK), Science Photo Library. (B) Copyright © 2001, The National Academy of Sciences, USA.

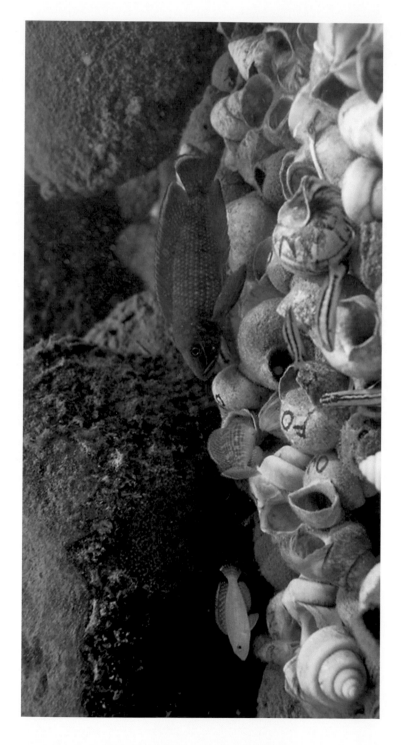

Figure 4.33 Nest of *Lamprologus callipterus* consisting of empty snail shells. From right to left: nest male (large, dark), female (inspecting a shell; mottled, seen from behind) and dwarf male (farthest left, pale). In the foreground (middle) there are three specimens of a different species (striped; *Telmatochromis vittatus*). (From Wirtz-Ocaña et al. 2013.) © 2013 The Authors. *Ecology and Evolution* published by John Wiley & Sons Ltd; open access.

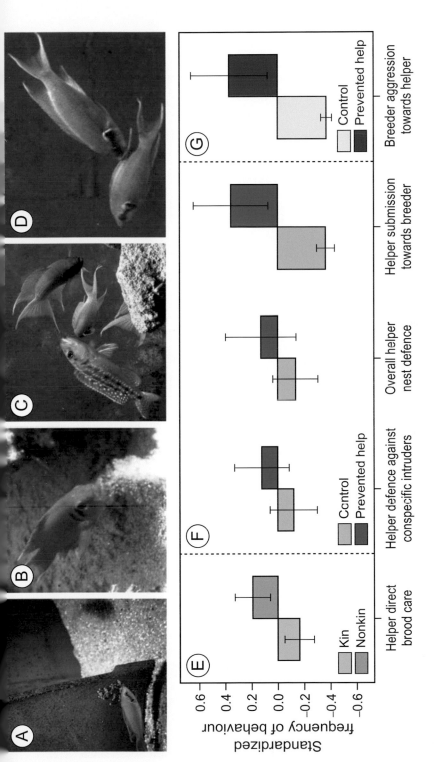

Figure D.1 Cooperative and aggressive behaviours of *N. pulcher*. Subordinate helpers show brood care by cleaning the eggs of breeders (A), by performing nest maintenance such as digging out sand from shelters (B) and by defending the territory against predators, such as *Lepidiolamprologus elongatus* (C). These helping behaviours are prompted by aggression from the breeders. In (D), a breeder (right) shows aggression towards a subordinate, and the subordinate responds with submissive behaviour (tail quiver). Panels (E–G) summarize the results of experimental manipulations from several studies. Bars show the mean of the standardized frequency of behaviour, with error bars denoting the standard error of the standardized behaviour frequencies. (E) Unrelated helpers (purple) provide more help than related ones (green; Zöttl et al. 2013a). (F) After subordinates have been prevented from giving help (dark blue), they compensate by increasing their previous help and submission level (light blue), presumably in an attempt to appease the breeder (Bergmüller & Taborsky 2005; Fischer et al. 2014). (G) Aggression levels in the group are normally very low (cream), but they increase considerably when subordinates are experimentally prevented from helping (red; Fischer et al. 2014; after Quiñones et al. 2016).

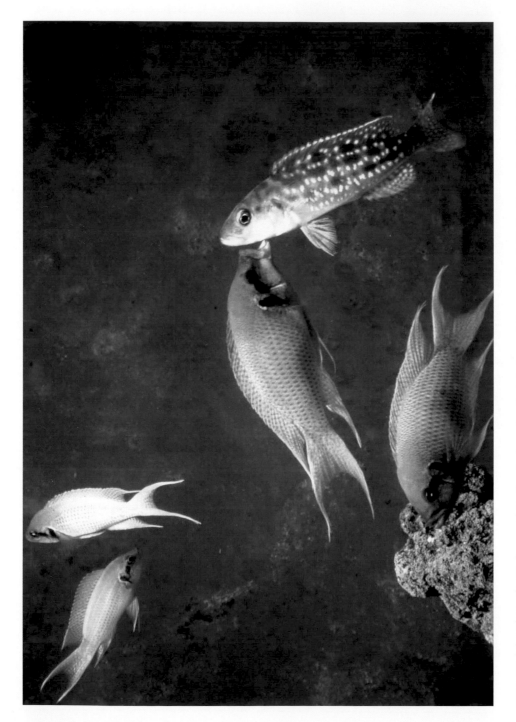

Figure D.3 A breeder male attacks a predator threatening subordinate helpers of the group (top left); the breeder female is in the foreground.

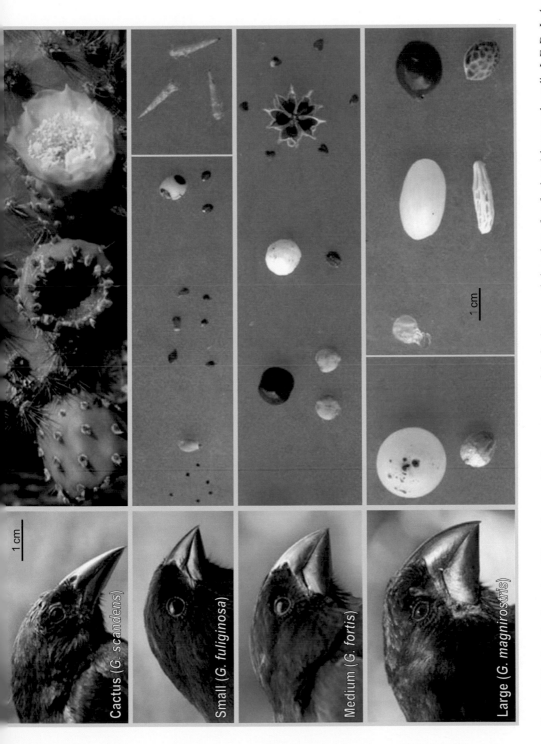

Figure 5.3 The four focal species of Darwin's ground finches and some of the food types and sizes they often feed on (photograph credit: L.F. De León; from De León et al. 2014). © 2014 The Authors. Journal of Evolutionary Biology © 2014 European Society For Evolutionary Biology.

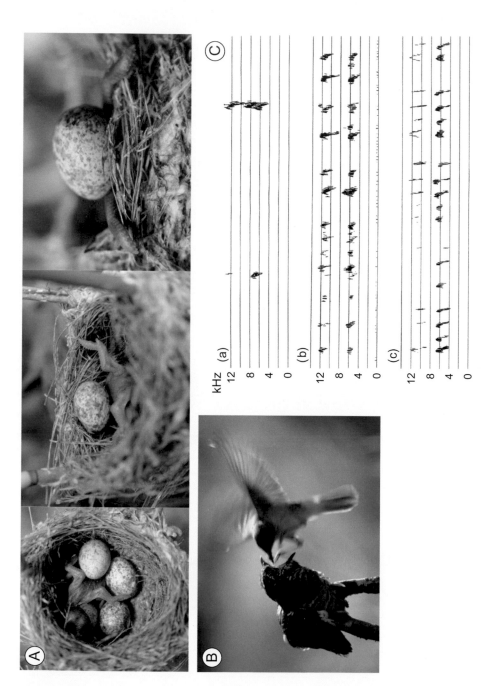

Figure 5.7 Cuckoo brood parasites destroy the reed warbler hosts' reproductive success without resistance. (A) Shortly after hatching, the cuckoo chick ejects the host eggs one by one, balancing them on its back and heaving them over the edge of the nest. (B) The reed warbler hosts continue to feed the young cuckoo even as it becomes significantly bigger than themselves (photographs credit O. Mikulica). (C) Sonograms (2.5 s) of the begging calls, recorded 60 min after feeding to satiation, of a single reed warbler chick, a brood of four reed warblers and a single cuckoo chick (from Davies et al. 1998).

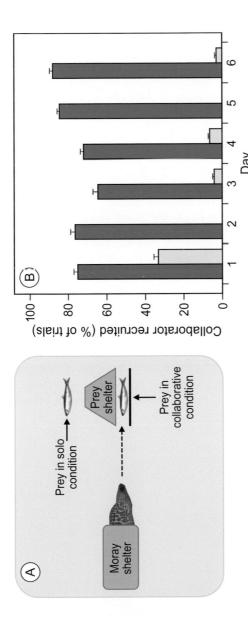

Figure 5.11 Experiment revealing that coral trout choose appropriately when and with whom to collaborate. (A) Bird's eye view of the experimental setup. (B) Results of experiment involving eight trout participating in up to four trials per condition per day for six days, with solo (prey in the open) and collaborative (prey in a crevice) trials alternated within test periods (dark green bars represent collaborative trials and light yellow bars represent solo trials; means and standard errors are shown; from Vail et al. 2014).

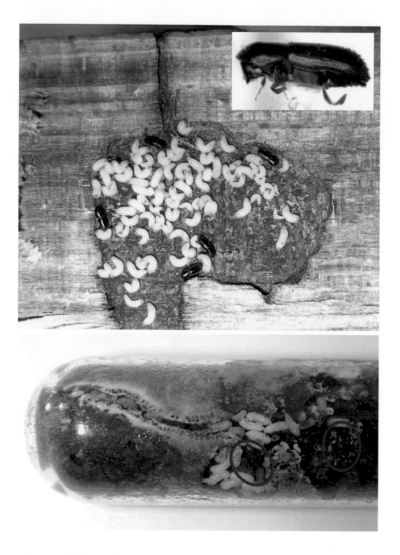

Figure E.1 Gallery of *Xyleborinus saxesenii* in the field (above; with adult female shown in the insert) and in the laboratory (below; adult females located amidst the white larvae are encircled). Photos: Peter Biedermann.

Box 4.5 Biological Markets and Cooperation

The exchange of goods and services between individuals often appears to be influenced by the law of supply and demand, similar to human market economy (Noë et al. 1991). Indeed, it has been postulated that biological markets pervade virtually any cooperative interaction between individuals, regardless of whether they belong to the same or different species and whether the same or different commodities are exchanged (Noë & Hammerstein 1994, 1995; Werner et al. 2014; Hammerstein & Noë 2016). Biological markets face the same difficulty as reciprocal cooperation, where the danger of being exploited by defectors and free-riders is a destabilizing influence on cooperation. The evolution of specialization and increased dependence of trading partners on each other can protect trade from cheating (Hammerstein & Noë 2016).

There are currently few examples where biological market theory has been tested conclusively with the help of appropriate experiments. One reason for this limitation is that conventional models from human economics are of limited value to biology, because human trade often entails binding contracts (Hammerstein & Noë 2016). Another limitation is that quantitative predictions are notoriously difficult to make where different commodities are exchanged. Examples where exchanges based on a biological market can be scrutinized include interspecific mutualisms and symbioses (Kiers et al. 2011), where the genetic separation between species facilitates the evolution of specialization among interspecific trading partners (Hammerstein & Noë 2016). At the intraspecific level, different commodities may be traded against one another if appropriate control mechanisms exist. In vervet monkeys, for example, there is evidence that exchanges fluctuate according to the law of supply and demand. Low-ranking females that provided food received more allogrooming than they themselves gave, and when a second food-providing female was introduced, the service to the original food provider declined (Fruteau et al. 2009). Even if this experiment did not test quantitative predictions regarding the traded commodities, these results suggest that exchanges among animals may follow somewhat similar rules as those applied in human market economy.

The idea of biological markets has become popular in behavioural studies, especially of non-human primates (Figure 4.9). Monkeys and apes often spend large amounts of time grooming each other, with the recipients gaining benefits in terms of hygiene and social stress reduction (van de Waal et al. 2013). There is some evidence that grooming is exchanged for other types of benefit such as coalitionary support (Seyfarth 1977), escape from aggression (Barrett et al. 2002), tolerance at feeding sites (Tiddi et al. 2011) and mating acceptance (Barelli et al. 2011; Table 4.1). In many primate species young offspring seem to constitute social value and are hence a source of great interest and attraction to non-parent group members, and there is evidence that females groom mothers in exchange for permission to handle their offspring (Henzi & Barrett 2003; Fruteau et al. 2011a, 2011b; Slater et al. 2007). The reasons why handling

Box 4.5 (*cont.*)

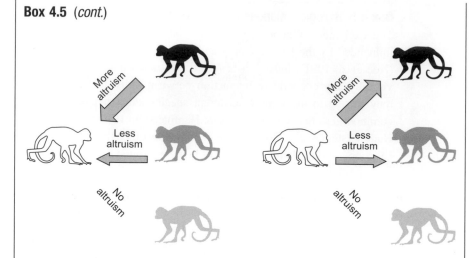

Figure 4.9 Partner choice based on received benefits. Arrows represent altruistic behaviours (or events). Animals can choose which partner to help how much. From Tiddi et al. (2011). Copyright © 2011, Oxford University Press.

offspring is valued so highly by non-mothers are still unclear. Mothers are often reluctant to allow access to their offspring, and it has been suggested that infant handling may in fact involve a subtle form of harassment (Silk et al. 2003). The grooming market in some primates is therefore a good example to illustrate the combination of both negotiation and subtle forms of coercion in reciprocal inter-actions. Nevertheless, for a rigorous test of quantitative predictions of market theory in this context the behavioural effects on fitness, or on good fitness correlates, would need to be determined, which is a worthwhile challenge for future studies.

An unfortunate misunderstanding of the application of market concepts to reciprocal trade among animals is that biological markets represent an *alternative* explanation to the four basic explanatory principles of the evolution of cooperation outlined above: (1) (by-product) mutualism; pay-offs correlated by (2) reciprocity or (3) shared genes; and (4) enforcement. In particular, biological markets have been misinterpreted as an alternative to the concept of reciprocity (Hammerstein & Noë 2016). However, the existence of a 'market', i.e. the availability of alternative options and the possibility to choose one's exchange partners, cannot by itself explain why goods and services are exchanged in the first place. To answer this question, one or the other of the four mentioned principles must be invoked, if the observed behaviour is a product of natural selection. The fact that individuals may choose from a range of potential partners to interact with may complicate the analysis of a cooperative interaction, but it cannot be an alternative explanation of cooperation. In other words, if individual A can choose to groom either individual

---

Box 4.5 (*cont.*)

B or individual C, both unrelated, evolutionarily speaking the decision to groom one of them depends on the expectation of future returns from that individual as opposed to those from the other partner. The underlying principle responsible for the cooperative act is hence *reciprocity* (Schino & Aureli 2010b).

---

functions by the application of simple decision rules produced by natural selection. In Table 4.1 we list 95 vertebrate species making use of reciprocal cooperation, and this list is not nearly comprehensive, even with respect to vertebrates. For instance, beyond the examples given in this table, male cooperation in reproduction following the principles of either mutualism or reciprocity has been described in 33 fish species reviewed in Taborsky (1994, 2008) and in 87 species of invertebrates, fishes, reptiles, birds and mammals reviewed in Diaz-Munoz et al. (2014). In the past, scepticism has been expressed regarding the importance of reciprocal interactions in nature because of alleged cognitive demands involved in such cooperation (Hammerstein 2003; Stevens & Hauser 2004; Stevens et al. 2005). This view has been contested (Ligon 1983; Wiley & Rabenold 1984; Rutte & Taborsky 2008; Schino & Aureli 2010c; Taborsky 2013; Carter 2014; Dolivo et al. 2016; Taborsky et al. 2016; Schweinfurth & Call 2019a; Kettler et al. 2021). Our review of the pertinent literature shows that reciprocity is neither rare in nature nor confined to taxa possessing large brains and highly advanced cognitive faculties. Even polychaete worms can exchange benefits reciprocally following conditional decision rules (Picchi et al. 2018). There is hence little doubt that virtually *any* animal has the potential to apply the decision rules of generalized and direct reciprocity, and the intriguing question is rather under which circumstances animals make use of this potential (Taborsky 2013; Carter 2014; Schweinfurth & Call 2019a).

4.1.2.1.9 *Negotiations and Trading*

Reciprocal exchange of goods and services usually involves some sort of negotiation between social partners. A context well illustrating the importance of negotiations in nature is biparental care (Houston & Davies 1985; McNamara et al. 1999). This form of parental invesment typically involves negotiations between mates that are interdependent on each other due to their common stakes – the shared offspring (Roberts 2005). Each pair member could gain if the respective partner assumed a higher share of parental effort. How much each of them invests in the care of their offspring may depend on an intricate negotiation process involving reciprocity, where continued effort in offspring care is contingent on previous investment of the partner (which is predictive of their future investment decisions), and coercion, whereby mates attempt to leave each other holding the baby by spending as little effort as possible without risking the brood, or by threatening outright desertion of the brood (Barta et al. 2002; Houston et al. 2005; Lessels & McNamara 2012; Johnstone & Savage 2019).

Studies of biparental care, primarily in birds and fish, revealed the difficulty for parents to find an optimal response to their partner's investment when attempting to maximize fitness by provisioning their offspring, while at the same time striving to minimize their own effort (Grüter & Taborsky 2005; Steinegger & Taborsky 2007; Johnstone et al. 2014; Iserbyt et al. 2015; Bebbington & Hatchwell 2016; Savage et al. 2017; Baldan et al. 2019; Smiseth 2019; Storey et al. 2020). Specialization of parents into different tasks may mediate the conflict between them, because of synergistic benefits of cooperation (Barta et al. 2014).

Such interactions between unrelated individuals (e.g. parents) involving a series of interactions in which social partners negotiate about how much to invest in a common interest (e.g. brood) suggest that natural selection may determine evolutionarily stable negotiation rules in a wide range of contexts (McNamara et al. 1999). In contrast to exchanging commodities voluntarily, negotiations between social partners may involve also a component of coercion (cf. Chapter 3 and Section 4.2.1). For instance, allogrooming may be demanded as a service by aggressively challenging another group member, as has been suggested by positive correlations determined between aggression given and grooming received in meerkats, *Suricata suricatta* (Madden & Clutton-Brock 2009), and Barbary macaques, *Macaca sylvanus* (Carne et al. 2011). Aggression and threats of eviction from the group may serve to generate a large variety of cooperative behaviours from subordinate group members ('pay-to-stay': Gaston 1978, Taborsky 1985), which will be outlined in Section 4.2.

In conclusion, the types of reciprocity that we should expect to find most often in nature may (i) involve an exchange of commodities that allows for immediate mutual adjustment of benevolence; this adjustment is facilitated if the exchange of services is either concurrent (e.g. coaction; van Doorn et al. 2014), or if it occurs among long-term social partnerships (e.g. attitudinal reciprocity: de Waal 2000; altruism as a signal: Roberts 1998; McNamara et al. 2008). Alternatively, (ii) reciprocal cooperation may be based on simple decision rules such as 'help anyone if helped by someone' (generalized reciprocity), which are not limited by constraints and costs of information acquisition and processing. There is ample evidence for the prevalence of the former, also including interspecific interactions (e.g. coral–zooxanthellae endosymbiosis) as outlined in Chapter 6, but it has not yet been scrutinized how widespread the latter mechanism is in biological systems, despite experimental demonstration of its functionality.

In some natural systems, the occurrence of apparent altruism is difficult to understand because the potential (future) benefit to the altruist is obscure. For example, altruistic brood care was observed in the Antarctic plunder fish (*Harpagifer bispinis*). Female plunder fish prepare nest sites, spawn and guard their eggs for 4–5 months until the eggs hatch, which is the longest brooding period reported for any fish (Breder & Rosen 1966). If the guarding female is removed, a second conspecific, usually a male, arrives to assume nest guarding, and in turn, if this guard is removed, another male assumes guarding. The reason that replacement guards are males is that in the Antarctic environment females are limited. The presence of a guard is necessary for egg survival. The guard prevents fungal growth that otherwise destroys unguarded nests within weeks, and protects the nest from major egg predators, such as starfish and sea urchins (Daniels 1978). When a starfish reaches the nest, the guard takes the lead arm in its mouth and removes the starfish from the nest. When a sea urchin approaches the nest, the guard lifts it up and pushes it away from the nest. The guarding behaviour by replacement guards does not seem to serve any selfish purposes. For example, it does not improve the chances of obtaining a protected nest site as these were abundantly present. Guarding behaviour by replacement males does not appear to serve parental or alloparental care, because replacement guards were often males from other locations, which were hence very unlikely to be related to the female and eggs they guarded. Moreover, replacement males cannot expect reciprocation, because the previous guard had permanently disappeared (Daniels 1979). Even generalized reciprocity seems unlikely to explain the observed behaviour, because the replacement guards may not have received a helpful act in the past. Given that guarding behaviour by replacement guards does not seem to result in any fitness benefits to the guarding male, replacement guarding has been assumed to be truly altruistic (Daniels 1979).

In the Antarctic plunder fish conditions for the development of altruistic behaviours seem to be favourable, as the costs of guarding are apparently low. The feeding rate, growth and body condition are similar for guarding and non-guarding males (Daniels 1979). However, a condition for the evolution of cooperation between unrelated individuals is that unilateral exploitation of the recipient is avoided. In other words, cooperation among unrelated individuals can only evolve when cooperators obtain a net fitness benefit from their actions, which can be achieved by (by-product) mutualism or correlated pay-offs as outlined above, or by enforcement, which will be outlined in Section 4.2. In the example of the Antarctic plunder fish, if the behaviour of replacement nest guards were indeed altruistic, a non-guarding mutant would benefit by the apparent abundance of altruists readily taking over their brood care duty. Even if cheap, it is hard to imagine that the behaviour does not involve any costs, because it apparently involves behavioural effort. To understand the ultimate cause of the behaviour of replacement guards in this species, more information is required, such as long-term data on potentially accrued fitness benefits by guarding versus non guarding males, and genetic information to reveal whether replacement guards were indeed unrelated to the brood and the guards they replaced. Importantly, the peculiar alloparental care behaviour of Antarctic plunder fish is not a one-off; it has been described in several fishes and other aquatic animals (e.g. Farmer & Alonzo 2008; Ramos et al. 2012; Stiver et al. 2012; see Taborsky 1994 for review). One possibility to explain the alloparental behaviour of replacement guards might be selfish fitness benefits by increased mating opportunities, as suggested to explain alloparental care, for instance, in the polychaete worm *Ophryotrocha diadema* (Premoli & Sella 1995), in the tessellated darter (*Etheostoma olmstedi*; Stiver & Alonzo 2011) and in cases where neighbours steal broods apparently to improve their mating chances (e.g. three-spined stickleback, *Gasterosteus aculeatus*: Mori 1995; Kraak et al. 1999), where female fish often prefer to spawn in nests already containing eggs (e.g. Ridley & Rechten 1981; Marconato & Bisazza 1986; Knapp & Sargent 1989; Goldschmidt et al. 1993; Kraak & Groothuis 1994).

4.1.2.2   Kin Selection

As outlined in Section 4.1, William D. Hamilton (1963, 1964) argued that the Darwinian fitness of an individual is correlated with the frequency of its genes that are present in future generations and which are identical by descent. This implies that if individuals do not reproduce themselves they can gain 'indirect fitness' by enhancing the reproductive output of related individuals. In other words, an individual that does not breed can help to pass on copies of its genes by assisting the reproduction of relatives. This can be accomplished by improving the survival of the young they help to raise, or by enhancing the reproduction of related social partners they assist (e.g. Brown 1987; Mumme et al. 1989; Emlen 1991; Cockburn 1998; Clutton-Brock 2002; Roulin 2002; Koenig & Dickinson 2004; reviewed by West et al. 2007c). In cooperative breeders, the presence of such helpers can enhance the food delivery to the young they have not produced themselves, their growth rates and survival and the survival and productivity of the parents of these young (Brown 1980; Taborsky 1984; Mumme et al. 1989; Clutton-Brock et al. 2001; Gilchrist 2004; Brouwer et al. 2005; Hodge 2005; reviewed by Brown 1987; Emlen 1991; Taborsky 1994; Cockburn 1998; Hatchwell 1999; Clutton-Brock 2002; Roulin 2002; Koenig & Dickinson 2004, 2016).

The indirect fitness gains of cooperative behaviours have been considered as the most important and general explanation for the evolution of altruistic behaviour, defined as behaviour that is costly to the donor and beneficial to the recipient. Hamilton (1963, 1964) proposed that the investment in altruistic help should be positively influenced by the degree of relatedness between the actor and the recipient. Such kin-selected cooperation requires that three conditions are fulfilled. (i) The recipient and donor are genetically related. (ii) The recipient benefits from the help of the donor, for example in terms of increased survival or production of young. (iii) The relationship between fitness costs to the donor, fitness benefits to the recipient and relatedness between them complies with Hamilton's rule

$$rb - c > 0$$

where r is the genetic relatedness between the actor and the recipient based on common descent, b is the accrued fitness benefit to the recipient, and c is the fitness cost to the donor of expressing cooperative behaviour. Hamilton's rule predicts that the probability and level of cooperation will be higher if the net fitness gain of cooperation (product of b times r) is higher than c. The formulation of Hamilton's rule has generated a strong focus on kin selection in studies of the evolution of cooperation (Hamilton 1964, 1972; Grafen 1984; Taylor 1992a; West et al. 2002; Komdeur et al. 2008; for a discussion of the significance of alternative explanations of evolutionary mechanisms underlying cooperation, see Trivers 1971; Lehmann & Keller 2006a, 2006b; Clutton-Brock 2009; Taborsky et al. 2016; Komdeur et al. 2017).

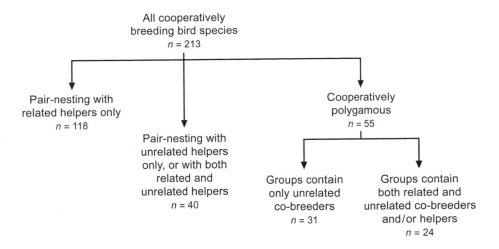

Figure 4.10 Classification of group composition and social mating system for all 213 species of cooperatively breeding birds for which data are available (from Riehl 2013). © 2013 The Author. Published by the Royal Society. All rights reserved.

The kin-selected or indirect fitness benefits accrued from helping have been used to explain the evolution of cooperative breeding systems observed in many arthropod and vertebrate species, particularly in birds (e.g. Brown 1987; Emlen 1997; Solomon & French 1997; Oli 2003; Koenig & Dickinson 2004; Wilson & Hölldobler 2005; Foster et al. 2006; West et al. 2007c; Bshary & Bergmüller 2008; Boomsma 2009; Cornwallis et al. 2010). However, in 213 cooperatively breeding bird species for which genetic relatedness of members of breeding groups and helping records were available, cooperative breeding by *unrelated* individuals was shown to be common, with 44 per cent of species breeding in social groups regularly including unrelated helpers, and in some cases social groups being composed entirely of unrelated adults (Figure 4.10; Riehl 2013). This suggests that helping behaviour may not only be driven by kin-selected (or indirect) fitness benefits.

Despite these observations of helping by unrelated individuals, the prevalence of helping in family groups, most conspicuously in eusocial hymenoptera, where haplo-diploid sex determination causes females to be more closely related to their sisters than to their own offspring, led to the assumption that kin selection is key to the evolution of altruism, cooperative breeding and eusociality (Trivers & Hare 1976; Queller & Strassmann 1998; Griffin & West 2003; Koenig & Dickinson 2004; Koenig et al. 2016). The explanation of the evolution of eusociality with permanently non-reproductive castes in haplodiploid organisms was originally based on the observation that females are more closely related to their full sisters ($r = 0.75$) than to their own offspring ($r = 0.5$) and to full brothers ($r = 0.25$; Hamilton 1964). By skewing the operational sex ratio towards more reproductive females through selective brood care, non-reproductive females could create a sex ratio in the brood that is favourable to their reproductive abstinence, which in turn would select for eusociality

(Trivers & Hare 1976). This is a reasonable assumption as workers, not queens, rear broods to adulthood. Several empirical studies on eusocial species have confirmed that workers bias their investment towards sisters (e.g. Crozier & Pamilo 1996; Queller & Strassmann 1998; Bourke 2005; West 2009) and subsequently bias brood sex ratios (e.g. Pamilo & Rosengren 1984; Pamilo 1990; Chapuisat & Keller 1999). A meta-analysis on social Hymenoptera reveals that workers bias colony sex allocation in their favour when relatedness asymmetry varies among colonies (Meunier et al. 2008). Another approach suggests that in species where dispersal is male-biased, implying female philopatry and non-local mating, haplodiploidy is in fact more favourable than diploidy to the evolution of reproductive altruism in females (Johnstone et al. 2012; Rautiala et al. 2019). However, a comparative analysis across all sexually reproducing eusocial taxa suggested that in general ecological factors are more important than haplodiploidy in favouring eusociality (Ross et al. 2013).

Two main hypotheses have been proposed by Hamilton (1964) by which individuals may derive indirect fitness benefits from cooperative behaviour. These are often considered as two forms of kin selection (Cant 2011). (1) Discriminate altruism in which the actor directs its cooperative behaviour only or preferentially to recipients that are genetically related (Hamilton 1964). Helpers can gain the most indirect fitness by directing help to the closest genetic relatives, which reflects 'kin discrimination'. As a consequence, the ability to assess the relatedness of individuals or groups of individuals, to discriminate between these individuals or groups of individuals, and to preferentially direct care towards kin are important determinants for the evolution of sociality (Komdeur & Hatchwell 1999). Only by responding differently to kin and nonkin can individuals obtain indirect fitness benefits. (2) Indiscriminate altruism may be favoured if dispersal is limited so that the average relatedness between actors and recipients of help is higher than that of the population at large. Under such circumstances, assessing the relatedness of individuals and discriminating between them is not a prerequisite for individuals to obtain fitness benefits (Berger-Tal et al. 2015). For example, individuals that live in viscous populations (i.e. populations with dispersal constraints) are more likely to interact with others that are more closely related than the population average, which does not involve any discrimination. Indeed, comparative studies provide evidence that individuals that live in groups consisting of close relatives are less likely to show discrimination between kin and nonkin. Kin discrimination was weaker when mean relatedness between individuals was higher (Figure 4.11; Cornwallis et al. 2009, 2010).

Although assortment and population viscosity provide conditions where altruism can spread even without the necessity to show kin discrimination, for instance by generalized reciprocity (Rankin & Taborsky 2009), this does not mean that kin discrimination cannot be effective under such circumstances. By recognizing relatives when living in viscous populations (i.e. by avoiding cooperation with individuals sharing relatedness below population average), higher kin-selected benefits can still be gained (Wolf & Trillmich 2008). As such, the two alternatives outlined above might be considered as two steps that can help the spread of altruism by kin selection with different intensity. First, the constraints on dispersal may lead to interactions among

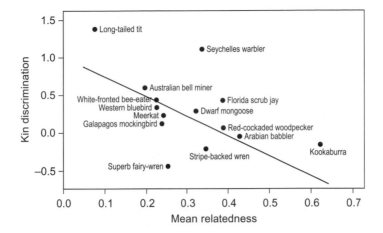

Figure 4.11 Kin discrimination in relation to average relatedness between individuals across 18 cooperatively breeding vertebrates. A positive value of kin discrimination corresponds to helpers preferentially helping closer relatives, whereas a negative value corresponds to the opposite pattern (mean relatedness: $F_{1, 10} = 7.80$, $P = 0.02$; solid line represents predicted relationship from the linear mixed model). From Cornwallis et al. (2009). © 2009 The Authors. Journal Compilation © 2009 European Society For Evolutionary Biology.

individuals that on average are more closely related than the rest of the population, and second, kin discrimination can occur within such viscous groups. Nevertheless, whether kin discrimination promotes cooperation depends on whether the optimal level of cooperation is a convex, concave or linear function of genetic relatedness (Faria & Gardner 2020).

A role of kin selection in the evolution of altruism can be tested, for instance in cooperative breeders, by determining whether helpers adjust their cooperative effort to the relatedness to recipients, i.e. the dominant breeders and their offspring. Usually, in such systems alloparental care is provided by subordinate group members. Studies of subordinate investment in species where estimates of relatedness between subordinates and nestlings are available provide mixed results regarding the evidence for discerning kin preference (Emlen 1997; Komdeur & Hatchwell 1999; Griffin & West 2003; Komdeur et al. 2007). Some studies have shown no relationship between the level of investment by subordinate helpers and kinship (Cockburn 1998; Clutton-Brock et al. 2000, 2001). Others have shown facultative adjustment of helping by subordinates toward close kin (Clarke 1984; Reyer 1984; Curry 1988; Emlen & Wrege 1988; Arnold 1990a, 1990b; Komdeur 1994b; Emlen 1997; Russell 2000; Sharp et al. 2005; Green et al. 2016), or help directed preferentially towards nonkin (Zöttl et al. 2013a).

In many situations where close genetic relationships were thought to exist (i.e. subordinates helping their 'social' parents), the occurrence of co-breeding by subordinates and of extra-group paternity (with young sired by males from outside the group) revealed lower levels of relatedness between subordinates and the offspring they help to raise than assumed from the social pedigree (e.g. Brooker et al. 1990; Mulder et al. 1994; Dickinson & Akre 1998; Richardson et al. 2001, 2003a, 2003b; Koenig & Dickinson 2004; MacColl & Hatchwell 2004; Dierkes et al. 2005; Covas et al. 2006; Wright et al. 2009). As a consequence, the reduced relatedness to recipients lowers the potential indirect fitness benefits of helping (see Riehl 2013 for review), which prompts a search for alternative explanations to kin selection (Cockburn 1998; McDonald 2014; Field & Leadbeater 2016; Gadagkar 2016).

Below we discuss several mechanisms through which cooperative and altruistic behaviour can spread or be maintained in populations by virtue of kin selection. We consider mechanisms allowing potential helpers to direct care preferentially to kin and between different classes of kin, and we discuss both the accrued fitness benefits and the evidence for apparent kin selected helping. We also discuss confounding effects that may mask accrued benefits and kin selected helping. We use cooperatively breeding species with 'helpers at the nest' (Skutch 1935) to illustrate the principles, but we discuss also other forms of social and cooperative behaviour in a variety of contexts.

4.1.2.2.1 *Evidence for Kin-directed Care in Social Systems*

Across a range of social animals the probability and amount of cooperation are associated with the degree of relatedness between helpers and recipients. Studies ranging from insects to mammals have demonstrated that brood care helpers exhibit a preference for joining and assisting close relatives (reviewed in Bourke et al. 1995; Crozier & Pamilo 1996; Emlen 1995, 1997; Komdeur & Hatchwell 1999; Griffin & West 2003; Koenig & Dickinson 2004, 2016; West et al. 2007c; Hughes et al. 2008; Cornwallis et al. 2009; Hatchwell 2009; Bourke 2011; Smith 2014; Green et al. 2016; Komdeur et al. 2017). For example, in some cooperative animals, when faced with a choice of potential nests to care for, helpers preferentially help the breeding pair to which they are more closely related (Table 4.2). Furthermore, some studies showed an effect of relatedness on the provisioning rate in cooperative breeders, with helpers showing higher levels of care for those to which they are more related (Table 4.2). A comparative analysis revealed that species-specific helper contributions to brood care in cooperatively breeding bird species increase with higher mean relatedness between helpers and recipients (Figure 4.12; Green et al. 2016). These results provide strong support for kin-selection driving the evolution of helping effort in cooperatively breeding birds (Green et al. 2016). Helpers apparently possess mechanisms by which they can assess relatedness to their social partners.

In contrast, at an intraspecific level, studies of several cooperatively breeding mammal, bird, fish and insect species have shown that helpers do not discriminate between kin and nonkin (Table 4.2). Although in insects such helpers often do distinguish between nestmates and non-nestmates, they do not distinguish among different degrees of relatedness among nestmates (Keller 1997; Queller et al. 2000; Leadbeater et al. 2011). Moreover, in some cooperative societies relatedness affects social interactions negatively (Table 4.2). The focus in this section will be first on kin-

Table 4.2. Examples showing (a) evidence for a preference to care for and about related individuals, (b) no correlation between relatedness and cooperation, i.e. no evidence for kin-directed care in cooperative breeders or kin-selected vigilance and sentinel behaviour, and (c) evidence for a preference to cooperate among less related or unrelated individuals in cooperatively breeding animals, i.e. relatedness negatively affects helping. Note: the dwarf mongooses studied in Serengeti National Park, Tanzania showed a preference to care for related individuals (Creel et al. 1991) whereas dwarf mongooses studied in the laboratory (Rasa 1977) and in the Taru Desert, Kenya (Rasa 1986) showed no preference to care for related individuals. The observed differences may be a consequence of different populations where different selection pressures operate.

Taxon	Reference
(a₁) Preference to care for related individuals	
Mammals	
Dwarf mongoose (*Helogale parvula*)	Creel et al. 1991
House mouse (*Mus domesticus*)	Rusu & Krackow 2004
Birds	
Bell miner (*Manorina malanophrys*)	Clarke 1984, 1989; Painter et al. 2000; Wright et al. 2009
Galápagos mockingbird (*Nesomimus parvulus*)	Curry 1988
White fronted bee-eater (*Merops bullockoides*)	Emlen & Wrege 1988; Emlen 1997
Pinyon jay (*Gymnorhinus cyamocephalus*)	Marzluff & Balda 1990
Florida scrub jay (*Apholecoma coerulescens*)	Mumme 1992
European bee-eater (*Merops apiaster*)	Lessells 1991
Seychelles warbler (*Acrocephalus sechellensis*)	Komdeur 1994b; Richardson et al. 2003a, 2003b
Western blue-bird (*Sialia mexicana*)	Dickinson et al. 1996
Carrion crow (*Corvus corone corone*)	Baglione et al. 2003
Sociable weaver (*Philetairus soci*)	Covas et al. 2006
Long-tailed tit (*Aegithalos caudatus*)	Russell & Hatchwell 2001; Sharp et al. 2005; Nam et al. 2010
Insects	
Polyembryonic wasp (*Copidosoma floridanum*)	Giron et al. 2004
(a₂) Kin-adjusted vigilance and sentinel behaviour	
Mammals	
Columbian ground squirrel (*Urocitellus columbianus*)	Carey & Moore 1986
Belding's ground squirrel (*Spermophilus beldingi*)	Sherman 1977
Round-tailed ground squirrel (*S. tereticaudus*)	Dunford 1977
Birds	
Siberian jay (*Perisoreus infaustus*)	Griesser 2003; Griesser & Ekman 2004, 2005
(b₁) No preference to care for related individuals	
Mammals	
Meerkat (*Suricata suricatta*)	Clutton-Brock et al. 2000
Dwarf mongoose (*Helogale parvula*)	Rasa 1977, 1986
African wild dog (*Lycaon pictus*)	Creel & Creel 2002
Banded mongoose (*Mungos mungo*)	Vitikainen et al. 2017
Birds	
Superb fairy-wren (*Malurus cyaneus*)	Dunn et al. 1995
White-browed scrubwren (*Sericornis frontalis*)	Magrath & Whittingham 1997; Whittingham et al. 1997
Galápagos hawk (*Buteo galapagoensis*)	DeLay et al. 1996

Table 4.2. (cont.)

Mexican jay (*Aphelocoma ultramarine*)	Brown & Brown 1980, 1990
Green woodhoopoe (*Phoeniculus purpureus*)	Du Plessis 1993
Stripe-backed wren (*Campylorynchus nuchalis*)	Rabenold 1985, Piper 1994
Red-cockaded woodpecker (*Picoides borealis*)	Walters 1990
Western bluebird (*Sialia mexicana*)	Dickinson 2004
Pied kingfisher (*Ceryle rudis rudis*)	Reyer 1980
Rifleman (*Acanthisitta chloris*)	Sherley 1990
White-winged chough (*Corcorax melanorhamphos*)	Heinsohn 1991
Florida scrub jay	Woolfenden & Fitzpatrick 1984
Arabian babbler (*Turdoides squamiceps*)	Zahavi 1990
Fish	
Lake Tanganyikan cichlid (*Neolamprologus pulcher*)	Le Vin et al. 2011
Insects	
European paper wasp (*Polistes dominulus*)	Queller et al. 2000

(b₂) No kin-adjusted vigilance and sentinel behaviour

Mammals	
Meerkat (*Suricata suricatta*)	Clutton-Brock et al. 1999
Columbian ground squirrel	Fairbanks & Dobson 2010
Degu (*Octodon degus*)	Quirici et al. 2013
Sooty mangabeys (*Cercocebus atys atys*)	Mielke et al. 2019
Birds	
Arabian babbler (*Turdoides squamiceps*)	Wright 1999

(c) Enhanced alloparental care by unrelated helpers

Mammals	
Dwarf mongoose (*Helogale parvula*)	Rood 1990
African wild dog (*Lycaon pictus*)	Creel & Creel 2002
Birds	
White-browed scrubwren (*Sericornis frontalis*)	Magrath & Whittingham 1997
Rifleman (*Acanthisitta chloris*)	Sherley 1990
Green woodhoopoe (*Phoeniculus purpureus*)	Ligon & Ligon 1978a
Fish	
Lake Tanganyika cichlid (*Neolamprologus pulcher*)	Stiver et al. 2005; Zöttl et al. 2013a

directed helping, continued with discussion of cases with no or negative social effect of relatedness on helping activities.

4.1.2.2.2   *Mechanisms to Promote Kin-directed Helping*

Helpers may preferentially benefit related recipients, by adjusting their investment using kin recognition mechanisms. There has been a long history of research on kin recognition (e.g. Holmes & Sherman 1983; Waldman 1988; Halpin 1991; Hepper

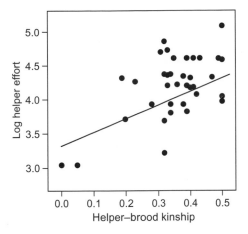

Figure 4.12 Helper effort (log-transformed) was positively related to helper–brood kinship across 36 bird species [log (effort) = 1.98 × kinship + 3.32; $t = 3.40$, $P = 0.002$, $R^2 = 0.23$]. The effect of kinship was still evident when excluding the two outlying species [cactus finch (*Geospiza scandens*) and pied kingfisher (*Ceryle rudis*)] with very low helper–brood kinship ($t = 2.03$, $P = 0.05$) (from Green et al. 2016). © The Authors 2016.

1991; Tang-Martinez 2001; Komdeur et al. 2008), but the proximate mechanisms underlying the discrimination of helper investment towards kin are not always clear. As outlined above, there are two principal mechanisms by which individuals can selectively assist related social partners: (i) inadvertent kin-directed care through spatial cues at the territory or population level caused by demographic population patterns, such as philopatry, sex-biased dispersal, high site fidelity, or high longevity; (ii) selective kin-directed care through using recognition mechanisms to discriminate between related and unrelated individuals. We discuss both mechanisms for kin-directed helping and elaborate on the importance of fine-scale genetic structure to the fitness consequences of individuals living in such structures and behavioural mechanisms by which animals reduce the negative fitness effects of among-kin competition.

4.1.2.2.3 Inadvertent Kin-directed Care

Kin-directed helping may not be based on an active differentiation between kin and nonkin (Clutton-Brock et al. 2001; Clutton-Brock 2002; Canestrari et al. 2005). There are several conditions and, sometimes, simple mechanisms by which inadvertent kin-directed helping may ensue. For example, if individuals live in social groups containing predominantly close relatives, or live in local clusters of related individuals, it is not necessary to recognize kin to gain indirect fitness benefits from being cooperative and no adjustment in helping effort is expected (Cornwallis et al. 2009). Local associations of close kin have been observed in populations of a large number of species across a wide range of taxa (Table 4.3).

Table 4.3. The presence of local genetic clusters resulting from philopatry. Examples include cooperatively breeding species in which young delay dispersal and remain on their family territories, and non-cooperatively breeding species also showing limited (natal) dispersal.

Non-cooperatively breeding species	Reference
Mammals	
Common marmoset (*Callithrix jacchus*)	Faulkes et al. 2003
Gundi (*Ctenodactylus gundi*)	Nutt 2008
Yellow mongoose (*Cynictis penicillata*)	Vidya et al. 2009
African wild dog (*Lycaon pictus*)	Girman et al. 1997
Mound-building mouse (*Mus spicilegus*)	Garza et al. 1997
Naked mole-rat (*Heterocephalus glaber*)	Reeve et al. 1990
Great gerbil (*Rhombomys opimus*)	Randall et al. 2005
Banded mongoose (*Mungos mungo*)	Nichols et al. 2012a
Birds	
Stripe-backed wren (*Campylorhynchus nuchalis*)	Yáber & Rabenold 2002
Grey-crowned babbler (*Pomatostomus temporalis*)	Edwards 1993
White-winged chough (*Corcorax melanorhamphos*)	Beck et al. 2008
White-throated magpie-jay (*Calocitta formosa*)	Berg et al. 2009
Cabanis's greenbul (*Phyllastrephus cabanisis*)	Vangestel et al. 2013
Apostlebird (*Struthidea cinerea*)	Woxvold et al. 2006
White-breasted thrasher (*Ramphocinclus rachyurus*)	Temple et al. 2006, 2009
Sociable weaver (*Philetairus socius*)	Covas et al. 2006
Superb fairy-wren (*Malurus cyaneus*)	Double et al. 2005; Harrisson et al. 2013
Guira cuckoo (*Guira guira*)	Lima et al. 2011
Karoo scrub-robin (*Cercotrichas coryphaeus*)	Ribeiro et al. 2012
Fish	
Lake Tanganyika cichlid (*Neolamprologus pulcher*)	Dierkes et al. 2005
Insects	
Ambrosia beetle (*Xylosandrus germanus*)	Peer & Taborsky 2005
Non-cooperatively breeding species	**References**
Mammals	
Pilot whale (*Globicephala melas*)	Amos et al. 1991
Dolphin (*Stenella coeruleoalba*)	Gaspari et al. 2007
Polar bear (*Ursus maritimus*)	Zeyl et al. 2009
Beaver (*Castor canadensis*)	Crawford et al. 2009
Dusky-footed woodrat (*Neotoma fuscipes*)	McEachern et al. 2007; Innes et al. 2012
Birds	
Manakin (*Manacus manacus*)	Shorey et al. 2000
Black grouse	Höglund et al. 1999
Barnacle goose (*Branta leucopsis*)	Anderholm et al. 2009
Cackling Canada goose (*Branta canadensis minima*)	A.C. Fowler 2005
Common eider (*Somateria m. mollissima*)	McKinnon et al. 2006; Hario et al. 2012
Vinous-throated parrotbill	Lee et al. 2010
Great tit (*Parus major*)	Garroway et al. 2013
Lesser kestrel (*Falco naumanni*)	Ortego et al. 2008
Fish	
Spotted eagle ray (*Aetobatus narinari*)	Newby et al. 2014
Trinidad guppy (*Poecilia reticulate*)	Piyapong et al. 2011
Squaretail coral grouper (*Plectropous arealoatus*)	Almany et al. 2013

Table 4.3. (cont.)

Non-cooperatively breeding species	Reference
Insects	
Red flour beetle (*Tribolium castaneum*)	Drury et al. 2015
Mycophagous beetle (*Phalacrus substriatus*)	Ingvarsson 1998
Fruit fly (*Drosophila melanogaster*)	Drury et al. 2009

Comparative analyses demonstrate that in species where the average relatedness between individuals in a group is higher and shows little variation between groups, kin discrimination is weaker (Griffin & West 2003; Cornwallis et al. 2009; Figure 4.11). This suggests that species that live in groups with closer relatives are less likely to show discrimination between kin and nonkin. High within-group relatedness can occur through low breeder turnover (high longevity), reduced dispersal (strong philopatry), or low levels of promiscuity (low extra-pair mating by the breeding pair). Below we will discuss the effect of each of these population characteristics on the occurrence of kin clusters and kin-directed behaviour.

4.1.2.2.3.1 *Longevity as a Driver for Inadvertent Kin-directed Cooperation*

Longevity affects kin structure and hence the potential that cooperation can entail kin-selected fitness benefits. In cooperatively breeding vertebrates, a dominant pair usually produces the majority of the offspring, while caring for the offspring is shared with non-breeding subordinate helpers (Skutch 1961; Brown 1987; Jennions & Macdonald 1994; Taborsky 1994; Solomon & French 1997; Cockburn 1998; Hatchwell & Komdeur 2000; Clutton-Brock 2002; Griffin & West 2003; Koenig & Dickinson 2004, 2016; Komdeur et al. 2017; Rosenbaum & Gettler 2018). Most cooperative breeding systems involve long-lived individuals that show a high degree of natal philopatry, with offspring delaying dispersal and deferring reproduction (Koenig et al. 1992; Arnold & Owens 1998). This results in an overlap of generations and in the formation of breeding groups consisting mainly of relatives. Long-lived individuals are often of higher quality than short-lived individuals (Gaillard et al. 2000; Cam et al. 2002; Beauplet et al. 2006), they may have higher reproductive success at all ages (Weladji et al. 2006; Hamel 2009a, 2009b) and high life-time fecundity (Hamel et al. 2009a). As such, long-lived and older individuals, which have produced several offspring, are more likely to live in kin associations than short-lived or young individuals (Johnstone & Cant 2010). Associated with longevity of parents that remain together as a breeding pair, delayed dispersal causes the formation of high local relatedness levels (all offspring being born to the same father and mother being siblings).

If parents are long-lived, offspring can develop a simple rule that does not require kin recognition: to help any individual on its natal territory to raise a subsequent brood, as these individuals are likely to be its parents or other close relatives and hence helpers will care for related beneficiaries. In the case when both parents remain alive, the focal individual will share half of its genes with its siblings and its potential offspring by common descent; helping to raise a sibling produced by the helper's parents is equivalent to breeding and raising offspring from the point of view of passing on genes to the next generation (Dawkins 1976). This allows helpers in long-lived species to gain kin-selected benefits without selective kin discrimination. This may work even if offspring have (temporarily) left their natal territory. For example, in the white-fronted bee-eater (*Merops bullockoides*) and the western bluebird, helpers are failed breeders and often return to their natal territory after dispersal to help their parents (Emlen & Wrege 1988; Dickinson et al. 1996). In the Galápagos mockingbird (*Nesomimus parvulus*), helping behaviour sometimes occurs among nonkin, and the care of helpers is better predicted by prior association with the parents than by kinship per se (Curry & Grant 1990). Similarly, in the Seychelles warbler (*Acrocephalus sechellensis*) the helping rule is based on the identity of parents rather than that of nestlings, and a rule such as 'help anyone who fed me as a nestling' (i.e. direct reciprocity) is the best predictor of care (Komdeur 1994b; Komdeur et al. 2004b).

The indiscriminate provisioning by helpers of those that are present on their natal territory is favoured if recognition errors are pervasive (Duncan et al. 2019), but it may be effective only under certain ecological, individual and social conditions. There are three major limitations of the underlying associative learning serving as a recognition mechanism. First, the rule outlined above – to help any individual that is present on the helper's natal territory to raise a subsequent brood – may lead to misdirected investment even in species that are relatively long-lived, because some parents may have lower survival resulting in a high turnover of breeders and consequently lower relatedness among group members. To put this differently, parents may die or disappear before the offspring have an opportunity to help them. Within species, there is often large variance in individual quality, and hence the local availability of kin in the population may vary as a function of correlates of individual quality (e.g. Beckerman et al. 2011). For example, individuals of better quality may settle in high-quality environments (high food abundance, absence of predators or parasites), have higher life expectancy and produce more offspring than individuals that are of inferior quality. Groups present in low-quality environments may exhibit higher breeder turnover, with a subsequent diminution of relatedness between helpers and recipients, which thus in case of indiscriminative helping may result in helping nonkin.

Second, many animal societies have extensive networks of kin of varying relatedness, which could either reduce selection for cooperation in the (natal) group, or increase selection for finer discrimination between different degrees of relatedness in order to enable cooperation among closer relatives. A kin structure with high variance in relatedness may be caused by high levels of promiscuity and infidelity, or high divorce rates among breeding pairs. Many cooperatively breeding species exhibit shared parentage of broods and extra-pair parentage (Cockburn 2004; Taborsky 2009). In cooperatively breeding birds, some of the highest promiscuity rates occur in the superb fairy-wren (with 76 per cent of offspring sired by extra-group fathers: Mulder et al. 1994), the Australian magpie (*Gymnorhina tibicen*, with 82 per cent of offspring sired by extra-group fathers: Hughes et al. 2003) and the Seychelles warbler (*Acrocephalus sechellensis*, with 44 per cent of offspring sired by extra-group fathers:

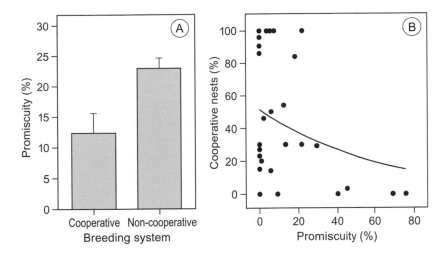

Figure 4.13 Promiscuity and cooperation. (A) Rates of promiscuity (percentage of broods with one or more offspring sired by an extra-group male) in cooperative and non-cooperative species. Promiscuity was significantly higher in non-cooperative than in cooperative species. Data shown are means ± SE. (B) The relationship between levels of cooperation (population with the lowest percentage of nests with helpers throughout the species range) and promiscuity in cooperative species. Helpers were present in a lower percentage of nests in species with higher rates of promiscuity. The line is the log-linear regression curve (from Cornwallis et al. 2010). Copyright © 2010, Nature Publishing Group.

Richardson et al. 2001; Hadfield et al. 2006). Theory predicts that high levels of promiscuity leading to low within-group relatedness may select against the occurrence of cooperation and altruism (Hamilton 1972; Charnov 1978a, 1982; Boomsma 2007, 2009). For example, if the mother in a sexually producing species mates with multiple males, the relatedness between an individual and its half-siblings will be lower than the relatedness to its own offspring, and selection for own breeding will be stronger than for helping. This is corroborated by the fact that, in general, the level of promiscuity in birds correlates negatively with the occurrence and amount of cooperative breeding. Furthermore, in cooperative species, helping is more common when promiscuity is low (Figure 4.13; Cornwallis et al. 2010). Nevertheless, helping does also occur for reasons other than supporting close kin, as revealed by a comparative analysis of cooperatively breeding birds (Kingma 2017).

However, promiscuity does not necessarily select against staying and cooperating in natal groups. For example, promiscuity in terms of shared parentage of broods may not have a major impact on a helper's relatedness to the brood provided that parentage is shared among relatives *within* the social group, as in acorn woodpeckers (Haydock et al. 2001) and superb fairy-wrens (Mulder et al. 1994). However, in those cases where parentage (usually paternity) is attributable to nonkin from *outside* the social group, a helper's kinship to the helped brood may be substantially reduced, e.g. in superb fairy-wren (Double & Cockburn 2003), Australian magpie (Hughes et al. 2003) and

Seychelles warbler (Richardson et al. 2001; Hadfield et al. 2006). It is intriguing that in these cases, cooperation and alloparental care are still the rule.

Third, in species with high longevity and breeding site fidelity, the proportion of groups or clusters consisting of relatives can also vary as a result of predation (Beckerman et al. 2011). If predation in viscous populations is centred on family groups where predators remove entire broods together with the breeders, rather than only a part of the brood, this may cause a skew of reproduction within a population, with few individuals having relatively high reproductive success. This also means that only a few individuals have the ability to produce clusters of recruited close kin resulting in higher levels of relatedness among adults in a population. This is the case in long-tailed tits, where corvids predate on whole broods together with the parents, causing a population structure with temporal increase in average relatedness among group members (Beckerman et al. 2011).

In the different scenarios outlined above, a helper may have few cues on its true relatedness to a brood. If the kin-selected benefits of helping are potentially larger than the direct benefits of helping that do not depend on kinship, it will be advantageous for potential helpers to employ selective kin discrimination through recognition, and preferential aid of relatives. This seems particularly important in eusocial insects such as ants, where non-reproductive workers have no direct fitness. In some ant species unrelated females join forces to found a colony. However, as soon as the first mature workers emerge, queens typically fight to the death until only one survives, thereby solving the problem of asymmetrical relatedness within the colony (Bernasconi & Strassmann 1999).

4.1.2.2.3.2 Limited Natal Dispersal

Hamilton (1964, 1972) proposed that high relatedness can arise in 'viscous' populations, which are characterized by low rates of juvenile dispersal from natal sites, leading to increased levels of relatedness between individuals in social groups or neighbourhoods within populations (see Section 3.3.1). Thereby, limited dispersal can be an important precondition for generating indirect fitness benefits of cooperation. Theoretical research has demonstrated that such population viscosity, which is often regarded synonymously to limited dispersal, results in kin-structured patches in which cooperative interactions may occur to gain kin-selected benefits (e.g. Queller 1992; Taylor 1992a, 1992b; Wilson et al. 1992; Balshine-Earn et al. 1998; Mitteldorf & Wilson 2000; Lehmann & Keller 2006b; Kümmerli et al. 2009a). In such populations, kin-directed helping might simply be a consequence of demographic viscosity rather than result from active choice (Clutton-Brock et al. 2001; Clutton-Brock 2002; Canestrari et al. 2005). Limited dispersal has been suggested as an important driving force for the evolution of cooperative breeding in vertebrates (Griffin & West 2002).

There is good support from empirical research for the importance of population viscosity in the evolution of sociality (e.g. Pope 1998; reviewed in Ekman 2004; Smith 2014). In most cooperative breeders, individuals are long-lived, defend permanent territories and show strong natal philopatry (e.g. Brown 1987; Stacey & Koenig 1990; Emlen 1991; Arnold & Owens 1998; Hatchwell & Komdeur 2000;

Cornwallis et al. 2009). Mature offspring typically delay dispersal and remain on their natal territory with their parents, or acquire territories close to their natal territory by a 'budding' process, creating a new territory situated partly in or adjacent to their natal territory (e.g. Woolfenden & Fitzpatrick 1978, 1984; Komdeur & Edelaar 2001; Dickinson et al. 2014). This results in an extended period of association between parents and offspring on the latter's natal territory (Brown 1987; Komdeur & Edelaar 2001; Fitzpatrick & Bowman 2016), which can lead to the formation of a spatial aggregation of extended kin groups.

Limited natal dispersal is often sex-biased. In many species, members of one sex disperse more frequently and over greater distances than members of the opposite sex (Lawson Handley & Perrin 2007). As a consequence, the non-dispersing sex may aggregate in kin groups (e.g. Queller & Goodnight 1989; de Ruiter & Geffen 1998; Tiedemann & Noer 1998; Surridge et al. 1999; Lawler et al. 2003), which can have profound consequences for the differential evolution of social behaviour in males and females. In cooperatively breeding birds and mammals with sex-specific dispersal, it is typically the philopatric sex which provides more help (Cockburn 1998; Russell et al. 2004). In social Hymenoptera dispersal is often male-biased, which, among other things, selects for helping to occur among females (Johnstone et al. 2012). Kin-selection benefits accrue under these conditions even without specific kin discrimination mechanisms.

An intriguing pattern is that natal dispersal is typically female-biased in birds and male-biased in mammals (Greenwood 1980; Dobson 1982; Wolff & Plissner 1998; Lawson Handley & Perrin 2007; Clutton-Brock & Lukas 2012). In the cooperatively breeding Karoo scrub-robin, which shows strong male natal philopatry, most males gain their first breeding position within a distance of two territories from their natal site. Once a male fills a breeding vacancy, it often stays in that territory. This high philopatry in males translates into a strong clustering of descendants around the natal site (Ribeiro et al. 2012). Such strong sex-biased philopatry and associated kin clustering of one sex has also been observed in other cooperative breeders, e.g. in the white-breasted thrasher (*Ramphocinclus brachyurus*: Temple et al. 2006), the superb fairy-wren (Cockburn et al. 2008) and the brown tree creeper (*Climacteris picumnus*: Doerr & Doerr 2006). In line with this male-biased philopatry, these species exhibit male-biased helping behaviour. Males can gain kin-selected benefits simply by helping any individual living on or near the natal territory, which may serve as a reliable indicator of kinship.

However, kin structures may also occur in species with sex-specific delayed dispersal, where the social group consists of more than one breeding pair and subordinates help several breeding pairs within the social group. This was demonstrated for the cooperatively breeding bell miner (*Manorina melanophrys*), which lives in colonies often comprising hundreds of individuals. Each colony consists of several coteries, containing multiple breeding pairs and non-breeders of both sexes. Within a coterie, individuals interact and help in raising young of more than a single breeding pair. Helpers do not assist in other coteries (Clarke 1989; Painter et al. 2000). Male offspring often remain in their natal coterie as helpers, whereas females disperse to neighbouring colonies to gain a breeding position (Clarke & Heathcote 1990). These characteristics determine the degree of genetic relatedness, especially among males within and between colonies. Within coteries, males are often highly related, whereas males present in different coteries, even within the same colony, show variable degrees of relatedness (Painter et al. 2000). In such situations, males may gain kin-selection benefits by remaining on the natal coterie to assist related coterie members, rather than by dispersing and helping in other coteries containing less related individuals. Bell miner helpers remaining in their natal coteries adjust their food provisioning effort according to their genetic relatedness to the broods they are provisioning, showing that individuals may correctly assess the genetic relatedness to breeding pairs within the coterie. Dispersing subordinates preferentially join coteries with highly related members, but once they have joined a new coterie, in contrast to helpers staying in their natal territory, dispersed helpers do not adjust their helping levels to the relatedness variation within their new group (Wright et al. 2009). Hence, the bell miner example demonstrates that the two described mechanisms, care based on kin discrimination and indiscriminate care within groups containing close relatives, may both operate within one species, depending on the natal philopatry of subordinates.

Limited (natal) dispersal either by one or both sexes also occurs in several species that do not breed cooperatively, where offspring remaining at home neither breed independently nor help others to raise young (e.g. Ekman et al. 2001; Ekman 2004, 2006; Komdeur & Ekman 2010; Table 4.4). In these species, limited dispersal may also have an effect on fine-scale genetic structuring. It is not fully understood why

Table 4.4. The occurrence of kin-structured populations as a consequence of joint dispersal of relatives in several cooperatively and non-cooperatively breeding species.

Cooperatively breeding species	References
Mammals	
Western gorilla (*Gorilla gorilla*)	Bradley et al. 2007
Red-fronted lemur (*Eulemur fulvus rufus*)	Port et al. 2009
Banded mongoose (*Mungos mungo*)	Nichols et al. 2012a; Thompson et al. 2017
Birds	
White-winged chough	Heinsohn et al. 2000
Tasmanian native hen	Goldizen et al. 2000
Long-tailed tit (*Aegithalos caudatus*)	Sharp et al. 2008
African lion (*Panthera leo*)	Packer et al. 1991; Packer & Pusey 1993
Acorn woodpecker (*Melanerpes formicivorus*)	Koenig et al. 2000
Brown jay (*Cyanocorax morio*)	Williams & Rabenold 2005
Insects	
Several species of polistine wasps	Peeters & Ito 2001
Non-cooperatively breeding species	**References**
Mammals	
Big brown bat (*Eptesicus fuscus*)	Metheny et al. 2008
Birds	
Vinous-throated parrotbill	Lee et al. 2009
Ground tit (*Parus humilis*)	Wang & Lu 2011

such species exhibiting delayed dispersal, which leads to family groups consisting of close relatives, lack helping behaviour of subordinate group members (Ekman et al. 2004; Ekman 2006, reviewed in Komdeur & Ekman 2010), but this form of family living is regarded as an essential stepping stone in the evolution of cooperative breeding (Griesser et al. 2017). In some species parents even seem to actively prevent offspring from helping (e.g. Verbeek & Butler 1981; Strickland 1991; Burt & Peterson 1993; Ekman et al. 1994). Delaying dispersal and living in genetic clusters can result in future direct benefits as a result of group augmentation, yielding either enhanced survival (e.g. by dilution effects, better predator defence or improved access to food) and/or enhanced (future) reproduction (Kingma et al. 2014). The direct benefits of living in genetic clusters obtained in non-cooperatively breeding species will be discussed below.

4.1.2.2.3.3 High Breeding Site Fidelity

Individuals may show strong breeding philopatry and return to breed in close proximity to their previous breeding or natal site. Where natal philopatry is coupled with long-term philopatry, breeding aggregations consisting of highly related individuals may form, which may facilitate the evolution of kin-selected cooperation. It has long been recognized that patterns of dispersal are related to the occurrence of cooperative breeding (Dickinson & Hatchwell 2004). However, not only limited natal dispersal as discussed above but also high breeding site fidelity may result in structured local kin structures as found in several cooperatively breeding species (Table 4.3).

Many waterfowl species are characterized by females that are philopatric not only to their natal area but also to their breeding sites (Anderson et al. 1992; Öst & Tierala 2011). Such philopatric behaviour may result in higher local relatedness among females within waterfowl populations, which may facilitate the evolution of kin-selected female cooperation (e.g. Andersson & Åhlund 2000; Semel & Sherman 2001; Nielsen et al. 2006; Waldeck et al. 2007; Jaatinen et al. 2009). Hitherto, this has rarely been examined in waterfowl. For example, in the colonially nesting common eider, females exhibit high levels of natal and breeding philopatry to breeding areas resulting in higher levels of genetic relatedness between females within breeding groups of a colony (McKinnon et al. 2006). Females escort their broods to the water shortly after hatching. They either raise their broods alone or form brood-rearing coalitions or 'crèches' with one to four other females, some of them non-breeders, which participate in protection of ducklings against avian predators such as gulls. Crèches may consist of a few up to over 150 ducklings. Once formed, a crèche tends to stay together throughout the brood-rearing period. Due to the relatedness structure, females that failed breeding may gain indirect fitness benefits by caring for related ducklings. In addition, the direct fitness benefits to coalition members are considerable, as the reproductive output of females in coalitions often exceeds that of solo parents (Öst et al. 2008).

It seems that eider duck coalitions are beneficial to females irrespective of whether they consist of kin associations. First, the kin-selected fitness benefits arising from cooperating with distant relatives seem less important than the substantial direct fitness benefits accrued to coalition-forming females due to the dilution of predation risk, improved predator detection and shared parental duties (Sharp et al. 2005; Nam et al. 2010). Second, there are costs associated with prolonged searching for suitable coalition partners, as predation on eider ducklings peaks in the first few days after hatching and prospective coalition partners need to hatch their broods within a week for successful cooperation (Öst et al. 2008).

A high breeding site philopatry and fine-scale genetic clustering has also been observed in other non-cooperatively breeding species, which may yield kin-selected benefits through, for example, nepotistic cooperation for vigilance, courtship and mate attraction (Box 4.6). Nepotistic tolerance on the breeding site during reproduction, nepotistic alarm-calling and vigilance behaviour in response to predators have been observed, for instance, in ground squirrels and the Siberian jay (*Perisoreus infaustus*). Compared to males, female ground squirrels exhibit strong natal and breeding site philopatry and hence they are more likely to be associated with close kin than males (Dunford 1977; Sherman 1977; Viblanc et al. 2009). Females are more tolerant to female relatives breeding nearby and they alarm-called more frequently than males, which may be explained by higher inclusive fitness benefits accrued to females compared to males resulting from living in closer kin associations (Box 4.6). In the Siberian jay, one offspring in three delays dispersal, but they do not take part in the care of younger siblings hatched from subsequent broods. Parents actively prevent older offspring from approaching the nest, apparently because given the high risk of nest predation, any activity around the nest is a major threat to reproductive success (Ekman et al. 1994). As for ground squirrels, females among Siberian jays gain higher indirect fitness benefits and exhibit more nepotistic vigilance behaviour than males (Box 4.6).

4.1.2.2.3.4 Lekking and Mate Sharing

Kin associations may also form among displaying males in lekking species, where males form aggregations or 'leks' to attract females for mating (Höglund & Alatalo 1995). Larger leks may be more attractive to females, thus enhancing each male's reproductive success (Alatalo et al. 1992; Balmford 1992; Lank & Smith 1992; Shelly 2001). However, leks are characterized by a high male mating skew, with few males achieving most copulations, and most males accruing little or no direct reproductive benefits (Mackenzie et al. 1995; Shorey 2002; Stein & Uy 2005). It has been suggested that lekking males that are unsuccessful in obtaining copulations may gain inclusive fitness benefits through kin selection (Kokko & Lindström 1996). Males may establish a courtship location in the vicinity of related males. Several studies have demonstrated that kin associations exist on bird leks, for example in black grouse (Höglund et al. 1999), capercaillie (*Tetrao urogallus*: Regnaut et al. 2006; Segelbacher et al. 2007), grouse (Höglund et al. 1999), peafowl (Petrie et al. 1999), white-bearded manakin (*Manacus manacus*; Shorey et al. 2000) and wild turkey (*Meleagris gallopavo*; Krakauer 2005). However, the mere presence of kin groups within leks does not necessarily mean that kin selection is the cause of cooperative lekking between relatives. High relatedness within leks may be caused by males and

---

Box 4.6 Nepotistic Cooperation in Alarm-calling and Vigilance

The Columbian ground squirrel (*Urocitellus columbianus*) forms female kin associations. These territorial squirrels are relatively long-lived (up to 10 years), dwell in burrows, have overlapping generations and exhibit strong female philopatry resulting in high relatedness among female neighbours (Viblanc et al. 2009). Females hold individual territories during reproduction and construct nest burrows a few days before birth. They are more tolerant to female kin than to nonkin (King 1989a), resulting in high concentrations of nesting burrows of close kin (Dobson et al. 2012). Females with more close female kin around them gain higher direct fitness than females with fewer kin present, as the former produce larger litters at weaning (Viblanc et al. 2009). This effect may be due to negative discrimination against offspring produced by nonkin female neighbours. Females differentiate between kin and nonkin by being less aggressive and more tolerant towards neighbouring maternal kin during the lactation period (King 1989b). Through this behaviour related females may gain more energy for reproduction and produce larger litters themselves (Viblanc et al. 2009). This results in considerable inclusive fitness benefits for female ground squirrels (Dobson et al. 2012).

The increased fitness in Columbian ground squirrels when kin are present might also be associated with kin-biased alarm-calling and vigilance behaviour, by which individuals scan the environment for potential predators and give advance warning. Individuals that spend more time on vigilance behaviour spend less time feeding (Carey & Moore 1986). Thus, more shared vigilance behaviour allows individuals to spend less time being vigilant, enabling them to increase their foraging time. However, cooperation in vigilance among kin was not observed (Fairbanks & Dobson 2010), but kin groups might invest more in alarm-calling, which needs further study.

Kin-biased alarm-calling in response to predators has been observed in other ground squirrels, for example in the Belding's ground squirrel (*Spermophilus beldingi*: Sherman 1977) and the round-tailed ground squirrel (*S. tereticaudus*: Dunford 1977). For both species calling is dangerous, and both species show a sex difference in calling behaviour, with females calling more frequently than males. It has been suggested that this is due to the fact that adult females exhibit strong natal and breeding site philopatry, whereas adult males dispersed greater distances, and as a result females are more likely to be associated with close kin than males (Dunford 1977; Sherman 1977). Furthermore, in the Belding's ground squirrel females called more often in the presence of descendants and other kin than in the presence of unrelated individuals (Sherman 1977). This suggests that female Belding's ground squirrels preferentially warn relatives and hence are nepotistic in their alarm-calling behaviour.

In the Siberian jay (*Perisoreus infaustus*) parents also show nepotistic vigilance behaviour (Griesser 2003) and alarm-calling (Griesser & Ekman 2004, 2005). Siberian jays live in year-round small groups, which may comprise the dominant breeding pair and retained offspring or unrelated immigrants, or both (Ekman et al.

Box 4.6 (*cont.*)

1994). Alarm-calling and vigilance is relevant because predation by sparrowhawks (*Accipiter nisus*) and goshawks (*Accipiter gentilis*) is an important cause of death (Griesser 2003; Griesser et al. 2006). As in the Belding's ground squirrel, dominant females but not dominant males are nepotistic in their alarm-calling and predator mobbing behaviour. Males give alarm calls when they are accompanied by unrelated as well as by related birds, whereas females call more frequently in response to predator attacks when accompanied by their retained offspring than when accompanied by unrelated immigrants (Griesser & Ekman 2004).

---

their male offspring returning to the same courtship location year after year. For kin-selected benefits to accrue, low-ranked males lekking with related dominant males should enhance the latter's reproductive success, which is possible simply because female visitation rate often increases with the number of males present on a lek (Kokko & Lindström 1996; Höglund 2003). Thereby, subordinate males that are hardly able to attract females for themselves may receive indirect fitness benefits by enhancing the attractiveness of related dominant males, which will raise the latter's mating success.

In lekking species the number of matings is often a useful proxy of paternity (e.g. Alatalo et al. 1996; Semple et al. 2001; Lank et al. 2002; Reynolds et al. 2007). In wild turkeys, two males typically pair up to attract more females. Both males display, but there is no reproductive sharing and only the dominant male produces offspring (Figure 4.14A; Krakauer 2005). The help provided to the dominant by the subordinate considerably increases the reproductive success of dominant males compared with non-cooperating, solitary males. Apparently, the higher reproductive output by assisted dominant males is not due to their better quality. Because both males are brothers or half-brothers (Figure 4.14B), the non-reproducing subordinate male partners benefit indirectly by helping their close relative to breed. Notably, cooperative subordinate males are unlikely to increase their future mating opportunities by assisting their brother, for example through an increased likelihood to inherit a display site or territory as observed in other lekking species (McDonald & Potts 1994), because turkeys do not defend display sites or breeding territories (Healy 1992). If subordinate males do not seem to gain direct (future) fitness benefits while clearly acquiring indirect fitness benefits, kin selection seems to provide the best explanation for the evolution of cooperative courtship in wild turkeys (Krakauer 2005).

Other lekking species exhibit cooperative courtship displays to gain future direct fitness benefits, as was demonstrated in the lance-tailed manakin (*Chiroxiphia lanceolate*: DuVal 2007a). Unrelated males form cooperative alliances of a dominant and a subordinate partner to perform synchronized courtship dances and duet songs in small leks situated in close proximity to each other (DuVal 2007a). Typically, leks are attended by alliances of one dominant and one subordinate male that both display towards females, but solo displays are also shown (DuVal 2007b). Dominant and

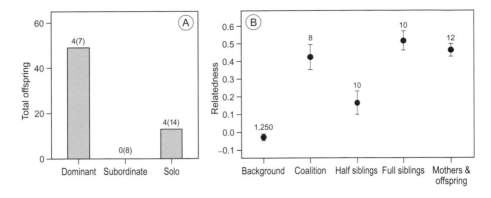

Figure 4.14 (A) Reproductive success of three male display strategies in wild turkeys. Males were classified as either dominant coalition member, subordinate coalition helper or non-cooperating solitary male. Reproductive success is shown as total number of offspring. The number of males assigned paternity, with total sampled males in parentheses, are indicated above the bars. None of eight subordinate males fathered any offspring compared with four out of seven dominant members of coalitions (Fisher exact test, $P = 0.026$) and four out of 14 solitary males. (B) Relatedness values calculated from microsatellite genotypes for all adult males ('background relatedness') and for subordinate males to their dominant partner ('Coalition'). Relatedness of three known genealogical relationships including half and full siblings, and mothers with offspring, reveal concordance with their predicted values based on pedigree. Dotted lines represent expected values for full and half siblings; unrelated individuals should have $r = 0$. Dots indicate means $\pm$ SE and numbers indicate sample sizes (from Krakauer 2005). Copyright © 2005, Macmillan Magazines Ltd; Springer Nature.

subordinate males do not switch behavioural roles. Females move freely among display areas to assess potential mates, and the subordinate male helps to create an attractive location for females ready to mate. Dominant males and their subordinate helpers are not related (Figure 4.15) and therefore the latter do not receive indirect fitness benefits from their cooperative behaviour (DuVal 2007c), in contrast to wild turkeys (Krakauer 2005). Moreover, subordinate males very rarely obtain copulations and thus do not gain important immediate direct fitness benefits (Figure 4.15), which is similar to other species of manakins with male courtship alliances (Foster 1977, 1981; McDonald 1993a, 1993b). In long-tailed manakins (*Chiroxiphia linearis*), it has been suggested that subordinate males may cooperate with dominant males in order to inherit the display perch after the death of the dominant male, thereby gaining delayed direct fitness benefits (McDonald & Potts 1994), similar to inheritance of the breeding position in cichlids (Balshine-Earn et al. 1998; Dierkes et al. 2005; Stiver et al. 2006), paper wasps (Field et al. 2006) and several other cooperatively breeding species (see below; reviewed in Kingma 2017).

The Tasmanian native hen (*Gallinula mortierii*) is a cooperatively breeding species in which mate-sharing regularly occurs. Monogamy, polyandry, polygyny and poly-gynandry occur in this species (e.g. Maynard Smith & Ridpath 1972; Gibbs et al. 1994). In most groups, males and females become co-breeders, and co-breeders of both sexes are usually close relatives. In polygynous and polygynandrous mating

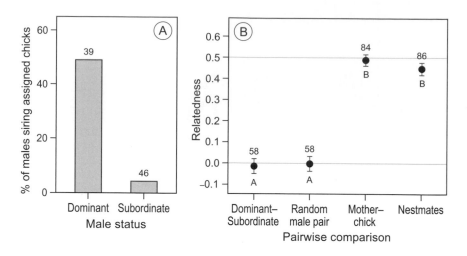

Figure 4.15 (A) Genetically determined reproductive success of male lance-tailed manakins in different status classes. Based on the assigned offspring, 49 per cent of alpha males sired chicks versus only 4 per cent of betas ($\chi^2 = 22.3$, $P < 0.001$). (B) Mean relatedness values of observed alpha–beta partners. Dotted lines indicate expected relatedness values for full siblings or parent–offspring comparisons (0.5) and unrelated individuals (0). Common letters denote groups that are not statistically different in relatedness but are significantly different from groups marked by different letters. Dots indicate means ± SE and numbers indicate sample sizes (from DuVal 2007c). © 2007 by The University of Chicago.

systems females lay joint clutches (Goldizen et al. 2000). A shortage of high-quality habitat prevents subordinate group members from dispersing from their natal territories for breeding elsewhere (Goldizen et al. 1998a). Male co-breeders share the number of copulations more equally than female co-breeders. It has been argued that males benefit more from mate sharing than females, and hence males should offer incentives to other males within the group. Males that shared mates had higher-quality territories than males that did not share mates, whereas no such relationship occurred for mate-sharing by females (Goldizen et al. 1998b). However, sex differences in reproductive cooperation could also result from sex-specific patterns of relatedness within groups, with males being more related to each other than females and thus being more tolerant of sexual behaviour by male social partners.

There are also remarkable examples of cooperative reproductive behaviour between male competitors in fishes (reviewed in Taborsky 1994, 2001, 2008; Díaz-Muñoz et al. 2014). Males may associate for some time during reproduction and cooperate in nest building, courtship and mate attraction and spawning without attacking each other. In most fishes it is unlikely that collaborating males are much closer related to each other to obtain kin-selected benefits than the population average, because males are unlikely to remain localized or stay together from their hatching until reaching reproductive status. This is particularly true for marine fishes exhibiting planktonic larval dispersal (Taborsky & Wong 2017). We are not aware of studies

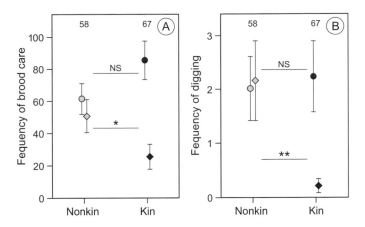

Figure 4.16 Effects of relatedness on helping effort in cooperatively breeding cichlids. Groups were experimentally established consisting of a pair and a female helper that was either related to the female breeder ('Kin') or not ('Nonkin'). Investment in direct egg care (A) and shelter digging (B) was significantly higher in unrelated than in related helpers (diamonds), whereas the egg care and digging effort of the female breeders did not differ between treatments (circles). Means ± SE are shown. Numbers indicate sample sizes. NS = non-significant; *$P < 0.05$; **$P < 0.01$ (from Zöttl et al. 2013a). Copyright © 2013, Nature Publishing Group.

showing that male cooperation in fishes is associated with genetic relatedness between social partners to gain kin-selected benefits. To the contrary, in highly social cichlids relatedness was shown to diminish cooperation (Figure 4.16; Stiver et al. 2005; Zöttl et al. 2013a). Apparently, in fish other reasons than kin-selected benefits explain the tolerance of and cooperation among competing males during reproduction, such as mutual benefits by increasing the attractiveness of a spawning site to females (Taborsky et al. 1987) or by jointly facilitating spawning (e.g. in sucker (Catostomidae) fish; Taborsky 1994), or reciprocal altruism by which males take turns in aiding each other (see above).

In lekking species, it is worth noting that many studies failed to find (i) kin-structured clustering within leks (Loiselle et al. 2007; McDonald 2009), sometimes with contrasting results between different study populations of the same species [e.g. manakin: kin structure (Concannon et al. 2012) versus no kin structure (Gibson et al. 2005)], and (ii) evidence for kin selection to be a major promoter of cooperation in lekking (e.g. Madden et al. 2004; Gibson et al. 2005; Knopp et al. 2008; Lebigre et al. 2008). Not only indirect fitness benefits but also immediate or delayed direct benefits to subordinate males may explain cooperative courtship displays. For example, the size of a male group on a lek may influence female visitation rate, as was demonstrated in Lake Malawi and Lake Tanganyika cichlid fish, where females prefer to visit large or dense male aggregations (Young et al. 2009). In some cooperatively lekking species subordinate males may gain access to reproduction, as was demonstrated in the ruff (*Philomachus pugnax*), where subordinate males help dominant males to attract additional females, while at the same time obtaining copulations with females when the dominant male is distracted (Lank et al. 2002). Males of the bluehead wrasse (*Thalassoma bifasciatum*), a coral reef fish, may spawn jointly in aggregations comprising dominant and additional males with one female (group spawning) which is attracted to such groups (Robertson & Warner 1978).

4.1.2.2.3.5 Dispersal in Kin Coalitions

Even when natal dispersal occurs, kin-structured populations may form if, for example, related individuals disperse together to settle in kin neighbourhoods. This has been observed in cooperatively and non-cooperatively breeding species (Table 4.4; see also Clutton-Brock 2002), creating a situation in which individuals can gain kin-selected benefits by helping to raise offspring produced by a member of the kin group. For example, in the cooperatively breeding white-winged chough (*Corcorax melanorhamphos*), new groups consisting of relatives may form by joint dispersal. Dominant males of such groups were always successful in gaining a breeding position when having supporting relatives. In contrast, many males without the support of relatives failed to gain a breeding position. However, dominant females in new groups nearly always gained a breeding position, independently of the presence of supporting relatives. Subordinates gained indirect fitness benefits by first assisting the related dominant male to secure a breeding territory and then helping him to raise young (Heinsohn et al. 2000). Eviction by dominant group members may also lead to dispersal of kin coalitions, as was observed in banded mongooses (Thompson et al. 2017b; see also Section 3.2.1).

Individuals may also disperse in coalitions of relatives to gain future benefits in case their own reproductive attempt fails. This has been observed for instance in long-tailed tit (*Aegithalos caudatus*: Sharp et al. 2008), wild turkey (*Meleagris gallopavo*: Krakauer et al. 2005) and lion (*Panthera leo*, e.g. Packer et al. 1991; Pusey & Packer 1987, 1994; see Box 4.7). Dispersing with relatives may be widespread in animals, as suggested by the observation that even when a pelagic larval stage is involved, relatives may stick together (e.g. in humbug damselfish, *Dascyllus aruanus*: Buston et al. 2009). Evidence for natal philopatry is scarce in marine fish populations, because of the difficulty of constructing multigenerational pedigrees with dispersing larvae. In the orange clownfish (*Amphiprion percula*) that lives in Papua Guinnea, a reconstruction of a multi-generational pedigree showed that longitudinal natal philopatry is recurrent even across generations. Larvae disperse before settlement into adult habitat, but larval offspring tend to return to their birth habitat and settle close to their parents, resulting in related individuals often sharing the same colony (Salles et al. 2016).

4.1.2.2.4 Kin Discrimination Involving Kin Recognition

According to Hamilton's rule, $rb - c > 0$, kin discrimination – the organism's ability to distinguish between kin and nonkin – becomes less important when the accrued fitness benefits from helping are much higher than the costs of helping (i.e. if b/c is high). Thus, Hamilton's rule predicts that when the ratio of benefits (b) and costs (c) of

Box 4.7 Fitness Benefits of Dispersing in Coalitions of Relatives

In the long-tailed tit (*Aegithalos caudatus*), offspring disperse in sibling coalitions and, because the recruitment rate is also high, siblings often become breeders in the next year in close proximity to each other (Sharp et al. 2008). When a nest fails, they may have the opportunity to help at a sibling's nest simply by aiding a nest close to their failed nest (Sharp et al. 2008; Figure 4.17A). However, long-tailed tits do not help neighbours indiscriminately, but have developed a mechanism for selective kin-discrimination on the basis of vocalizations (Sharp et al. 2005; see main text).

In wild turkeys, brothers or half-brothers disperse in sibling coalitions to form a team in courtship displays to attract females (Krakauer 2005; Figure 4.17B). Both males display, but there is no reproductive sharing and only the dominant male produces offspring. Subordinate males may receive indirect fitness benefits by enhancing the attractiveness of related dominant males to females (Krakauer 2005).

Female lions often disperse with other females from their natal prides to form a pride consisting of relatives (Pusey & Packer 1987). Adult females often breed synchronously and give birth simultaneously, and they form crèches with other mothers in their pride (Packer & Pusey 1983). Females rear their young communally, lactating their own young and also other young produced in the pride (Figure 4.17C). Lactation is energetically costly (Hanwell & Peaker 1977) and can increase mortality rates of female mammals (Clutton-Brock et al. 1989). Therefore, non-offspring nursing might be expected among females that are close kin, which is the case in lions (Pusey & Packer 1994). However, cubs reared in crèches do not receive more milk than cubs reared alone. It has been suggested that non-offspring nursing occurs as a

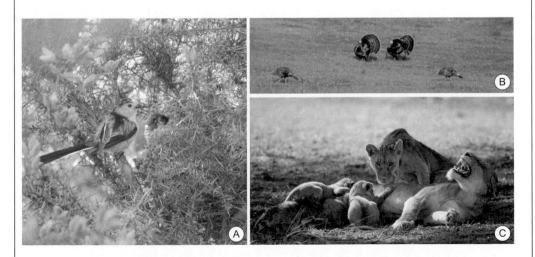

Figure 4.17 (A) Long-tailed tit feeding young at the nest (photo by Ben Hatchwell). (B) Dominant male wild turkey (left) and his subordinate brother display their tail fans and bright heads and throats to attract so-far uninterested females (photo by Alan Krakauer). (C) Female lions rearing and lactating their young communally (photo by Craig Packer).

Box 4.7 (*cont.*)

by-product of females forming crèches to better defend their cubs from infanticide by invading males (Packer & Pusey 1983; Packer et al. 1990). Male lions also disperse from their natal prides often in coalitions of relatives (Packer et al. 1991). After taking over a pride of females, reproductive sharing among males is lower when male coalitions are made up of relatives, possibly because of kin-selected benefits accrued to non-reproducing males.

---

helping is low, kin discrimination and the ability to preferentially direct help towards relatives becomes more important. Individuals may discriminate kin from nonkin on the basis of cues that reliably predict kinship (which is termed 'kin recognition'). Where individuals within a group differ in how much they are related to each other, active kin discrimination will be important if individuals are to maximize the indirect fitness benefits gained through helping. Preferential aiding according to relatedness occurs in both cooperatively and non-cooperatively breeding species, which indicates that individuals may often use kin recognition to achieve kin discrimination.

Given that in many social species groups contain mainly closely related individuals, there is a good opportunity to cooperate with kin without the need for kin recognition. When parents are long-lived, young from previous broods may often have an opportunity to care for related offspring in their natal territories. Subordinates may apply a simple rule: help any individual that cared for you when you were in need of help, as this individual is likely to be your parent or sibling. For example, in white-fronted bee-eater (Emlen 1997), Florida scrub jay (Mumme 1992) and Seychelles warbler (Komdeur 1994b; Richardson et al. 2003a, 2003b), the proportion of non-breeders that helped raising offspring produced by the dominant breeders decreased when unrelated step-parents took over the territory.

In groups where individuals differ in relatedness to each other and to the brood, for instance because of a high rate of breeder turnover or immigration, or because of sexual infidelity, active kin discrimination will be required if potential helpers are to maximize their indirect fitness benefits. Positive kin discrimination and kin-directed helping have been demonstrated in several cooperatively breeding vertebrates (Komdeur et al. 2008), even though negative kin discrimination may also occur (Zöttl et al. 2013a; Quinones et al. 2016). A meta-analysis including cooperatively breeding birds (16 species) and mammals (two species) revealed that often helpers discriminate between kin and nonkin, and that the helpers' propensity to assist more related individuals increases when greater indirect fitness benefits can be gained, which explained roughly 10 per cent of the variation in helping behaviour (Griffin & West 2003; Cornwallis et al. 2009). Positive kin discrimination was experimentally demonstrated in Seychelles warblers, where subordinates adjust their care according to the presence of the mother and their likely relatedness to a brood (Komdeur 1994b; Richardson et al. 2003a, 2003b; see also Case Study A). Kin discrimination was also shown in the cooperatively breeding cichlid *Neolamprologus pulcher* (Le Vin et al. 2010), but here helping did not increase with relatedness (Le Vin et al. 2011).

In contrast, direct egg care was even higher if helpers and beneficiaries were unrelated to each other (Zöttl et al. 2013a).

Other studies of cooperative breeding found that helping behaviour did not co-vary with relatedness (Table 4.2). In some cooperative breeders, related subordinates do not help (Cockburn 1998), or helpers are unrelated to the young but still help as much as close relatives (Cockburn 1998; Clutton-Brock 2002; Wright et al. 2009; Riehl 2011, 2013). Among other possibilities, such behaviour might result from recognition errors. In some cases, helpers even actively compete for access to unrelated offspring, for example in meerkat (Clutton-Brock et al. 2000), superb fairy-wren (Dunn et al. 1995) and white-browed scrubwren (Magrath & Whittingham 1997). Thereby helpers may foster to form 'social bonds' with recipient young that later benefit the helper, either by becoming a helper for them in turn, or by promoting development of coalitions beneficial in competition for breeding positions (Ligon 1983; Emlen 1991; Emlen et al. 1991). Also, ecological conditions such as the availability of future breeding options for subordinate group members may strongly influence cooperation propensity independent of relatedness between helpers und beneficiaries, as suggested by comparative analyses of cooperatively breeding birds (Kingma 2017).

Notably, the standard prediction of kin selection theory can also be reversed, leading to negative kin discrimination as shown in the banded mongoose (*Mungus mungo*). Here, dominants often violently evict subordinates from the group. Eviction attempts are highly aggressive and involve biting, chasing and wrestling. The evicted individuals often suffer from serious injuries and sometimes die (Thompson et al. 2016). Dominant females target especially closely related subordinate females for violent eviction from the group (see Case Study B, Figure B.2A). At first glance, this is contrary to the expectation that both tolerance in the territory and resistance against eviction should diminish with increasing relatedness between dominants and subordinates. However, if the resistance against eviction is indeed higher when dominants and subordinates are unrelated, negative kin discrimination might be explained by reduced eviction costs when attacker and attacked are closely related (Thompson et al. 2017b). Negative kin discrimination also occurs in other social systems and situations, for instance in polyembryonic wasps where soldiers preferentially attack more closely related larvae (Dunn et al. 2014), in staged encounters of sea anemones (Foster & Briffa 2014) and in reciprocal cooperation between Norway rats (Schweinfurth & Taborsky 2018a).

In most cooperatively breeding species, kin-directed helping occurs before dispersal. Therefore, a decision rule 'care for any offspring in my natal territory' could suffice as a reliable discriminator between kin and nonkin. In such systems helpers may not need to discriminate between kin and nonkin when making helping decisions. In contrast, kin recognition may be much more important in species where help is redirected, i.e. where helpers are failed breeders who, after dispersal, choose to help at a nest of another pair (Emlen & Wrege 1988; Emlen 1997; Russell & Hatchwell 2001; Griffin & West 2003; Krakauer 2005; Foster et al. 2006; Komdeur et al. 2008; Sharp et al. 2008). For example, in long-tailed tits all mature individuals try to breed independently each year, but if their breeding attempt fails, some of these failed breeders become helpers and usually assist at the nest of a relative. Experiments showed that long-tailed tits are able to discriminate between nests with kin and nonkin using vocal cues for kin recognition (Hatchwell et al. 2004). By helping at nests of related individuals subordinate long-tailed tits gain substantial kin-selected fitness benefits (Russell & Hatchwell 2001; Hatchwell et al. 2004; MacColl & Hatchwell 2004; Box 4.7). Active kin discrimination in this species was demonstrated experimentally by providing failed breeders with a choice between broods of related or unrelated neighbours that were situated at equal distances from the potential helpers. Failed breeders chose to help related broods more often than unrelated broods, discriminating between kin and nonkin by vocalizations learnt from adults during the nesting period (Hatchwell et al. 2001; Sharp et al. 2005), which is a reliable cue for kin recognition (Sharp et al. 2005) as mate infidelity is rare in this species (Hatchwell et al. 2002). Despite the apparent kin preference in provisioning of young (see Figure 4.21), by far the most important component of inclusive fitness in long-tailed tits is evidently direct and not indirect (kin-selected) fitness, irrespective of whether philopatric resident birds (born within population) or immigrant birds (dispersed into population) are concerned. The contribution of indirect fitness to inclusive fitness was estimated to be merely 13.4 per cent for males and 1.5 per cent for females (Figure 4.18; Green & Hatchwell 2018). Also in Seychelles warblers (see Case Study A, Figure A.2; Richardson et al. 2002) and in Tanganyika cichlids (Figure 4.19; Jungwirth & Taborsky 2015), subordinates gain much higher direct fitness benefits of cooperative breeding than indirect fitness benefits, which is the case for both male and female helpers in both species. A comparative analysis of 44 species

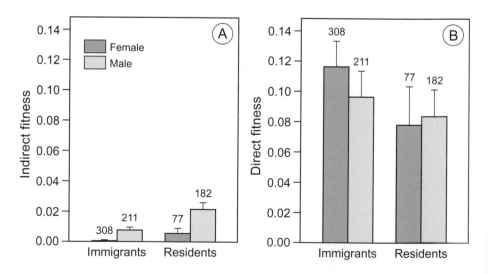

Figure 4.18 Mean ± SE. (A) Indirect fitness and (B) direct fitness accrued by female and male long-tailed tits in relation to whether they were immigrants or philopatric residents in the study population. Lifetime reproductive success data (as genetic offspring) were used to quantify the direct and indirect components of fitness on an individual basis. Numbers indicate sample sizes (from Green & Hatchwell 2018).

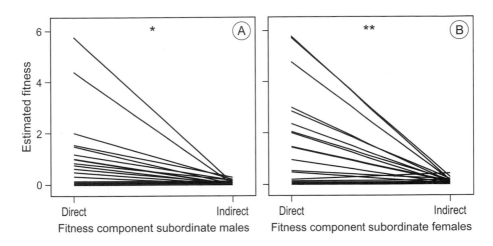

Figure 4.19 The estimated direct and indirect fitness of cooperative breeding gained by female and male subordinates in Tanganyika cichlids. Each line represents an individual fish and connects the estimate of its direct fitness with the estimate of its indirect fitness. Asterisks indicate significance levels from Wilcoxon tests (*$P < 0.01$; **$P < 0.001$; from Jungwirth & Taborsky 2015). © 2015 The Authors.

of cooperatively breeding birds suggested that direct fitness benefits might be generally more important than kin-selected fitness effects, even if kin selection can explain helping behaviour in some species (Kingma 2017).

Strong evidence for kin recognition also comes from species that are less social and do not live in kin-clusters. The red squirrel (*Tasmiasciurus hudsonicus*) is a non-social species living in year-round territories. Females with a litter occasionally adopt an orphaned juvenile of similar age to their own young before weaning, which is nursed together with their own offspring. Females suffer fitness costs of adoption through reduced survival of their own juveniles, but gain indirect fitness benefits when the adopted juvenile is closely related to them. Adoptions were confined exclusively to circumstances in which the benefits to the adopted juvenile (*b*) multiplied by the degree of relatedness between the surrogate mother and the orphan (*r*) exceeded the fitness costs of adding an extra juvenile to her litter (*c*), as predicted by Hamilton's rule ($rb > c$) for the evolution of altruism (Figure 4.20). Female red squirrels demonstrated active kin discrimination and kin recognition. Females significantly preferred to adopt related juveniles and refrained from adopting unrelated juveniles, even when there was an opportunity to do so. The mechanisms by which female red squirrels assess their relatedness to juveniles are yet unknown (Gorrell et al. 2010).

Some cooperative breeders exhibit fine-scale kin discrimination by helpers leading to an increase of the provisioning rate of helpers with increasing genetic relatedness to nestlings, as shown in Seychelles warbler (Richardson et al. 2003a, 2003b), long-tailed tit (Figure 4.21; Nam et al. 2010) and bell miner (Wright et al. 2009). However,

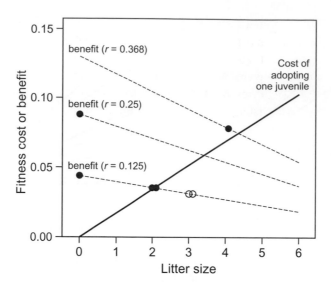

Figure 4.20 Adoptions of an orphaned juvenile by female red squirrels of similar age to their own young increase inclusive fitness, consistent with Hamilton's rule. Predicted fitness cost (solid line) of adoption to the surrogate dam increases, while fitness benefit (dashed lines) to the adopted juvenile decreases with litter size. Dashed lines represent three different degrees of relatedness calculated from a maternal genetic pedigree and multiplied by the benefit to the juvenile (rb). Adoptions (closed circles) increased inclusive fitness, whereas unadopted litters (open circles) would have reduced inclusive fitness if adopted (from Gorrell et al. 2010). Copyright © 2010, Nature Publishing Group.

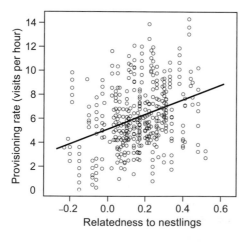

Figure 4.21 The provisioning rate of helpers in long-tailed tits in relation to their mean genetic relatedness to the nestlings they provisioned. The line shows predicted values ($\chi^2 = 9.72$, $P = 0.002$) (from Nam et al. 2010). © 2010 The Royal Society.

in most species helpers do not seem to adjust the amount of help to their relatedness with recipients, even if relatedness varies quite markedly within groups. This does not necessarily mean that kin selection is unimportant. A failure to discriminate between different degrees of kinship may result from employing a simple recognition rule that categorizes conspecifics as either related or unrelated in accordance with group membership, for example, which may on average lead to adequate decisions.

4.1.2.2.5 *Mechanisms Underlying Active Kin Discrimination*

Even if the ability to recognize kin has been demonstrated in many species, the mechanisms underlying kin recognition are often less clear. Four different types of mechanisms have been proposed: spatially based recognition, familiarity or recognition through association, recognition alleles (green-beard genes) and phenotype matching. However, it should be noted that more than one mechanism can work in combination.

Spatially based recognition. As outlined above, kin-directed helping may occur in the absence of active kin discrimination. For example, if individuals live in social groups containing predominantly close relatives, or in local clusters of related individuals, they do not need to recognize kin in order to obtain indirect fitness benefits; it may be sufficient to just help social partners in close proximity. Indeed, comparative studies provide evidence that individuals living in groups that typically consist of close relatives are less likely to show discrimination between kin and nonkin (Cornwallis et al. 2009, 2010).

Familiarity or recognition through association. Learning through association is the most widespread mechanism of discriminating kin from nonkin in vertebrate societies (Blaustein et al. 1987; Komdeur et al. 2008). It works reliably whenever there is a significant correlation between genetic relatedness and association. Imprinting of offspring onto parents or vice versa, where recognition results from a period of association, is an obvious example of such associative learning. The requirement of a period for familiarization with relatives is likely to be satisfied in any species with an extended period of parental care. Many cooperative breeders have a relatively long period of parental care, during which they associate with family members (e.g. Stacey & Koenig 1990; Emlen et al. 1991; Arnold & Owens 1998; Hatchwell & Komdeur 2000; Cornwallis et al. 2009). The crucial difference from spatially based kin recognition is that kin recognition through associative learning is a much more dynamic process; during the period of association an individual can learn the cues or labels identifying its putative kin, which can then be used to recognize kin outside of the association context. For example, long-tailed tit nestlings learn the calls of the adults feeding them, which provide cues for discrimination. This enables them at a later stage to assess the degree of kinship to breeders and to decide about help (Nam et al. 2010). However, recognition gained through only familiarity provides no basis for recognizing relatives that were never encountered before. For example, subordinate Seychelles warblers discriminate between kin and nonkin based on association, which is achieved through learning the identity of parents (Komdeur et al. 2004b). Cross-fostering experiments of nestlings between nests have confirmed that the subordinate's decision to help is based on the identity of the parents, rather than a direct assessment of the genetic relatedness to the nestling (Komdeur et al. 2004b).

Green-beard genes. This mechanism requires that a gene (or gene complex) confers an identifiable phenotype on its carrier that can be recognized by conspecifics (e.g. a 'green beard'; Dawkins 1976), which enables the carrier to perceive that phenotypic trait and to discriminate accordingly (Hamilton 1964). An allele encoding cooperation that is linked to such discrimination abilities can be expected to spread more rapidly through a population by natural selection than other alleles without this discriminatory capacity. If a linkage disequilibrium exists between genes encoding a phenotypic trait used for recognition and genes responsible for helping, altruism can be selected irrespective of genealogical relationships between social partners (Hamilton 1964; Dawkins 1976; Gardner & West 2010). If recombination can break down the linkage between recognition and altruism genes, which is likely if complex, polygenic traits and sexual reproduction are involved, green-beard effects will be unstable over evolutionary time (Lehmann & Keller 2006b), except if a tight linkage disequilibrium between recognition and altruism genes would be kept by strong correlational selection on another trait (Sinervo & Clobert 2003). Hence, cooperation based on green-beard effects is probably a rare phenomenon. In the red fire ant (*Solenopsis invicta*), workers bearing a green-beard allele kill all queens not bearing this allele (Keller & Ross 1998). In side-blotched lizards (*Uta stansburiana*), genetically similar but unrelated blue male morphs prefer to settle on territories next to each other and to cooperate. These clusters form apparently on the basis of the blue throat, and they are not predicted by whole-genome relatedness. Blue-throated male fitness improves in the vicinity of other blue-throated males through providing a buffer against aggressive orange males. Neighbouring blue-throated males are more successful at mate guarding their female partners against larger and aggressive orange males, and orange males are less likely to usurp territories of blue males if the latter's territories are not adjacent to orange males. In this species blue males seem to share key genes for signalling, recognition and cooperation (Sinervo et al. 2006), suggesting the coexistence of multiple green-beards (Nonacs 2011).

Phenotype matching. Kin recognition through phenotype matching involves the learning and assessment of phenotypes (e.g. odour, song, or visual cues) of relatives. An individual's phenotype, or that of closely related conspecifics, forms a phenotypic 'template' against which the phenotypes of unfamiliar individuals can be compared. The degree of matching reflects kinship, enabling appropriate kin-directed behaviour. Kin recognition by phenotype matching was experimentally demonstrated, for instance, in meerkats, where encounters between individuals of varying relatedness levels are common. Kin recognition is also important to avoid the negative effects of inbreeding, i.e. reproducing with close relatives

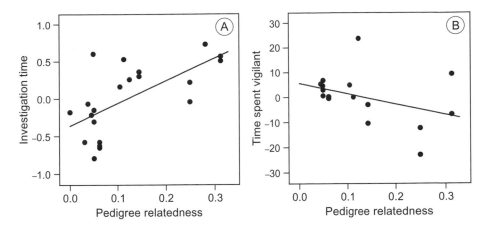

Figure 4.22 (A) Investigation time [residuals of a generalized linear mixed model (GLMM)] of dominant females to the scent of unfamiliar subordinate male meerkats with varying degrees of pedigree relatedness ($F_{1, 7.42} = 22.26$, $P = 0.002$). (B) Time spent vigilant (residuals of a GLMM) by dominant females in response to the scent of unfamiliar subordinate males with varying degrees of pedigree relatedness ($F_{1, 12} = 7.23$, $P = 0.020$) (from Leclaire et al. 2013). © 2012 The Authors.

(Nielsen et al. 2012). Dominant female meerkats presented with anal gland secretions from unfamiliar males varying in relatedness were able to discriminate the scent of anal glands of unfamiliar kin from unfamiliar nonkin, in that they spent more time investigating the scent of unfamiliar males and spent more time vigilant when offered scents of more genetically related but unfamiliar males (Figure 4.22; Leclaire et al. 2013). Similarly, male rats distinguished the odour of unfamiliar related conspecifics from that of unfamiliar unrelated conspecifics (Schweinfurth & Taborsky 2018a). In many fishes olfactory cues are also used to recognize relatives independently of familiarity. Female sticklebacks presented with olfactory cues from familiar and unfamiliar brothers are capable of distinguishing both familiar and unfamiliar brothers from nonkin males (Mehlis et al. 2008). Females showed a preference for nonkin males possibly to avoid mating with a brother, in order to avoid the negative effects of inbreeding, such as reduced egg and fry survival (Frommen et al. 2007).

It should be noted that these mechanisms of kin recognition are not mutually exclusive. For example, recognition by phenotype matching as found in meerkats does not exclude the use of green-beard genes causing the expression of phenotypic cues that allow intrinsic recognition (Leclaire et al. 2013). Moreover, in small families of cooperative animals, recognition of specific individuals can be relatively straightforward, but it may be a challenge for larger family groups consisting of kin of varying relatedness. Finer discrimination might be possible by, for example, combining several recognition mechanisms. This occurs in the cooperatively breeding bell miners. These birds live in highly social colonies comprising several hundred individuals, and they constitute one of the best examples of fine-scale facultative adjustment of helping effort according to kinship (Wright et al. 2009). Helper investment is costly and adaptive adjustment of effort occurs according to relatedness to the brood (Wright et al. 2009). Bell miner helpers use a fine-scale kin discrimination mechanism based on the similarity of mew call structure, which indicates genetic relatedness between individuals. Variation in helper effort was best explained by helper mew call similarity to the calls of breeding males, and not to breeding females, which is indicative of genetic relatedness to the brood (McDonald & Wright 2011). This makes sense because the majority of helpers are male and breeding females are always unrelated immigrants having a shorter life-span than breeding males; in addition, extra-pair fertilizations in this species are rare (Conrad et al. 1998). The characteristics of mew calls are inflexible and innate, reliably indicating relatedness between individuals. This provides an effective mechanism by which helpers can assess their relatedness to any group member (McDonald & Wright 2011).

The described kin recognition mechanisms are not always effective. This is not only true for discrimination between kin- and nonkin, but especially for discrimination among various degrees of kinship, for several reasons. (a) The recognition system may not be perfect if, for example, the cues used in discriminating kin from nonkin are not clear, leading to recognition errors and the potential acceptance of unrelated individuals. (b) There can be recognition errors if nonkin are present during the 'associative-learning period' of relatives, which will then be regarded as kin, whereas true kin who are absent during this period will be regarded as nonkin. (c) A kin recognition mechanism can be exploited by cheats, which has been referred to as 'kinship deceit' (Connor & Curry 1995). For example, in the white-winged chough, an obligate cooperative breeder in which reproductive success is positively related to group size, groups kidnap unrelated fledglings. Because of recognition through association, kidnapped young who survive subsequently become imprinted on their new group members and apparently regard them as relatives when becoming (unrelated) helpers in their adoptive groups (Heinsohn 1991). This is reminiscent of slave-making ants, where the pilfered larvae of the slaves learn the cues of the slave-making species (Delattre et al. 2012). Slave-maker ants are brood parasites that capture the broods of other ant species to increase the worker force for their own colony. After emerging in the slave-makers' nest, the host larvae are imprinted on and integrated into the mixed colony, and they work as if they were in their own colony, including to help rearing the slave-makers' brood, to feed and groom the slave-makers' workers and to defend the slave-makers' nest against aliens (Delattre et al. 2012). Oddly, they defend the slave-makers' nest even against members of their original colony (Miramontes 1993). Altruistic acts of slaves are thus directed towards unrelated individuals, i.e. the slave-makers. In such cases, a fine-tuning of the recognition system would be useful, but its evolution might be frequency-dependent and subject to cognitive ability and to the relative costs of recognition failure (Reeve 1989; Sherman et al. 1997). Another reason for a lack of recognition is that in cooperatively breeding species, helpers may gain higher *direct* fitness benefits than non-helpers (e.g.

by superior protection in the territory of successful breeders; Quinones et al. 2016), implying that kin recognition is not required.

4.1.2.2.6 *Ecological Determinants of Kin-clustering and Cooperation*

To some extent, dispersal is a plastic response to local ecological and social conditions (Baglione et al. 2002, 2006; Galliard et al. 2003; Shen et al. 2017). Several ecological and social conditions may constrain or delay juvenile dispersal and lead to the formation of kin-clustering, such as the scarcity of required resources outside of the natal territory, a lack of suitable breeding vacancies, shortage of mates, high predation risk, competition with superior rivals, or parental facilitation. However, it should be noted that delayed dispersal is not a prerequisite for the formation of kin clusters. As discussed above, individuals may also form kin-clusters through joint natal dispersal with relatives (see Table 4.4). A common factor resulting in delayed dispersal is the limitation of suitable breeding vacancies as a consequence of habitat saturation. When the entire habitat is occupied by territories of breeders or groups, juveniles often delay dispersal and stay in their natal territories until a breeding vacancy arises (Arnold & Owens 1999; Hatchwell & Komdeur 2000; Koenig & Dickinson 2016). Constraints on delayed juvenile dispersal have been demonstrated by experimentally creating breeding vacancies (Komdeur 1992; Walters et al. 1992), and breeding vacancies with a potential mate already present (Pruett-Jones & Lewis 1990; Ligon et al. 1991). Experimental evidence for the causal relationship between habitat saturation and delayed dispersal was shown in the carrion crow (*Corvus corone corone*) and the Seychelles warbler. In most carrion crow populations, offspring leave their natal territory to fill a breeding vacancy elsewhere. However, some populations have limited breeding opportunities and are cooperative, with juveniles often delaying dispersal and remaining with their parents. Carrion crow eggs that were transferred from nests in a non-cooperative population and raised in nests in a cooperatively breeding population resulted in juveniles mostly delaying dispersal, and some becoming brood care helpers (Baglione et al. 2002). Also, in the cooperatively breeding Seychelles warbler, the frequency of delayed dispersal and cooperative breeding is influenced by habitat saturation. Until recently, the entire world population of this species was confined to one small island in the Seychelles. Although warblers can breed independently in their first year, in this population some individuals remained in their natal territory to become helpers with their parents. When individual adult birds were transplanted to previously uninhabited islands, they produced offspring that did not delay dispersal, but filled up breeding vacancies immediately after reaching independence. Only after the new populations also reached saturation in the novel habitats did offspring start to delay dispersal and help to care for the offspring of the dominant breeders in their natal territory (Komdeur 1992; Komdeur et al. 1995).

A shortage of potential breeding partners or high predation pressure can also result in delayed dispersal. For example, a shortage of potential breeding partners resulting in delayed dispersal was revealed in several bird species where the removal of a breeder from a territory caused philopatric adult offspring from neighbouring territories to rapidly move in and take over the vacant breeding position. This happened in the acorn woodpecker (Hannon et al. 1985), the red-cockaded woodpecker (Walters et al. 1992), the superb fairy-wren (Pruett-Jones & Lewis 1990; Ligon et al. 1991) and the Seychelles warbler (Komdeur 1992). In the cooperatively breeding cichlid princess of Lake Tanganyika, dispersing young risk being predated by piscivorous fish during dispersal. If predation pressure was increased experimentally, helpers were less likely to disperse from their home territory where they receive protection against predators (Heg et al. 2004a), and instead they continued to care for the offspring of dominant breeders in their natal territory (Heg & Taborsky 2010).

Another factor that can cause delayed juvenile dispersal is that some groups may control high-quality territories, for instance with abundant food resources, creating an incentive to stay in such a group. This scenario can be illustrated by the formerly endangered Seychelles warbler. In 1968, when the entire world population consisted of only 26 remaining individuals, habitat restoration programmes were implemented. Over the following 30 years, the population grew very fast. No family groups were reported among warblers until 1973, roughly the time at which all suitable breeding habitat had become occupied (Figure 4.23). In subsequent years family groups formed and became the norm (Komdeur 1992). The population of mature birds has consistently exceeded the number of occupied territories. To enhance the numbers of Seychelles warblers, birds were introduced onto nearby, previously unoccupied islands. The quality of all territories was evaluated in terms of adult survival and nesting success. Consequently, the vacancies created by the translocation of breeders from the source population were filled only by offspring from territories of equivalent or poorer quality (Komdeur 1992). Offspring from families residing on high-quality areas thus had fewer acceptable outside opportunities, and as such remained on their natal territory for longer periods of time (Figure 4.23). Other evidence for the role of resources in the natal territory on dispersal behaviour comes from experimental manipulations of food levels, which revealed that offspring may be more likely to stay when territories are of high quality. In the western bluebird (*Sialia mexicana*), the natural food resources were experimentally depleted in family territories. In winter, the bluebird is dependent mainly on berries of the oak mistletoe (*Phoradendron villosum*) for food. By reducing half of the mistletoe abundance, sons (the philopatric sex) of the breeding pair left the depleted territory (Dickinson & McGowan 2005). Likewise, offspring in a cooperatively breeding population of the carrion crow that were given additional food in their natal territory were more likely to delay dispersal (Figure 4.24; Baglione et al. 2006).

However, often constraints on delayed dispersal alone cannot explain why juveniles stay on their natal territory. In some species offspring delay dispersal even in the absence of constraints on dispersal (Komdeur et al. 1995; Macedo & Bianchi 1997; Heg et al. 2008a), either because the natal site provides clear direct fitness benefits, for example through enhanced protection and survival in family groups (Heg et al. 2004a, 2005a, 2005b), or helping to care for related group members yields sufficient indirect fitness benefits. In addition, breeders may manipulate the dispersal decision of their mature offspring to enhance survival or future reproduction (e.g. parental facilitation; Brown & Brown 1984). Breeders are often more tolerant of offspring than of nonkin

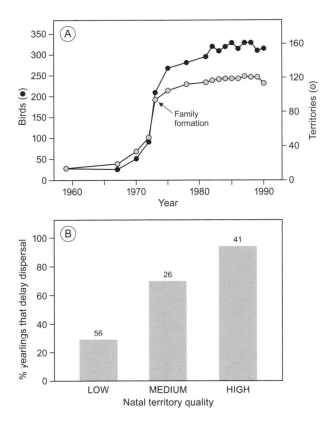

Figure 4.23 Ecological constraints and family formation in Seychelles warblers. (A) The number of individuals and occupied territories on Cousin Island between 1959 and 1990. Family formation was first observed when all available territories became filled. (B) The likelihood that yearlings stay at home, plotted as a function of the quality of their natal territories. Sample sizes of yearlings in each territory quality are given above bars (from Komdeur 1992). Copyright © 1992, Nature Publishing Group.

group members (e.g. Scott 1980; Barkan et al. 1986; Black & Owen 1989; Ekman et al. 1994; Pravosudova & Grubb 2000; Dickinson & McGowan 2005). Parental facilitation allows offspring to remain in their natal territory to benefit from protection and privileged resource use. In the Siberian jay, parents give alarm calls primarily when in company with related offspring (Griesser & Ekman 2004, 2005). In several species retained offspring do disperse when their parents disappear or have been removed (Balcombe 1989; Ekman & Griesser 2002; Galliard et al. 2003; Eikenaar et al. 2007), suggesting a potential role of parental facilitation of delayed dispersal.

The determinants of delayed dispersal can also differ between sexes. For example, if females benefit more from kin cooperation than males, females should show a higher tendency to delay dispersal. Individuals may benefit from kin cooperation either for breeding or for resource acquisition (Lawson Handley & Perrin 2007).

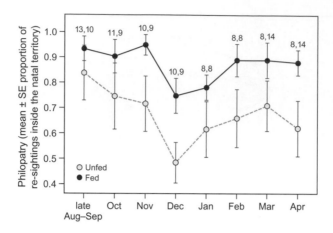

Figure 4.24 Philopatry, measured as average proportion of re-sightings ($\pm$ SE) inside the natal territories, in fed (filled circles) and unfed (open circles) juvenile crows throughout the study period. Sample sizes are given above bars for fed and unfed individuals, respectively (from Baglione et al. 2006). © 2006 The Royal Society.

The benefits of sex-specific kin clustering and concomitant delayed dispersal, or high site philopatry, have been shown in several species (as discussed above).

4.1.2.2.7 *Kin Selection and Sexual Conflict Resolution*

Above we have illustrated that sexual cooperation among related males may reduce competition for matings and improve the fitness of cooperating males. However, the fitness consequences for females resulting from sexual cooperation among related males have received less attention. A higher relatedness between males may not only increase cooperation among males over matings as outlined above, but also reduce sexual conflict. Sexual conflict may arise because males and females have divergent fitness interests. Thus, behaviours that are beneficial to members of one sex may result in costs to members of the opposite sex (Trivers 1972; Parker 1979, 2006; Johnstone & Keller 2000). For instance, sexual conflict may arise over mating frequency, as males usually benefit from mating with more than one female, resulting in higher reproductive success (Bateman 1948). However, females that mate multiply may suffer from fitness costs through reduced fecundity or survivorship (Arnqvist & Rowe 2005). This is because males may harm females after copulation to prevent them from mating with other males. The damage occurring to females will often be higher than the gain to males from extra matings (e.g. Morrow & Arnqvist 2003; Edvardsson & Tregenza 2005). For example, in the bed bug (*Cimex lectularius*) males pierce the abdominal wall of females with their external genitalia to inseminate into her body, where spermatozoa migrate to the ovaries (e.g. Stutt & Siva-Jothy 2001; Figure 4.25). The female's genital tract is not used for copulation but functions only for egg laying (Carayon 1966). This pattern of insemination carries a fitness cost for females, as repeated copulatory wounding results in reduced longevity without a

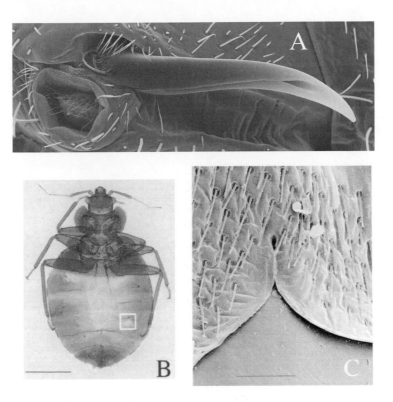

Figure 4.25 (A) The intromittent organ, specialized to deliver sperm during copulation, of the male bed bug (modified paramere). The groove in which the paramere sits when not in use is visible underneath the paramere (bar = 0.1 mm). (B) The site of copulation on the ventrum of the female's abdomen. The male always copulates at this site (bar = 1.5 mm; from Stutt & Siva-Jothy 2001). (C) Detail of the copulation site on the female's abdomen showing the incurving of the female's sternite, which acts as a guide for the male's intromittent organ (bar = 0.1 mm). (A) and (C) © Andrew Syred (Microscopix, UK), Science Photo Library. (B) Copyright © 2001, The National Academy of Sciences, USA. (A black and white version of this figure will appear in some formats. For the colour version, please refer to the plate section.)

compensatory increase in egg-laying rates (Stutt & Siva-Jothy 2001). Females from an experimental group in which their mate's intromittent organ was made inoperable so that he was unable to pierce her but showed similar mounting frequencies to unmanipulated males (low-mating group) died at a significantly lower rate than females mated with unmanipulated males (control group; Figure 4.26A). Females produced fertile eggs at the same rate regardless of which group they were from (Figure 4.26B). In turn, by harming females, males may reduce the number of females available for mating, resulting in even more male–male competition. There is high variability in the expression of female harm observed across and within taxa (Pizzari & Gardner 2012).

Kin selection cannot only reduce competition for mates among male relatives, but also inhibit the evolution of male harm to females (Rankin 2011; Wild et al. 2011). Relatedness among male reproductive competitors may arise, for example, through limited male dispersal (Johnstone & Cant 2008; Gardner 2010), or when only a few

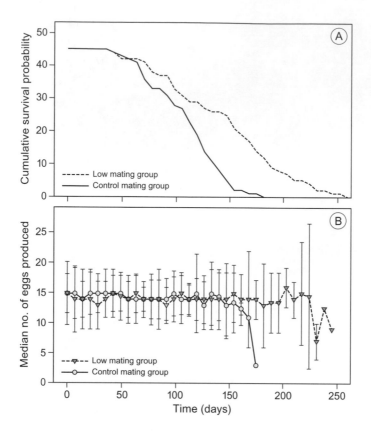

Figure 4.26 (A) Survival curves for female bed bugs in the low-mating and the control mating groups. The cumulative survival probability is the number of females alive at the end of a given sampling period (7 days). (B) Median egg production of females from the low-mating and control mating groups. Bars show the interquartile range (from Stutt & Siva-Jothy 2001). Copyright © 2001, The National Academy of Sciences, USA.

males produce most of the male offspring in a population (McDonald & Pots 1994; Francisco et al. 2009). A reduction in female harm by associations of related males then results from kin selection diminishing competition for access to mates. Few studies have considered the influence of relatedness on the outcome of sexual conflict (Queller 1994b; Chapman 2006; Bourke 2009) or on the evolution of sexual conflict over mating (Eldakar et al. 2009). In groups of *Drosophila melanogaster*, genetic relatedness among males was experimentally manipulated, and subsequently these males were allowed to compete for copulations with females. As predicted, males in groups consisting of brothers fought less with each other, courted females less intensively and lived longer than males in groups of unrelated males (Figure 4.27). Moreover, females that were exposed to groups of brothers were significantly less harmed and had higher lifetime reproductive success compared to females exposed to groups of unrelated males, when both types of groups were unrelated to the female (Figure 4.28; Carazo et al. 2014). This shows that variation in relatedness and

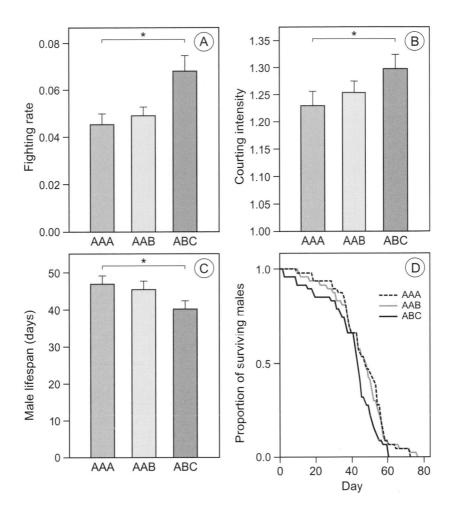

Figure 4.27 The effect of male–male relatedness on male sexual behaviour and longevity in *Drosophila melanogaster*. (A) Triplets of unrelated males (ABC) had a significantly higher frequency of male–male fighting than triplets of brothers (AAA) (proportion of focal scans in which male–male fighting was observed). (B) Compared to triplets of brothers (AAA), triplets of unrelated males (ABC) were characterized by higher courting intensity (number of courting males when courting was observed). (C) Male longevity was significantly lower in unrelated triplets (ABC) than among full-sibling brothers (AAA). (D) Male mortality risk was significantly different across treatments, and post-hoc direct comparisons between the treatments indicated that this effect was due to males in unrelated triplets (ABC) being more likely to die than in AAA triplets and AAB triplets. Error bars represent means $\pm$ SE; asterisks represent significant post-hoc comparisons. *$P < 0.05$; $n_{AAA} = n_{AAB} = n_{ABC} = 47$ (after Carazo et al. 2014). Copyright © 2014, Nature Publishing Group.

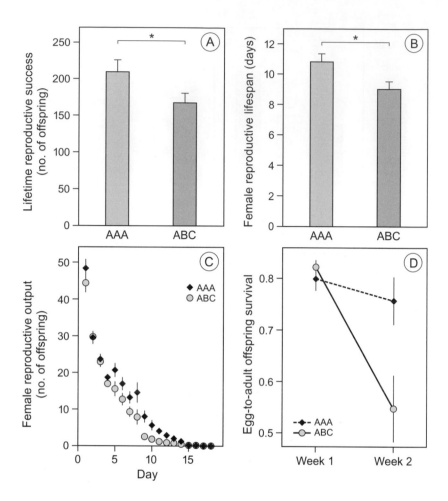

Figure 4.28 The effect of male–male relatedness on female fitness in *Drosophila melanogaster*. (A) Female lifetime reproductive success was higher in the high male-relatedness treatment (AAA) than in the low male-relatedness treatment (ABC). This difference was highly significant when female reproductive lifespan and its interaction with treatment as factors were included in the analysis. (B) Female reproductive lifespan was longer in the high-male relatedness treatment (AAA) than in the low-male relatedness treatment (ABC) and the probability to cease reproducing at any given time was lower. (C) Female reproductive rates declined more sharply in individual females exposed to ABC rather than to AAA males (average number of offspring produced by AAA and ABC females over successive days of their life). (D) Offspring viability (egg-to-adult survival) declined more sharply over time in females exposed to ABC rather than AAA males. Error bars represent mean $\pm$ SE; *$P < 0.05$; $n_{AAA} = 61$, $n_{ABC} = 60$ unless stated otherwise (after Carazo et al. 2014). Copyright © 2014, Nature Publishing Group.

respective responses to kin are possible key factors triggering the harm competing males may inflict on females, which may affect the evolution of sexual conflict over matings in general.

Furthermore, in species where males can harm females during mating, females may prefer males related *to them* as mates above unrelated males, as related males may be less inclined to inflict damage. For example, in the Japanese quail (*Coturnix japonica*) courtship and mating are physically harmful to females through male harassment, which includes chasing and pecking at a female, seizing feathers at the back of her head and dragging her around by her head feathers before copulating (Mills et al. 1997). This may be the reason that female quails have a strong preference for selecting cousins as mates over unrelated males (Bateson et al. 1982). Nevertheless, it is presently unknown whether related males cause less damage to females, as are the potential fitness consequences of inbreeding in this species.

4.1.2.2.8 *Kin Associations Do Not Always Lead to Cooperation*

The examples discussed above suggest that associations among kin may enhance the evolution of cooperative behaviour among relatives. However, this is not always the case (reviewed in Cockburn 1998; Clutton-Brock 2002, 2009; Dickinson & Hatchwell 2004; Riehl 2013; Wilkinson et al. 2019). Many species living in kin-structures do not show a correlation between relatedness and kin-selected behaviours, such as helping, vigilance and sentinel behaviour (Table 4.2). For instance, a meta-analysis on kinship, association and social complexity across bat species showed that relatedness is not a prerequisite for cooperation to arise among individuals (Figure 4.29). Although kinship was predictive of social associations among individuals of the same sex in a few species, it did not predict the occurrence of various types of cooperation, such as information exchange, huddling for warmth, social grooming and communal nursing and food sharing. It should be noted that relatedness among group members was very low (except in one species, the disk-winged bat *Thyroptera tricolor*), and hence perhaps too small to generate selection for a correlation between relatedness and cooperation. Instead, complex social behaviour in bats appears to require frequent interactions among a small number of individuals that roost together for multiple years (Wilkinson et al. 2019).

In fact, theory also suggests that limited dispersal and the formation of kin groups does not necessarily lead to cooperation (cf. Section 3.3.1). This is the case because the benefits of cooperation may be offset by the costs of increased competition with relatives for resources or reproductive opportunities, hence competition between individuals of a kin group can be similarly strong to that among unrelated group members (e.g. Hamilton 1971, 1975; Queller 1992, 1994a; Frank 1998; Taylor 1992b; Wilson et al. 1992; West et al. 2001, 2002; Griffin & West 2002; Griffin et al. 2004; Lehmann & Rousset 2010; Cant 2012; Rodrigues & Gardner 2012). This largely results from local density-dependent effects, as the increased productivity of relatives also increases future local competition between relatives (Gardner & West 2004; Cant 2011). A clear example of how relatedness and competition may influence the evolution of altruistic cooperation comes from experimental research on a pathogenic

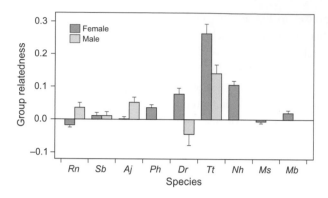

Figure 4.29 Average within-community relatedness for each sex in nine species of bats. Standard errors obtained by bootstrapping. Only one species, the disk-winged bat *Thyroptera tricolor* (family Thyropteridae), exhibits relatively high relatedness levels among group members, and only in this species is relatedness a strong predictor of associations among both males and females. Species names from left to right: *Rn*: *Rhynchonycteris naso*, *Sb*: *Saccopteryx bilineata*, *Aj*: *Artibeus jamaicensis*, *Ph*: *Phyllostomus hastatus*, *Dr*: *Desmodus rotundus*, *Tt*: *Thyroptera tricolor*, *Nh*: *Nycticeius humeralis*, *Ms*: *Myotis septentrionalis*, *Mb*: *Myotis bechsteinii* (from Wilkinson et al. 2019). Copyright © 2019, Springer-Verlag GmbH Germany, part of Springer Nature.

bacterium (*Pseudomonas aeruginosa*). This bacterium depends on iron for growth and parasite virulence (damage as a result of parasite infection). Iron is a limiting factor for bacterial growth, because most iron in the environment is present in the insoluble form. However, the bacteria produce siderophores scavenging insoluble iron for bacterial metabolism (Ratledge & Dover 2000). The production of siderophores is essential for bacterial growth, but also metabolically costly to the individual cell. At the same time it provides a benefit to the local group, because other individuals can take up the siderophore–iron complex without incurring any production costs (Ratledge & Dover 2000), hence creating a public goods dilemma (defined as a situation in which the whole group can benefit if some members give something for the common good, but individuals benefit from the public goods without paying for them if enough others contribute; Allison & Kerr 1994). To investigate how relatedness and competition between individuals affect cooperation, both were independently manipulated using populations containing a mixture of individuals either belonging to the wild-type strain that produces siderophores, or to the mutant strain that does not (Griffin et al. 2004). The experiments were conducted using closed populations in the absence of local dispersal of individuals (no immigration and emigration), which may have affected local relatedness and competition and thus the outcome of the experiment. In this bacterium, a higher relatedness between interacting individuals leads to higher levels of cooperative siderophore production. However, an increase in local competition between relatives selected for lower levels of cooperative siderophore production between relatives (Figure 4.30; Griffin et al. 2004). In other words, the degree of relatedness between individuals has less effect on cooperation when the

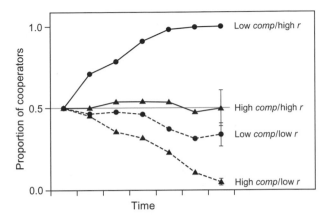

Figure 4.30 The evolution of cooperation in response to relatedness and the scale of competition. The proportion of cooperative individuals who produce pyoverdin siderophores is plotted against time. The different lines represent relatively high (solid lines) and low (dashed lines) relatedness. The different symbols represent relatively low (circle) and high (triangle) amounts of competition between relatives. Each of the four treatments was replicated four times, and standard errors are shown for the final time point. Cooperation is favoured by higher relatedness and lower competition between relatives (from Griffin et al. 2004). Copyright © 2004, Macmillan Magazines Ltd.

scale of competition increases. This study is important, because both relatedness and competition were manipulated independently in the absence of dispersal behaviour, demonstrating that relatedness and competition can both matter for the quantity of cooperation exhibited.

In addition, manipulation of dispersal behaviour showed a significant effect on siderophore production. When dispersal behaviour was manipulated through culturing bacteria in media with different degrees of viscosity, increasing viscosity of the growth medium significantly limited bacterial dispersal and the diffusion of sidero-phore molecules, and increased the fitness of individuals that produced siderophores relative to mutants that did not. Under these circumstances, the benefits of siderophore production are more likely to accrue to relatives (i.e. greater indirect benefits) and, at the same time, the bacteria are more likely to gain direct fitness benefits by taking up siderophore molecules produced by themselves (i.e. the trait becomes less coopera-tive; Kümmerli et al. 2009b).

In natural populations, relatedness and the degree of competition often emerge as a result of population demography, so they are usually not independent from each other. When in viscous populations competition becomes more local, this may lead to increased competition between neighbouring individuals which are relatives, con-comitantly reducing the amount of cooperation between them (Grafen 1984; Taylor 1992a, 1992b; Queller 1994a; Frank 1998). This was also demonstrated in the above-described pathogenic bacterium. When the amount of local relatedness between individuals was simultaneously manipulated with the amount of local competition, the effects of dispersal cancelled out the intensity of local competition between relatives, just as predicted for saturated viscous populations (Taylor 1992a, 1992b). Dispersal resulted in both lower local relatedness among individuals and reduced local competition, hence the combination of relatedness and competition had no influence on the net level of cooperation (Griffin et al. 2004; Kümmerli et al. 2009a). In other words, in viscous populations that are saturated, the effect of limited dispersal per se does not favour cooperation, except if patch quality is heterogeneous (Rodrigues & Gardner 2012). Importantly, the scale of competition among social partners affects selection for cooperation between relatives. For example, competition for food is an important determinant of the investment in communal care for pups in the banded mongoose (*Mungos mungo*). Juvenile helpers and non-breeding female helpers invest less in caring for pups when food is scarce and hence resource competition is high, while adult males and breeding females do not change their investment (Nichols et al. 2012b).

However, it should be noted that high interaction levels between individuals may lead not only to higher competition, but also to changes in reproduction, survival and dispersal, which may also affect selection for cooperation (Lehmann & Rousset 2010). Disproportionate effects of increased relatedness and local competition on the evolution of altruistic traits and toleration were demonstrated for fig wasps. Fig wasps develop within the fruit of fig trees, and in many species males are wingless, do not disperse and remain lifelong in the fruit where they were born. Males mate locally, resulting in increased density and relatedness between males (Molbo et al. 2004) and consequently increased competition between related males over mating. Across fig wasp species, the level of aggression between non-dispersing males varies greatly. The main weapons used in fights are the mandibles, which vary greatly in size between species (Cook et al. 1997), as does the average relatedness between males. This is associated with the number of females producing (male) offspring in each fig. In some species, only one female lays eggs in a fruit, resulting in male offspring being brothers, whereas in other species several females lay eggs in the same fruit, resulting in lower relatedness among males. Unexpectedly, across fig wasp species there is no relationship between relatedness among males and male–male competition for females (Hamilton 1979; Cook et al. 1997; Bean & Cook 2001; West et al. 2001), as well as male aggression levels (measured as the injuries obtained during the wasps' lifetimes: West et al. 2001; or the probability of fighting: Nelson & Greeff 2009). Instead, males fight less when more future mating opportunities are available, i.e. when the number of females developing in the fruit is high (West et al. 2001).

Similar results were found within species. Males of the fig wasp *Sycoscapter australis* differ considerably with respect to their mandible size, which increases with the level of mating competition between males (Bean & Cook 2001). This suggests that with limited dispersal the competition between relatives becomes severe and local. Any increase in reproduction of an individual raises the costs to its neighbours, thereby reflecting competition between relatives, which may rule out the effects of increased relatedness in favouring kin-selected behaviours (West et al. 2001).

If fitness benefits decline through increased competition among relatives, this should select for dispersal to reduce competition between relatives (Hamilton & May 1977; Taylor 1988; Frank 1998; Gandon & Rousset 1999; Ronce et al. 2000; Rousset & Gandon 2002; Leggett et al. 2011). This may increase reproduction of the remaining, related individuals, by which effect the dispersing individuals gain indirect benefits (Clobert et al. 2001; Ridley et al. 2003). Indeed, dispersal by male fig wasps *Platyscapa awekei* seems to be a means for avoiding competition among close kin. As predicted by models of kin competition avoidance, male dispersal increased with lower density of foundresses, which caused higher relatedness within the natal fig (Moore et al. 2005). Nevertheless, dispersal strategies driven by kin competition are apparently phenotype-dependent in this species, with smaller males being more prone to disperse with higher kin competition than larger and stronger males that win more fights for mates (Moore et al. 2005).

One way to reduce local competition between relatives is to disperse in groups of relatives ('budding dispersal') to areas with lower density (Gardner & West 2006). In this scenario, high relatedness is maintained because kin disperse together, settle in close proximity to each other in a new area with lower competition, and hence they may benefit from cooperation among relatives at lower levels of competition. As outlined above, dispersal in small groups of close kin has been observed in a number of cooperative and non-cooperative species, including insects, birds and mammals (Table 4.4). In several species of polistine wasps, for example, as colonies get larger and aggression among reproductive females increases, groups of related adults may move to new nest sites (Jeanne 1991). However, clear empirical support that dispersal of relatives to areas of lower competition would favour cooperation among both the remaining individuals and the dispersing group members is hitherto missing.

Close relatedness between breeders and adult helpers that could potentially breed themselves also may reduce the conflict over reproduction. For example, cooperatively breeding acorn woodpeckers live in polygynandrous groups in which nearly all group members are close relatives, consisting of co-breeding males and joint-nesting females, but also offspring from prior years that delay dispersal and act as non-reproductive brood care helpers. Co-breeders are often close relatives. Consequently, within-group relatedness between co-breeders and non-breeding helpers is very high, which may reduce conflict over reproduction. Nevertheless, most breeder females are unrelated to breeder males, so incestuous matings between close relatives are uncommon (Haydock et al. 2001). Despite the high relatedness among most group members, when a reproductive vacancy arises within a group through the death of a breeder, which is often replaced by an unrelated immigrant, intense reproductive competition develops among mature offspring of the same sex as the disappearing parent (Koenig et al. 1998). Helpers can inherit the dominant position and breed following the disappearance of related adults of the opposite sex, but not of their own sex, which entails incest avoidance. As a consequence of sex-specific reproductive competition among adult subordinates, the time required to fill breeding vacancies was significantly longer for groups with helpers of the same sex as the disappearing breeder compared with groups experiencing vacancies that did not contain helpers of the same sex as the disappearing breeder (Koenig et al. 1998).

4.1.2.2.9 Inbreeding and Kin-selected Benefits

Mating with kin may result in direct fitness benefits, such as higher offspring survival, reduced sexual conflict and higher lifetime fitness (Peer & Taborsky 2005; Carazo et al. 2014). Theoretical studies predict also long-term benefits of close inbreeding, because mating with kin can increase an individual's future inclusive fitness, as there will be more copies of common genes in future generations (e.g. Bengtsson 1978; Parker 1979, 2006; Lehmann & Perrin 2003; Kokko & Ots 2006). By choosing close relatives, females may ensure genetic compatibility (Bonneaud et al. 2006) and perpetuate their own alleles (Kokko & Ots 2006). Prolonged inbreeding can also result in the eradication of recessive deleterious alleles from a population, thereby improving long-term population persistence (Quilichini et al. 2001). However, close inbreeding can also reduce fitness due to increased expression of deleterious alleles, and thus cause inbreeding depression (Charlesworth & Charlesworth 1987; Lynch & Walsh 1998; Keller & Waller 2002). Inbreeding can reduce heterozygosity, offspring fitness and population size. Because the benefits of inbreeding often appear to be lower than the costs, many animals avoid mating with close kin (e.g. Pusey & Wolf 1996; Frommen & Bakker 2006; Gerlach & Lysiak 2006; Ilmonen et al. 2009; Välimäki et al. 2011; Sanderson et al. 2015a).

Nevertheless, some species actively engage in inbreeding, i.e. selection of more closely related mates when a choice is available (e.g. Thünken et al. 2007, 2012). Species with a long history of inbreeding are expected to have few negative effects of inbreeding due to purging of deleterious alleles (Lubin & Bilde 2007). Instead, they may suffer from an outbreeding depression, for instance because of incompatible genetic variation between lineages. Ambrosia beetles, with limited male dispersal and almost inevitable incestuous mating among full siblings (Keller et al. 2011), suffer from outbreeding depression, but not from inbreeding depression. Experimentally created inbred breeding pairs did not produce offspring with reduced fitness. In contrast, experimentally created outcrossed breeding pairs suffered from greatly reduced hatching rates of their offspring (Peer & Taborsky 2005). Active inbreeding has also been reported in a range of other animals. For example, in the Peron's tree frog (*Litoria peronei*) females fertilize more eggs with sperm of more closely related males (Sherman et al. 2008). Female wire-tailed manakins (*Pipra filicauda*) preferentially select related males as mates (Ryder et al. 2009). In the biparental great frigatebird (*Fregata minor*), females choose mates that are genetically similar, which may provide an incentive for both parents to care better (see below). However, the performance of offspring of more genetically similar parents was not better than that of less genetically similar parents, which does not exclude that offspring performance might be affected at a later point in life (e.g. adult fecundity), which was not yet measured (Cohen & Dearborn 2004).

In species with biparental care, inbreeding between male and female partners may result in better offspring performance as a result of a reduction of conflict between parents over care. This was demonstrated in *Pelvicachromis taeniatus*, a socially monogamous cichlid fish from West Africa showing biparental brood care (Thünken et al. 2007). Reproductive males live solitarily and aggressively defend small caves as breeding shelters against rivals, while females compete for access to males. Males with caves are limited and competition for mates among females is strong, with some females being prevented from breeding due to this limitation. Both parents guard the free-swimming offspring against predators. There is preferential inbreeding between males and females, both in wild populations (Langen et al. 2011) and in the laboratory (Thünken et al. 2007). A mate-choice experiment showed that males and females in breeding condition are able to discriminate between unfamiliar kin and unfamiliar nonkin of the opposite sex, and actively prefer kin over nonkin as mating partners (Figure 4.31; Thünken et al. 2007). The observed preferences are mediated by self-derived olfactory cues (Thünken et al. 2014b). Inbreeding pairs were more cooperative and invested more time into parental care than unrelated pairs. Males of inbred pairs spent significantly more time guarding the caves than males of outbred pairs (Figure 4.31). Furthermore, when the fry swam free, inbreeding males spent significantly less time attacking their mates and more time guarding the young than outbreeding males (Figure 4.31). Females did not differ with respect to their guarding and aggressive behaviours. Overall, inbred pairs showed less within-pair aggression during care and they spent more time caring, while young of inbred and outbred pairs did not differ in survival.

Given the absence of negative effects of inbreeding on offspring performance, inbreeding in *P. taeniatus* seems to be an advantageous strategy with respect to diminishing conflict between parents over care, and through increasing the inclusive fitness to both parents by producing more highly related offspring (Thünken et al. 2007). However, the benefits resulting from inbreeding seem to differ between the sexes. For females, relatedness gained greater importance than body size, whereas the opposite was true for males. When both sexes were given the choice between two mating partners differing in relatedness as well as body size, females preferred related males but their relative kin preference decreased with increasing male size (Thünken et al. 2014b). When choosing a large male as partner, females benefit because large males outcompete smaller males (Thünken et al. 2012). However, if only small males are available, females gain from choosing a related and more cooperative partner. Males, on the other hand, preferred large females even if unrelated, because female body size is correlated with fecundity and thus male fitness. Males therefore rejected related females of low quality, preferring unrelated, high-quality females as partners (Thünken et al. 2014b). Inbreeding can also entail behavioural effects in partners of inbred individuals. For example, in the burying beetle (*Nicrophorus vespilloides*) partners of inbred parents (the latter having an inbreeding history) increased the amount of care provided to offspring compared to partners of outbred parents (Figure 4.32; Mattey & Smiseth 2015). Thus, partners of inbred parents increased the amount of direct care they provided despite the fact that there was no difference in the amount of care provided by inbred and outbred parents (Figure 4.32). As a consequence, the total amount of direct care by the two parents was higher when at

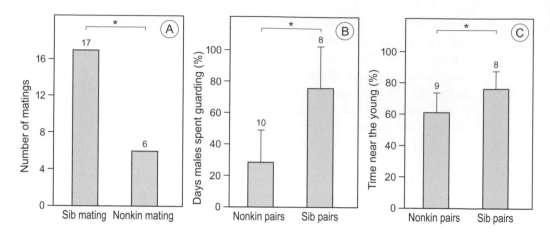

Figure 4.31 (A) Spawning experiment in *Pelvicachromis taeniatus*. Number of matings between sibs and nonsibs in spawning experiments with one male and two females, one related and the other unrelated to the male. (B) Cave guarding of in- and outbreeding males. The average proportion of days (in per cent ± SD) in which males of in- and outbreeding pairs guarded the cave where the female cared for the eggs. (C) Young guarding of in- and outbreeding parents. The average proportion of parent–offspring associations (in per cent ± SD) of related and unrelated parents. Sample sizes are given above bars, *$P < 0.025$ (from Thünken et al. 2007). Copyright © 2007 Elsevier Ltd. All rights reserved.

least one parent was inbred than when both parents were outbred, indicating that partners of inbred parents responded by overcompensation rather than incomplete or no compensation (Mattey & Smiseth 2015). Given that inbreeding in the burying beetle has no detrimental effects on offspring fitness (Mattey & Smiseth 2015) and enhanced parental care may cause fitness benefits, e.g. through better offspring performance, inbreeding seems to be adaptive in this species.

Sex-biased dispersal may not always decrease the likelihood of encounters and matings between relatives, and thus lower inbreeding. The cooperatively breeding Lake Tanganyika cichlid fish *Neolamprologus pulcher* exhibits male-biased dispersal (Stiver et al. 2007), and mean relatedness between social mates was not different from expected if pairs had mated randomly, suggesting neither active avoidance nor preference for pairing with relatives (Stiver et al. 2008). However, highly related pair members showed more aggression against each other than less-related pair members (Stiver et al. 2008). This matches with experimental results revealing costs of inbreeding in this species due to lower offspring survival, even though parental performance was not affected by relatedness between pair members (Ermeidou 2016; Ermeidou et al., 2021). The reason why individuals do not seem to avoid related individuals as mates in this species may reflect limited breeding opportunities in the field. In *N. pulcher*, breeding independently is dangerous because of high predation risk (Heg et al. 2004a; Groenewoud et al. 2016) and individuals may do better by breeding with relatives than by breeding without brood care helpers, which rarely occurs in

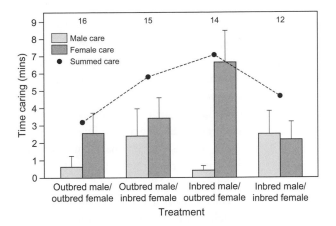

Figure 4.32 Effects of inbreeding on biparental cooperation in *Nicrophorus vespilloides*. Comparison of the amount of time spent providing care by inbred or outbred male (open bars) and inbred and outbred female (grey bars) parents caring for outbred offspring during a 30-min observation (mean $\pm$ SE). The total amount of care offspring received from both parents (filled circles) is shown for each treatment (mean). Male partners of inbred females spent significantly more time providing care than male partners of outbred females ($Z = 3.90$, $P < 0.001$), and female partners of inbred males spent significantly more time providing direct care than female partners of outbred males ($Z = 4.08$, $P < 0.001$). Numbers of pairs are given above bars (from Mattey & Smiseth 2015). © 2015 Blackwell Verlag GmbH.

nature (Wong & Balshine 2011; Taborsky 2016). The negative effects of inbreeding may be circumvented by producing broods of mixed paternity, with extra-pair young being produced by nonrelated males. *N. pulcher* indeed produce broods of mixed paternity (Dierkes et al. 1999, 2008; Heg et al. 2008b; Bruintjes et al. 2011), but it is currently unknown to what extent this reduces potential inbreeding costs of pairs consisting of related mates.

Selective, kin-directed brood care may be important where breeders face a mixture of related and unrelated young. It can be achieved, for instance, through (partial) filial cannibalism of nonkin young. Filial cannibalism, the consumption of offspring, either eggs or young, occurs in many animal species ranging from insects (Thomas & Manica 2003), fish (Klug & Bonsall 2007) and birds (Gilbert et al. 2005) to mammals (Elwood 1991). It is often associated with parental care (Manica 2002). In many species, reproductive parasitism is common, and caring for foreign eggs or young that do not share the breeders' genes has detrimental fitness effects. Therefore, eating offspring can be adaptive if the probability of own parentage is low. Several studies have shown that breeders adjust their parental investment to the amount of foreign eggs or young (e.g. Neff 2003; Maan & Taborsky 2007; reviewed by Kempenaers & Sheldon 1997; Sheldon 2002; Alonzo 2010; Alonzo & Klug 2012; Box 4.8). Moreover, reduced paternity may trigger cannibalism of entire clutches, as shown by caring males in several fish species (e.g. Frommen et al. 2007; Mehlis et al. 2010; Box 4.8).

Box 4.8 Selective Paternal Care and Cannibalism in Fish Males

In bluegill sunfish (*Lepomis macrochirus*), nest-tending males prefer caring for broods that contain a high number of closely related fry (Neff 2003). This was demonstrated experimentally by manipulating the paternity of eggs immediately after spawning through swapping part of the clutches between nests. Males do not adjust paternal care to paternity at the egg stage, but once the larvae have hatched, suggesting that they can only distinguish their own from foreign offspring after the larvae have hatched. It has been suggested that males may use urinary cues released by the hatched fry to distinguish them (Neff 2003), which are not present during the egg phase (Neff & Sherman 2003).

In three-spined sticklebacks (*Gasterosteus aculeatus*) males care for the eggs by fanning oxygen towards the clutch and defending eggs from predators, which is energetically costly. Parasitic fertilizations are common (Le Comber et al. 2003), which may result in males caring for eggs that were fertilized by their competitors. Males may minimize the fitness costs resulting from reduced paternity by cannibalizing their entire clutch. The higher the proportion of foreign eggs in a clutch, the higher the probability of cannibalism by caring males (Frommen et al. 2007). This was experimentally demonstrated by manipulating the percentages of own fertilized eggs in a clutch while keeping the absolute number of eggs before and after manipulation similar (Mehlis et al. 2010). Although males seem to estimate the percentage of foreign eggs in the nest and adjust the probability of complete clutch cannibalisms accordingly, they do not direct cannibalism specifically towards foreign eggs. Males may assess the proportion of foreign eggs in their nests by olfactory cues from the eggs (Mehlis et al. 2008). The odour profile of an egg changes during its development. Paternal genes might influence the odour profile of an egg, with paternal odours being only or more clearly expressed in the later stages of embryonic development. Total filial cannibalism (consuming the complete clutch) occurred always during later embryonic stages (Mehlis et al. 2010).

In the polygynous African cichlid *Lamprologus callipterus*, females breed in empty snail shells collected by nest-building males. Because competition for shells is severe, males frequently steal shells from occupied nests or take over entire nests. In addition, reproductive parasitism by males pursuing alternative fertilization tactics is common (Figure 4.33; Taborsky 2001; Sato et al. 2004; Wirtz Ocana et al. 2014; Taborsky et al. 2018). This causes males to sometimes possess shells containing breeding females that had spawned with other males. Nest owners recognize young they have not produced from the odour contained in the shell, and they attempt to expel the brood-caring female from the shell if the number of foreign young in the shell is high (Maan & Taborsky 2007). Like in bluegill sunfish, males respond to the presence of foreign offspring only after the larvae have hatched. Males expel females from such shells either by burying the shells under sand, or by repeatedly taking the shell up with the mouth and turning it until the female leaves, which entails infanticide (the loss of all offspring present in

Box 4.8 (*cont.*)

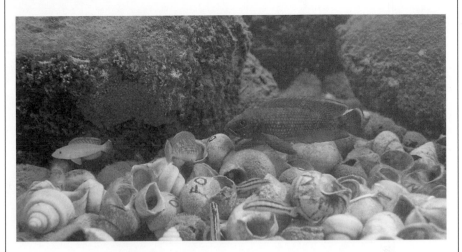

Figure 4.33 Nest of *Lamprologus callipterus* consisting of empty snail shells. From right to left: nest male (large, dark), female (inspecting a shell; mottled, seen from behind) and dwarf male (farthest left, pale). In the foreground (middle) there are three specimens of a different species (striped; *Telmatochromis vittatus*). (From Wirtz-Ocaña et al. 2013.) © 2013 The Authors. *Ecology and Evolution* published by John Wiley & Sons Ltd; open access. (A black and white version of this figure will appear in some formats. For the colour version, please refer to the plate section.)

the shell). Infanticide appears to serve a different purpose here than in the three-spined stickleback. It is adaptive for males because female expulsion results in emptying shells, which makes them available for new females and thereby increases male reproductive success (Maan & Taborsky 2007). Territorial males do not remate with the expelled females, because these need several weeks to replenish resources to be able to produce new eggs (Schütz et al. 2006). As the breeding success of females that are taken over by a different male is significantly reduced, females seem to prefer mating with large males, which may reduce the risk of shell stealing and hence infanticide (Maan & Taborsky 2007). Interestingly, female choice of shells for spawning is not influenced by this apparent male–female conflict and both sexes prefer different shell characteristics for reproduction (Mitchell et al. 2014).

In the tessellated darter (*Etheostoma olmstedi*) some males move and spawn at several nests, whereas others care for these nests that also contain foreign eggs. In contrast to *L. callipterus*, nest-takeover here is not a result of limited resources. Males prefer to take over nests with eggs fertilized by another male above empty nests (Farmer & Alonzo 2008) and females prefer to spawn in nests containing eggs compared to empty nests (Stiver & Alonzo 2011). By providing care in a nest that already contains eggs, males increase their attractiveness and hence mating

Box 4.8 (*cont.*)

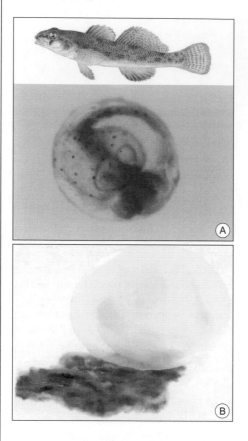

Figure 4.34 Tessellated darter embryo (A) and egg (B) recovered from the stomachs of cannibalistic nesting males (insert). Such remains suggest that the embryos were generally in good health before being eaten and probably had been free of fungal disease. (From DeWoody et al. 2001.) Copyright © 2001, The National Academy of Sciences, USA.

success. In addition, males prefer to care for nests containing foreign eggs in early developmental stages, because females prefer to spawn in such nests. This reduces the chance that their offspring hatch considerably later than the young from eggs already present, which affects the risk of being cannibalized by older young (Stiver & Alonzo 2011). Nevertheless, male nest owners were shown also to cannibalize healthy eggs they have fertilized themselves (Figure 4.34; DeWoody et al. 2001).

In many fish species with paternal care, males may steal nests or preferentially take over nests from other males that already contain eggs or young sired by the previous owner (e.g. Daniels 1979; Taborsky et al. 1987; Stiver & Alonzo 2011), or they may kidnap eggs from neighbouring nests and rear them (Rohwer 1978), which would entail brood care of unrelated offspring. Nevertheless, nest takeovers and egg kidnapping can be adaptive for males if females prefer to spawn in nests that already contain eggs. Experimental evidence showing that the presence of eggs has a positive influence on female choice exists for example in three-spined stickleback (Ridley & Rechten 1981; Goldschmidt et al. 1993), river bullhead (Marconato & Bisazza 1986), fathead minnows (Unger & Sargent 1988), fantail darter (Knapp & Sargent 1989) and sphynx blenny (*Aidablennius sphynx*: Kraak 1996). Females apparently prefer to spawn in nests with eggs already present irrespective of the quality of the nest owner. In experiments where males of various qualities were given eggs or no eggs, females did not differentiate on the basis of male quality, but between eggs or no eggs present (Ridley & Rechten 1981; Groothuis & Kraak 1994). In addition, females often prefer nests with many eggs over those with few (e.g. Ridley & Rechten 1981; Sikkel 1989; Goldschmidt et al. 1993; Forsgren et al. 1996), but this is not always the case (see Östlund-Nilsson 2002). Two reasons in particular may explain why females prefer to spawn in nests containing (many) eggs. (i) Females may show a preference for males that have already accumulated many eggs because these males are likely to provide superior parental care as a consequence of the high fitness value of their broods (Vestergaard & Magnhagen 1993; Östlund-Nilsson 2002). (ii) A high number of eggs may raise the survival probability of each egg, because the risk of predation for any one egg decreases with the number of eggs present in the nest (predation dilution: Kraak 1996). However, not only egg presence or the number of eggs in a nest is important for female choice, but also the developmental stage of the eggs, because eggs laid late in the sequence run a greater risk of being cannibalized. This may happen because earlier hatched young consume the remaining eggs, or males may consume the last laid eggs of a brood as an investment in future broods. Therefore, females should not lay eggs in nests with eggs in advanced stages because their eggs would be more likely to be consumed (Rohwer 1978). Accordingly, female garibaldi fish (*Hypsypops rubicundus*) prefer to spawn in nests containing eggs in early stages of development to spawning in empty nests or in nests with eggs in advanced stages of development (Sikkel 1989).

4.1.2.2.10 *Absence of Adjustment of Social Behaviour to Kinship*

Several of the examples given above may suggest that the formation of kin groups will lead to more cooperation among group members, and that whether to cooperate is a self-chosen decision of the individual. However, as we have already seen, relatedness is not necessarily the main reason for cooperation. Several studies have shown that even if indirect benefits are important and helpers help more closely related kin, they do not always adjust their helping effort to the degree of kinship (Komdeur & Hatchwell 1999; Griffin & West 2003; Komdeur et al. 2008; Cornwallis et al. 2009; Green et al. 2016; see Figure 4.35). The relative importance of kin selection in favouring helping behaviour varies greatly across species. Nevertheless, the higher the benefits of helping, the more kin-biased helping was found in a comparison of cooperatively breeding vertebrate species (Figure 4.35). As discussed above, one reason for a weak or missing correlation between relatedness and cooperation can

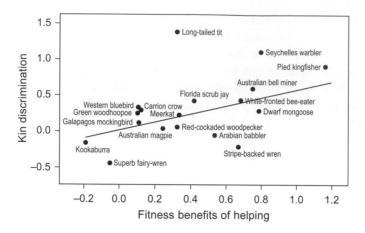

Figure 4.35 Correlation between kin discrimination and the benefits to offspring of helping across 18 cooperatively breeding vertebrates. The effect size of the relationship between helping level and relatedness is plotted against the effect size of the relationship between helping level and the benefit of helping. A positive value of kin discrimination corresponds to helpers preferentially helping closer relatives, whereas a negative value corresponds to the opposite pattern. The positive relationship between these two variables ($P = 0.05$) indicates that preferential helping of relatives (kin discrimination) is more likely in species where there are greater fitness benefits from helping (from Cornwallis et al. 2009). © 2009 The Authors. Journal Compilation © 2009 European Society For Evolutionary Biology.

be the potential negative fitness effects of among-kin competition (e.g. Hamilton 1971, 1975; Queller 1992, 1994a; Taylor 1992b; Wilson et al. 1992; Frank 1998; West et al. 2001, 2002; Griffin & West 2002; Griffin et al. 2004; Lehmann & Rousset 2010; Rodrigues & Gardner 2012). But there are in fact several potential reasons why social behaviour may not be adjusted to kinship:

Inability to discriminate relatedness. As outlined above, if unrelated individuals cooperate as readily as related ones, as shown by helpers in several cooperative breeders (Cockburn 1998; Clutton-Brock 2002; Wright et al. 2009; Riehl 2011a, 2013; Vitikainen et al. 2017), such behaviour might result from recognition errors or the inability to discriminate relatedness.

Large direct fitness effects. Direct fitness benefits may be sufficient for the maintenance of cooperation, regardless of any kin-selected fitness benefits (Lehmann & Keller 2006b; West et al. 2007c; Clutton-Brock 2009; Quinones et al. 2016; Taborsky et al. 2016; Kingma 2017; see Section 4.1). In this case kin discrimination may not be expected. For example, in cooperative breeders helping may lead to higher status within the group and consequently to a higher probability to successfully compete for a territory after the death of its owner (Zack 1990; Koenig et al. 1992; Balshine-Earn et al. 1998; Leadbeater et al. 2011). Alternatively, helping can result in higher productivity and thus a larger group size ('group augmentation'). This may raise the fitness of group members, for instance if larger groups are better at finding food, competing with other groups or deterring predators (Kokko et al. 2001;

Kingma et al. 2014). Such mutualistic benefits of cooperation may be prominent where benefits of group living are large (e.g. in meerkats and Lake Tanganyika cichlids; see Kingma et al. 2014). This concept is further supported by the 'kidnapping' of members of other groups as observed in several cooperative breeders, for example in white-winged choughs and banded mongooses, where adult 'kidnappers' herd young from another group into their own territory (Heinsohn 1991; Müller & Bell 2009).

In cooperatively breeding birds where the prospects of territory inheritance are good, subordinates providing help do not preferentially direct their care towards related offspring (Figure 4.36; Kingma 2017). If the group increases the size of its territory by outcompeting neighbouring groups, the helper may eventually be able to

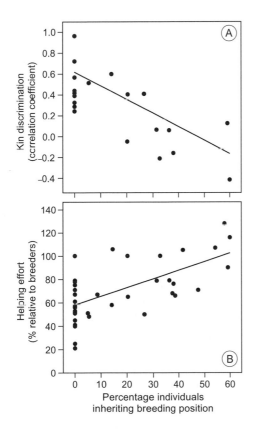

Figure 4.36 The likelihood of territory inheritance drives helping decisions in cooperatively breeding birds. (A) Helpers with a high likelihood of inheriting their resident territory do not invest more in more related offspring (low levels of kin discrimination), whereas when prospects of territory inheritance are limited, subordinates mainly direct help towards related offspring (*n* = 20 species). (B) Helpers provision offspring on average more (mean per cent offspring food provisioning per helper, relative to breeders) when the probability of inheriting their resident territory is larger (*n* = 38 species). Dots reflect species averages, and model-predicted regression lines are plotted (from Kingma 2017). Open access.

take over a portion of the breeders' territory for own breeding (Emlen 1991). This happens, for example, in males of the Florida scrub jay (Woolfenden & Fitzpatrick 1978, 1984) and the Seychelles warbler (Komdeur & Edelaar 2001), where helpers may inherit the territory (Kingma 2017) or disperse together with other group members, so that younger subordinates can help former helpers in return (delayed reciprocity: Ligon & Ligon 1978; Kingma et al. 2014). Other direct reproductive benefits that may be gained by helping have been proposed. Helpers may gain breeding experience, which allows these individuals to be more productive when they obtain a breeding position themselves. For example, in the Seychelles warbler, individuals with helping experience produced their first fledgling as fast as experienced breeders and significantly faster than individuals without helping experience (Komdeur 1996c). In the Mexican jay (*Aphelocoma ultramarine*), individuals that helped with brood care also improved their success of their first own broods (Brown 1987).

Punishment. Dominant individuals may force subordinate group members to provide help in brood care and other important duties, which the latter may obey if they do not have better outside options. As discussed in Chapter 3 and in Section 4.2 below, individuals in kin groups can be socially forced by dominants to cooperate through coercion, punishment and policing (Balshine-Earn et al. 1998; Lehmann & Keller 2006a; Ratnieks & Wenseleers 2008; Fischer et al. 2014; Ågren et al. 2019). As a result, the relative costs of refraining from helping become greater compared with the option of helping. However, it should be noted that such enforcement is more likely to happen among unrelated social partners than among related ones, because of the latter's shared fitness interests based on genetic similarity (Quinones et al. 2016; Ågren et al. 2019).

Inherent individual variation. Differences in personality traits or behavioural types may explain variance in helping behaviour better than relatedness (Heinsohn & Legge 1999; Schürch & Heg 2010b). For example, among group members in the Lake Tanganyika cichlid *N. pulcher*, individual differences in helping effort are better explained by personality differences than by relatedness to the dominant breeding pair (Le Vin et al. 2011). Although subordinates can recognize kin (Le Vin et al. 2010), relatedness to the breeding pair had no effect on the amount of helping performed. In contrast, helping was linked to personality traits, with aggressive individuals participating more in territory defence than submissive individuals (Le Vin et al. 2011). This results from the development of different individuals in alternative 'social niches' (Bergmüller & Taborsky 2007, 2010).

Condition-dependent helping. Absence of kin-selected helping could also be explained if individuals make condition-dependent decisions on whether to become a helper. This is because helping is energetically expensive (Grantner & Taborsky 1998; Taborsky & Grantner 1988; Heinsohn & Legge 1999) and the amount of help given may, therefore, depend on the helper's physiological condition; this may in turn influence the costs of helping (e.g. the probability of survival and future breeding). If the costs of helping are high, it is expected that only subordinates in sufficiently good physical condition can afford to help. For example, in meerkats and Seychelles

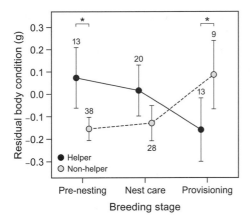

Figure 4.37 Variation in body condition for helping and non-helping subordinate Seychelles warblers (white) throughout the breeding season. Dots indicate mean ± SE and numbers indicate sample sizes. *$P < 0.05$ (from van de Crommenacker et al. 2011b).

warblers, there is evidence that helping results in a decline in body condition and that only subordinates in sufficiently high condition can afford to help (Russell et al. 2003; van de Crommenacker et al. 2011b). In Seychelles warblers prior to breeding, subordinates that did not subsequently help (non-helpers) had significantly lower body condition than subordinates that did subsequently help. During the later stages of breeding (incubation and provisioning of nestlings) body condition declined in helpers but not in non-helpers, and at the end of the helping period body condition of helpers was lower than that of non-helpers (Figure 4.37; van de Crommenacker et al. 2011b). This indicates that only subordinates with a sufficiently good body condition can afford to help, as they need reserves to be used up by costly brood care (Figure 4.37). Hitherto, condition-dependence of helping activity has rarely been incorporated into models of helping strategies (e.g. Heinsohn & Legge 1999; Russell et al. 2003; Covas & Griesser 2007; Lawson Handley & Perrin 2007). However, it is important to realize that not only the costs of helping but also trade-offs incorporating both the costs of helping and potential future benefits need to be considered when attempting to understand the decision rules underlying helping.

4.2 Forced Cooperation

One individual may help another due to the latter's manipulation, even against its own fitness interests (Clutton-Brock & Parker 1995; Ågren et al. 2019; Engelhardt & Taborsky 2020). This may involve open force or surreptitious manipulation. Evolutionarily speaking, what may look like 'purposeful cooperation' is in fact exploitation of one partner by the other, i.e. parasitism. If keas (*Nestor notabilis*) are exposed to a situation where food can be obtained only with the help of others, these birds do not reciprocate help in series of repeated interactions, as would be predicted by the concept of reciprocal altruism, but instead dominants force subordinates to produce food for them (Tebbich et al. 1996). Well-known examples of enforced cooperation include food sharing in primates (Gilby 2006) and the policing observed in social insects, where workers remove the eggs of other workers by egg cannibalism (Ratnieks 1988; Wenseleers & Ratnieks 2006b; Zweden et al. 2007). In this case, policing takes the form of damage limitation, after the eggs have been laid. As outlined in Section 3.2.3, policing may also take more subtle forms, where the mere threat of infanticide causes subordinates to refrain from reproduction (Cant et al. 2014). In cooperatively breeding species such as meerkats and Lake Tanganyika cichlids, the fact that breeders usually gain higher inclusive fitness than their subordinate helpers may also indicate a form of enforcement (Sharp & Clutton-Brock 2011; Jungwirth & Taborsky 2015). Surreptitious manipulation of help, on the other hand, is exemplified conspicuously by brood parasitism, both at intra- and interspecific levels. Host parents raising a cuckoo chick exhibit what might be viewed as the ultimate form of altruism; they spend enormous effort involving substantial fitness costs at the benefit of a heterospecific with which they share neither interests nor pay-off (Davies et al. 1989; Davies 2000, 2015; cf. Section 5.3).

Here we distinguish two mechnisms by which cooperation may be forced by one partner upon another: coercion and surreptitious exploitation.

4.2.1   Coercion

Individuals may coerce others either to do something in favour of their direct or indirect fitness, or to refrain from doing something that is against their fitness interests. The possibilities for open enforcement depend on the relative power and alternative options of the interacting partners.

4.2.1.1   Power Symmetry

Typically, forced helping is not expected among individuals of similar strength because the costs of coercion are likely to be high and threats of punishment are unlikely to be credible (Section 3.3.3). However, worker policing appears to be a case where a group of equal-ranked individuals can enforce reproductive restraint among potential cheats (Ratnieks & Wenseleers 2005, 2008). It is still unclear whether policing among workers can also serve to increase work rate (such as food provisioning), or whether it merely serves to suppress selfish reproduction, i.e. the production of worker eggs (see Box 4.9 for potential reasons). In the social wasp *Ropalidia marginata*, workers that do not apparently differ from others take over the reproductive role when the resident queen dies or disappears, subsequently forcing the other workers to care for their eggs by hyperaggressively acquiring dominance (Bang & Gadagkar 2012; Gadagkar 2016). Even if power asymmetry characterizes the relationship between this new queen and her former peers, before the takeover of the queen role the relationship between the upcoming 'potential queen' and the other

Box 4.9 When Does Punishment Create Cooperation, and How Common is it in Nature?

Negative feedback such as punishment is well suited to suppress the unwelcome behaviour of subordinates. Nevertheless, the prevalence of punishment in natural interactions among animals is controversial. While some regard punishment as common in social animals (also referred to as 'retaliatory aggression' or 'negative reciprocity'; Clutton-Brock & Parker 1995), others bewail its apparent rarity (Raihani et al. 2012). Partly, this is due to differences in how punishment is defined. Some define punishment broadly as as 'a behaviour that inflicts a net cost on, or removes net benefits from, a target individual in response to a specific behavior by that target individual' (Singh & Boomsma 2015). Others prefer a narrower definition which requires that punishment must be costly to the punisher (Raihani et al. 2012); such type of behaviour otherwise has been referred to as 'altruistic punishment' in public goods games (Fehr & Gächter 2002; Boyd et al. 2003; Fowler 2005). The narrow definition implies that both interaction partners suffer costs of punishment, but the idea is that the costs of the receiver exceed those of the actor, and that the latter's costs are offset by future benefits resulting from the punishment. This conception excludes, for instance, cases where social control delivers immediate benefits to the actor, such as when ant workers eat the eggs of other workers, which ultimately ensures reproductive skew in the colony ('policing'; Ratnieks et al. 2006). As consuming an egg provides immediate nutritional benefits, it may be regarded as 'self-serving' and hence does not qualify as punishment according to the narrow definition (in Raihani et al.'s 2012 terms this corresponds to a 'sanction').

As outlined above, we prefer using operational definitions that do not run counter connotations of everyday language. Therefore, in our understanding, punishment refers to actions directed against an individual contingent on harm it had caused; these actions typically are costly to the punished individual, and they may or may not entail costs to the punisher (cf. Singh & Boomsma 2015). If punishing causes costs to the actor at a benefit to others, this is termed 'altruistic punishment' in accordance with earlier literature (e.g. Fehr & Gächter 2002; Boyd et al. 2003).

Punishment may be a response to a social partner's behaviour causing adverse effects, or to its abstention from cooperation. As we are dealing with cooperation in this chapter, we shall here confine discussion to the latter aspect. In vervet monkeys (*Chlorocebus aethiops pygerythrus*), for instance, females may aggressively punish males that have abstained from participating in intergroup warfare, which increases the likelihood that they will take part in future fights about resources with neighbouring groups (Arseneau-Robar et al. 2016). In the highly social naked mole-rats (*Heterocephalus glaber*), the dominant female may increase the working propensity of lazy non-reproductives by aggressively pushing them through the tunnel system ('shoving'; Reeve & Sherman 1991; Reeve 1992), but the contingency between received aggression and an increase in work seems to be

Box 4.9 (*cont.*)

context-dependent (Jacobs & Jarvis 1996; Clarke & Faulkes 2001). The propensity of non-reproductive individuals in this species to engage in work, for instance in digging out the gallery system, may be triggered by odour cues of the dominant female reproductive (Kutsukake et al. 2012). In social paper wasps, *Polistes fuscatus*, dominant queens attack inactive workers, which induces cooperative behaviours such as food collection (Reeve & Gamboa 1983, 1987; Gamboa et al. 1990; Sumana & Starks 2004). In other wasp species, work may be regulated partly by aggression exhibited among workers (*Polybia occidentalis*: O'Donnell 2001; *Polistes versicolor*: De Souza & Prezoto 2012). An experiment with the bacterium *Pseudomonas aeruginosa* showed that punishment of non-cooperative strains by cooperators evolved if traits responsible for punishment and cooperation were genetically linked (Inglis et al. 2014). Punishment occurring in the context of negotiations and trading between members of different species will be discussed in Chapter 5.

Theoretical models have shown that aggression can be a useful tool to cause helping by a behavioural mechanism called 'pay-to-stay' (Gaston 1978; Kokko et al. 2002; Hamilton & Taborsky 2005b; Quinones et al. 2016; Hellmann & Hamilton 2018). This works when subordinates benefit from group membership but cause costs to dominants by competition for resources and reproduction. It implies that dominants demand compensation of these costs by subordinates, comparable to 'payment of rent' for group membership and the use of resources monopolized by the group. In addition to the evidence for regulation of cooperative work in mammals and insects discussed above, there is experimental and observational evidence that helpful behaviour of subordinates is triggered by aggressive actions of dominants also in birds (superb fairy-wrens, *Malurus cyaneus*: Mulder & Langmore 1993; sociable weavers, *Philetairus socius*: Leighton & Vander Meiden 2016) and fish (Princess of Lake Tanganyika, *Neolamprologus pulcher*: Taborsky 1985; Balshine-Earn et al. 1998; Bergmüller & Taborsky 2005; Bergmüller et al. 2005a; Heg & Taborsky 2010; Zöttl et al. 2013a; Fischer et al. 2014; Naef & Taborsky 2020a, 2020b). Experimental evidence for the pay-to-stay mechanism comes from manipulation of (i) the presence of helpers (Mulder & Langmore 1993; Balshine-Earn et al. 1998; Fischer et al. 2014), (ii) the need of help (Taborsky 1985; Bruintjes & Taborsky 2008; Heg & Taborsky 2010; Zöttl et al. 2013b), and (iii) the behaviour of subordinates (Bergmüller & Taborsky 2005; Zöttl et al. 2013c; Fischer et al. 2014; Naef & Taborsky 2020a, 2020b). Additional evidence results from the experimental manipulation of outside options for helpers, which affects their propensity to engage in cooperative behaviour within their original group (cichlid fish: Bergmüller et al. 2005a; paper wasps: Grinsted & Field 2017). Payment for group membership may also occur through hygienic behaviour such as allogrooming directed towards dominants (meerkats: Kutsukake & Clutton-Brock 2010), or through help shown by subordinates in

Box 4.9 *(cont.)*

response to reacceptance in the group (antipredator defence in cichlids: Taborsky 1985; allonursing in meerkats: MacLeod et al. 2013).

Other studies searching for evidence that helpers pay to stay have been less successful (acorn woodpecker, *Melanerpes formicivorus*: Koenig & Walters 2011; meerkats, Santema & Clutton-Brock 2012; chestnut-crowned babbler, *Pomatostomus ruficeps*: Nomano et al. 2015; El Oro parakeet, *Pyrrhura orcesi*: Kramer et al. 2016). The absence of evidence for the aggressive manipulation of cooperative behaviour may have several reasons. (1) Coercion may be difficult to detect because it usually involves threats; punishment is only necessary when a threat fails to cause the desired response (Johnstone & Cant 1999; Cant & Johnstone 2009; Cant 2011). Typically, restrained aggression (in the form of threats) occurs much more frequently than overt attacks. As threats are usually much less conspicuous than outright assaults, coercion and punishment may often remain undetected. (2) Negotiations between social partners may render coercive interference unnecessary (Taylor & Day 2004; Quinones et al. 2016; Ito et al. 2017; see also McNamara 2013). Again, negotiations can involve threats, but also offers, and the administration of overt aggression and punishment for non-cooperative responses may be rare and difficult to detect. (3) Conditions conducive to coercive manipulation of social partners might in fact be rather uncommon. They require a combination of a clear dominance asymmetry among the involved parties with the availability of only somewhat undesirable outside options to the subordinate partner. For instance, if subordinates are quasi 'trapped' in a group because leaving would mean almost certain demise, such as in *N. pulcher* (Taborsky 1984; Heg et al. 2004a), dominants may demand compensation from subordinates for the costs they cause (Hamilton & Taborsky 2005b). If the attractiveness of outside options increases in comparison to the situation in the home territory, however, subordinates may resist the demands of dominants and choose the more favourable alternative (Bergmüller et al. 2005a, 2005b; Zöttl et al. 2013d; Jungwirth et al. 2015a), i.e. they may threaten to end the interaction and exit the group (Cant & Johnstone 2006). Subordinates should accept enforcement of help only to a level where the costs of paying for being allowed to stay exceed the costs of leaving the group (Kokko et al. 2002). (4) Social partners often may not withhold cooperation due to own, synergistic benefits (Riehl & Frederickson 2016). If uncooperative individuals have lower, not higher, fitness than cooperators, cheating will be absent, which makes punishment redundant. Conflicts of fitness interests in tightly knit social groups might in fact be rarer than commonly assumed (Bshary et al. 2016). (5) Last but not least, the rarity of aggressive manipulation of cooperative behaviour by social partners may be ostensible rather than actual due to a dearth of suitable studies. For instance, in cooperative breeders a conclusive test of a pay-to-stay mechanism requires experimental manipulation of the behaviour of dominants and subordinates, which has rarely been conducted

---

Box 4.9 (*cont.*)

(cf. Taborsky 1985; Bergmüller & Taborsky 2005; Fischer et al. 2014; Naef & Taborsky 2020a, 2020b).

In eusocial insects, pay-to-stay is an unlikely mechanism because workers typically do not have 'outside options' due to sterility; hence, their fitness interests are congruent with those of the reproductive (i.e. queen), which means that there is no need for being made to work by enforcement. Nevertheless if the concept of cooperation is extended to the abstention of selfish acts (or 'acquiescence': Wenseleers et al. 2004a), enforced altruism may in fact be widespread in eusocial insects exhibiting behavioural, morphological and physiological differentiation among reproductive and non-reproductive castes, especially through the suppression of worker reproduction by aggression or egg cannibalism (Ratnieks & Wenseleers 2005, 2008; Wenseleers & Ratnieks 2006a). It might be argued that non-reproductive group members like insect workers are not 'individuals' in the functional sense, but rather comparable to organs in a multicellular organism (Wheller 1911; Queller & Strassmann 2009). Hence, their fitness interests are so highly correlated with those of their other group members, particularly the reproductives or 'queens', that even if their behaviour is manipulated by others, this occurs in their own fitness interest, i.e. policing reflects an adaptive, regulatory process for the policed. As policing provides strong incentives for nest mates to refrain from own, 'selfish' reproduction and instead help to raise sisters, this is also favoured by kin selection (Wenseleers et al. 2004a, 2004b; Wenseleers & Ratnieks 2006a; Ratnieks & Wenseleers 2008). In effect, a eusocial insect queen makes herself incapable of caring for her offspring, thereby prompting daughters to care for their sisters, which is chemically enforced by queen pheromone (Oi et al. 2015a). As the daughters are highly related among one another – if they are full sisters even higher than they would be to their own daughters – altruism is also favoured by kin selection (Oi et al. 2015b). However, while policing may not reflect a response to diverging fitness interests in some circumstances (van Zweden et al. 2007; Meunier et al. 2010), this may not apply in others (Brunner & Heinze 2009).

---

workers seems to be rather symmetrical (Lamba et al. 2007; Bhadra & Gadagkar 2008).

A different form of 'enforcement' of cooperation that does not rely on asymmetry in strength is self-handicapping. In hornbills of the genus *Tockus*, females self-handicap to force males to help by sealing themselves up in the nesting cavity with their clutch and moulting their feathers (Kemp & Woodcock 1995; Klaassen et al. 2003). By credibly removing the ability to forage for herself, a female forces her male partner to perform all the work involved in provisioning both her and their shared brood. This form of coercion is effective so long as males get a higher pay-off by staying to work than they would from desertion. Self-handicapping can occur also on an evolutionary timescale, through changes in morphology or life history. In some eusocial insects, queens have evolved to become so specialized for egg production that they are incapable of surviving without the help of workers, as exemplifed by mound-building termites *Macrotermes* (Bignell et al. 2011). In resident killer whales, males become more dependent on the presence of their mother the older and bigger they get (Foster et al. 2012). One hypothesis is that intrasexual selection for large size in males has left them unable to catch fast-moving salmon prey, and due to this size handicap they depend on food sharing by their mother (D. Croft, pers. comm.). As in eusocial insects, here self-handicapping, a form of coercion enforcing cooperative behaviour of social partners with aligned fitness interests due to shared genes, seems to select for altruistic behaviour in conjunction with kin selection.

4.2.1.2 Power Asymmetry

Clear power asymmetries among social partners may make it easier and more rewarding for a dominant individual to demand cooperation of a subordinate by force. This applies in particular if subordinates have limited outside options or none at all. In that case, subordinates cannot gain more fitness by leaving their current group, for instance because of a lack in competitive power as exemplified by low-quality males partaking in reproductive coalitions (McDonald & Potts 1994; DuVal 2007c; Rubenstein & Nuñez 2009), or because the habitat suitable for breeding is saturated (Koenig et al. 1992), or because dispersal is too risky (Heg et al. 2004a). In such a case, a dominant individual can demand helping effort for amenities provided to the subordinate. This is the case, for instance, when subordinates must pay to stay in the territory of dominants (Bergmüller et al. 2005a; Zöttl et al. 2013d). A special situation applies in eusocial insects, where subordinates may not have an outside option at all because they are not able to reproduce on their own (see Section 3.3.2). In such a case, the fitness interests of dominants (the queen) and subordinates (the workers) may fully overlap, rendering coercion of help unnecessary (Korb & Heinze 2004; Bourke 2011). If there is division of labour between divergent castes, workers typically determine the caste fate of larvae by different feeding regimes, and reproductive individuals are produced approximately in proportion to colony needs (Wilson 1971; Wenseleers et al. 2003; Ratnieks et al. 2006). However, in many social insects manipulation of subordinates by a dominant queen is implemented by use of chemical signals and/or aggressive dominance to prevent subordinate reproduction (e.g. Lüscher 1961; Fletcher & Ross 1985; Gadagkar 2001; Bhadra et al. 2010; Holman et al. 2010; Matsuura 2012; Saha et al. 2012; Oi et al. 2015a; Brahma et al. 2018, 2019). Strong reproductive skew based on dominance asymmetries and manipulation is a common characteristic also of vertebrate societies (Hager & Jones 2009; see Section 3.2.3).

In cooperative breeders, if staying in a group or access to a territory is important for individuals unable to monopolize essential resources by themselves, they may be selected to pay for being allowed to stay with conspecifics that have power over the required facilities (Gaston 1978; Kokko et al. 2002; Hamilton & Taborsky 2005b; see Box 4.9). In such a situation, payment can be either enforced by aggression or by a credible threat of eviction (Cant 2011; Section 3.2.3). In cooperatively breeding fish,

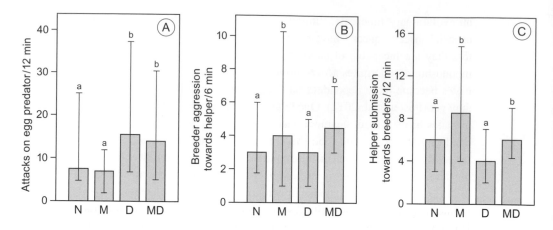

Figure 4.38 Effect of prevensting helping behaviour on (A) subsequsent compensation by increased cooperative defence against an egg predator in the social cichlid *N. pulcher*. When defence had been prevented by experimental manipulation (treatment D), helpers roughly doubled their defence effort against an egg predator compared with a situation in which either no helping had been previously prevented (treatment N), or only territory maintenance (digging out a common shelter) had been prevented (treatment M). In the situation in which both defence and territory maintenance had been previously prevented (treatment MD), helpers also greatly increased their cooperative defence effort during the subsequent test period. (B) Effect of preventing helping to dig out a common shelter (territory maintenance, M) on aggression of breeders towards helpers directly after the manipulation, and (C) on submissive behaviour of helpers towards breeders. These results suggest that in contrast to defence against egg predators, a lack of cooperative territory maintenance in helpers is punished by breeders, which leads to increased submission by the helpers. Medians and interquartile ranges are shown, different letters within graphs denote statistical significance (GLMM, $P < 0.05$; after Naef & Taborsky 2020a, 2020b).

birds and mammals, there is indeed evidence that helping by subordinates can be triggered by aggression of dominants or by the threats of eviction (Box 4.9). Dominant females among naked mole-rats, for instance, may forcefully activate lazy workers (Reeve & Sherman 1991; Reeve 1992), whereas temporarily removed helpers among superb fairy-wrens are attacked upon their return, which seems to make them work harder (Mulder & Langmore 1993). Payment of 'rent' may explain cooperative behaviour of helpers in bird species in which they lack opportunities to leave and breed elsewhere due to habitat saturation (Cockburn 1998), but this needs further study. Helpers of cooperatively breeding cichlids are made to work for others by frequent aggressive enforcement by dominant group members (Taborsky 1985). After subordinates were temporarily prevented from helping, they are exposed to increased aggression by dominants (Fischer et al. 2014; Naef & Taborsky 2020a, 2020b) and may attempt to pre-emptively appease dominants by submission and increased help, such as cooperative territory defence (Bergmüller & Taborsky 2005; Naef & Taborsky 2020b; Figure 4.38). Helping in these fish mainly serves to pay rent for being allowed to stay in a safe territory, which is essential for subordinates because survival outside of a group is hardly possible (Taborsky 1984; Heg et al. 2004a). Natural groups are mixed between related and unrelated individuals (Dierkes et al. 2005), and experiments have revealed that pay-to-stay creates higher helping levels than relatedness (Stiver et al. 2005; Zöttl et al. 2013a; the general importance of the pay-to-stay mechanism in different systems is discussed in Section 3.2 and Box 4.9).

For dominant breeders, in turn, subordinates provide important help in brood care and other duties, which may result in load lightening (Johnstone 2011). An experiment in which *N. pulcher* breeders were randomly assigned to have helpers or not showed that the presence of helpers enhanced the reproductive rate of dominant females (Taborsky 1984). In the field, experimental manipulation of helper numbers revealed significant positive effects of helpers on offspring survival (Brouwer et al. 2005), which may be the ultimate reason why females with many helpers produce smaller eggs than females with few helpers, apparently saving energy for an increasing number of offspring at the expense of their quality (Taborsky et al. 2007). Important load-lightening effects for breeders caused by the action of helpers have been identified also in a closely related cooperatively breeding cichlid, *N. obscurus* (Tanaka et al. 2018a, 2018b, 2018c), and in several cooperatively breeding birds (Crick 1992; Hatchwell 1999; Heinsohn 2004; Brouwer et al. 2014; van Boheemen et al. 2019). In both cooperatively breeding cichlids and birds, contributions of helpers have been shown also to cause additive effects on the breeders' Darwinian fitness (i.e. when the latter do not or only partially reduce their parental investment in response to the helpers' aid, and hence total investment in brood care increases; Hatchwell 1999; Bruintjes et al. 2013; Zöttl et al. 2013c; Brouwer et al. 2014; Liebl et al. 2016; van Boheemen et al. 2019).

In cooperatively breeding northern paper wasps *Polistes fuscatus*, subordinate females are prompted to make foraging trips by the behaviour of the dominant female, as revealed by manipulation of the latter's ability to interfere with them. The dominant's manipulation of subordinates involves various behaviours, including aggression (Reeve & Gamboa 1987). Male helpers among meerkats are subject to more aggression by dominants if being lazy, and they seem to be punished by dominants if they pretend to supply the latters' offspring with food while in fact consuming it themselves (Clutton-Brock et al. 2005). Female subordinates are often evicted before the dominant female gives birth to her litter (Clutton-Brock et al. 1998) but may be reaccepted, which coincides with reduced aggression of the dominant female (Young et al. 2006; Clutton-Brock et al. 2008). Such females are more likely to allonurse the dominant's offspring, which might serve payment for reacceptance in the territory (MacLeod et al. 2013). Nevertheless, playback experiments using begging calls to imply a perceived increase of need did not reveal that the dominant female adjusts its aggression towards helpers to increase their provisioning (Santema & Clutton-Brock 2012). In contrast, aggression towards helpers is clearly contingent on need in *N. pulcher*. In these cichlids, helpers are expelled from territories when not needed, and they are reaccepted when demand is experimentally increased (Taborsky 1985). Experimental enhancement of demand even causes acceptance of unrelated, previously unknown individuals in the territory, which subsequently engage in intense helping (Zöttl et al. 2013b).

Asymmetries may not only exist in power, but also with regard to outside options or situational knowledge. In a prisoner's dilemma situation, if a player realizes that its behaviour can influence its partner's response, it can extort the latter's behaviour to its own benefit (Press & Dyson 2012). With certain probabilistic strategies smart individuals may thereby exploit the response of less-informed partners that by their behaviour still maximize own fitness returns which, however, will not match the benefits of the players determining the rules. In other words, one player can force the other to accept a less-than-equal share of the pay-off. If players have similar strategic possibilities, extortion may be only a transient phenomenon that lacks long-term evolutionary stability (Adami & Hintze 2013; Hilbe et al. 2013), but with partners differing in strategic power or outside options, extortion may emerge more easily (Hilbe et al. 2014, 2016). As extortion in the iterated prisoner's dilemma benefits from asymmetrical information, this strategy leads smoothly over to 'surreptitious exploitation' as discussed in the subsequent section.

4.2.2   Surreptitious Exploitation

Individuals may exploit the effort of a social partner surreptitiously, for instance by evading recognition mechanisms. This is exemplified by intraspecific and interspecific brood parasitism and by parasitic mating tactics of males producing offspring that are tended by nest owners. Such behaviour will select for counter-measures of the exploited party, such as greater recognition power, which may result in an arms race between involved players (Dawkins et al. 1979; see Chapter 5). This form of altruism, which clearly opposes the fitness interests of the deceived partner and hence is commonly called *social parasitism*, is widespread and most impressively illustrated by species subject to brood parasitism (Andersson et al. 2019; especially conspicuous at the interspecific level: Davies et al. 1989; Davies 2000; Kilner & Langmore 2011; see Section 5.3.3) and alternative mating tactics (Oliveira et al. 2008; Taborsky & Brockmann 2010; see Section 2.6.3).

Intraspecific brood parasitism, where individuals deposit eggs or young in a conspecific's nest, mouth or den to leave their offspring in the latter's custody, is common in insects, fishes and birds (Yom-Tov 1980, 2001; Andersson 1984; Tallamy 1985, 2005; Yanagisawa 1985; Petrie & Moller 1991; Wisenden 1999; Ochi & Yanagisawa 2005; Schaedelin et al. 2013; Andersson et al. 2019). Interestingly, the degree of social parasitism differs between the sexes. In males, individuals may specialize in parasitic reproduction lifelong (Taborsky 1994, 1988; Alonzo et al. 2000), which can reflect a genetic polymorphism (Lank et al. 1995; Shuster & Sassaman 1997; Tsubaki 2003; Wirtz-Ocaña et al. 2014). This is apparently not the case in females, where specialization in lifelong brood parasitism of conspecifics has not been found (Andersson et al. 2019). Nevertheless, interspecific brood parasitism (see Section 5.3) likely starts with females parasitizing conspecifics (Davies et al. 1989; Davies 2000), but the evolutionary transition from intraspecific to interspecific brood parasitism is difficult to observe. A remarkable case in point is the African honeybee. South Africa is home to two subspecies of honeybee, the Cape bee (*Apis mellifera capensis*) and the African honeybee *A. m. scuttelata*. Workers of the former subspecies can successfully invade colonies of the latter and produce parthenogenetic diploid daughter eggs which evade policing by host workers, most likely by mimicking the pheromonal profile of queen-laid eggs (Martin et al. 2002; Beekman & Oldroyd 2008). These daughters are reared by the host colony and produce yet more parasitic daughters themselves, some of which disperse to infect other colonies. The end result is a disaster for the host colony and a massive loss of colonies in the wider *Scuttelata* population (the so-called Capensis calamity; Beekman & Oldroyd 2008).

4.3   Conclusions

When considering the four alternative mechanisms responsible for the evolution of cooperation, by-product mutualism, reciprocity, shared genes, and coercion or deception, a burning question is their relative importance for the explanation of cooperative behaviour as found in nature. The importance of correlated fitness pay-offs becomes clear immediately when considering the most widespread altruistic cooperation in nature – offspring care or, more generally, parental investment. Offspring are in demand of help because their survival competence is typically inferior to that of their caregiver, hence the benefits, b, of help to them are high. Due to the inherent competence asymmetry, parents can often provide such required help by paying rather small costs, c. In addition, parents and offspring have correlated pay-offs due to their high share of (potentially causal) genes, which is denoted by r. Therefore, correlated pay-offs are undoubtedly a – if not *the* – major cause of cooperation in nature (Hamilton 1964), which often extends beyond the interaction between parents and their offspring by involving alloparental care (Bourke 2011).

The role of *mutualistic* cooperation has been revealed mainly in the interspecific context, where this field of research has a long history (Boucher 1985; Thompson 1994; Stadler & Dixon 2008; Douglas 2010). In contrast, the evolution of mutualistic interactions between conspecifics has received comparatively little attention, both regarding the development of theory (e.g. Bednekoff 1997; Kokko et al. 2001; Lehmann & Keller 2006a) and empirical studies (for review, see Dugatkin 1997; Clutton-Brock 2002, 2009; Kingma et al. 2014). However, as we have outlined in this chapter, mutualistic cooperation based on by-product benefits cannot be cheated. Due to this and the obviously widespread situation that behaviour benefitting an actor directly will also prove advantageous to a social partner, cooperation based on (by-product) mutualism is expected to be widespread (Stevens & Gilby 2004). The prototype of intraspecific behavioural mutualism is cooperative hunting, which has been studied in many taxa (see Packer & Ruttan 1988; Clutton-Brock 2002, 2009 for review).

Potential evolutionary mechanisms causing cooperation on the basis of *reciprocity* have received much theoretical attention, due to their inherent complicacy. Importantly, fitness pay-offs are also somewhat correlated between reciprocating interaction partners, albeit in this case not due to shared genes but to a shared future

(Taborsky et al. 2016). The standard paradigm used to test for the potential evolutionary stability of decision rules to cooperate or to defect is the prisoner's dilemma, especially in its iterated variant, together with some other game theoretic models of social dilemmas (Axelrod & Hamilton 1981; Nowak & Sigmund 1993; Killingback & Doebeli 2002; Doebeli et al. 2005; Pfeiffer et al. 2005). As outlined in this chapter, the behavioural rules characterizing the three different forms, generalized, direct and indirect reciprocity, imply increasing demands in the involved cognitive mechanisms. Hence, the simplest decision rule 'help anyone if helped by someone', which represents *generalized reciprocity*, involves the least demands on the acquisition, processing and keeping of information. Various theoretical models have shown that despite the vulnerability of this decision rule to selfish exploitation, cooperation based on this simple mechanism can be evolutionarily stable (Hamilton & Taborsky 2005a; Pfeiffer et al. 2005; Nowak & Roch 2007; Rankin & Taborsky 2009; Barta et al. 2011; van Doorn & Taborsky 2012). In addition, several studies using controlled experiments have revealed that humans and other animals are using this decision rule (Bartlett & DeSteno 2006; Rutte & Taborsky 2007; Stanca 2009; Leimgruber et al. 2014; Claidiere et al. 2015; Gfrerer & Taborsky 2017). However, the natural occurrence of cooperation based on generalized reciprocity is still unclear. Despite many scenarios where it could explain social behaviour of animals, alternative explanatory mechanisms, such as kin selection if cooperation happens between relatives, or a hidden involvement of enforcement or deception, are notoriously difficult to exclude. However, if this mechanism will be studied experimentally in a greater number of taxa, this might bring to light that generalized reciprocity often causes cooperation also in nature.

Indirect reciprocity, in contrast, might be too demanding to be an important cause of cooperation in nature outside of humans (Milinski & Wedekind 1998). Even if animals have the ability to acquire, process and memorize the required information, it is probably too costly and prone to errors to be an efficient strategy of cooperation. As opposed to indirect reciprocity, where interactions between third parties determine an individual's cooperation propensity, *direct reciprocity* has frequently been shown to explain the cooperative behaviour of animals, against the belief of sceptics (de Waal & Brosnan 2006; Schino & Aureli 2009, 2010a, 2010c, 2017; Carter 2014; Taborsky et al. 2016; Freidin et al. 2017; Schweinfurth & Call 2019b; Table 4.1). Nevertheless, the role of trading and negotiations about the same or different commodities in such reciprocal interactions of animals is currently little understood. The potential to generate high levels of cooperation by such negotiation processes has been shown to be even greater than by correlated pay-offs based on relatedness (Carter & Wilkinson 2013, 2016; Zöttl et al. 2013a; Quinones et al. 2016; Schweinfurth & Taborsky 2018a). This opens exciting opportunities for future research in order to reveal the extent to which negotiations and trading explain cooperation among animals in their natural environment.

According to Hamilton's rule (Hamilton 1964), altruistic cooperation should be selected in dependence of the degree of *relatedness* between an actor and the recipient of a helpful act. This is perhaps most obviously demonstrated by the evolution of parental care (Clutton-Brock 1991; Royle et al. 2012); costly investment of parents benefits their progeny, thereby propagating genes responsible for the cooperative investment. Notably, such costly cooperation may be favoured by natural selection also if it benefits the progeny of others, as long as these share the respective genetic machinery either by common descent (kin selection; Hamilton 1964) or combined with a recognition mechanism identifying the responsible genetic architecture ('green-beard genes'; Dawkins 1976). Hence associations among kin may enhance the evolution of cooperative behaviour among relatives. However, this is not always the case (Lehmann & Rousset 2010), partly because kin typically also compete for resources (Taylor 1992b; Wilson et al. 1992). Therefore, it may not be surprising that many species living in kin-structured groups do not show a correlation between relatedness and cooperation. Moreover, if other mechanisms selecting for cooperation apply as well, such as reciprocity or enforcement, relatedness may actually reduce cooperation instead of favouring it (Zöttl et al. 2013a; Schweinfurth & Taborsky 2018a). It is hence important to identify the demographic conditions and the different selection mechanisms involved before making clear predictions about how relatedness will affect the evolution of cooperation in a particular system and context (Frank 1998). For the empiricist, the relative importance of nepotism and reciprocity may be difficult to disentangle (Carter et al. 2019).

Forced cooperation is probably widespread, because asymmetries in capabilities and pay-offs are the rule rather than the exception (Phillips 2018), which sets the stage for manipulations based on exerting power over social partners. Policing in eusocial insects, pay-to-stay in social vertebrates, and other forms of imposed help are illustrating the potential importance of enforcement in apparently cooperative interactions. Typically, these asymmetrical interactions also include an element of negotiation and trading. It is probably rare that a dominant individual has full power over the behavioural and other traits of a subordinate. If there are outside options, the subordinate should only submit to pressure up to the point where leaving the interaction provides higher fitness benefits (Kokko et al. 2002; Cant & Johnstone 2006). In eusocial insects featuring castes, in which morphological modifications have degraded workers and soldiers to mere supporting organs of the reproducing queen, the lack of outside options may select for complete submission of subordinates to the fitness interests of the entire 'organism' containing reproductive (queen) and other functional units (workers, soldiers; Queller & Strassmann 2009).

A different selection regime underlies the evolution of altruistic help elicited among conspecifics by surreptitious deception, as in the intraspecific brood parasitism observed in insects, fishes and birds. Interestingly, even if typically this runs against the fitness interests of the parasitized hosts, they may sometimes also be beneficiaries of supplemented broods, implying that their cooperation is not always entirely altruistic (Andersson et al. 2019).

Probably the most captivating challenge for future research is the clarification of multiple and multicomponent selection mechanisms in the causation of cooperation. Multifarious selection mechanisms are usually involved in the evolution of biological traits, and cooperative behaviour is no exception to this rule. Currently, we are far away from understanding how different mechanisms such as kin selection, mutualism, reciprocity and social manipulation interact in creating the terrific diversity and complexity of cooperation and social structure found in nature, but there is no doubt that typically several different selection mechanisms concur in their origin and maintenance (Alexander 1974; Dugatkin 1997; Lehmann & Keller 2006a; West et al. 2007c; Quinones et al. 2016). In the next chapter we shall outline that, apart from shared genes, all selection mechanisms causing cooperation among conspecifics can generate cooperation also among individuals of different species and organisms, which can be instrumental in creating entities of higher organizational levels.

The Evolution of Social Complexity in the Princess of Lake Tanganyika

Summary

Cooperatively breeding cichlids of Lake Tanganyika constitute a unique model for the study of ultimate and proximate mechanisms underlying social complexity and cooperation. Groups of *Neolamprologus pulcher*, aka the 'Princess of Lake Tanganyika', consist of a mixture of related and unrelated individuals of both sexes and a wide range of sizes, reproductive and life-history stages. They all collaborate in one way or another to maintain shelters and defend a territory, and to care for the brood that is produced largely by a dominant pair. This enabled unravelling the relative importance of relatedness and of reciprocal trading of services for the evolutionary ecology of cooperative breeding in this model system.

Both experimental evidence and a comparison of distinct populations revealed that *one* environmental factor – predation risk – is the fundamental ecological driver of this social system. Subordinates obtain protection by antipredator defence of territory owners and by obtaining access to a safe shelter, which is essential for their survival. In turn, they help in maintaining the breeding shelter and in the care and protection of young produced by the territory owners. If helpers are not fulfilling their duties, they are punished through dominants' attacks. If their help is not needed, they are expelled from the territory. Moreover, if helpers are related to the beneficiaries of their aid, they show less investment than if they are unrelated. Hence, kin selection cannot explain the high degree of cooperation in this system. Instead, group members are trading services among each other.

All parties involved, whether dominant or subordinate, have alternative options if the costs of cooperation start exceeding the benefits. The resulting interaction is an evident example of cooperation based on reciprocity. Due to the inherent dominance asymmetry, there is an element of coercion involved in this relationship. By attacking idle helpers, dominants can modify the cooperative propensity of subordinates through imposing costs resulting from neglect, but they cannot make subordinates help if they do not provide benefits in return: helpers have outside options and can always leave for good. Hence, the pay-to-stay scenario observed in *N. pulcher* clearly reflects reciprocal trading, which is an alternative explanation of cooperative breeding to kin selection, as frequently supposed in similar social organizations in mammals and birds.

Introduction

At the Max-Planck-Institute for Behavioural Physiology in Seewiesen, the Masters student Klaus Kalas observed that in a cichlid fish named *Lamprologus brichardi*, the young of previous broods would not disperse but instead stay in their natal territory and help in rearing subsequent broods. Wolfgang Wickler, head of the institute and a profound expert in both evolutionary biology and cichlid behaviour, immediately realized the spectacular nature of this observation. At that time, in vertebrates such 'cooperative breeding syndrome' was only known from birds and mammals. Wickler's insight spawned a cascade of studies, over the years making these fish one of the best-studied social vertebrates to date. The diversity of their behavioural repertoire, their intricate ways of communicating among group members and the cooperative sharing of tasks all seem appropriate for highly social primates, but not for an unremarkable fish of some 6 cm in size. The striking social complexity of these fish opened up unique opportunities to study the fitness costs and benefits of social behaviour in a vertebrate experimentally and in nature, thereby addressing some of the 'big questions' in evolutionary and behavioural ecology: how can apparently altruistic cooperation evolve? What is the relative importance of direct and indirect fitness effects of cooperation? Which mechanisms prevent unilateral exploitation and consequent instability of social interactions? Which ecological conditions select for cooperation and reproductive restraint? What are the synergisms generated by advanced levels of teamwork and coordination?

Group Living and Cooperation

Groups of these cooperative cichlids consist of a dominant pair of breeders and a variable number of subordinate individuals ranging widely in size. On average, groups contain 5–6 subordinate helpers, which includes immature and mature fish of both sexes. In some cases, helper numbers may go up to 30. Pairs without helpers almost never occur as their chances to survive and successfully reproduce would be small; hence, this species can be categorized as an obligatory cooperative breeder (Taborsky & Limberger 1981; Balshine et al. 2001; Heg et al. 2005a). Within groups there is a strict dominance hierarchy, with rank determined by body size, even if size differences may be small (Dey et al. 2013). Teleost fish grow throughout life, so size is a dynamic variable of fundamental importance in social interactions. Aggressive displays, overt attacks, affiliative and submissive behaviours help in maintaining the dominance relationships among group members (Taborsky 1984, 1985; Hamilton et al. 2005; Reddon et al. 2011a), which involve visual and chemical signals (Hirschenhauser et al. 2008; Balzarini et al. 2014, 2017; Bayani et al. 2017).

Young as small as 1.5 cm in length may already help cleaning the eggs produced by the dominant pair. A little later they start helping to dig out the breeding shelter, and if other fish approach the territory too closely, they will set out defending it (Figure D.1). They will continue to share in these

duties during all their continued presence in the natal territory, way beyond sexual maturity. Importantly, this help increases the productivity of breeders – experimental variation of group structure showed that breeders with helpers produce larger clutches than those lacking such collaboration (Taborsky 1984). Further, later experiments revealed that breeders base their investment in each egg upon the prospective receipt of help during subsequent brood care, laying smaller eggs the larger the group of subordinates and hence the more help they can anticipate (Taborsky et al. 2007).

Observing and manipulating animals under controlled conditions in the laboratory is one thing, but the significance of what we find by such procedure needs checking in nature. Only when the ecological conditions affecting Darwinian fitness are considered can the selection mechanisms underlying social behaviour be elucidated. The first attempt to unveil the social behaviour in the context of the natural environment of these fish focused on a population at the northern tip of Lake Tanganyika near Magara in Burundi, some 40 km south of Bujumbura. Fortunately, the group structure and behaviour, everything known from previous aquarium studies, looked exactly the same at the lake, except that territories were sometimes quite far apart, dependent on suitable breeding shelters. Importantly, the philopatric nature of the social structure was also confirmed. Helpers stayed in their territory and continued helping even if provided with attractive vacancies in nearby territories. Instead, foreign individuals from nearby aggregations took over any breeding vacancies experimentally created. This was interesting, because it meant that the relatedness within these groups was abated by the occasional exchange of dominant breeders. It meant that the older (larger) helpers are, the less they are related to their beneficiaries because of the enhanced chances that since their own birth, one or both breeders had already been replaced by foreign individuals (Taborsky & Limberger 1981; Dierkes et al. 2005; Figure D.2).

Another similarity to the aquarium situation was that breeder males often monopolized more than one group – a harem – each consisting of a dominant

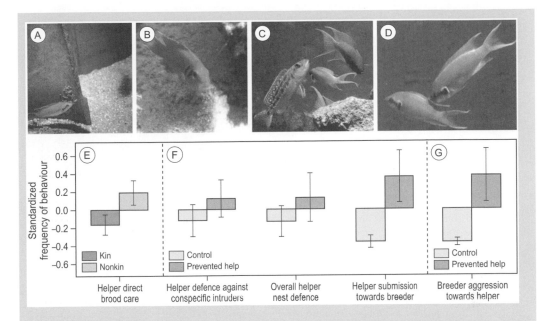

Figure D.1 Cooperative and aggressive behaviours of *N. pulcher*. Subordinate helpers show brood care by cleaning the eggs of breeders (A), by performing nest maintenance such as digging out sand from shelters (B) and by defending the territory against predators, such as *Lepidiolamprologus elongatus* (C). These helping behaviours are prompted by aggression from the breeders. In (D), a breeder (right) shows aggression towards a subordinate, and the subordinate responds with submissive behaviour (tail quiver). Panels (E–G) summarize the results of experimental manipulations from several studies. Bars show the mean of the standardized frequency of behaviour, with error bars denoting the standard error of the standardized behaviour frequencies. (E) Unrelated helpers (purple) provide more help than related ones (green; Zöttl et al. 2013a). (F) After subordinates have been prevented from giving help (dark blue), they compensate by increasing their previous help and submission level (light blue), presumably in an attempt to appease the breeder (Bergmüller & Taborsky 2005; Fischer et al. 2014). (G) Aggression levels in the group are normally very low (cream), but they increase considerably when subordinates are experimentally prevented from helping (red; Fischer et al. 2014; after Quinones et al. 2016). (A black and white version of this figure will appear in some formats. For the colour version, please refer to the plate section.)

female breeder and a number of subordinate helpers (Limberger 1983). Such polygynous males regularly visited their different territories, which were up to 7 m apart (quite remarkably for a fish 7 cm in size; see figure 16.1 in Taborsky 2016 for illustration). When comparing the relative effort in territory maintenance and defence between group members, large helpers were the major investors in defence against other species threatening the shelters and brood (Taborsky & Limberger 1981). Other duties, including digging away sand, removing snails

(potential egg predators) and particles, and defence against conspecifics, were more equally shared among the group.

Knowing that groups in nature consist of related and unrelated individuals alike, the obvious question emerged how relatedness between helpers and beneficiaries affected behaviour and cooperation. Remarkably, the helpers least related to the beneficiaries of their aid, i.e. the largest and hence oldest subordinates in the group (cf. Figure D.2), invested most in the demanding and risky business of territory

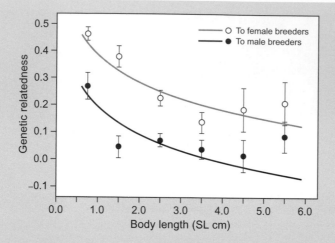

Figure D.2 Relatedness between helpers and breeders in a Zambian population of *N. pulcher*. Relatedness between auxiliaries and beneficiaries declined significantly with advancing body size and age of helpers, reflecting that when a breeder is exchanged by colony members from outside the group, which are usually unrelated, subordinates remain in the group and continue aiding the new territory owner. Depicted are mean values ± SEM per 1 cm class, with two regression lines from a GLMM [$N = 264$ (relatedness to male breeders) and $N = 260$ (relatedness to female breeders), respectively; from Dierkes et al. 2005]. © John Wiley & Sons Ltd/CNRS.

defence. This made sense only if relatedness was not the main driver of such cooperation. Would helpers prefer to stay in the territory of dominants irrespective of relatedness and 'pay rent' to the latter for this opportunity? A series of experiments in the aquarium scrutinized the propensity of helpers to stay in the territory when they could choose between staying as helpers in a group with unrelated breeders, or leaving the territory for good to breed independently. Surprisingly, subordinates usually preferred the helper role. However, they were not always welcomed by dominant breeders: if there was no environmental challenge, e.g. no defence was required, large helpers were evicted from the territory. When space competitors were released in the tank, the ousted helpers were immediately reaccepted, which they rewarded by immediately engaging in fierce defence against the intruders (Taborsky 1985). This suggested mutual trading of important services – access to a territory and its resources against taking up arms to help defend the group.

Fitness Costs and Benefits

Which essential benefits can helpers derive from their group membership? It cannot be food, because these fish feed on plankton mainly outside of the territory. Could it be protection? To test this possibility, helpers of a dominant pair and same-sized control individuals were experimentally exposed to the main predators of this species, *Lepidiolamprologus elongatus*. Helpers clearly survived better than their size-matched controls, and they did so because of the protection obtained from the defence of the dominant breeders (Taborsky 1984; Figure D.3).

Would this fitness benefit of staying in a safe territory as subordinate helper also hold in nature? To answer this question a population at the southern end of Lake Tanganyika was chosen for study, because the north of the lake was inaccessible in the meantime due to political uproar. An ideal study site at the southern end of the lake emerged at a place called Kasakalawe Point, 4 km west of Mpulungu. To avoid confusion, it should be noted that since its

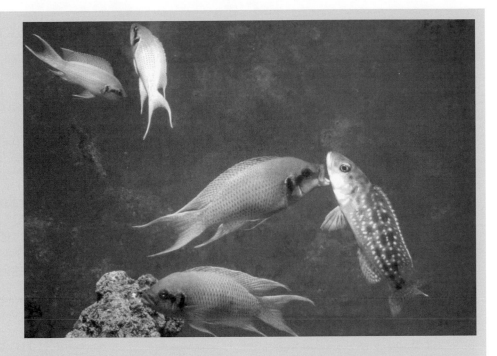

Figure D.3 A breeder male attacks a predator threatening subordinate helpers of the group (top left); the breeder female is in the foreground. (A black and white version of this figure will appear in some formats. For the colour version, please refer to the plate section.)

discovery as a cooperative breeder, the species name has changed by taxonomical rearrangement. *Lamprologus brichardi* was transferred into a different genus, *Neolamprologus*. Furthermore, the species originally studied at the north of the lake was found to have been described earlier by a different name in the south, *Neolamprologus pulcher*. A comparison of populations all along the shorelines of Lake Tanganyika revealed that despite superficial differences in colour markings, these fish should all be viewed as belonging to one and the same species, which, by taxonomic priority, should be referred to as *Neolamprologus pulcher* (Duftner et al. 2007). Due to its lake-wide distribution, the popular name of these fish, 'Princess of Burundi', was misleading as well, and 'Princess of Lake Tanganyika' was an obvious alternative.

The habitat of the southern population of *N. pulcher* differed from that in the north. Wide stretches of sand were interspersed with scattered stones, which by diligent excavation provided the burrows needed by the fish for shelter and breeding. Nevertheless, the territory structure and social units looked very similar between these populations, and the fish's behaviour as well. *N. pulcher* territories consist of a breeding shelter and a variable number of additional shelters, which may be monopolized by individual group members but are typically shared by several of them (Taborsky 1984; Balshine et al. 2001; Werner et al. 2003). A small space around these shelters is also part of the defended area (≤ 0.33 m^2; Taborsky & Limberger 1981). Depending on habitat, shelters consist either of natural holes and crevices in rocks, or they are dug out by group members from underneath stones. In the former case, there may be competition for space because the number and size of shelters cannot be augmented by group members, so group size may be limited to some extent by the availability of shelter space. In the latter case, the possibility to excavate and expand shelters creates a tragedy of the commons, because the digging effort of individuals can be exploited by defectors refraining from participating in digging while using the shelters created or enlarged by others. An experimental study of digging effort of helper-sized fish showed, however, that helpers resolve this conflict of interest through coordinating their digging effort by reciprocal cooperation (Taborsky & Riebli 2020). If digging out a common shelter was experimentally manipulated in one of two similar-sized fish of helper size, its partner economized on its own digging activity in response to concurrent burrowing effort of the manipulated subject. In the subsequent time period, however, the partner adjusted its collaborative digging effort to the digging activity the manipulated fish had shown before, i.e. it reciprocated received help.

With a new population at hand at the southern end of Lake Tanganyika that could be easily studied both in the field and laboratory, important questions of species-specific and general interest could be addressed. Was it possible to obtain experimental proof for the trading of group membership against alloparental care? Would helpers increase group productivity also under natural conditions, and would they receive essential protection from predators in return? What was the importance of group size, which can vary between 3 and 30 in the natural groups? In addition, it was obvious that group living was not the only important social condition, because groups were assembled in colonies, without obvious environmental discontinuities explaining such a pattern. What are the benefits of assembling in colonies, and is this a by-effect of some non-randomly distributed ecological variable or a result of active choice? What is the effect of predators on group size and composition, and on the behaviour of different types of group members? Last but not least, the role of relatedness for interactions among group members and for their cooperation propensity needed experimental scrutiny.

The Trading of Services Among Group Members

Temporary removal experiments in the field suggested that upon return, helpers were punished for failing to contribute to accruing duties (Balshine-

Earn et al. 1998), implying that helpers pay to stay. The logic of this mechanism is that subordinate group members entail costs to dominants, for instance due to resource competition, which may be compensated by cooperative behavior of subordinates. This amounts to alloparental care serving as 'rent payment' (Gaston 1978; Kokko et al. 2002). In *N. pulcher*, the costs helpers incur to dominants include competition for shelters, behavioural expenditure diminishing growth and reproductive competition (reviewed in Taborsky 2016). The last is also indicated by a positive correlation of the testis mass of male breeders with the number of male helpers in their group (Fitzpatrick et al. 2006). If accepting subordinates is costly to dominants, the latter will be selected to demand compensation (Kokko et al. 2002; Hamilton & Taborsky 2005b). The ensuing pay-to-stay mechanism has been elucidated with the help of various experimental approaches.

In aquarium experiments, helpers were prevented from participating in territory defence while staying with the group by depriving them of the information that an intruder was present. This prescribed idleness caused them to compensate later by enhancing their cooperative defence at the next occasion at which they were enabled to do so (Bergmüller & Taborsky 2005; Figure D.4). When helpers were prevented from cooperating in the field by being constrained in a transparent container, they were subsequently punished for being idle; in small groups they were attacked by the dominant breeders, whereas in large groups other helpers attended to this disciplinary measure (Fischer et al. 2014). When the dominant breeders punished lazy helpers, the latter increased their cooperative defence, confirming a pay-to-stay negotiation process.

Interestingly, the bargaining between dominants and subordinates about the latter's payment involves divergent regulatory processes for different cooperative tasks. When the participation in shelter digging of helpers was experimentally inhibited, dominants punished such idleness by aggressive attacks, which triggered a submissive response in the helpers (Naef & Taborsky 2020a). Subordinates also received more aggression from dominants after they had abstained from defending the territory against egg predators, and they strongly increased their defence effort against such intruders when it was subsequently enabled. In contrast, when a fish predator was presented to the group, breeders reduced their attacks on helpers irrespective of the latters' participation in antipredator defence (Naef & Taborsky 2020b). Hence, the participation of helpers in defence against predators of adults might be triggered by mutualistic benefits rather than rent payment.

The interaction between dominants and subordinates in *N. pulcher* is clearly a win–win situation. Apart from enhancement of the breeders' reproductive rate by the helpers' cooperation as outlined above, the breeders benefit also from the protective function of their subordinate group members. When in the field helpers were removed from groups with small dependent young for a week, the mortality rate of the young more than doubled in comparison to control groups (Brouwer et al. 2005), which confirmed the significant role of helpers for the Darwinian fitness of breeders. Helpers in return benefit from the protective function of breeders, as shown in the laboratory experiments outlined above. In a series of field experiments employing 8 m^3 large cages that enclosed parts of local *N. pulcher* populations, critical environmental parameters could be experimentally manipulated, such as the presence of predators of adults or eggs, or the global food abundance in the water column. Results showed that when predation risk was experimentally raised, large and medium-sized helpers survived better in large groups, and they increased their cooperative defence and shelter digging (Heg et al. 2004a; Heg & Taborsky 2010). Large helpers, in particular, increased their cooperative investment per aggression received from breeders when dangerous predators were present, suggesting they were prepared to pay a higher prize if the value of their group membership was enhanced. Global food reduction, on the other hand, reduced the helping effort of subordinates, apparently due to a trade-off between foraging effort and cooperation (Bruintjes et al. 2010). Aquarium experiments revealed that subordinates expand helping effort according to demand, and that

large helpers generally pay more than small ones, which enables them to be tolerated in the dominant's territory despite the costs they occasion (Bruintjes & Taborsky 2008).

Stay or Leave

The experimental manipulation of predation risk in the field revealed that helpers were only prepared to disperse from their home territory when predators were absent (Heg et al. 2004a). But how would, in benign conditions, a decision to leave affect their cooperative effort at home? Experimental facilitation of dispersal by providing independent breeding opportunities revealed that helpers that are prepared to disperse reduce their work load at home (Bergmüller et al. 2005a), which also happens under natural conditions (Zöttl et al. 2013d). Interestingly, helpers establish a network of relationships with fish from neighbouring groups by visiting them periodically and interacting with them in their home territories. When the conditions at home deteriorate, for instance by experimental disturbance, or when other groups provide better opportunities to enhance personal fitness, they make use of these relations by dispersing into other groups (Bergmüller et al. 2005b). Prospecting other groups prepares large helpers for potential between-group dispersal, and it increases survival chances (Jungwirth et al. 2015a). If dominants need additional help, they accept immigrants working for their group membership (Zöttl et al. 2013b). When dispersing into another group, helpers prefer to join large over small groups and groups containing large, more dominant individuals (Jordan et al. 2010; Reddon et al. 2011b), which enhances safety from predators and again illustrates the importance of group membership for individuals beneath breeder size.

This preference for large groups also hints at the relative importance of benefits from protection, which are greater in large groups, and the inheritance of the territory, which might be enhanced in small groups. Even if most helpers disperse at some stage when surviving to breeder size, not all of them do (Stiver et al. 2004). In particular, large female helpers may inherit their natal territory when the dominant breeder female disappears (Stiver et al.

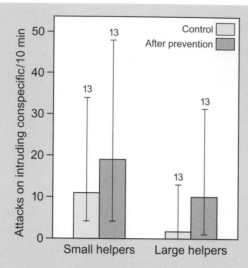

Figure D.4 Preemptive appeasement. Results from an experiment in which helpers were experimentally prevented from participating in defence by depriving them of information about a territory challenge. Subsequently, they were allowed to help defend the territory. After they had been made idle (black columns, 'After prevention'), both small and large helpers significantly increased their defence effort against an intruder as compared to the control condition (white columns, 'Control'), in which they could participate in defence in the previous period. Medians and interquartile ranges are shown and numbers represent sample sizes (after Bergmüller & Taborsky 2005). Copyright © 2004 The Association for the Study of Animal Behaviour. Published by Elsevier Ltd. All rights reserved.

2006), causing matrilines to occur in roughly a fifth of natural groups in the Kasakalawe population at the south of the lake (Dierkes et al. 2005).

The Importance of Relatedness

Cooperative breeding is so interesting – evolutionarily speaking – because it involves apparently altruistic behaviour, but it falls short of the genetic altruism characterizing eusocial organization. In the latter case, i.e. when individuals (usually the majority of group members) completely forfeit reproduction over their entire lifetime, kin selection, or the preferential support of non-descendant close relatives, is the only mechanism explaining this ultimate degree of cooperation. This is not so in cooperative breeders, where reproductive abstinence is temporary. Hence, in cooperative breeders we can ask which possible selection mechanism, kin selection or individual selection, is responsible for the

occurrence of alloparental care and cooperation in general. *N. pulcher* provides the unique opportunity to study this aspect experimentally because of the possibility to combine groups to your liking regarding size, age, sex, relatedness and the number of members. This is so because in nature, groups are also mixtures of individuals differing in all these factors, hence a natural (selected) response to such experimental variation can be expected.

It is important to know that these fish can recognize individuals, which they do by visual cues (Hert 1985; Balshine-Earn & Lotem 1998; Kohda et al. 2015), and relatives, which occurs by chemical means (Le Vin et al. 2010), and they apparently make use of this ability. In both the laboratory and the field, relatedness between helpers and breeders explains the cooperative behaviour performed by subordinate group members, albeit in a somewhat unexpected direction (Stiver et al. 2005). In a laboratory experiment involving groups made up of helpers either related or unrelated to both breeders, the work effort of helpers in the unrelated treatment exceeded that of helpers in the related treatment roughly 10-fold (Stiver et al. 2005). A crucial experiment tested for the importance of relatedness for the propensity to show alloparental egg care, which is a truly altruistic behaviour without immediate fitness returns to the alloparent. This experiment revealed that relatedness indeed *reduced* the alloparental investment of helpers. When a female helper was experimentally combined with a pair containing either her mother or full sister, or alternatively an unrelated female breeder, *un*related helpers invested more in direct egg care, which involves egg cleaning and fanning (Zöttl et al. 2013a; see Figure 4.16). This contrasts with predictions from kin selection theory, but it can be plausibly explained by the pay-to-stay mechanism governing the interactions between helpers and dominant breeders in this species. In fact, a theoretical model revealed that by negotiations between dominant breeders and subordinate helpers higher levels of altruistic cooperation can evolve than by kin selection (Quiñones et al. 2016).

When estimating the relative importance of direct and indirect fitness benefits for the evolution of cooperative breeding in this species, direct fitness effects were found to outweigh indirect fitness effects by far, i.e. kin selection is apparently of secondary importance (Jungwirth & Taborsky 2015; see Figure 4.18). Accordingly, when providing *N. pulcher* of various sizes with an opportunity to join related or unrelated group members, they preferentially settled with unrelated ones (Heg et al. 2011). Contrary to the secondary importance of relatedness for these cooperative cichlids, the social organization beyond group level has substantive impact on individual fitness in addition to intragroup relationships. To have many conspecifics around you seems paramount for these fish. Both large group size and a high density of territories in the colony enhance group persistence (Heg et al. 2005a; Jungwirth & Taborsky 2015). This also explains why territory vacancies experimentally provided at the edge or amidst a colony differ greatly in their attractiveness to group founders: whereas territories at the colony edge were largely ignored, those created in the midst of the colony were readily occupied by dispersing group members (Heg et al. 2008a). Predator exposure experiments in the field revealed a clear advantage of having close-by neighbours: the required defence effort is shared by members of neighbouring groups, thereby reducing their individual investment (Jungwirth et al. 2015b).

Predation Risk and Conditional Division of Labour

This again points to the fundamental importance of predation pressure in the evolutionary ecology of these fish. A comparison of eight populations of *N. pulcher* in the south of the lake revealed a significant influence of predation on the social structure (Groenewoud et al. 2016; Figure D.5). Remarkably, the intensity of predation affects group structure more strongly than group size, with inverse effects on small and large group members. High predation risk and limited shelter numbers lead to groups containing few small but many large group members, and vice versa. Apparently, enhanced safety from predators by cooperative defence and shelter maintenance are the primary benefits of cooperative breeding in this species. In addition, all group members benefit from synergistic effects of cooperation, particularly through division of labour between individuals differently suited to perform alternative duties. Tasks are shared unequally among them, dependent on their respective size, sex and status, and on current demands (Taborsky & Limberger 1981; Taborsky 1984, 1985; Desjardins et al. 2008a, 2008b; Bruintjes & Taborsky 2011; this is similar in other social cichlids: Tanaka et al. 2018c; Josi et al. 2020a, 2020b). If several demands emerge concurrently, helpers specialize in territory maintenance, whereas female breeders focus on direct brood care and both breeders engage in defence (Taborsky et al. 1986). Depending on the type of intrusion pressure, large helpers may focus especially on territory defence (Taborsky & Limberger 1981), or they may specialize in digging while smaller helpers defend the breeding shelter against egg predators (Bruintjes & Taborsky 2011).

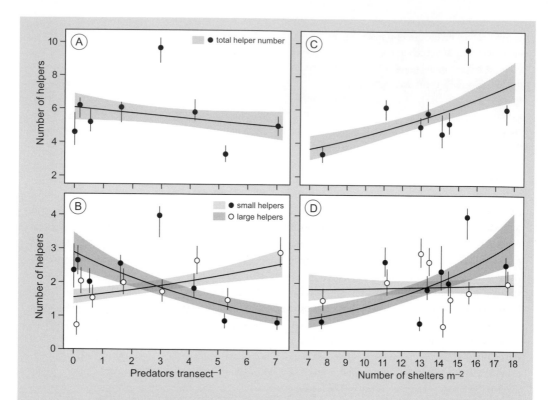

Figure D.5 Predation risk affects group structure. A comparison of eight populations of *N. pulcher* diverging in predator and shelter densities revealed a positive effect of shelter number on total group size (C), whereas the latter did not vary significantly with predation risk (A). However, when considering differently sized helpers separately, the numbers of small helpers decreased while the numbers of large helpers increased with rising predation risk (B). Furthermore, a higher number of shelters was associated with a greater number of *small* helpers, whereas the number of large helpers seemed unaffected by shelter number (D). Population means and bootstrapped 95 per cent confidence intervals are given for total helper number (filled circles in A and C), small helpers (filled circles in B and D), and large helpers (open circles in B and D). Data points are slightly offset horizontally to avoid overlapping confidence intervals. Solid regression lines represent the model predicted values with bootstrapped 95 per cent confidence intervals for total helper numbers (grey), small helpers (dark), and large helpers (light; after Groenewoud et al. 2016).

Reproductive Competition

As medium and large helpers are reproductively mature, they may share in reproduction (Dierkes et al. 1999; Heg et al. 2006, 2008b; Bruintjes et al. 2011; Hellmann et al. 2015). A meta-analysis from six studies showed that the proportion of broods in a territory in which a male helper sired offspring (19 per cent) is on average slightly higher than the proportion of broods produced by female helpers (14 per cent), but at the level of produced young, female helpers have the edge over male helpers (15 per cent vs. 5 per cent; Taborsky 2016). Due to sperm competition with the male territory owner, male helpers can apparently sire only a small number of young in their territory (on average roughly 5 young per brood), whereas female helpers produce on average 40 young per brood *if* they do lay a clutch. This occurs more rarely, however (Heg 2008). In any case, the proportion of offspring produced by helpers in a group lies roughly between 5 per cent and 15 per cent (Dierkes et al. 1999; Hellmann et al. 2015; Taborsky 2016). Hence, the reproductive skew is high within groups, and the participation of helpers in reproduction reflects limited control rather than concessions (Heg & Hamilton 2008; Mitchell et al. 2009a; Taborsky 2009). Helpers partly compensate for the costs inflicted to dominant breeders by their reproductive participation through increasing their cooperative investment when siring own offspring in the territory (Heg et al. 2008b, 2009; Bruintjes et al. 2011). Nevertheless, male breeders suffer higher fitness costs from the reproductive participation of male helpers than female breeders do from egg laying female helpers (Mitchell et al. 2009b); each egg fertilized by the sperm of a male helper means one offspring fewer for the male breeder, whereas a clutch produced by a female helper does not affect the number of eggs the dominant female can lay.

The higher reproductive competition among male members of a group than among females is also reflected by gender differences in growth, in dependence of size differences between the dominant breeder and the respective largest, same-sex helper. Experiments varying the size gap between the dominant male and the largest male helper revealed that a difference in body size of about 15 per cent is constantly kept by the helper, which is enforced by continual aggression of the male breeder towards the male helper (Heg et al. 2004b). In contrast, female size differences are unimportant for the growth speed of female helpers (Hamilton & Heg 2008; Heg 2010). Apart from this strategic growth adjustment of male helpers, the speed of growth is also affected by the energetic investment in helping duties (Taborsky 1984). Some of the helping behaviours enhance basal metabolic rate up to sixfold, i.e. they are almost as energetically demanding as bird flight (Grantner & Taborsky 1998). This affects the behavioural energy budget of subordinates substantially (Taborsky & Grantner 1988).

Developmental Plasticity

The environment that helpers encounter early in life influences their behavioural and life history decisions as adults. Group size in early ontogeny, for instance, impacts their unfolding of social skills fundamentally by affecting brain development (Fischer et al. 2015). The presence of large adults early in life seems particularly important, because it can alter the programming of the stress axis by changing the expression of genes of the hypothalamic–pituitary–interrenal (HPI) axis at the adult stage (Taborsky et al. 2013). Thereby, fish growing up with large adults develop a better social competence lifelong, responding more adequately and economically to social challenges than fish lacking this early experience (Arnold & Taborsky 2010; Taborsky et al. 2012).

Growing up in a complex social environment can trigger persistent individual differences (Taborsky & Oliveira 2012), as adopting a specific social niche may generate positive feedback (Bergmüller & Taborsky 2007, 2010). Individuals responding in a certain way to competitive or cooperative interactions, for example, will get better and better in that response the more often it is performed, both because of a training effect and because the other individuals in the group learn the individual's role and react correspondingly. This can result in adaptive social niche specialization (Bergmüller & Taborsky 2010). In *N. pulcher*, differences in behavioural type or 'personality' persist over life and they show a heritable component, hence they are subject to natural selection (Chervet et al. 2011). These behavioural type differences affect dominance, growth, resource allocation, exploration and dispersal propensity, group joining preferences and the establishment of social networks and cooperation decisions (Begmüller & Taborsky 2007; Schürch & Heg 2010a, 2010b; Schürch et al. 2010; Witsenburg et al. 2010; Heg et al. 2011; Riebli et al. 2011, 2012; Hamilton & Ligocki 2012). Remarkably, personality differences affect cooperation decisions in these fish distinctly more than relatedness does (Le Vin et al. 2011).

Towards New Frontiers

It is of great interest to know how unique the social structure and level of cooperation is of the Princess of Lake Tanganyika. There are about 25 species of the tribe Lamprologini, all endemic to Lake Tanganyika, that apparently show variations of the theme (Taborsky 1994, 2009, 2016; Awata et al. 2005; Heg et al. 2005b, 2006; Kohda et al. 2009; Tanaka et al. 2015, 2016, 2018a–2018c). They belong to the genera *Julidochromis*, *Chalinochromis*, *Lepidiolamprologus* and *Neolamprologus*, and it seems from preliminary analyses that cooperative breeding has arisen several times in Lake Tanganyika (Dey et al. 2017; Tanaka et al. 2018d). There are other fishes showing varieties of cooperative breeding, some of which are again cichlids (Taborsky 1994, 2009; Martin & Taborsky 1997). However, the biology and ecology of cooperative breeding in fish hitherto has been studied extensively only at Lake Tanganyika. Exciting variations of cooperative breeding in fishes lurk beneath the surface only to be unearthed by future generations of enthusiastic researchers.

From a humble student project conducted at an idyllic lake in Bavaria, the study of cooperatively breeding cichlids has spread through many a laboratory throughout the world. *Neolamprologus pulcher* has become a popular model for the study of social evolution, and other cooperatively breeding cichlids are increasingly joining the limelight. Presently, the endocrine, neurophysiological, developmental, genetic and epigenetic mechanisms involved in the social behaviour of cooperative cichlids are being scrutinized by a number of different research groups. This and the expansion of eco-evolutionary research on cooperative cichlids are predestined to further enhance our understanding of evolutionary mechanisms of sociality at large.

5   Interspecific Relations

In nature, conflict and cooperation are prevalent not only between individuals of the same species, as discussed in Chapters 2–4, but also between individuals belonging to different species. If thinking of interspecific relations, what perhaps first crosses one's mind are the salient relations between predators and prey, or between parasites and hosts. However, different organisms also cooperate with each other, which in fact may lead to entirely new organisms (Kiers & West 2015). Here we focus on the behavioural responses of individuals to competition with individuals of other species, based on the concepts we outlined in the introduction to this book: non-interference rivalry (*race*), conflict (*fight*), or cooperation (*share*).

Cooperation between unrelated individuals, in particular, remains a key topic in evolutionary biology that can be perfectly scrutinized in interactions between members of different species (Barker et al. 2017). While kin selection provides an important conceptual framework for the evolution of cooperation between related individuals, as outlined in Section 4.1.2.2, cooperation between unrelated individuals of the same or different species generally cannot be explained by this mechanism. The concepts underlying cooperation between unrelated individuals belonging to the same species can thus form the basis for studies of the evolution of cooperation between individuals of different species, and vice versa. In fact, as relatedness effects can be excluded as a cause for evolved decision rules in interactions between organisms belonging to different species, interspecific interactions provide a unique opportunity to test predictions of evolutionary theory that go beyond kin selection (cf. Sections 4.1 and 4.2).

In general, altruistic behaviour directed towards unrelated individuals can only be favoured by selection if it increases the donors' direct fitness (Lehmann & Keller 2006a; West et al. 2007c), or if it is caused by coercion or deceit, i.e. against the fitness interests of the actor. As such, the study of interspecific interactions provides excellent potential for investigating general mechanisms of cooperation. As we have argued in Chapter 4, this includes (i) mutualism, i.e. the trait under selection has positive direct fitness effects on its bearer independently of the returns it might receive from others, (ii) reciprocity, i.e. the trait under selection bears immediate fitness costs to its bearer at a benefit to others, which provide return benefits compensating for such costs, and (iii) coercion or deceit, where one party exploits another against the latter's fitness interests. It should be stressed here once again that we refer to 'mutualism' as an evolutionary concept (see Glossary); in ecology, this term is often used for any seemingly non-exploitative interspecific relationships with apparent positive fitness effects to the involved parties, irrespective of the underlying evolutionary mechanism (Bronstein 2015).

The ecological significance of interspecific relations in nature is substantial and ubiquitous, both in antagonistic (e.g. predator–prey, parasite–host interactions) and cooperative contexts (e.g. symbiosis; reviewed in Bronstein 2015; Kiers & West 2015; West et al. 2015; Barker et al. 2017). Cooperation between different species can involve parties providing benefits to each other such as resources boosting growth (Douglas 2010) and other crucial fitness components, which may cause mutual dependencies. For example, several species of catenulid flatworms (belonging to the genus *Paracatenula*) are colonized by bacterial symbionts that provide chemical resources of energy to the host. The symbionts constitute a substantial proportion of the worms' biomass; up to 50 per cent of the body volume of the various worm species consists of bacterial symbionts. The hosts have evolved a high level of dependency on the symbionts, because they have lost their mouths and digestive systems. The symbionts, in turn, are highly dependent on the genomes of their host, because they have reduced genomes that are integrated in the genome of the flatworms (Gruber-Vodicka et al. 2011). The symbiont transmission through host generations leads to a high relatedness between the symbionts within a host, across host generations, causing the linking of the symbiont fitness to host performance, which reduces conflict among symbionts (Bright & Bulgheresi 2010).

For interspecific cooperation to evolve, the partners of an interaction have a shared purpose which should benefit both and, accordingly, the degree of conflict may seem to be low. At first glance, one might assume that the same factors that lead to a high potential for cooperation also lead to low potential conflict. However, the levels of cooperation and conflict may not be strongly correlated. Like in the case of intraspecific relationships (see Chapters 3 and 4), most co-active interactions among different organisms are not entirely cooperative but also contain some degree of conflict. The levels of conflict and cooperation in an interaction can be imagined as a relationship represented by two perpendicular axes denoting the degree of cooperation and conflict among the partners (Figure 5.1; Queller & Strassmann 2009; see also Section 3.1 for similar considerations at the intraspecific level). Many mutualistic species pairs perform essential services for each other and an intriguing question is how much ongoing conflict there is among them. For example, in which cases, and by which processes, does conflict become so much reduced that the relationship is essentially organismal, like among host cells and mitochondria?

Interspecific cooperation can also involve more than two species (Mueller et al. 1998, 2005; Little & Currie 2007; Kiers et al. 2011; Biedermann et al. 2013; McFall-Ngai 2014), but most studies considering the costs and benefits involved in mutual cooperation have focused on the interaction between individuals belonging to two species only (two-way interactions between unrelated individuals). This approach facilitates the study of the evolution of interspecific cooperation, because the underlying mechanisms may differ between interacting species and the fitness effects may be subject to complex multi-way interactions.

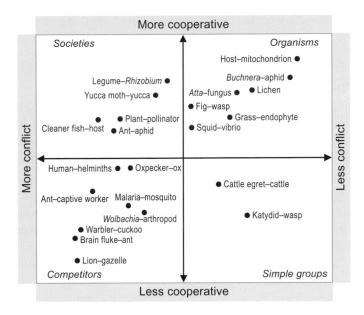

Figure 5.1 Cooperation and conflict in two-partner groups involving different taxa along two perpendicular axes of tendencies towards cooperation and conflict (from Queller & Strassmann 2009). © 2009 The Royal Society.

We should be aware that the evolution of interactions between species can also involve transmission mechanisms forcing pairs of species to cooperate across generations (Dawkins et al. 1979; Yamamura et al. 2004; Gardner et al. 2007; Fletcher & Doebeli 2009). For example, if offspring of a symbiont interact with offspring of the host, the symbiont could gain a greater advantage by helping rather than exploiting the host species, otherwise it might harm the future prospects of its own progeny in future generations. The evolution of indiscriminate cooperation between species can also be favoured by population viscosity alone (Wyatt et al. 2013). The donor species may cooperate with cooperative individuals of the other species, because the reproductive success of the recipient species is enhanced and associated with an increase in the population frequency of the donor species' genes. This is reminiscent of generalized reciprocity among individuals of the same species and may involve similar evolutionary mechanisms (Rankin & Taborsky 2009).

Given the plethora of examples of interspecific interactions (e.g. in ecosystems) in the literature, in this book we focus on interspecific interactions at the level of behaviour, and discuss their functional significance for the involved interaction partners. In this chapter, we discuss various types of interactions between species. As we are interested in evolutionary aspects of interspecific interactions, we especially focus on how species interact with other species, discuss whether and in which way such interactions have the potential for interspecific conflict or cooperation, and ponder which of the involved parties benefit or suffer.

Furthermore, we discuss the underlying conditions that might be essential to achieve different forms of interspecific interactions.

5.1   Types of Interspecific Interactions

Interspecific cooperation and conflict based on commensalism, mutualism or reciprocity are widespread in nature, but often it remains unclear how such relationships have evolved and how they can be maintained (e.g. Doebeli & Knowlton 1998; Herre et al. 1999; Hoeksema & Bruna 2000; Sachs et al. 2004; Foster & Wenseleers 2006; West et al. 2007c; Leigh 2010). In keeping with the central concept of our book, we shall distinguish among three types of interspecific interactions: (i) non-interference rivalry (*race*), where several species have similar access to resources but try to outcompete others by being 'quicker' or more efficient than others at exploiting those resources (Case & Giplin 1974); (ii) conflict (*fight*), where competitors directly interfere with each other for access to resources, which may result either in coexistence characterized by steady struggle between the parties, or in the displacement of a party by another (Case & Gilpin 1974; Schoener 1983); and (iii) cooperation (*share*), where interests are shared between species.

5.2   Non-interference Rivalry

When species occurring in the same area use similar resources, they are likely to compete for access to them, which may ultimately lead to competitive exclusion of one species by the other. However, it may also lead to coexistence characterized by continual scramble for resources. Here we discuss two main mechanisms underlying such coexistence of species through non-interference rivalry: character displacement and competition among specialists versus generalists.

5.2.1   Character Displacement

Character displacement refers to differences in resource acquisition or morphologies between species, which arise as a consequence of competition between species for limited resources (e.g. food, habitat, shelter, etc.; Brown & Wilson 1956). Character displacement plays an important role in structuring communities. Competing species can only coexist persistently in the same environment if they somewhat differ in their ecological niche, because without niche differentiation, competition between species will result in one species being eliminated. This may select for a shift in resource use, which will ultimately result in character displacement at the population or species level, i.e. species will adjust their demands to reduce competition. Niche shifts due to interspecific competition have been observed, for example, in European tits. In coniferous forests in Sweden, where willow tit (*Parus montanus*), crested tit (*Parus cristatus*), coal tit (*Parus ater*) and goldcrest (*Regulus regulus*) occur sympatrically, willow and crested tits forage in the inner parts of trees, whereas coal tits and goldcrests feed on the outer parts. On the island of Gotland in Sweden, where willow and crested tits are absent, the foraging niche of coal tits encompasses mainly the inner, needle-free parts of trees. This niche divergence of coal tits in different populations appears to be a consequence of the presence or absence of interspecific competition with willow and crested tits (Alerstam et al. 1974). Goldcrests on Gotland, on the other hand, do not use different foraging niches than on the mainland (Alerstam et al. 1974). Coal tits are socially dominant over goldcrests (Morse 1978) and because coal tits on Gotland occur in high numbers, interspecific competition for the inner tree foraging sites may not be relaxed for goldcrests on this island.

To test experimentally whether the foraging site selection by coal tits and gold-crests is influenced by interspecific competition with willow tits and crested tits, the density of the latter species was reduced in some forest plots by more than half. Both coal tits and goldcrests responded to the reduction in densities of willow tits and crested tits by expanding their foraging niches into the inner canopy, compared to unmanipulated forest plots (Figure 5.2; Alatalo et al. 1985), which confirms that interspecific competition affects foraging site selection. The observed niche shift may have been caused by 'interference competition', because coal tits and goldcrests are relatively small and subordinate compared to the larger willow and crested tits (Morse 1978). However, niche shifts could also occur through scramble or 'exploitation' competition, if changes in profitability of different tree sites caused by one species can produce shifts in foraging behaviour of another. For example, the profitability of inner tree parts as foraging sites for coal tits and goldcrests can be modified by the quicker or more efficient removal of food by the other tits.

This may have important fitness effects for another fitness component: mortality risk. Tits foraging among twigs and needles are more exposed to avian predators than if they were feeding in the centre of trees. Avian predators were observed to prey most heavily on the needle-foraging coal tits and goldcrests, whereas crested tits were never preyed upon (Suhonen 1993a). Apart from increased predation risk, the twig- and needle-foraging tits may also spend less time with feeding because more time is needed for vigilance (Suhonen 1993a, 1993b). Scramble or exploitation competition may, like interference competition, also involve asymmetries between competitors, even if they do not interact aggressively. For example, if the inner tree parts are clearly better (e.g. because they are safer), the species that are more successful in the scramble should not move to the less-optimal areas (twigs and needles).

Related species with broad niche overlap can coexist in sympatry also through the ability to feed on different resources (i.e. different diets). When competition between species becomes very high, on an evolutionary timescale species may reduce competition by undergoing morphological character displacement. This was demonstrated for four Darwin's ground finch species (*Geospiza* spp.) in the Galápagos that live in sympatry and have similar and overlapping diets, typically feeding on seeds. Overall, competition among these finch species is weak, but diet overlap and competition for similar resources occur. All ground finches use a diversity of overlapping resources, such as arthropods and seeds. When conditions are favourable (during high rainfall),

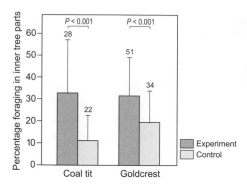

Figure 5.2 Mean percentage (± SD) of foraging in inner tree parts (without needles) for coal tits and goldcrests in experimental plots, where the densities of competing willow tits and crested tits had been reduced by more than half, compared to control plots without manipulation (drawn after data from Alatalo et al. 1985).

all species feed mostly on arthropods, the best resource. However, each species also exploits its own resources for which they are superior competitors because they have developed different beak morphologies: the large ground finch (*Geospiza magnirostris*) has the largest beak and highest bite force, and feeds on large seeds, the medium ground finch (*G. fortis*) has intermediate beak size and bite force, and feeds on intermediate-sized seeds, the small ground finch (*G. fuliginosa*) has the smallest beak and lowest bite force, and feeds on small seeds, whereas the common cactus finch (*G. scandens*) has the longest beak, and probes on flowers of cacti (Figure 5.3; e.g. Schluter & Grant 1984; Sulloway & Kleindorfer 2013; De León et al. 2014). The use of these divergent resources becomes more important when the availability of the preferred shared arthropod foods is reduced during dry periods. When conditions are poor (during dry periods or years), the species use those resources for which their beak morphologies are best adapted, causing greater divergence in diet use (Figure 5.4). Thus, the ground finches use overlapping resources under benign conditions and less-preferred resources under adverse conditions, allowing the coexistence of closely related species (De León et al. 2014).

5.2.2   Specialists versus Generalists

Coexistence of species using the same resources may also be possible because one species is a specialist and the other a generalist. The main characteristics of specialist species are that they use a limited variety of resources efficiently and survive only under special environmental conditions, whereas generalist species use a great variety of resources less efficiently, but can occur in a wide variety of environments. When a joint food resource becomes scarce, the specialist will be more efficient in exploiting it than the generalist, but both species can still coexist as the generalist can use alternative forage without competing with the specialist. To minimize competition, the strategy of a subordinate generalist competitor often includes avoidance of the

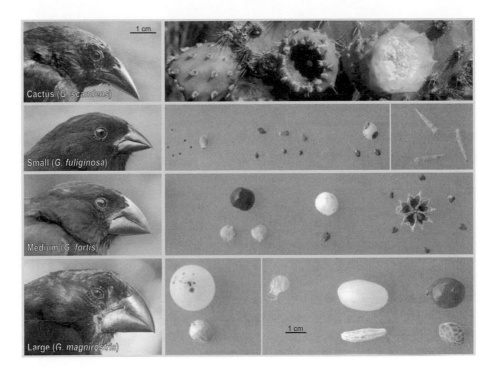

Figure 5.3 The four focal species of Darwin's ground finches and some of the food types and sizes they often feed on (photograph credit: L.F. De León; from De León et al. 2014). © 2014 The Authors. Journal of Evolutionary Biology © 2014 European Society For Evolutionary Biology. (A black and white version of this figure will appear in some formats. For the colour version, please refer to the plate section.)

dominant specialist. For example, red foxes (*Vulpes vulpes*) and coyotes (*Canis latrans*) are sympatric over much of North America and often share the same prey species. Coyotes are superior over foxes, displacing the latter from certain areas (e.g. Voigt & Earle 1983). However, both species coexist in the same areas simultaneously in good numbers in south-west Yukon, a subarctic montane environment with limited prey abundance. There, both species prey on snowshoe hares (*Lepus americanus*), which occur in fluctuating abundance. During the peak of the hare cycle, both species had similar diets and preyed intensively on hares. However, after the peak of the hare cycle, coyotes took more hares than foxes did, and foxes often took alternative prey such as Arctic ground squirrels (*Spermophilus parryii*), which may be less profitable but were abundant (Theberge & Wedeles 1989). Hence, red foxes seem to be able to coexist with coyotes due to their ability to use alternative prey, which is required by non-interference competition with the more successful competitor, coyotes. On the other hand, the success of the latter may be caused at least partly by their physical dominance over foxes, by which they can keep away foxes from areas where hares are most abundant (i.e. interference competition; Theberge & Wedeles 1989).

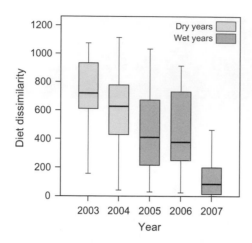

Figure 5.4 Analysis of diet disparity of four species of Darwin's ground finches (common cactus finch; small, medium and large ground finch) for years differing in rainfall, including two dry years (2003, 2004) and three wet years (2005–2007, with 2007 being particularly wet). Diets diverged much more between species in dry years with poor food conditions than in wet years with reduced food competition. Box plots show the median (solid bar), interquartile range (box) and full range (whiskers) of the data (from De León et al. 2014). © 2014 The Authors. Journal of Evolutionary Biology © 2014 European Society For Evolutionary Biology.

This example demonstrates the different responses of specialists (coyotes) and generalists (red foxes), which influence each other's coping with competition for prey, perhaps by a combination of interference and non-interference competition.

In addition to selecting different prey, species may also coexist by selecting different habitats within the same location. For example, in the Rocky Mountains of southern Alberta, Canada, a community of three small rodent species coexists. The mix of mesic and xeric habitats has different effects on habitat preferences and spatial regulation of these three species. The deer mouse (*Peromyscus maniculatus*) prefers the xeric habitat, whereas the red-backed vole (*Clethrionomys gapperi*) prefers the mesic habitat (Morris 1996). In contrast, the pine chipmunk (*Tamias amoenus*) is a generalist with no preference for either habitat. Competitive interactions between the deer mouse and the vole may be responsible for different habitat use. However, shared predators might have a greater impact. Predators should preferentially exploit the habitat with highest prey density (higher energy return; Korpimäki et al. 2005). In other words, when deer mice are rare and voles are abundant, predators should preferentially forage in the mesic habitat, and vice versa they should switch to xeric habitats when voles are rare and deer mice abundant. The switching of predators between prey types may facilitate the coexistence of prey species, resulting in a predator-mediated coexistence of the two specialist prey species through their control of prey densities. However, it remains to be tested whether the predator is actually responsible for the distinct habitat preferences of both species. Another possibility is that an increase in one prey type has a negative effect on the other prey type indirectly via a shared predator (Holt 1977). The coexistence of the chipmunk with the two specialized rodent species can be explained by the fact that the chipmunk responds to habitat quality at a larger scale than the specialists do, exploiting areas that are only marginally used by the two specialist species. Competition by both specialists may drive the chipmunk into separate habitats, where, being a generalist, it can still survive. It is worth noting that coexistence may also be facilitated by other factors, such as differences in diurnal activity patterns (Morris 1996).

5.3   Conflict

In contrast to non-interference rivalry, interference competition implies that competitors directly interfere with each other when struggling for access to resources, which may result in coexistence characterized by steady conflict between the parties, or in the displacement of one species by the other (Case & Gilpin 1974; Schoener 1983). It has been hypothesized that species specialized in a particular habitat or resource are more competitive than generalist species. As a consequence, specialist species can exclude more generalist, opportunistic competitors from their optimal habitats. It should be noted that even if interactions are basically cooperative, there is potential for conflict, not the least because of asymmetries in abilities and pay-offs (Phillips 2018). At the intraspecific level, individuals can compete for instance for a disproportional share of reproduction (see Section 3.2.3). However, living and cooperating in groups may also affect how individuals of a species interact with individuals of other species. In this section we will discuss how conflict may arise between individuals of different species, how conflicts are resolved, and who benefits. In so doing, we shall focus on interspecific resource monopolization, and on relations characterized by predator–prey and host–parasite interactions.

5.3.1   Interspecific Resource Monopolization

While many species defend resources only against conspecifics, sometimes individuals defend their territories against competitors from other species. This may happen when competition for the same resources is intense between species that have similar requirements. Such interspecific territoriality is found, for example, between the chaffinch (*Fringilla coelebs*) and the great tit (*Parus major*) on some Scottish islands, which contrasts with the situation in the mainland populations of Western Scotland. On the islands, the territories of these two species do not overlap, and both species aggressively defend them against each other and respond to both great tit and chaffinch song play-back. When chaffinches were removed from part of the island, great tits expanded into the vacated sites rapidly. It has been suggested that chaffinches and great tits have similar feeding habits and areas, and this has resulted in interspecific territoriality on the poorer island habitats compared to the richer mainland (Reed 1982). Interspecific territoriality may have been caused by the recent arrival of the great tit and insufficient time to evolve even more morphological divergence between the competing species, which would allow them to change their resource use in order to reduce resource overlap (ecological character displacement) and competition. However, theoretical studies have shown that high levels of resource overlap are not always required for interspecific territoriality to be adaptive (Grether et al. 2009).

North American wood warblers (Parulidae) show a high incidence of interspecific territoriality (39 per cent of species) among two or more species. Here, interspecific territoriality is not restricted to poor habitats. Most wood warblers breed in complex and rich habitats. Furthermore, all wood warbler species are insectivorous and insects are abundant throughout their habitats, suggesting that here interspecific territoriality might be unrelated to competition for food. These observations do not seem to support the long-standing hypothesis that interspecific territoriality occurs when resource overlap between species is very high. However, wood warbler species showing interspecific territoriality have more recent common ancestors and are more similar phenotypically than sympatric species not defending interspecific territories. By taking phylogenetic relationships into account, similarity between species in plumage and territorial song were shown to be significant predictors of interspecific territoriality (Losin et al. 2016).

It has been argued that interspecific territoriality should only occur between species competing for resources that cannot be partitioned, or in cases of recent sympatry (Orians & Willson 1964). For several species it is common for males to compete for mates with males from closely related species, i.e. males court and attempt to mate with heterospecific females (reviewed in Wirtz 1999; Gröning & Hochkirch 2008; Grether et al. 2009, 2013; Drury et al. 2015). As male gametes are relatively cheap, the benefits for males of mating with heterospecific females may outweigh the costs. Males may benefit from interspecific fertilizations, which cause hybridization, because they may produce viable offspring and thereby successfully transfer genes to the next generation. However, we should be aware that the occurrence of interspecific mating does not necessarily imply adaptive behaviour. It may also be maladaptive, resulting merely from recognition errors of males. For example, in *Hetaerina* damselflies, interspecific aggression between males occurs in most sympatric species pairs, and in most cases territory holders are equally aggressive to conspecific and heterospecific male intruders. However, the level of interspecific aggression varies across species pairs. Male *Hetaerina* damselflies compete for small mating territories along rivers where females oviposit in submerged vegetation. Males have conspicuous, species-specific colouration, but females are cryptic in colouration and resemble each other. Females that are more similar to heterospecific females in wing colouration are more likely to be clasped by heterospecific males. Hence the overlap between species in female colouration appears to be a major cause of reproductive interference by males of different species. Females, on the other hand, do distinguish males of their own species from those of others. They remate until they copulate with a conspecific male, at which point the eggs are fertilized by that male's sperm and oviposition occurs. In other words, sperm transfer only takes place when mating occurs between a conspecific pair. This means that it is costly for males to mate with a female belonging to another species, because the latter refrain from egg laying and no fertilizations will take place. The prolonged tandem flights during copulation pose opportunity costs, hampering the male from finding a conspecific female to mate with. This may explain why the more divergent the females are, the lower the interspecific aggression between males and the less frequently they attempt to mate with a heterospecific female. Basically, when males are less able to distinguish females of sympatric species, females become a shared resource. As such, interspecific competition and thus interspecific aggression increase, but this is apparently a result of recognition errors by males, which are maladaptive (Drury et al. 2015).

In some species, either males or females may even prefer mating with heterospecific partners, which also affects interspecific competition. In males this was obser־verd, for instance, in ground-hoppers (grasshopper), where *Tetrix ceperoi* males prefer copulating with *T. subulata* females (Hochkirch et al. 2007). In contrast, females of the spadefoot toads (*Spea bombifrons*) prefer to mate with heterospecific males, which actually may yield benefits from hybridization. Spadefoot toads breed in ponds which are temporarily filled with water and tadpoles often fail to metamorphose before the ponds dry out (Pfennig 1992). Tadpoles produced by *S. bombifrons* develop slower than those produced by *S. multiplicata*, and hybrid tadpoles metamorphose sooner than *S. bombifrons* tadpoles (Pfennig & Simovich 2002). However, hybrid offspring also have lower fertility and fecundity. So the fitness effects of hybridization depend on the pond characteristics in which offspring develop. As a consequence, female *S. bombifrons* adjust their choice for conspecific versus heterospecific mates depending on how long the breeding pond will be stocked with water. In deep water, females chose conspecific calls significantly more frequently than random, and more frequently than they did in shallow water. In shallow water, females showed no preference for conspecific calls (Figure 5.5). This demonstrates nicely that switches in mate choice can evolve in response to the adaptiveness of hybridization (Pfennig 2007).

Some species exhibit serial territoriality, wherein the boundary at which an intruder is attacked varies and depends, at least partially, on the intruder's degree of resource competition (Myrberg & Thresher 1974). Serial territoriality depends on the existence of a generic dominance order to exploit and defend a resource. For example, some herbivorous marine damselfishes of the genus *Pomacentrus* that live on coral reefs protect algae as their food resource in a fiercely defended territory. They discriminate potential intruders based on their food habits and attack herbivorous fish that represent strong food competitors further outside their algae gardens than other fishes (Syrop 1974; Thresher 1976; Ebersole 1977; Kohda 1997). Some carnivorous species feeding on eggs and fry are tolerated until close to the centre of the territory, where they are attacked near the defender's brood. As a result of this context-specific defence pattern the standing crop of filamentous algae, which represent the major food source of the territory owners, was greater within the protected feeding space compared to the surrounding unprotected areas (Syrop 1974). The occurrence and form of serial territoriality not only depends on the type of competitor, but also on the degree of competition with them. The fiercer the competition for defended resources, the bigger the defended area. For example, herbivorous fish defended larger territories on a reef with a great number of herbivorous competitors present (Syrop 1974). Interspecific

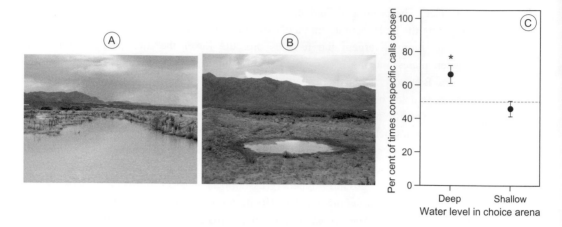

Figure 5.5 *S. bombifrons* breeding ponds vary in depth (2 to 66 cm) and longevity (7 days to several months between years, depending on the amount of rainfall). (A) and (B) show the same pond in different years. (C) The mean percentage (± SE) of times that conspecific calls were chosen by sympatric *S. bombifrons* females differed between deep and shallow pools in repeated preference tests (Wilcoxon signed rank = 245, $n = 52$ females, $P = 0.009$; from Pfennig 2007). © David Pfennig.

hierarchies also exist in certain cichlids and coral-reef surgeon fishes, where the occurrence and form of serial territoriality may depend on the fishes' diet, but in part also on their body size, physical environment and the effect of predation (Barlow 1974). The above examples highlight that many species can coexist through serial territoriality, despite a broad overlap in feeding habits and resource requirements.

A demonstration that serial territoriality can be driven by dietary overlap with other species was achieved for *Neolamprologus tetracanthus*, a shrimp-eating Lake Tanganyika cichlid. Females defend territories against a variety of intruding fish species, but they show different levels of aggression based on the degree of competition with them. Females repelled conspecific females, heterospecific benthivores, which are also shrimp eaters, and omnivores near the edge or even outside of their swimming ranges, whereas piscivores, algae and detritus feeders and herbivores were attacked only inside their usual home ranges (Figure 5.6). Soon after removal of the resident females, many food competitors invaded their foraging areas to feed on prey, suggesting that the territories are indeed maintained for the protection of the food resource from these competitors. Females apparently discriminate intruding fishes and change their territorial defence primarily on the basis of the degree of dietary overlap, resulting in serial territoriality (Matsumoto & Kohda 2004).

5.3.2   How to Deal with Predators: Interspecific Associations

Predators exploit prey, which is probably the most drastic example of interspecific conflict of interest. This is a major topic in ecology that goes far beyond the subjects we wish to discuss in this book. However, the risk of predation may also influence

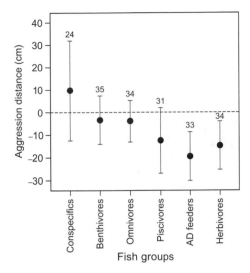

Figure 5.6 Aggression distance of each fish group. Aggression distance is the distance between the edge of the undisturbed swimming range (distance zero, marked by dotted line) of female *Neolamprologus tetracanthus* and the points where approaching fishes were attacked by the territory owners. Dots mark means ± SD, with sample sizes given above; 'AD feeders' refers to 'algae and detritus feeders' (from Matsumoto & Kohda 2004).

how individuals behave in order to minimize predation risk, and this may again involve interactions between different species. To reduce the risk of predation, for instance, individuals may form groups and cooperate, either to benefit from safety in numbers or from grouping around an 'umbrella' species that helps to protect them from mutual predators (reviewed by Haemig 2001; Quinn & Ueta 2008). For example, Bullock's orioles (*Icterus galbula bullockii*) prefer to cluster their nests in areas that contain nests of larger and more aggressive yellow-billed magpies (*Pica nuttali*), as they afford protection against other corvids predating on nests. Oriole nests built near magpie nests benefit from a reduced predation rate. Interestingly, despite the fact that orioles also defended their nest against magpies, no predation of oriole nests by magpies was observed (Richardson & Bolen 1999). Oriole colonies tended to be larger when associated with magpies, which provides older males with a greater opportunity to gain extra-pair paternity at the expense of younger males (Richardson & Burke 2001). This example shows that nesting associations may not only result in protective benefits when nesting near birds of prey, but that these may also have consequences for other fitness components such as fertilization opportunities for males. It has not yet been experimentally shown, however, that defence behaviour by magpies caused the higher reproductive success in orioles, and it is not known whether the magpies might benefit in turn from the presence of orioles, e.g. by enhanced predator detection, more efficient mobbing, or safety in numbers (dilution effects; Richardson & Bolen 1999).

An experimental demonstration that nest defence intensity by another, 'protective' species can reduce predation rates of heterospecific beneficiaries involved dummy nests consisting of two quail eggs (*Coturnix japonica*) positioned near individual nests of Eurasian hobbies (*Falco subbuteo*). A higher nest defence intensity by hobbies was associated with lower predation rates on eggs in the dummy nests (Sergio & Bogliani 2001). Pairs of hobbies with the highest breeding success protected a greater proportion of dummy nests (Sergio & Bogliani 2001). This might be a reason why the number of woodpigeons (*Columba palumbus*) nesting near hobbies was positively correlated with the degree of aggression of individual hobbies (Bogliani et al. 1999). The risk of predation on adult woodpigeons by hobbies is not a major cost of nesting near hobbies, as this is extremely low (Bogliani et al. 1999).

In fishes, temporary group formation of individuals belonging to different species for the purpose of joint brood care has been observed, for instance, in cyprinids (hornyhead chub, *Hybopsis biguttata*) with common shiner (*Notropis cornutus*: Hankinson 1920), and between cichlids and catfish (McKaye 1985; McKaye et al. 1992). As discussed above, mixed species broods occur frequently in cichlids, sometimes also between cichlids and catfish (see Taborsky 1994 for review; Box 5.1).

In general, many studies on protective nesting associations in birds and fishes show that such associations occur by active choice and not because the involved species choose similar habitat. Species benefitting from the protection by others may apparently select actively whom to join, which is probably based on a trade-off between the costs and benefits of nesting with, or near to, aggressive species potentially helping to protect one's own offspring. For example, red-breasted geese (*Branta ruficollis*) prefer to settle near peregrine falcons (*Falco peregrinus*) in areas with high abundance of predators such as Arctic foxes (*Alopex lagopus*), which are attacked by falcons when approaching nests closely (Quinn et al. 2003). Most geese apparently nest at those places where the combined risks of predation by foxes and falcons are minimized. In contrast, when the predation risk by Arctic foxes is low, geese nest further away from the falcons (Quinn & Kokorev 2002).

For most 'protective species' nesting associations there is still little information on fitness consequences (Quinn & Ueta 2008) and hence the potential role of interspecific mutualism or parasitism is little understood in this context. A good example of an interspecific mutualism in which both the protective and protected species benefit may be the association between the merlin and the fieldfare. The merlin (*Falco columbarius*), a protective species, produces better by nesting near fieldfares (*Turdus pilar*), which are themselves aggressive nest defenders (Wiklund 1979). Fieldfares, in turn, also produce better when associating with merlins, and there is no predation by merlins on fieldfares. Aggression was considered to be the main strategy used by fieldfares to deter attacks by the merlins with which they associate (Wiklund 1982).

Nevertheless, 'protecting species' can also pay a cost, which implies that they are parasitized. For example, sand-coloured nighthawks (*Chordeiles rupestris*) nest in the vicinity of three protective species: large-billed tern (*Phaetusa simplex*), yellow-billed tern (*Sterna superciliari*) and black skimmer (*Rvnchops niger*). Costs and benefits of the association were distributed asymmetrically among the species. The nighthawks

Box 5.1 Interspecific Brood Mixing in Cichlids Through Passive or Active Processes

Interspecific brood mixing may occur through passive or active processes. The mixing of parentally protected fry is common in several cichlid fish species, including mouthbrooders. In the latter, eggs are picked up by one parent, usually the female, immediately after oviposition, and they are subsequently incubated in the buccal cavity. The fry stay in the buccal cavity for varying lengths of time until the young are either released and guarded for some additional time, or until they have reached complete independence (Barlow 2008; Sefc 2011). Guarded fry feeding outside of the parent's mouth frequently return to it in case of danger, using the parent's mouth as a refuge when threatened by predation until they become independent (Barlow 2008). Orally incubating parents may sometimes transport some or all of their free-swimming young in the mouth to neighbouring parents and put them under their custody, which has been called 'brood farming out' (Yanagisawa 1985). Cichlid mouthbrooders may also actively farm out their offspring into broods of catfish (McKaye et al. 1992). Interspecific brood mixing may not only occur before independence of young (e.g. Baba et al. 1990; Ochi & Yanagisawa 1996; Katula & Page 1998; Ochi et al. 2001) but also thereafter, through autonomous intrusion of independent young into other, still guarded broods (Ribbink et al. 1980; Ochi et al. 2001).

Cichlid donor parents apparently select host species for their fry that have similar foraging requirements to themselves, but mostly they seem to avoid host species with highly aggressive young (Ochi & Yanagisawa 1996), suggesting that donors select host parents prudently in order to benefit from the latter's alloparental effort while at the same time avoiding the costs of suffering from fierce intrabrood competition. It is often less clear why host parents adopt fry, which will be discussed further down.

There are various benefits members of donor species can gain from foisting their young on alloparents. First, it will reduce the costs of parental care for the donors, like in cuckoos and other brood parasites (Clutton-Brock 1991; Keenleyside 1991). Parental care often causes considerable energy, mortality and opportunity costs (Clutton-Brock 1991; Smith & Wootton 1995). In Lake Tanganyika cichlids, for instance, some species care for their brood for three months or more (e.g. *Perissodus microlepis*: Yanagisawa 1983; Ochi et al. 1995; *Lepidiolamprologus attenuates*: Nagoshi & Gashagaza 1988; *L. elongates*: Ochi & Yanagisawa 1996; *Boulengerochromis microlepis*: Koblmüller et al. 2015). In mouthbrooders, care is expensive because the parent cannot feed for extended periods of time (they may lose a third of their body weight; e.g. Smith & Wootton 1994; Okuda 2001; Schürch & Taborsky 2005). In substrate brooders, cleaning and fanning of eggs and larvae, maintaining the nest or burrow and defence against predators are energetically demanding (Chellappa & Huntingford 1989; Grantner & Taborsky 1998; Taborsky & Grantner 1998; Steinhart et al. 2005; Cooke et al. 2010). Such intensive parental care may cause long-term costs, such as nest loss (Horak et al.

Box 5.1 (*cont.*)

1999) and reduced future reproductive success and survival (Steinhart et al. 2005). Therefore, a reduction of the costs of parental care by foisting offspring on alloparents may provide high fitness gains (McKaye & McKaye 1977; Yanagisawa 1986; Wisenden 1999).

The donor species may also take advantage by reducing the costs of nest preparation when using a nest prepared for spawning by the host species. In a case of brood-mixing between two catfish species in Lake Tanganyika, the host bagrid catfish *Auchenoglanis occidentalis* prepares a nest by gathering large amounts of shells and gravel, which are scarce in the nesting area. The donor catfish *Dinotopterus cunningtoni* dumps its eggs into the host nest, by which it takes advantage of the host's nest preparation and from the fact that its brood will be safe from attacks by predating cichlid fishes (Ochi et al. 2001). However, an additional predatory function cannot be excluded, because donor young were observed to prey on smaller host young (Ochi et al. 2001).

Second, in mouthbrooders an increase in buccal cavity space after farming out seems to be a major benefit to the donor, which may also reduce intrabuccal competition. This may be particularly important in mouthbrooding species in which young eat food within the parent's mouth. It has been suggested that such intra-buccal feeding of young can be costly to the (foster) parents, because young intercept food in the buccal cavity before it is ingested by the parents (Yanagisawa et al. 1996). When young are large enough to be farmed out, they begin to appear as adopted young in other broods both of the same species (e.g. Ochi et al. 1995; Kellogg et al. 1998) and of other species of cichlids (e.g. Ochi & Yanagisawa 1996). Mouthbrooding females create a situation that seems to be highly susceptible to brood mixing (Wisenden 1999; Ochi & Yanagisawa 2005). In most cases, however, it is unknown how the transfer of fry to foster parents takes place. Therefore, the process of adoption of heterospecific fry in mouthbrooders has been assumed to be sometimes caused by an accidental mixture of fry (Ribbink 1977), which led to the hypothesis that interspecific adoption might be maladaptive altogether (Lewis 1980).

Third, by brood-mixing, the donor's offspring may benefit from reduced mortality risk by a 'safety in numbers' effect, i.e. due to predation risk dilution (McKaye & McKaye 1977; Wisenden & Keenleyside 1994) and predator confusion (Milinski 1977), or if the foster parents can provide more efficient protection against predators, which may depend on the size and aggressiveness of the parents, the relative size of adopted and foster parents' young, or on spatial variation in predation risk (Wisenden & Keenleyside 1992; Wisenden 1999). For instance, if the donor's young are larger than those of the foster parents, they may have better chances to escape a predator (Wisenden & Keenleyside 1992). In environments with high predation pressure, donor individuals may also benefit from a bet-hedging strategy when placing offspring with multiple foster parents which may ensure that some will survive (Kellog et al. 1995; Roy Nielsen et al. 2008).

Box 5.1 (*cont.*)

Young have also been shown to sometimes join foster broods of smaller young on their own, which makes them less vulnerable to predators (Krause & Godin 1994), as smaller fry are predated before larger ones (Wisenden & Keenleyside 1992, 1994; Wisenden 1999).

The benefits to the host species of adopting foreign young are often less clear, and it may well be that in many cases the brood 'donors' actually parasitize the brood care effort of the host. However, this is not always the case. Typically, the size of young is crucial for the host species' adoption decision (Wisenden & Keenleyside 1992; Espmark & Knudsen 2001). Only young of matching size or young smaller than own offspring of the host are usually accepted, whereas larger young are commonly rejected or eaten by the host parents, providing them with nutritional benefits (McKaye & McKaye 1977; Wisenden and Keenleyside 1992; Fraser et al. 1993; Espmark & Knudsen 2001). On the other hand, hosts may adopt young from other species to increase the survival of their own young due to predation risk dilution. Brood-caring parents may also adopt smaller young for the benefit of serving as food for their own offspring. Apart from the fact that predators may selectively feed on the smallest young in a group (Wisenden 1999), size-selective adoption may also reflect potential predation risk within a group of young. For example, in the convict cichlid parents do not adopt young that are larger than their own, and it has been shown that such large, non-descendant young can predate on their own, smaller offspring (Fraser et al. 1993). Hosts of foreign young may also increase the survival of their young by allowing donor parents to co-protect the mixed brood. For example, when cichlid parents remained present with catfish and their mixed broods, no attacks by predators were observed upon the catfish, but mainly on the cichlids. When catfish parents were experimentally removed, the cichlid young were consumed first and then the catfish young. When cichlids were present the catfish young survived significantly better than if no cichlid parents were there. Parental catfish increase the survival of their own young by allowing young from cichlids into their brood, which is further enhanced by accepting the joining of the cichlids' parents (McKaye 1985).

never defended their own nest, whereas the terns actively defended their nests by chasing predators, which incidentally also protected the nearby nests of nighthawks. Nighthawks had higher nesting success when nesting near terns and skimmers, but their presence forced the terns and skimmers to spend more time being vigilant and defending the colony from predators. Hence they had less time available to engage in parental care, which resulted in lower reproductive success when nesting among many nighthawks (Groom 1992). This illustrates that an apparently 'mutualistic relationship' in fact reflects parasitism, where one species benefits from the other whereas the latter is paying a cost. Why terns and skimmers tolerate nighthawks nesting in close proximity is unclear, but it could be that they are unable to prevent nighthawks from nesting nearby except by paying even higher repulsion costs. Nighthawks nest later than terns and skimmers, and therefore terns and skimmers cannot choose nesting sites without nighthawks when not abandoning their clutches (Groom 1992).

It is an important consequence of interactions with other species that the selection regime for social behaviours among conspecifics can be strongly affected. For example, individuals may form aggregations to avoid predation, which may then facilitate social interactions and the evolution of cooperation. As we have outlined in Chapter 4, female eider ducks (*Somateria mollissima*) either raise their broods alone or form brood-rearing coalitions or 'crèches' with 1–4 other females to protect the ducklings from gull predation. The presence of other group members increases total vigilance and contributes to improved predator detection (Öst et al. 2007). A high offspring predation risk increases the propensity of females with ducklings to form coalitions with other females (Öst & Tierala 2011), and the reproductive output of females in coalitions often exceeds that of single parents (Öst et al. 2008). Such crèches formed for the protection of offspring can also involve members of different species. For example, in mixed colonies of Chinese crested tern (*Thalasseus bernsteini*) and greater crested tern (*Thallasseus bergii*), chicks of the former often join chicks of the latter. These crèches are guarded against predators by a few adults of both species (Chen et al. 2011). Both species breed synchronously at the same colony. However, whether crèching results in higher chick survival is presently unknown.

Interference competition involves agonistic interactions between competitors that may, for example, fight over scarce resources. In this case, more-specialized competitors may displace less-efficient or more-generalized ones (Case & Gilpin 1974). In such relations, third parties such as predators and parasites may interfere with the interactions among competing species. A classic example of interference of a predator with a multi-species prey dynamic is the interaction between the stoat (*Mustela erminea*) and several prey species, including field voles (*Microtus agrestis*) and bank voles (*Myodes glareolus*) in northern Fennoscandia. The larger field voles are dominant over bank voles through aggressive interference (Eccard & Ylönen 2002). When stoat numbers are low, their preferred (i.e. larger) prey, field voles, occurs in high numbers, which results in much interference competition with bank voles. When predator numbers increase, field vole abundance consequently declines and interference competition with bank voles becomes less severe (Korpimäki et al. 1991; Oksanen & Henttonen 1996). This causes bank voles, which are better able to avoid predators, to increase in numbers (Eccard & Ylönen 2002).

5.3.3   Host–Parasite Relations

Parasitism is a relationship between species where individuals of one species, the parasite, live on or use individuals from another species, the host, who suffer some harm. We may distinguish two types of host–parasite relations. (i) Exploitation, where the parasite uses a host without modifying the host traits. Exploitation also occurs between conspecifics in the form of social or reproductive parasitism (as described in Chapter 3). (ii) Manipulation, where the parasite changes traits of the host in its own fitness interest. This is more likely to occur *between* species than among conspecifics, due to a lag in evolutionary responses of the exploited. However, manipulation does also occur in intraspecific interactions, for instance by forced cooperation or intraspecific brood parasitism (see Chapter 4).

We should like to stress that the margin between cooperative (mutualistic) and parasitic relationships can be narrow, which often prevents conclusions about the underlying selection mechanisms when observing interspecific relations. This will be illustrated below by examples of joint brood defence in fishes. Therefore, incorporating fitness consequences of interspecific relations is important for distinguishing cases of parasitism from those reflecting cooperation. In the following section we focus on host–parasite relationships at the level of brood care.

Brood care of young from other species is widespread in mammals, birds, fishes and social insects (Wilson 1975; Riedman 1982; Taborsky 1994; Wisenden 1999). Several fish species raise mixed-species broods, and some also raise pure heterospecific broods (reviewed in Taborsky 1994; Wisenden 1999). Such interspecific brood mixing may occur through passive or active processes (Box 5.1). An example illustrating potential benefits of interspecific adoption for the donor species and the potential costs to the host species has been provided by a study of brood mixing between spinynose sculpin (*Asemichthys taylori*) and buffalo sculpin (*Enophrys bison*: Kent et al. 2011). Spinynose sculpins do not provide parental care and instead deposit their eggs into nests from other fish species. Thereby, they often lay eggs on top of buffalo sculpin eggs, and the male buffalo sculpin nest owners care for and guard the mixed cluster of eggs. This entails costs, as the nest owners need to raise their fanning effort for the enlarged broods. In addition, the spinynose eggs benefit more from fanning, as they lie on top of those of the host. The covering spinynose eggs are tightly packed and hamper oxygen flow to the covered buffalo eggs, which slows down the development of the buffalo embryos and likely reduces their survival. This brood parasitism of spinynose sculpins in buffalo sculpin nests provides obvious benefits to the parasite at the expense of the host: the spinynose eggs, which are smaller, hatch faster than the earlier laid buffalo eggs, and the survival of buffalo eggs is apparently reduced; in addition, buffalo sculpins were never observed to lay their eggs on top of eggs of spinynose sculpins deposited in their nests. In spite of these obvious fitness costs, no aggression by buffalo sculpin toward spinynose sculpin was observed (Kent et al. 2011). The rare occurrence of the spinynose sculpin (Coffie 1998) and its limited geographic distribution may be responsible for the fact that no countermeasures against this nest parasitism have yet evolved in buffalo sculpin (Kent et al. 2011), similarly to an avian host species that is rarely parasitized by the common cuckoo (*Cuculus canorus*; Davies et al. 1989).

Another intriguing example of the diverging costs and benefits for interaction partners involved in brood mixing is provided by the parasitism by a catfish species of some mouthbrooding cichlids in Lake Tanganyika. The mochokid catfish *Synodontis multipunctatus* is an obligatory brood parasite of several species of mouthbrooding cichlids (Sato 1987). Female catfish dump their eggs at the time when the cichlids spawn (Sato 1987; Schrader 1993). The parasitized cichlid female picks the deposited egg(s) up together with her own eggs. Once inside the buccal cavity, the parasite's offspring develop faster than those of the host (Sato 1987), so that the catfish eggs hatch earlier and the young catfish feed on the host's offspring in the foster mother's mouth. The mouthbrooding cichlid hosts have apparently not developed efficient mechanisms to avoid being parasitized, probably because of the low parasitism rate by catfish, which partly results from their use of many different host species (at least 11; Sato 1987). Thereby, the selection pressure to develop efficient antiparasite behaviours may not be strong enough, just like in the (temporary) hosts of European cuckoos (Davies et al. 1989). Nevertheless, host species coevolved with the parasitic catfish show much higher rejection rates than evolutionarily naïve allopatric cichlid species (Blazek et al. 2018).

Such brood parasitism is also well known from birds. As in the catfish–cichlid relationship, the host species suffers a cost of raising foreign young, which typically goes at the expense of their own young. For example, some species of the cuckoo family (Cuculidae) are brood parasites. The common cuckoo has several genetically distinct host races or 'gentes', of which each specializes on a particular host species in the nests of which they lay an egg typically matching the eggs of the species they parasitize. During the egg-laying period by the host, a female cuckoo observes the nests of potential hosts for extended periods of time before she approaches a nest and removes one host egg, which she consumes, and surreptitiously and quickly lays her own egg in its place (Davies & Brooke 1988; Honza et al. 2002). The whole process may take less than 10 seconds. The host species often accept the cuckoo egg, but sometimes reject it. The cuckoo chick usually hatches first because despite its larger size, the cuckoo egg needs a shorter period of incubation than the host eggs. A couple of hours after hatching the cuckoo chick balances each of the host eggs one by one on its back and ejects them from the nest, until all have been ejected (Figure 5.7). The host adults never act to prevent this. The cuckoo chick remains on its own in the nest and is fed and raised by the host parents. The cuckoo nestling exploits its host stepparents through vocal trickery to enhance brood care. Cuckoo nestlings beg at much higher rates than single host chicks would do; they even call similarly, often as a whole brood of reed warblers would (Figure 5.7), which raises the provisioning rate of the stepparents (Davies et al. 1998). This is a dramatic example of the costs of interspecific brood parasitism, as the hosts not only lose their entire brood, but in the seasonal environments where European cuckoos are common the hosts may completely miss out on reproducing in a given year, which is detrimental for short-lived songbirds, the usual hosts of cuckoos. This strongly selects for counter-adaptation, which in the case of cuckoo hosts is the ability to discriminate between their own and parasitic eggs, in order to be able to reject the cuckoo egg from their nest. This reflects a coevolutionary arms race between cuckoos and hosts, involving the cuckoo's tricks to get their eggs accepted by hosts, and correspondingly host defences to reject them. This arms race implies the following coevolutionary sequence (Davies 2000; see Figure 5.8). Stage 1: at the start of the arms race, a new host exhibits little or no rejection of foreign eggs and there is no selection on cuckoos to develop similarity of their eggs to the eggs of this host (egg mimicry). Stage 2: in response to parasitism, the host then evolves egg rejection and/or more distinctive variation in egg

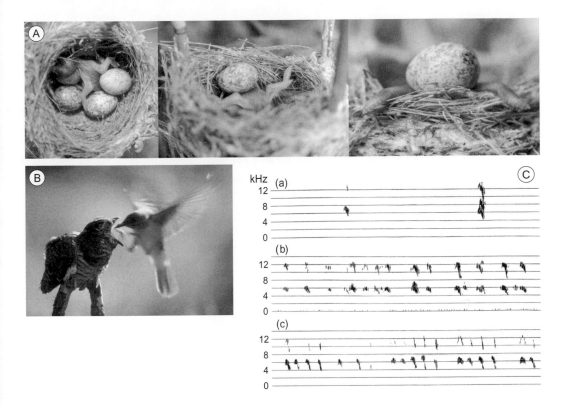

Figure 5.7 Cuckoo brood parasites destroy the reed warbler hosts' reproductive success without resistance. (A) Shortly after hatching, the cuckoo chick ejects the host eggs one by one, balancing them on its back and heaving them over the edge of the nest. (B) The reed warbler hosts continue to feed the young cuckoo even as it becomes significantly bigger than themselves (photographs credit O. Mikulica). (C) Sonograms (2.5 s) of the begging calls, recorded 60 min after feeding to satiation, of a single reed warbler chick, a brood of four reed warblers and a single cuckoo chick (from Davies et al. 1998). (A black and white version of this figure will appear in some formats. For the colour version, please refer to the plate section.)

markings. Stage 3: in response to host rejection of cuckoo eggs, cuckoos can either persist using the same host, in which case natural selection will favour those cuckoos that lay eggs resembling the host eggs (mimetic eggs), or they may switch to a different (new) host that does not reject non-matching eggs. Stage 4: if the egg mimicry is very good and parasitism levels are not too high, selection may favour hosts that accept cuckoo eggs to avoid the cost of erroneously rejecting their own eggs (Davies & Brooke 1989a, 1989b; Davies et al. 1989; Davies 1992, 2000).

When a host species cares for pure heterospecific broods, it is difficult to imagine an adaptive cause. The herbivorous Nicaragua cichlid *Cichlasoma nicaraguense* performs brood care of the fry of the predatory cichlid *Cichlasoma dovii* together with the *C. dovii* parents, mainly by protecting them against attacks from other predatory fishes (McKaye 1977, 1979). The benefits of such behaviour to the *C. dovii*

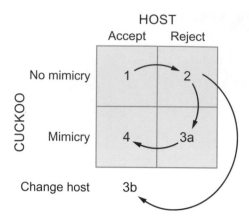

Figure 5.8 A scheme of the coevolutionary sequence depicting the arms race between cuckoos and their hosts, divided into four stages with stage 1 as starting point of the arms race and stage 4 as its end point (from Davies 2000).

parents are evident, as predation on their fry and defence effort can be reduced by this help. However, how can this altruistic help of *C. nicaraguense* be maintained in the population? It has been argued that this interspecific brood care of *C. nicaraguense* has evolved to raise the population density of *C. dovii*, which also predates a nest site competitor of *C. nicaraguense*, *Neetroplus nematopus* (McKaye 1977, 1979). However, it is dubious whether this can really work out as hypothesized (Coyne & Sohn 1978), as there is no obvious way that the resulting 'tragedy of the commons' can be overcome. All *C. nicaraguense* in a population might possibly benefit from the increased population density of their competitor's predator, but it is unclear why any particular *C. nicaraguense* should decide to bear the costs of helping to raise the predator's young instead of leaving this duty to another conspecific, thereby only reaping the benefits of this interspecific cooperation without paying the cost. In other words, such cooperative behaviour would not be cheat-proof (Dawkins et al. 1979; Nakazawa & Yamamura 2009). It seems more plausible that the altruistic behaviour of *C. nicaraguense* might be a consequence of breeders having lost their brood and instead caring for foreign juveniles due to lacking the ability to distinguish these different young (Coyne & Sohn 1978). If this holds true, this brood care would be misdirected and maladaptive, suggesting that the behaviour would only persist in the population if the situation releasing it is relatively rare. This in fact seems to be the case (Barlow 2008).

5.4   Cooperation

If pondering about cooperation, we might intuitively think of interactions between conspecifics, but there is no reason to believe that cooperation is confined to the intraspecific context, or that it is even rarer or less important in interactions among different species. In fact, cooperation among different species is extremely widespread in nature, and it can be of the essence. Cooperation between species may arise through shared interest. Symbioses, for instance, reflect a situation where both partners of an interaction depend on each other's disposition to cooperate (Kiers et al. 2011). Such cooperation can be based on mutualism or reciprocity, like in the interactions among conspecifics that are not merely based on kin selection, i.e. the preferential support of relatives resulting in enhanced indirect fitness.

Cooperation between different species, just like cooperation between unrelated individuals of the same species as discussed in Chapter 4, presents an evolutionary dilemma, if any change in behaviour in one species serves exclusively for the benefit of another species. An important focus of evolutionary research in cooperation is to understand the evolution of seemingly altruistic behaviour. In other words, how can costly acts performed by one individual to benefit another be maintained by natural selection? A methodological problem in the endeavour to understand the evolution of altruism is that return benefits to a cooperator may be delayed, rendering a full cost–benefit analysis of mutual cooperation difficult.

In this section we discuss cooperation through commensalism, mutualism and reciprocity. The evolutionary mechanisms underlying these different forms of cooperation are assumed to be identical to the forms of cooperation discussed at the intraspecific level.

5.4.1   Commensalism

Commensalism is a term in ecology referring to interactions in which traits exhibited by one species benefit that species directly, but in addition also have positive side effects on another, 'recipient' species. In the logic of evolutionary theory as outlined in Chapters 1 and 4, this bears one important component of mutualism: a trait will be selected by its direct positive effects on the actor's fitness; even if there is no additional gain accrued from the benefitting partner, the trait will be positively selected. However, in commensal relationships there is no feedback whatsoever from the affected receiver to the donor, making it truly a one-way interaction. Such relationship may turn into a mutualism, if potential additional benefits to the donor accrue from traits of the receiver, which may modify the intensity or speed of selection for the respective trait, but not necessarily its direction.

Grouping with other species can, for instance, improve foraging success. Various birds and mammals tend to follow foraging primate groups. The benefits of these loose associations seem to be asymmetrically distributed. Benefits for birds and non-primate mammals from following primates can be substantial, including, for example, consumption of dropped leaves and fruits, and flushed prey. They also consist of antipredation benefits through eavesdropping on primate alarm calls and vigilance. Primates, on the other hand, do not seem to benefit from associating with other species (reviewed in Heymann & Hsia 2015). In the Ethiopian highlands, Ethiopian wolves (*Canis simensis*) prey on rodents among groups of grazing gelada monkeys

(*Theropithecus gelada*). The wolves stay in close proximity to gelada herds without attempting to catch juvenile monkeys. In the presence of geladas, the wolves spent more time foraging and preyed more successfully than when foraging alone. Groups of geladas increase the vulnerability of rodents to predation, probably by disturbing the vegetation and driving rodents to the surface. The wolves habituate gelada herds to their presence by refraining from attacking them. In the rare cases where wolves were observed attacking juvenile geladas, wolves were mobbed by adult geladas, which reduced their foraging success. Wolves forgo foraging opportunities upon geladas to enable more effective feeding on rodents (Venkataraman et al. 2015). This may illustrate that non-primate species can gain benefits from associating with primates, without providing any benefits in return to the primates they associate with.

Commensalism is also a frequent phenomenon in synanthropic species making use of resources provided by human civilization. Such species have developed a commensal relationship with humans, in which urban development creates opportunities for them to obtain useful resources. As a result, they thrive alongside areas inhabited by humans. Renowned examples include the house sparrow, raccoon, house mouse and Norway rat, all of which have successfully adapted to human environments, benefitting from what humans leave behind. As humans are typically not affected by this incidental resource use (as long as rats and mice do not become pests), this is exemplifying a one-way relationship.

5.4.2   Mutualism

Mutualistic relationships between species, where both partners obtain immediate benefits from their behaviour (or other trait; West-Eberhard 1975; Brown 1983), are common in nature. Here the benefits to each partner accrue directly from their behaviours, which means that mutualistic cooperation cannot be cheated (there is no free-riding). Renowned examples of mutualistic relationships include the interaction between pollinators and flowers. Bees, for example, fly from flower to flower to collect nectar which they need to feed the brood and dependent members of their hive. In that process, the bees get some pollen attached to their bodies, which after being transported to the next flower may lead to successful pollination of the visited plant. The bees benefit from the plant to obtain a food resource and the plant benefits from the bees to enable fertilization.

An example illustrating mutualistic interspecific relationships between different animal taxa is provided by some species of burrowing shrimp (*Alpheus* spp.) associating with gobiid fishes that cohabit the same burrow, which is constructed by the shrimp (Karplus & Thompson 2011). The shrimp has poor eyesight, so individuals are prone to predation when outside their burrow foraging. Therefore, the shrimp depend on the presence of the goby fish for protection when leaving their burrow in order to forage efficiently. The goby warns their shrimp partners via a tactile warning system when predators are close (Jaafar & Zeng 2012). The benefit for the goby from this association derives from the extensive digging activity of the shrimp, which constructs complex burrow systems providing ample refuge from predators for both themselves and the gobies. Often, the goby stands guard outside the burrow, while the shrimp scoops out chambers to enhance the burrow. If the fish notices a predator, it flaps the shrimp with its fins to send it back into the burrow and then follows (Magnus 1967). This illustrates the functionality of mutualisms. The shrimp needs a burrow to hide, so burrowing is under positive selection independently of any effects on the goby. The goby needs to be vigilant about predators for its own safety, so its vigilance will also be positively selected independently of any effects on the shrimp. However, this system also seems to provide potential for reciprocity due to the partner-directed behaviours of both parties. The gobies seem to warn the shrimp with special behaviours providing tactile information, and the shrimp might enhance its digging activity if a goby is present, i.e. in the latter's favour. These potential reciprocal aspects of the shrimp–goby relationship need to be studied in more detail to check whether traits are expressed for the partner at a cost to the actor, making them vulnerable to being cheated, which is a prerequisite of reciprocity as outlined in Chapter 4 and Section 5.4.3.

A mutualistic interaction between birds and mammals is exemplified by the association between the oxpecker (*Buphagus* spp.) and the zebra (*Equus quagga*). The oxpecker is an African passerine bird that finds its food almost entirely on the skin of ungulates, such as zebra. Oxpeckers provide a cleaning service by removing ticks and other parasites from the zebra, which constitutes a valuable food source for them. In addition to tolerating oxpeckers riding on their body, the zebra may expose certain parts of its body with wounds to the oxpecker, which may then consume blood and pieces of dead skin and scar tissue of the zebra (Plantan et al. 2013). It is currently unclear whether this behaviour benefits or harms the zebra. In the first case, the relationship between oxpecker and zebra would be purely mutualistic, as both derive immediate (net) benefits from their behaviour. In the second case, this would reflect reciprocity, because the zebra provides an incentive to the oxpecker in order to continue its hygienic service, albeit at an immediate cost (e.g. blood loss or delayed wound healing). Some researchers have suggested that wound-feeding benefits mammals because the oxpecker cleans the wound of dead tissue and maggots (e.g. Breitwisch 1992; Weeks 1999), but there seems to be no evidence that oxpeckers really clean wounds and improve healing time (Weeks 1999). Oxpeckers may even reopen healed wounds or create new ones, which would prolong healing time and thereby occasion costs to the zebra (Plantan et al. 2013). Hence similar to the shrimp–goby case, the interaction might shift from mutualistic either to reciprocal or to parasitic.

Interspecific mutualisms may occur also in the context of brood care. In Lake Malawi, bagrid catfish (*Bagrus meridionalis*) parents and cichlid parents (several species) jointly guard their young from predators in mixed shoals. The parental catfish guard their young as well as the young of the cichlids, whereas the parental cichlids guard the periphery of these mixed broods from predators (McKaye & McKaye 1977; McKaye 1985). The young of both species benefit from reduced mortality risk by enhanced guarding effects by parents of both species (McKaye & Oliver 1980; McKaye et al. 1992) and by a 'safety in numbers' effect due to predation risk dilution

(Lewis 1980; Johnston 1994; Wisenden & Keenleyside 1994). Mutual benefits can thus select for interspecific joint brood care in environments with high predation pressure. Some Lake Malawi cichlids always seem to associate with catfish broods, as the young of some species (*Cyrtocara pleurostigmoides* and *C. pictus*) were always observed among a catfish brood, suggesting that this mutualism may have turned into an obligatory relationship (McKaye 1985).

5.4.3   Reciprocity

Natural selection will disfavour interspecific cooperation if cheating cannot be prevented (West et al. 2007c; Ghoul et al. 2014). Hence, cooperation between species may arise due to correlated pay-offs or 'shared interests' (Taborsky et al. 2016), or when partners have some control over each other, such as by punishment or by the adoption of outside options. Such forms of discriminative cooperation may easily evolve between species, owing to return benefits for the donor or the donor's relatives (Doebeli & Knowlton 1998; West et al. 2002; Foster & Wenseleers 2006). Frequently, cooperation between species involves the reciprocal exchange of commodities and services among each other. Like in the context of intraspecific interactions, when members of different species behave according to the rules of direct reciprocity, the principle is that a donor performs a costly act to benefit a recipient while in turn receiving a benefit from that recipient. This reflects a form of trading. Such interspecific cooperation through direct reciprocity can be illustrated by the interactions of the cleaner wrasse (*Labroides dimidiatus*), which removes and eats ectoparasites from other reef fish and clients such as the striated surgeonfish (*Ctenochaetus striatus*). The majority of reef fish actively visit cleaner fish in their territories ('cleaning stations'), which induces reciprocal exchange and negotiation.

The cleaner invests in a cleaning service (attending to the client and inspecting its surface) and receives food, whereas the client fish occasions opportunity costs (forgoing the possibility of spending time in other activities such as foraging, searching for mates or defending a territory) and receives a service. Although the ectoparasite removal by the cleaner fish is beneficial to both the cleaner (food) and the client (hygiene), this behaviour is prone to cheating, as the cleaner can eat skin and mucus instead of parasites, which is more profitable to the cleaner but costly to the client, and the client can attack the cleaner or move off, thereby making the cleaner move and depriving it of food, which is costly to the cleaner (Bshary & Grutter 2002). Hence, this interaction involves a conflict of interest between the partners and so does not conform with the concept of by-product mutualism but instead with reciprocity. Interestingly, the responses of clients to the cheating of cleaners differ in dependence on their alternative opportunities to receive hygienic service. Client fish that have access to only one cleaning station tend to respond to cheating by attacking the cleaner, which makes the latter more cooperative, i.e. less likely to feed on mucus and scales during the next interaction with the same client (Bshary & Grutter 2002, 2005). In contrast, client fish that have access to several cleaning stations to choose from respond to cheating by swimming off to another cleaning station, and they prefer to attend cooperative cleaners (Bshary & Schäffer 2002). Both control mechanisms force cleaners to mainly feed on parasites instead of skin (Bshary & Grutter 2002, 2005).

The cleaner and client fish association shows that cooperation can be promoted even when both parties can eventually do better by ending the cooperation or by cheating. This puts both partners in control of the outcome of the interaction: if the alternative option renders greater rewards than the act of cooperation, the respective agent does better in cheating or adopting the 'outside option'. If the cleaner obtains a higher long-term benefit by biting off a chunk of skin instead of searching for a parasite on the client's body, it should take the opportunity. If the client is thus cheated, or if the hygienic service of the cleaner is not satisfactory, it should leave the cleaning station and take a better opportunity. This results in a sort of negotiation involving an element of mutual enforcement by both partners, which has been referred to as 'partner control'. If the respective partner is not performing in a way beneficial to the other, the cooperative interaction can be ended either by cheating (i.e. exploiting the trust of the partner), or by abandoning the interaction. This resembles the reciprocal cooperation among conspecifics in cooperative breeders where helpers pay to stay in the territory of dominants (Quinones et al. 2016; Taborsky 2016).

Interestingly, interactions resembling indirect reciprocity may also occur in the relations between cleaners and clients. Bshary (2002; Bshary et al. 2006) and co-workers observed that if bystanders witness a cooperative or defective act of a potential partner with another individual, in a subsequent encounter they may respond towards the observed actor according to this observation. Eavesdropping clients spent more time next to 'cooperative' than to 'unknown cooperative level' cleaners, suggesting that clients may engage in some form of 'image-scoring' (Figure 5.9; Bshary & Grutter 2006). However, one could also expect the opposite: If the cooperation level is 'unknown', one should spend more not less time obtaining information through eavesdropping than if the cooperation propensity of the cleaner is already known to be high. In any case, this surveillance and response of third parties is beneficial to all three parties involved. Observant client fish potentially benefit from checking out and selecting cleaner fish that are cooperative instead of defective. Clients observed while being cleaned benefit because cleaners behave more cooperatively when being observed. Finally, cleaners benefit because by acting cooperatively they can increase their chances of being invited by other clients for future cleaning services (Bshary 2002; Bshary & Grutter 2002).

Interspecific reciprocity may also involve humans. For instance, in Kenya the greater honeyguide (*Indicator indicator*) maintains a reciprocal relationship with the native Boran people. In many parts of Africa, people searching for honey are guided to the bees' nests by the greater honeyguide. The Boran people developed a well-structured relationship with the honeyguide. Isack and Reyer (1989) showed that in unfamiliar areas the search time to locate a beehive was 8.9 hours when not guided, but only 3.2 hours when guided by a honeyeater. The honeyguide benefits as well, because bees' nests located in tree holes are only accessible to the birds after being opened by humans. After destruction of the hive to collect the honey, not all honey can be collected, and some pieces of honeycomb are left behind for the honeyguides.

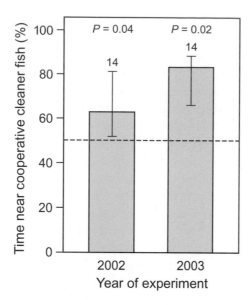

Figure 5.9 Potential clients of cleaner fish spent more than 50 per cent of experimental time near a cleaner feeding from the surface of a fish model (50 per cent would be expected if the time was distributed equally among both sides of the choice compartment; on the other side the presented cleaner did not feed from the contained fish model). The same experiment was conducted in two years. Medians and interquartile ranges are given; numbers indicate sample sizes (from Bshary & Grutter 2006). Copyright © 2006, Nature Publishing Group.

Given their mutual benefit, the humans and honeyguide have developed a sophisticated interspecific communication system. To draw the attention of the bird, the Borans use a specific whistle sound which doubles the encounter rate with the bird. The honeyguide, on the other hand, attempts to guide humans if there is a bees' nest nearby, and informs the people through its flight pattern and distinct calls about the direction and distance to the bee colony. In northern Mozambique, it was experimentally shown that the specialized vocal sound made by local honey-hunters seeking bees' nests elicits elevated cooperative behaviour from honeyguides. This sound reliably signals to honeyguides that a prospective human partner is specifically seeking honey and has the intention, tools and skills to open a bees' nest. The production of this sound increased the probability of being guided by a honeyguide from about 33 per cent to 67 per cent and the overall probability of finding a bees' nest from 17 per cent to 54 per cent, as compared with other animal or human sounds of similar amplitude (Figure 5.10). These results provide experimental evidence that a wild animal in a natural setting responds adaptively to a human signal of recruitment towards cooperative foraging (Spottiswoode et al. 2016). These communication tools of birds and humans are obviously intentionally directed towards members of the respective partner species, which occasion immediate costs and delayed benefits. Honeyguides associate the honey-hunting sound with successful collaboration. Such partner choice should be adaptive by allowing honeyguides to improve their net

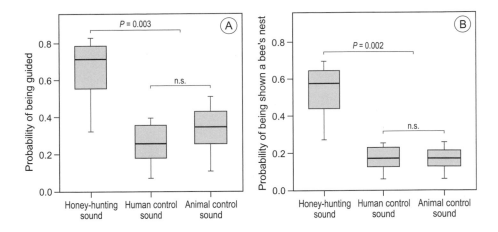

Figure 5.10 Probability of honeyguides leading humans to bees' nests in dependence on different sound playbacks. Values are probabilities of (A) being guided by a honeyguide and (B) being shown a bees' nest on a 15-min search. Compared to presented control sounds, the specific vocal sound produced by human honey-hunters significantly increased the probability that honeyguides would lead them to a bees' nest. Boxplots show medians, quartiles and ranges ($n = 24$ trials per treatment group; P values show planned comparisons; n.s. = not significant; from Spottiswoode et al. 2016). Copyright © 2016, American Association for the Advancement of Science.

benefit from interacting with humans. It is important to note that the immediate costs are probably low in comparison to the future reward, as they involve small amounts of wasted time (opportunity costs) and effort (energy costs) at a rather substantial future nutritional benefit. This exactly accords with what the theory of reciprocal altruism predicts (Trivers 1971).

Reciprocity resembling the interaction between honeyguides and humans also occurs among different species of predatory fish. In the red sea, the grouper (*Plectropomus pessuliferus*) hunts cooperatively with the giant moray eel (*Gymnothorax javanicus*: Bshary et al. 2006). Both fish species adopt complementary hunting strategies. Groupers usually hunt in open water, but an efficient strategy to avoid the risk of predation by potential prey fish is to hide in corals when a grouper appears. Moray eels, on the other hand, hunt prey in the crevices of corals, so to avoid being predated by moray eels, reef fish escape into the open water. Given the complementary hunting strategies of the predators, it is almost impossible for the prey to evade both predators simultaneously. Hence, if both predators team up, they can exploit this impracticable situation for the prey. Indeed, cooperative hunting between groupers and moray eels occurs more often than expected by chance, which hints at an intended association, and both species increase their foraging success when hunting together. The benefit for the grouper is that the moray eel flushes prey out into the open water, whereas the benefit for the moray eel is that the grouper guides it to prey hidden in the corals. The grouper initiates the joint hunt by visiting the resting place of the moray eel and providing head-shake signals close to the eel's head to attract and

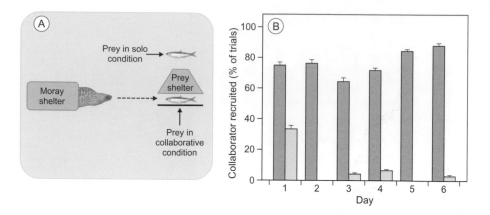

Figure 5.11 Experiment revealing that coral trout choose appropriately when and with whom to collaborate. (A) Bird's eye view of the experimental setup. (B) Results of experiment involving eight trout participating in up to four trials per condition per day for six days, with solo (prey in the open) and collaborative (prey in a crevice) trials alternated within test periods (dark green bars represent collaborative trials and light yellow bars represent solo trials; means and standard errors are shown; from Vail et al. 2014). Copyright © 2014 Elsevier Ltd. All rights reserved. (A black and white version of this figure will appear in some formats. For the colour version, please refer to the plate section.)

subsequently lead the eel to prey hidden in the corals (Bshary et al. 2006; Vail et al. 2013). This behaviour resembles the behaviour of the honeyguide attempting to catch the attention of humans to guide them to a bee nest. Joint hunting was significantly more likely to occur if a grouper signalled than if it did not signal before a hunt, and if the grouper was hungry. A similar relationship exists between coral trout (*Plectropomus leopardus*) and the giant moray eel in the Red Sea. Like the grouper, the coral trout uses gestural communication to initiate a collaborative hunt with a moray eel (Vail et al. 2013) and it was experimentally demonstrated that it recruits a moray collaborator more often when the situation requires it. To determine whether coral trout can determine when to collaborate, they were presented in a situation where prey was either in a crevice (collaborative condition) or in the open (solo condition; Figure 5.11). The correct choices (respectively) were to recruit a nearby model moray that would flush the prey out into the open or attack alone, after which the coral trout was fed a reward to simulate a successful hunt. Experimental subjects quickly learnt to choose effective collaborators and recruited the moray significantly more often in the collaborative than solo condition on all six testing days (Figure 5.11; Vail et al. 2014). If we consider the cost/benefit relations of the involved behaviours, groupers and trout pay a marginal cost in recruiting a moray eel partner, but they may reap a substantial future nutritional benefit from prey made available by the moray's hunting behaviour. Conversely, moray eels probably pay only a marginal cost by changing their activity pattern from hiding to following the grouper or trout, again at a potential high reward when catching prey indicated to them. Trivers' (1971) predictions of when reciprocal altruism should occur are hence again met.

Evidence for reciprocal exchanges among species also exists in taxa that are usually not on our radar when thinking of cooperation, such as among microorganisms. Bacteria are found everywhere and frequently live in densely populated multi-species communities, rather than as isolated cells (Tolker-Nielsen & Molin 2000). This propensity to live in communities suggests a strong adaptive value of an aggregated lifestyle. Bacteria commonly release metabolites into the external environment. Accumulating pools of extracellular metabolites create an ecological niche that benefits auxotrophic mutants, which have lost the ability to synthesize the corresponding metabolites for their growth and need to obtain metabolites as nutrient or energy source from their external environment. Metabolic cross-feeding interactions involving multiple bacterial species are common in nature (Schink 2002; Morris et al. 2013). Evolutionary theory, however, predicts that interactions, in which the production and exchange of metabolites incurs fitness costs, should be prone to the invasion of non-cooperating individuals, which reap cooperative benefits without reciprocating (Herre et al. 1999; Sachs et al. 2004; Travisano & Velicer 2004). Thus, such secreted metabolites behave as cooperative public goods: they can be exploited by non-producing organisms (or cells) in the vicinity. If these secretions are costly to create, public-good-producing bacteria should avoid being exploited by auxotrophic mutants.

The occurrence of cooperative cross-feeding interactions hinges on the existence of mechanisms resolving such conflicts of interests. Spatially structured environments should enhance partner fidelity feedbacks resulting in a positive assortment among cooperative individuals. Pande and co-workers (2015) tested the hypothesis that metabolic cross-feeding may be evolutionarily stable if the involved bacterial species reap mutual benefits through reciprocating, and non-cooperative species would be withheld from invasion. This was tested by experiments in which two bacterial species, *Acinetobacter baylyi* and *Escherichia coli*, were engineered in a way to reciprocally exchange essential amino acids. Experimental communities were created consisting of all possible combinations of two interspecific cross-feeders (cooperators) and one auxotroph (non-cooperator). Despite an initially random distribution of auxotrophs and cross-feeders, non-cooperating genotypes were selectively favoured in spatially unstructured (liquid culture), whereas they were selected against in spatially structured environments (agar plates). Segregation of cooperators, which may exchange cytoplasmic materials with help of nanotubes, and non-cooperators within a single bacterial colony can result in a spatial isolation of non-cooperating types, thus limiting their negative impact on the cross-feeding consortium. Increased amino acid concentrations in cooperator-rich regions were observed, whereas amino acid concentrations were generally low in areas populated with non-cooperators. These results accord with theoretical predictions of models testing for the effects of environmental heterogeneity and assortment on the evolution and maintenance of cooperation (Pepper & Smuts 2002; Hamilton & Taborsky 2005a; Hochberg et al. 2008; Estrela et al. 2019). They show that spatial structure can stabilize cooperative cross-feeding interactions between two bacterial species by spatial segregation of cooperating and non-cooperating genotypes, which limits the access of non-cooperators to cooperative benefits (Pande et al. 2015).

5.4.4   Manipulation

In some cases of apparent mutualistic relationships between different species, one partner manipulates the other to obtain a greater share than it is supposed to get. An example illustrating this possibility involves acoustic interactions in the context of predator deterrence, which occur between the fork-tailed drongo (*Dicrurus adsimilis*) and the ground-dwelling pied babbler (*Turdoides bicolor*). Drongos follow babblers and direct alarm calls to them when predators are nearby. Consequently, babblers reduce vigilance behaviours and increase their foraging success (Radford et al. 2011). This functional relationship was also experimentally demonstrated by playback of alarm calls of drongos to babblers (Ridley & Raihani 2007; Flower 2011). The alarm call causes the babblers to abandon their collected food and to flee in order to hide, which allows the drongo to obtain the food the babblers had collected once the danger is over (Ridley & Raihani 2007). Hence the babblers benefit from the presence of drongos due to enhanced safety, whereas the drongos benefit by obtaining food when alarmed babblers flee. At first sight this seems to imply interspecific mutualism (see below). However, this is not completely true because the drongos can cheat, which turns the case into an example of manipulation. Drongos sometimes provide false alarm calls if no predator is around that are identical to true alarm calls uttered when a predator is present. As babblers also flee when they hear false alarm calls, drongos can consequently feed on the food collected by the babblers. Deceptive alarm calls may evolve relatively easily because of the high cost to receivers of not responding when a predator is indeed present (e.g. Searcy & Nowicki 2005). Eventually, the presence of drongos can thus be costly to babblers. Babblers foraging in large groups with more own sentinel behaviour are less tolerant of drongos than babblers in small groups, which may point in this direction (Ridley & Raihani 2007).

5.5   Conclusions

The evolution of cooperation between individuals of different species provides an opportunity to explore and test predictions of evolutionary theory that go beyond kin selection. As Darwin (1859) already noted, cooperation between different species would present an evolutionary dilemma, if any change in the behaviour of one species served exclusively the benefit of another species. How can costly acts performed by a species that apparently benefit another be established and maintained by natural selection? The study of interspecific interactions including commensalism, mutualism and reciprocity provides excellent potential for investigating general mechanisms of cooperation. As we have seen in the previous chapters dealing with social behaviour among conspecifics, even interactions with a shared purpose that benefit all involved partners typically imply conflicting fitness interests. By the same token, the mere coexistence of different species that compete for resources can help us to unravel the functionality of conflict and non-interference rivalry.

Species competing for similar and limited resources can coexist without direct conflict through non-interference rivalry. Further, competing species can coexist in the same environment through character-displacement by which species adjust their resource demands and usage to reduce competitive pressure. When competition increases species may reduce competitive pressure by changing their mode of resource acquisition, for example by using alternative foraging strategies, which may be accompanied by morphological divergence and eventually allow different species to coexist.

There are also mechanisms of species coexistence involving conflict behaviour. For example, when species intensively compete for the same food resources which cannot be partitioned, they can succeed by developing interspecific territoriality or serial territoriality, wherein the boundary at which an intruder is attacked depends on the intruder's degree of competitive resource overlap.

Interspecific associations and cooperation may arise for different reasons, for instance to minimize predation risk. Individuals belonging to different species may associate to benefit from safety in numbers. Alternatively, members of a species may group around a protective species that helps to protect them from predators. Such associations occur through active choice, which is based on a trade-off between costs and benefits of settling near aggressive species. It remains unclear whether such associations are based on interspecific mutualism or parasitism because the fitness consequences for protective species of forming associations with protected species have been little investigated.

Interestingly, cooperative relationships between different species can occur through commensalism, in which traits exhibited by one species benefit that species directly and have a positive side effect on another species, which – at the intraspecific level – characterizes by-product benefits or mutualism (see Section 4.1.1). For example, in species sharing the same predator, one species may gain safety benefits through eavesdropping on alarm calls and vigilance of another species. Such mutualistic relationships cannot be cheated, because the behaviour of each partner improves their own fitness even without any response from the associate.

Cooperation between species often involves reciprocity by exchanging commodities and services among each other, where each species benefits from performing a costly act to the benefit of a recipient species, which leads to receiving a benefit from that recipient in return. This involves trading and negotiations between partner species, which works out due to shared interests. The widespread symbioses of all kinds provides striking evidence that cooperation through reciprocity can develop at low costs to each partner, which at the same time gains a high reward from this association.

Obviously, there are various pathways by which interspecific cooperation can evolve, but it is challenging to establish resulting fitness costs and benefits of the involved parties, especially in wild populations. Interspecific cooperation can be particularly suited to unravelling the evolutionary mechanisms underlying cooperation in the absence of kin selection. However, the margin between mutualistic and parasitic relationships can be narrow and return benefits to a cooperator may be delayed. This makes a representative cost–benefit analysis of mutual cooperation difficult. Research on these processes requires studies monitoring fitness (survival and breeding success) of substantial numbers of individuals in dependence on their behaviour towards other species for a long term. Such observations should be supplemented by experimental interventions, for instance by the removal of one of the species or by manipulating resources, in order to determine cause and effect. These are the worthwhile challenges for future studies.

The Evolution of Division of Labour and Agriculture

Summary

Agriculture was invented by insects ages before we humans got the knack of it. It involves the production of different public goods serving the community by specialized classes of individuals that are particularly apt to deal with their tasks. In eusocial insects, this often involves morphological differentiation into castes. Xyleborine ambrosia beetles do not have castes and they are not eusocial, meaning that they do not have lifelong reproductive division of labour. All individuals can reproduce at some time. Nevertheless, they perform highly specialized cooperative duties during certain stages of their life, from larval wood digging to adult fungus care and gallery guarding. Adult females delay their dispersal to help rear the brood of their mother, just as in many cooperatively breeding vertebrates. This allows experimental testing of the evolution of the two major constituents of cooperative breeding, delayed dispersal and alloparental care. Results from multi-generation, long-term experiments showed that when selecting for delayed dispersal, the cooperation propensity in these selection lines increased significantly, which raised the productivity of their natal galleries. This came at the cost of reduced reproductive competence after dispersal. Apparently, there is a genetic trade-off between a specialization in delaying dispersal and showing alloparental care, or in dispersing early and producing own offspring. But why delay dispersal and show alloparental care if this hampers own reproduction? In ambrosia beetles, this can be plausibly explained by kin selection. The relatedness between sisters is exceedingly high due to haplodiploidy and nearly obligate full-sib mating. Outbreeding in these beetles reduces fitness. Hence, in contrast to many cooperative breeders in fish, birds and mammals, where groups consist of a mixture of related and unrelated individuals, in ambrosia beetles the genetic conflict within groups is low and raising close relatives before trying one's own luck in reproduction seems the best bet.

Introduction

Agriculture is a major source of success for humankind (Smith 1998). Nevertheless, we are not the only ones that invented this vital technology. Tens of millions of years before us, several insect lineages evolved the ability to cultivate crops. Diverse ant species cultivate plants by growing seeds, weeding, and fertilizing. Others keep domestic animals such as aphids, which they protect, herd and breed (Hölldobler & Wilson 1990). Perhaps most remarkable among these techniques is the ability to cultivate fungus gardens, which is shown by a fungus-growing tribe of ants (Attini; ~220 species; Mueller et al. 2005), a subfamily of termites (Macrotermitinae; ~330 species; Aanen et al. 2002) and the ambrosia beetles (Scolytinae and Platypodinae; ~3400 species; Farrell et al. 2001). Typically, fungus-farming insects rely largely or completely on their crops for nutrition. Fungus farming involves the transport and planting of fungal spores, the excavation of tunnels and cavities, the preparation of suitable substrate for fungal growth, the cleaning and tending of the fungal garden, provisioning and fertilizing fungi, parasite removal, disease prevention and cure, the harvesting and consumption of the crop, and the removal of waste. It is obvious that all this cannot be done easily on one's own. Hence, these tasks are usually shared among members of a group, which engage in cooperative care of their garden and in elaborate division of labour.

If we are interested in the evolution of sociality and cooperation, agricultural insects are an obvious study target. It is hence surprising that until recently, work on the behavioural ecology of these unique models of social complexity had been done only on leaf-cutter ants and termites; the 10 times larger and much more variable group of ambrosia beetles had been strangely neglected for a long time. This is all the more astounding as fungus farming has apparently evolved 10 times independently in ambrosia beetles (Farrell et al. 2001; Jordal & Cognato 2012), whereas it has evolved only once each in the ants and termites (Aanen et al. 2002; Aanen & Eggleton 2005; Mueller et al. 2005).

Nevertheless, some of the nine xyleborine ambrosia beetles in Europe have been studied intensively over the last 15 years, establishing a novel model for the study of ultimate and proximate mechanisms of social evolution. In addition, a long-lived platipodid ambrosia beetle has been investigated in Australia, although the biology of that species hitherto precluded experimental approaches. Most of the experimental work on fungus-farming beetles has hence involved two European species, *Xylosandrus germanus* and *Xyleborinus saxesenii*. Luckily, these beetles can be lured pretty easily by putting up ethanol traps in the forest, and subsequently they can be studied in artificial medium in the laboratory.

Way of Living

Xyleborine ambrosia beetles colonize freshly dead trees. Living trees apparently possess appropriate means to ward them off, e.g. with the help of resin, which may be facilitated by the small size of most xyleborine ambrosia beetles. The species hitherto studied are all between 1.5 and 2.5 mm in length. If a fertilized female settles on a freshly dead tree, she excavates a small hole, infects it with fungi she carries with her in special organs (mycangia) and lays a few eggs after the fungus has started to grow. After hatching, the larvae excavate a tunnel and brood chamber while the female continues laying eggs. The adults emerging from pupae stay in the natal gallery and help tend to the fungi, cleaning the other group members, removing waste and guarding the gallery entrance.

Apparently, ambrosia beetles combine all the different components supposed to select for eusociality (Kirkendall et al. 1997). They live in a safe and stable environment, which at the same time provides ample substrate for their nutrition. Being small and dwelling in a huge tree, the available resources seem limitless. Cooperation is beneficial because of the many different tasks involved in agriculture. In addition, all roughly 1200 species of Xyleborini are haplodiploid (Normark et al. 1999; Kirkendall et al. 2015). As such they resemble the eusocial hymenoptera, where sisters are more closely related to each other than mothers with daughters. Therefore, one might expect ambrosia beetles to be eusocial. In the only Australian ambrosia beetle studied so far, which is a platypodid colonizing living trees, eusociality has been assumed (Kent & Simpson 1992; Smith et al. 2018). So there was every reason to suppose that the haplodiploid xyleborine ambrosia beetles had reached the most highly developed, lifelong altruistic social stage characterizing eusociality.

Perhaps it is not too surprising that these beetles have kept their social organization a secret until fairly recently. Ambrosia beetles live in the heartwood of trees (Figure E.1), which is not an easy substrate to uncover. Earlier information about the life of these beetles resulted mainly from the form of their cavity systems and from instantaneous collections of gallery members when a tree was cut at the appropriate position (Ratzeburg 1839; Eichhoff 1881). So, to study these beetles in any detail, first a laboratory medium had to be developed to keep and observe the beetles under controlled conditions. A medium based on sawdust (Saunders & Knoke 1967; Norris & Chu 1985) was refined with a number of goodies so that both the beetles and their fungi flourished in clear glass tubes (Peer & Taborsky 2004; cf. Biedermann et al. 2009), which allowed quantification of behaviour under the microscope (Biedermann & Taborsky 2011; Biedermann et al. 2012; Nuotcla et al. 2014).

Sex Ratio and Mating

As all xyleborini are haplodiploid, the sex ratio is at the discretion of the mother. Mated females can

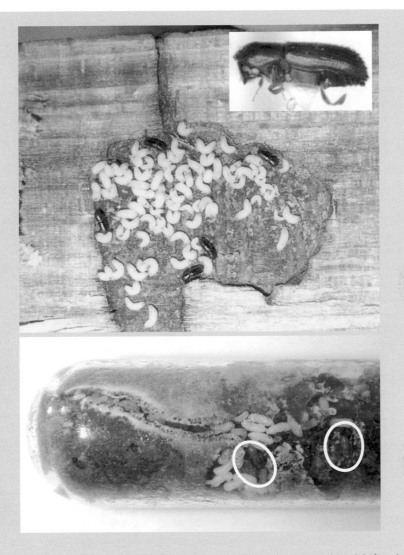

Figure E.1 Gallery of *Xyleborinus saxesenii* in the field (above; with adult female shown in the insert) and in the laboratory (below; adult females located amidst the white larvae are encircled). Photos: Peter Biedermann. (A black and white version of this figure will appear in some formats. For the colour version, please refer to the plate section.)

fertilize an egg before it is laid with sperm stored in her spermatheca, which results in a daughter. Or, they can lay an unfertilized egg, which results in a son. If females can thus determine their offspring's sex ratio, Hamilton's concept of local mate competition (LMC; Hamilton 1967, 1979) predicts that sex ratios should depart from equality given that mating takes place among related individuals. Taking the extreme case of obligatory full-sib mating, female fitness would be maximized if she produces only as many sons as can fertilize all her daughters. Any additional sons would be wasted. In xyleborini, mating usually occurs between full siblings within their natal gallery, and the sex ratio in these beetles is indeed strongly biased toward females, just as predicted by LMC theory (Kirkendall 1993; Biedermann 2010).

Nevertheless, complete inbreeding is rare. Sons usually have *some* mating chances beyond fertilizing their sisters, despite being flightless. On strongly infested trees where gallery density is high, males have been observed wandering on the bark surface to visit different gallery entrances (Schneider-Orelli 1913). This apparent outbreeding opportunity for males should affect the sex ratio optimization of females: the better the outbreeding opportunities for their sons, the more sons should be produced relative to daughters. Hence, the prediction of sex ratio optimization under LMC conditions can be ideally tested by experimentally varying the density of foundresses of xyleborine ambrosia beetles. To that end one, two or three foundresses of *X. germanus* were placed on suitable substrate in the laboratory, keeping substrate quantity per female constant. As predicted, the brood sex ratio of experimental females varied significantly with foundress number (between 0.06 and 0.1; Peer & Taborsky 2004). Females produced more sons if the latter's opportunities to obtain fertilization outside their natal gallery increased, and they produced sons early in the laying sequence. This was corroborated by field data. Dispersing individuals were caught with emergence traps attached to gallery entrances, and at the end of the season the galleries were extracted from the logs with hammer and chisel to collect remaining individuals. This revealed that two-thirds of the males produced in the surveyed galleries dispersed at some stage, apparently in search of additional mating opportunities. Twenty-seven of such dispersing males were individually marked and their paths were surveyed for up to 4 days. They passed foreign gallery entrances on average every 20 min and persistently tried to enter every other one of them, especially if the galleries contained many females. Often they interacted with the female blocking the entrance, including copulation attempts (Peer & Taborsky 2004).

Apparently, the key to the mating system of ambrosia beetles is regular inbreeding (Kirkendall 1993). This typically involves pre-dispersal mating in the natal gallery, which means that fertilized females can disperse and found new colonies independently. Males mainly serve to fertilize their full sisters before dispersal, with some chances to obtain additional matings elsewhere after this task was accomplished. Genetic analyses of *X. germanus* from three different populations in Switzerland revealed an outbreeding degree of 3 per cent (Keller et al. 2011). In other words, 97 per cent of matings occurred between full siblings. How can these beetles cope with the typically deleterious effects of inbreeding?

To compare the fitness effects of inbreeding and different degrees of outbreeding, females were crossed either with their full brothers or with males from the same or a different (distant) population. No deleterious effects of inbreeding were found in any life-history trait measured, but instead a marked *outbreeding* depression emerged, regardless of whether the males were from the same or a different population as the females (Peer & Taborsky 2005). On average, the hatching rate of outbred offspring was reduced by 11 per cent in comparison to full-sib matings. Apparently, through a long evolutionary history of inbreeding, recessive deleterious alleles have been purged, a process enhanced in haplodiploid organisms in male hemizygotes (Antolin 1999; Henter 2003), thereby removing any negative effects of full-sib inbreeding. The detected outbreeding depression might result from cytoplasmatic incompatibility caused by endosymbionts such as *Wolbachia*; different genetic strains of *Wolbachia* were determined in *X. germanus* (Kawasaki et al. 2010).

Group Structure and Social Life

Thus, group members within a gallery are highly related due to haplodiploidy and inbreeding. Only one to three sons are usually produced by the gallery foundress in the species hitherto studied, which suffice to fertilize all their sisters. Males typically disperse when all females have been fertilized. But what happens to the daughters – do they disperse as well, and if so, when? To answer this question, dispersal of *X. saxesenii* was determined in the field by putting up ethanol-baited traps, and by monitoring some 400 galleries through a combination of

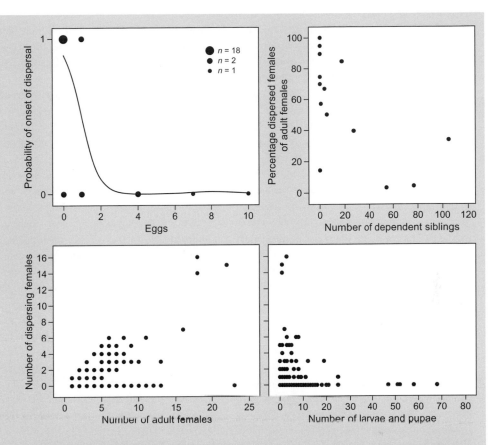

Figure E.2 Female dispersal in *X. saxesenii* in dependence on the number of dependent offspring and the total number of adult females in the gallery. Upper graphs: field data; left: probability of the onset of dispersal in dependence on egg numbers in 28 galleries; right: percentage of dispersed females in dependence on the total number of dependent offspring in 20 galleries (some points overlap; from Peer & Taborsky 2007). Lower graphs: laboratory data; left: number of females dispersing in relation to the number of adult females in the gallery; right: number of dispersing females in dependence on the number of larvae and pupae in the gallery. Each point represents data from a different gallery (after Biedermann & Taborsky 2011).

deploying emergence traps mounted around the gallery entrances and carving out and dissecting galleries at different stages of gallery development (Peer & Taborsky 2007; Figure E.2). This revealed that adult females stay for some time in their natal gallery. There they apparently refrain from reproduction, because the number of eggs produced in a gallery was independent of the number of adult females present. Instead, at some stage most adult females disperse from their natal gallery to found a new colony. However, on average one-quarter of females die in their natal gallery, i.e. they do not disperse and reproduce at all (Peer & Taborsky 2007). For females leaving the natal gallery, the timing of dispersal depends on the number of dependent siblings present: if no new eggs are produced and if the number of care-dependent sisters declines, females are more likely to disperse (Figure E.2). This was confirmed by both correlative and experimental data obtained from colonies in the laboratory (Biedermann & Taborsky 2011). When galleries were experimentally infected with pathogen spores, adult females further delayed dispersal and increased hygienic service, reflecting social immunity (Nuotcla et al. 2019), which previously had been demonstrated in eusocial insects (Cremer et al. 2007). In addition, in field colonies the number of adult females correlates positively with the number of larvae and pupae, suggesting that dispersal is delayed when daughters are needed for alloparental care (Peer & Taborsky 2007). Taken together, these data suggest that females (1) do not (or only rarely) participate in reproduction in their natal gallery, (2) stay home as long as they are needed for brood care of siblings and (3) have a positive effect on the production/survival of siblings. All this reflects cooperative breeding, but not eusociality; females are totipotent and disperse to reproduce independently at some stage if they survive until then.

Division of Labour

Given that females stay in their natal gallery as long as dependent sisters are there to be cared for, the obvious question is how they can actually help to raise them. What is the alloparental function of philopatric females? This question cannot be answered in the field, because the collection method of beetles and galleries is destructive. For this purpose, the beetles were kept in glass tubes and custom-made glass casings filled with culturing medium, in which the beetles' behaviour could be observed inside their gallery under an incident light microscope (Bischoff 2004). Adult females of *X. germanus* spent most of their active time cleaning the gallery walls and fungal gardens (37 per cent of total time). Larvae, instead, mainly engaged in enlarging the gallery by digging out and taking up substrate (25 per cent of total time). Both larvae and adult males spent also some time with cleaning gallery walls and fungi (11 per cent and 12 per cent of time, respectively). Males were the most active group members, often observed moving through the tunnels and cleaning females. Most copulations (80 per cent) happened with females during the first two days after their eclosion, a time period that can be recognized by the females' light cuticula. The

female foundress spent most of her time blocking the gallery entrance. Otherwise, she also engaged in cleaning gallery walls and fungal gardens (17 per cent of time).

Such division of labour was also confirmed in colonies of *X. saxesenii*. In this species, the task specializations also include all different classes of individuals present within a gallery: the foundress, which specializes in guarding the gallery entrance; larvae that dig out substrate, thereby enlarging the gallery system; adult females that mainly tend the fungal gardens; and males, which engage most extensively in allogrooming others (Figure E.3; Biedermann & Taborsky 2011). Interestingly, adult females of *X. saxesenii* spent more effort with fungus care and allogrooming the more care-dependent offspring were present in the gallery, and they tended to increase their digging effort, which otherwise is the major duty of larvae, after the last larvae had pupated. In addition, larvae and adult females are responsible for waste removal. This includes the compression of dispersed waste into compact balls ('balling') and the removal of these balls from the gallery ('shuffling'). Waste disposal requires cooperation between these different life stages: larvae are the only life form able to compress waste into compact balls because of their body flexibility. These waste balls can then be pushed to certain areas of the gallery or out of the entrance by adult female offspring, which sometimes accomplish this task by a chain of workers propelling the waste through the gallery tunnels. Video clips showing balling and shuffling are available at: www.pnas.org/lookup/suppl/doi:10.10 73/pnas.1107758108/-/DCSupplemental/sm01.mpg www.pnas.org/lookup/suppl/doi:10.1073/pnas.110 7758108/-/DCSupplemental/sm02.mpg

Occasionally, diseased or dead colony members are cannibalized, which is probably an important measure to prevent the spread of diseases and parasites (e.g. mould).

The functional significance of the different tasks performed by colony members seems obvious for most behaviours, but what in fact is the benefit of grooming others, or being groomed by them? Keeping pupae together either with one or six larvae

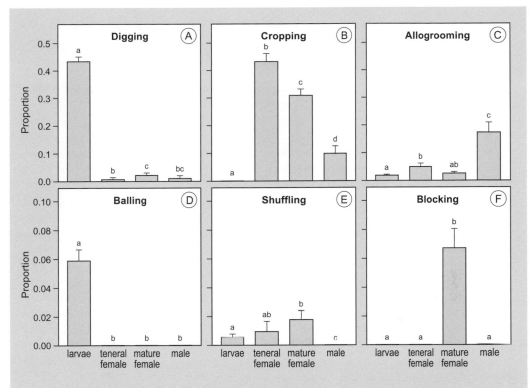

Figure E.3 Division of labour and age polyethism between age and sex classes in *X. saxesenii*. Bars show the mean (± SE) proportions of time larvae, teneral females, mature females and males performed different cooperative tasks. Statistically significant differences between the classes are denoted by different letters ($P < 0.05$; GEE). Note scale differences between A–C and D–F (from Biedermann & Taborsky 2011).

showed that survival significantly depended on the cleaning effort of the larvae; one larva usually did not suffice to prevent the pupa from being overgrown and killed by fungi (Biedermann & Taborsky 2011). Within a humid and enclosed tunnel system loaded with fungi and other microorganisms, mutual hygiene is obviously essential. This was corroborated by the observation that during the founding stage of a gallery, when the foundress is still on her own, she may be covered by fungi due to a lack of being groomed, which causes her death. In colonies artificially infected with pathogens, adult females significantly increased hygienic behaviours (Nuotcla et al. 2019). For males, allogrooming fulfils an additional function – the detection of

unfertilized adult females. Mating attempts are always preceded by allogrooming. If an unfertilized female founds a new gallery, she can only produce sons, which happens in about 2 per cent of *X. saxesenii* gallery foundations (Biedermann et al. 2009; Biedermann 2010). In such cases, males perform all the required duties, which demonstrates their universal behavioural abilities.

If we compare the division of labour shown in ambrosia beetle colonies with that exhibited by eusocial hymenoptera, there is an important difference. In social hymenoptera, the larvae are rather inactive receivers of help, which never participate in any cooperative tasks in the colony – with the sole exception of weaver ants (*Oecophylla, Polyrhachis*), where adults use larval silk production for nest construction. Rather, the division of labour between larvae and adults in ambrosia beetles is reminiscent of the sharing of tasks between different age classes in termites and social aphids (Biedermann & Taborsky 2011). However, these insects are hemimetabolous, i.e. lacking metamorphosis, which means that adults and juveniles resemble each other. Another important difference is that in ambrosia beetles, the different tasks including digging out tunnels (larvae), waste compacting (larvae), waste removal (adult females), fungus care (adult females) and gallery guarding (foundress) are all shown by the same individuals, in different stages of their life – a temporal transformation called 'polyethism'. This is known also from eusocial hymenoptera, e.g. honeybees, but there larvae are not involved.

There seems to be good reason that the hard work of digging out the gallery is almost exclusively performed by larvae. The mandibles used for this grind are used up by the hardness of the wood they penetrate. If adults were to do this task extensively, they would soon forfeit their capacity to dig due to their worn out mandibles. Larvae, instead, can just moult – they have three successive larval stages before pupation – emerging with pristine new mandibles each time. In addition, only larvae of *X. saxesenii*, but not adults, produce xylanolytic enzyme, which helps the (pre-)digestion of cell walls (De Fine Licht & Biedermann 2012). This digging may also provide nutrients to the larvae if the wood is already permeated by fungus hyphae, but the main purpose clearly is enlargement of the gallery system, which enhances fungus growth and productivity (Farrell et al. 2001).

Fungus care, instead, is probably best performed by adult offspring because of their greater mobility. Adult females constantly move through the gallery, screen the fungal garden with their antennae and move their comb-like mouthparts through the fungus (Biedermann & Taborsky 2011). This may serve to clean the fungus and to brush off fruiting bodies, which serves nutrition. At the same time this enhances fungus growth (Batra & Michie 1963; Francke-Grosmann 1967). In addition, this type of fungus care probably prevents invasions of the ambrosia garden by detrimental fungi and other microbes (Schneider-Orelli 1913; Biedermann et al. 2013).

Blocking the gallery entrance, which serves to guard the colony against predators, parasites, pathogens and, especially, foreign males, is primarily performed by the foundress. Unrelated males should be kept out of the gallery due to the described outbreeding depression. In addition, blocking serves to prevent larvae from falling out of the gallery entrance (Biedermann & Taborsky 2011), and the blocking female may actively push larvae approaching the gallery entrance back into the tunnel (Bischoff 2004). Blocking may also serve to regulate the gallery's microclimate. It makes sense that blocking is the foundress's specialized task, because only one individual is needed for this duty and it might be difficult to organize regular alternation if several individuals (daughters) were involved in this business. Daughters do take over this duty for short periods of time, though, when the foundress is otherwise busy.

Cooperation and Conflict

In ambrosia beetle colonies the potential for genetic conflict is low. Due to haplodiploidy and, especially, virtually obligate inbreeding, colony members are almost clones. This was corroborated by the observation that in the crossing experiment of *X. germanus* described above, there were highly significant matriline effects on several reproductive parameters, such as the number of eggs laid, hatching and pupation rates, offspring fecundity, and also on parameters of the fungal garden of the F_1 generation that are subject to the beetles' care behaviour, such as ambrosia growth and fungal contamination. The existence of an outbreeding depression even on a local scale may further suggest that populations of these beetles consist of highly differentiated inbred lines; intrinsic coadaptation may lead to an outbreeding depression whenever two different genotypes cross (Peer & Taborsky 2005).

This low potential for genetic conflict between colony members may explain the high degree of division of labour among them. It seems as if the amazing functionality of task sharing in these colonies results from the fact that each individual performs the tasks that serve the colony best. In addition, as we have seen above, adult females adjust their dispersal timing to the need of care-dependent offspring in their natal gallery (Figure E.2). This is remarkable because an experiment on *Xyleborus affinis* showed that females accumulate direct fitness costs from staying and helping. The longer they stay home, the smaller is their own reproductive success after dispersal (Biedermann et al. 2011). This apparently altruistic 'stay and help' can only be plausibly explained by kin selection – by the preferential investment in the promotion of close relatives, at the expense of own future reproduction.

But is there really no scope for conflict in these societies? Some observations might suggest otherwise. First, a few females reproduce in their natal gallery, which could induce reproductive competition. In a sample of 16 *X. saxesenii* galleries continuously monitored with dispersal traps and finally collected in the field, 4 (25 per cent) contained between 1 and 3 egg-laying daughters, as determined by dissection that revealed ovarioles containing oocytes (Biedermann & Taborsky 2011; Biedermann et al. 2012). In contrast, the ovarioles of dispersing females never contained oocytes. Egg laying of philopatric daughters only occurred after dispersal had already started in their natal gallery. The numbers of offspring produced (eggs, larvae and pupae) were positively correlated with the number of egg layers found in a gallery. In spite of this potential for reproductive competition, it should be noted that despite extensive behavioural monitoring under the microscope, no aggressive interactions were ever observed among colony members.

Second, focal animal sampling revealed that foundresses showed more cooperative behaviours than their daughters (Biedermann & Taborsky 2011). These are behaviours that benefit other group members, implying production of a public good. Behaviours in which foundresses invested more than their daughters included blocking behaviour, fungus care and shuffling of waste. Nevertheless, digging and allogrooming were more often exhibited by the daughters, and cannibalism, which is shown by

larvae and adult daughters, was never observed in one of the focal foundresses.

Finally, experimental removal of the foundress increased daughter dispersal (Biedermann & Taborsky 2011). On the one hand this may reflect inclusive fitness optimization of daughters, because if there is no longer an egg-laying female in the natal gallery, the need for alloparental care declines. On the other hand, it might indicate that blocking the gallery entrance by the foundress not only serves to prevent accidental loss of larvae, but also dispersal of adult daughters that are ready to leave for their own reproduction. As alloparental care was shown to reduce the personal fitness of females (in *X. affinis*; Biedermann et al. 2011), their dispersal delay may at least to some extent reflect a fitness interest conflict between the foundress and her daughters, which the foundress can turn in her favour by blocking the gallery entrance (i.e. exit).

In any case, even if there is some scope for conflict within the highly related ambrosia beetle colonies, the evolution of sociality and cooperation seems to be primarily based on kin selection. This clearly differs from many cooperative breeding systems of vertebrates, where the importance of individual selection prevails as outlined with our case studies of fish, birds and mammals.

Why Not Eusocial?

Let's now get back to our original question based on the fact that ambrosia beetles possess virtually all ecological and biological preconditions attributed to the evolution of eusociality. Apparently, high relatedness in combination with lifetime monogamy (Boomsma 2013), life in a safe and stable environment providing virtually unlimited resources and high benefits of cooperation due to the demanding workload involved in agriculture together do not suffice for the evolution of complete reproductive division of labour, the fundamental characteristic of eusociality (Boomsma 2007). Even if in the social insect literature the type of sociality shown by ambrosia beetles is referred to as 'primitive eusociality', this term is somewhat misleading if all or most individuals reproduce by themselves at some stage of their life. 'Cooperative breeding' is clearly the concept applying to this type of social organization, which is characterized by a combination of delayed dispersal, alloparental care and reproductive totipotency (Peer & Taborsky 2007).

An unsolved question in the evolutionary ecology of cooperative breeding is whether its essential components, delayed dispersal and alloparental care, evolve independently from each other. Due to their experimental tractability, short generation times and combination of traits ambrosia beetles provide a unique chance to unravel this question experimentally. Peter Biedermann established two selection lines of *X. saxesenii* for either early or late dispersal with 30 colonies each. Within each replicate, the first third of dispersing females ('early') and the last third, i.e. the longest staying females ('late'), were chosen for further breeding. For the 'late' samples, the galleries were augmented with additional medium to increase their potential for philopatry. After five successive generations bred with this regime, the two selection lines were kept under the same, non-augmented substrate conditions. A comparison of behavioural and life-history traits and their fitness effects revealed that females of the 'late' line dispersed on average 5 days later than females selected for early dispersal (Figure E.4). Remarkably, females of the two selection lines showed consistent behavioural differences: females selected for late dispersal showed significantly more cooperative behaviour in their natal galleries, including gallery protection (blocking) in females and allogrooming in males. This resulted in much higher offspring numbers in these selection lines. In contrast, fungus care and feeding was enhanced in females selected for early dispersal. The increased productivity of home colonies generated by the cooperative behaviour of females selected for late dispersal traded off against the success in founding an own gallery. Whereas 69 per cent of breeding attempts of females selected for early dispersal were successful, only 32 per cent were in the selection lines for late dispersal (Biedermann & Taborsky unpubl. ms).

The described selection regime obviously resulted in divergent specialization of beetles either (1) in enhanced cooperation and promotion of the success and productivity of the natal colony, or (2) in early dispersal and optimization of independent breeding. This implies genetic linkage between dispersal propensities and the decision to either enhance cooperation or own reproduction (Biedermann & Taborsky unpubl.), somewhat reminiscent of the genetic linkage between cooperation and punishment in bacteria (Inglis et al. 2014). Apparently, despite the high degree of inbreeding and resulting low degree of heterozygosity in ambrosia beetles (Peer & Taborsky 2005; Keller et al. 2011), the traits responsible for cooperation and for 'selfish' reproduction show sufficient genetic variance and responsiveness to selection that the evolution to higher degrees of sociality seems possible. So why on earth are ambrosia beetles not eusocial?

Perhaps the most plausible answer to this question is the rather ephemeral nature of the environment in which these beetles dwell. Freshly dead trees are a bonanza resource. When colonization happens, the freshly dead tree provides a virtually unlimited amount of resources to a millimetre-sized beetle. However, dead wood is not a substrate persisting in its original state for a long time. It dries out or gets soaked, dependent on microclimate, and it is consumed by a host of different microorganisms. At the beginning, beetles may successfully fend off detrimental fungi and other microorganisms, but with increasing time this seems to get harder, perhaps through a change with time of the microclimate (Biedermann et al. 2013; Nuotcla et al. 2021). If the usability of a gallery is rather short, there is only one method by which transgenerational sociality can persist: joint dispersal. This is successfully demonstrated by some hymenoptera, such as army ants and honeybees, but ambrosia beetles here seem to be subject to an insurmountable obstacle. If dispersing on foot, like males do after fertilizing their sisters in search of nearby colonies on the same tree, females might have a difficult time finding another suitable dead tree in the vicinity and, being virtually defenceless, they would be vulnerable to all sorts of predators. If dispersing on the wing, as females actually do (singly), it would likely be impossible to remain as a group. Bees are good flyers and

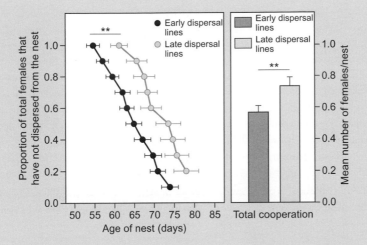

Figure E.4 Results from experimental selection on early or late dispersal. Left: dispersal of females in the late dispersal selection lines was delayed against the early dispersal selection lines by a factor of 1.96 (gallery means $\pm$ standard errors; Cox model: $z = 2.8$, $p = 0.005$). Right: the mean number of cooperating females was higher in the delayed dispersal selection lines than in the early dispersal selection lines (means $\pm$ standard errors; GLMM, $p < 0.01$; Biedermann & Taborsky, unpubl.).

therefore can disperse jointly, but for a millimetre-sized beetle any puff of wind can destroy group cohesion.

Towards New Frontiers

To test whether the ephemeral nature of freshly dead trees is indeed the ecological cause limiting the social organization of ambrosia beetles to the level of cooperative breeding instead of evolving eusociality, the social organization of ambrosia beetles colonizing *living* trees should be explored. The platypodid ambrosia beetle *Austroplatypus incompertus* (Kent & Simpson 1992; Smith et al. 2018) seems a good candidate for such investigation. At first glance, these beetles do seem to show even more congruence with eusocial insects than the xyleborine ambrosia beetles described above. Most remarkably, colonies of these beetles are extremely long-lived and can persist for several decades (Harris et al. 1976; Kent & Simpson 1992). The fact that daughters collected from 12 colonies had partly lost tarsi has been interpreted as evidence that they had committed to alloparental care for life, because mating and establishing an own, independent gallery was assumed to be difficult if tarsi are missing

(Smith et al. 2018). However, evidence for this assumption is currently missing. Furthermore, the comparison of 16 females younger than 6 months with 12 females from colonies ca. 10 years of age or older revealed that in the latter sample, no female of 12 had more than 1 leg without tarsal segment loss, whereas in the former sample, 5 of 19 females had more than 1 leg without tarsal segment loss. In the sample of gallery founding females, 13 of 19 females had all, or all but 1, tarsal segments missing in the majority of their legs, whereas the corresponding number was 8 of 13 in older females (supplementary tables 2 and 3 in Smith et al. 2018). This rather modest difference was interpreted as evidence that the loss of tarsi results from 'wear and tear' associated with work effort exhibited in the colony, predestining these females to forsake dispersal and to remain 'workers' in their home galleries for life (Smith et al. 2018). Nevertheless, females in dispersal traps were also sometimes found to have lost tarsi, questioning this interpretation. Furthermore, all females possess mycangia, specialized structures to transport symbiont fungus, which only makes sense if they disperse and found a new gallery at some stage in their life.

Hence it is currently unclear whether the platypodid ambrosia beetles colonizing living trees indeed evolved eusociality with a lifelong reproductive division of labour, or whether they are cooperative breeders similar to the described xyleborine ambrosia beetles. This riddle needs to be further explored. Apart from *A. incompertus*, candidates for such studies include other platipodid species such as *Trachyostus ghanaensis* (Roberts 1960), *Doliopygus dubius, Dendroplatypus impar* (Browne 1961, 1965) or *Megaplatypus mutates* (Santoro 1963), and the scolitid ambrosia beetles *Corthylus columbianus* (Crozier & Giese 1967a, 1967b) and *C. zulmae* (Jaramillo et al. 2011). In addition, some xyleborine ambrosia beetles from the tropics and subtropics are known to colonize living trees (Kirkendall 2006; Stilwell et al. 2014; for review see Hulcr & Dunn 2011; Kirkendall et al. 2015). Clearly, if ambrosia beetles can overcome tree defences successfully and colonize living trees, these should provide a sufficiently long-lived resource for eusociality to evolve. Ambrosia beetles hence provide a unique model to study the ecological conditions and adaptations leading to the most advanced levels of social organization known: eusociality.

6   Synopsis

In this book, we have aimed to make two major points.

(1) Life is social, which entails competition. This selects for efficient individual strategies to outcompete others in the struggle for survival and reproduction.
(2) Success can be achieved by being quicker than others (strategy *race*), stronger than others (strategy *fight*), or by cooperating with them in one way or another (strategy *share*).

6.1   Race

The behaviour that evolves in response to competition depends on the ecological distribution of resources, and the physical and social attributes of competing organisms. In Chapter 2 we explored the ecological and social factors that influence the form and intensity of competition, and the consequences of competition for animal distributions and social behaviour. We have focused on scramble competition – a *race* for resources – which is the most basic of social interactions and generally involves the least-complicated behaviour. By contrast, contest competition – a *fight* for resources – which we addressed in Chapter 3, leads to more varied, durable and complex social relationships.

Theoretical models elucidate how the distribution of resources in time and space affects selection for scramble versus contest competition (Parker 2000). Scramble competition occurs where resources are widely scattered, scarce and unpredictable in time and space. These ecological features combine to determine the economic defensibility of the resource. In Chapter 2 we showed how economic defensibility (or lack thereof) can provide a unifying explanation for patterns of territoriality, competitive foraging and mating system variation.

Another type of theoretical model targets the relationship between scramble effort and the number of competitors. These models help to predict the distribution of animals in their habitat, depending on the value of resources, the nature of competition and the information they have about the distribution of resources in their environment.

Competition can also lead to remarkable examples of group coordination, as exemplified by collective movement. In Chapter 2 we reviewed evidence that complex group behaviour can emerge as the result of individuals competing to find food or mates, or to avoid predation, by employing simple decision rules. Individuals often compete for information, and it is intriguing to see how selection to transmit or parasitize information can lead to the formation of social groups and to complex strategies of signalling and deception.

In addition to the ecological factors, the type of competitive behaviour favoured by natural selection is influenced by the social environment. The simplest social factor influencing competition is population density (Grant 1993). Both theory and empirical work suggest that population density can shift the nature of competition from scramble to contest. A second key social factor influencing the type of competitive behaviour observed within populations derives from individual variation. Differences in size or quality can cause individuals to adopt divergent competitive strategies to maximize their fitness. The type of competitive behaviour that evolves depends on how fitness of alternative strategies varies with their frequency in the population. Interestingly, competition combined with variation in quality can lead to the evolution of stable polymorphisms in behaviour and the formation of social alliances.

In Chapter 2 we also discussed the coevolution of behaviour in exploitative social relationships where one individual seeks to exploit or utilize another. Females, for instance, represent a resource over which males compete, but at the same time they have their own genetic incentives and are selected to avoid exploitation or monopolization by males if this is not in their own fitness interests. In these cases the type of competition observed among members of one party depends on the counterstrategies evolving among members of the other party. For example, females can shift the nature of male–male competition by synchronizing reproduction, or by mating at particular sites, which exacerbates male contest behaviour.

Our consideration demonstrates that both ecological and social factors may shift the nature of competition from scramble to contest. In contest competition, individuals may come into repeated, extended contact and be bound together by ecological constraints. This sets the stage for the evolution of complex social behaviours of negotiation, threats and reciprocity. The parties can be said to be involved in social conflict, i.e. '*fight*', rather than simple scramble competition, i.e. '*race*'.

6.2   Fight

In animal societies, an important source of conflict is membership of the group. Individuals can gain from grouping, but will be selected to join groups beyond optimal group size, depressing the fitness pay-offs of insiders. Insider–outsider conflict theory helps to explain patterns of aggression and eviction among group members. In groups that have stable membership, another source of conflict arises among individuals about their social status. Dominance hierarchies form as a means of reducing the frequency of repeated conflict among individuals that interact repeatedly. However, an important question is what keeps hierarchies stable, given that individuals may vary over time in strength and considering the costs and benefits of remaining at a given rank. In Chapter 3 we reviewed theory and data suggesting that observed patterns of aggression act as honest indicators of the resource holding potential of individuals (RHP; Parker 1974) or of their motivation, which helps maintain the stability of dominance hierarchies.

A conspicuous source of conflict is the competition for reproduction, which in animal societies includes the competition among females over offspring production. This is illustrated by numerous examples of infanticide and egg policing, which hints on the subtle strategies that females may employ to maximize their reproductive success in competition with co-breeders, for example via developmental effects on offspring. Furthermore, salient conflicts exist between males and females over mating, which is demonstrated by the divergent strategies that both sexes employ to control the distribution of paternity (Parker 2006). For example, in many animal societies males attempt to mate-guard females to prevent them mating with other males, but females may successfully resist this effort as they can gain genetic benefits by mating with males from outside the group. Finally, there are obvious conflicts of interest over the amount of parental care provided to developing offspring (Trivers 1972). Mothers, fathers and brood-care helpers often have differing interests in the current brood versus future broods, depending on patterns of kinship and the probability that the female will remate in the future. Apparently, such conflicts over parental and alloparental care are often resolved by a process of back-and-forth negotiation, rather than overt aggression.

Social conflict can lead to the evolution of complex strategies of competition. In some circumstances individuals may be selected to put their differences aside and work together as a team to outcompete other teams. Such transitions from outright conflict to cooperation have been called 'major transitions in evolution' (Maynard Smith & Szathmary 1995). The theory of major transitions tries to explain how and why many forms of life have become more complex over time, from self-replicating molecules to animal societies. Understanding how major transitions occur requires explaining how individual conflicts of interest can be suppressed for the good of the group. Major transitions in evolution often happened hundreds of millions of years ago, and are difficult to study (Levin et al. 2020). Probably the most recent major transition occurred with the evolution of cooperative animal societies from solitary ancestors. These societies are ideal systems to examine how strategies of conflict and cooperation coevolve. In Chapter 3 we explored the forms of conflict that arise in cooperative societies and the social behaviours that individuals use to shift the resolution of conflict in their own favour, from aggression and escalated fighting to more subtle forms of negotiation. This research also shows how selection can lead to the suppression and peaceful resolution of conflict among social partners, uniting their fitness interests and paving the way for the final stage of a major transition, the evolution of a new higher level of biological complexity.

Three different theoretical approaches have been used to understand the evolution of social conflict in cooperative groups. The first approach is based on classic population genetic models. In Chapter 3 we described how these structured population models can be used to predict the strength of selection for 'helping' and 'harming' traits, that increase or decrease the fecundity of local group members, as a function of patterns of mating and dispersal. The second approach uses evolutionary game theory to examine the coevolution of fixed genetic conflict strategies on an evolutionary timescale. These models examine how relatedness and differences in RHP influence the predicted effort invested in conflict, and the outcome of conflict in terms of resource partitioning (or skew). We showed how the assumed form of contest success function has a dramatic impact on the predicted outcome of competition, and how these models provide one explanation for how costly conflict can be suppressed in animal societies, despite apparent conflicts of interest. The third general approach focuses explicitly on the sequences of behaviour involved in conflict. Three behavioural mechanisms, threats, negotiation and assessment, can be used to resolve conflict on a behavioural timescale.

An interesting question is which forces can shift groups towards peaceful conflict resolution, which may set the stage for the emergence of a new tier of complexity (Packer et al. 2001). We identified three evolutionary routes to conflict reduction: kin selection, reproductive levelling and life-history segregation. Obviously, conflict between groups can unite the fitness interests of group members, which may lead to the emergence of cooperation even among non-relatives. However, empirical studies of the role of intergroup conflict suggest a wide range of within-group responses to intergroup interactions, from increased within-group cooperation to elevated aggression. These patterns suggest that our current understanding of the role of intergroup interactions in social evolution is at an early stage. An outstanding question is what can lead to cooperation between groups, rather than conflict. This problem is a repeat of the problem of cooperation between individuals, which we considered in Chapter 4. Understanding how the inherent 'looseness' of groups can be overcome to permit coordinated conflict, such as warfare, or coordinated cooperation is a particularly promising area for future research.

6.3   Share

In Chapter 4 we asked which evolutionary mechanisms can be responsible for the production of costly behaviours that apparently benefit individuals other than the actor, if the interacting partners inherently compete. This question puzzled Charles Darwin when proposing the theory of evolution by means of natural selection more than 150 years ago (Darwin 1859) and it is still one of the fundamental questions in biology today. At the 125th anniversary of the journal *Science*, the evolution of cooperation was classified as one of the 'Top 25 big questions facing science over the next quarter-century' (*Science* 2005). So, what is the playing field, what do we (think we) know and especially, what do we not yet understand?

In theory, if the restricted conditions favouring cooperation by group selection do not apply as we have outlined in Section 4.1, evolutionarily stable levels of cooperation can be selected either through positive fitness effects on the performer of a helpful act, or through manipulation of the actor by a receiver. Positive fitness effects can result (i) from the action itself, which may at the same time create benefits for somebody else, thereby creating a by-product benefit characterizing mutualism. As the action itself is positively selected even without considering effects on others, it is not altruistic but selfish and hence its evolution can be easily explained by the gain in the actor's direct fitness. Or, they may result from correlated pay-offs, either due to (ii) reciprocity or (iii) shared genes. As we have shown, these two mechanisms can explain altruistic traits, i.e. actions causing immediate fitness costs that are compensated for by future direct or indirect fitness benefits. Finally, cooperation can evolve even if the actor faces on average negative lifetime fitness effects, if (iv) the actor is manipulated by the receiver of the benefit. Examples taken from different taxa have demonstrated that such manipulation can involve either enforcement or deception.

The principles of these mechanisms are inherently simple (Figure 4.2). If an act benefitting someone else is positively selected due to direct fitness effects to the actor, i.e. without the necessity of a positive feedback from the receiver, the benefit to the receiver can be seen as a mere by-effect of the actor's behaviour. If this applies to both partners of an interaction, the resulting mutualism will generate cooperation without involving conflict of (fitness) interests. As in this case the actor is benefitting from its behaviour directly, i.e. the probability is irrelevant to sharing genes (which cause the behaviour) with a potential receiver, fitness benefits to the actor simply need to be higher than their fitness costs ($b > c$; Lehmann & Keller 2006a). If in contrast the act itself causes more costs than benefits to the performer, these costs can be compensated by correlated pay-offs between actor and receiver (Taborsky et al. 2016). Correlated pay-offs result either from the sharing of genes between actor and recipient, or by a conditional payback which denotes reciprocal cooperation between actor and receiver.

If fitness pay-offs are correlated by the sharing of genes between interacting partners, cooperative acts will benefit both sides and hence be selected for if the relationship between costs (c), benefits (b) and the likelihood of sharing the responsible genetic cause by common descent (relatedness; r) accord with Hamilton's rule ($rb > c$; Hamilton 1964). This facilitates the evolution of altruistic cooperation through kin selection. As we outline in Chapter 4, a role of kin selection in the evolution of altruism can be tested in cooperative breeders, for instance, by determining whether brood-care helpers adjust their cooperative effort to their relatedness with the recipients of their generosity. This is apparently the case in cooperatively breeding bird species (Green et al. 2016). Nevertheless, while helpers often seem to possess mechanisms by which they can assess relatedness to their social partners, in several cooperatively breeding mammal, bird, fish and insect species, helpers do not discriminate between kin and nonkin (Table 4.2), and negative kin discrimination also occurs. Interestingly, species that live in groups with close relatives, which may result, for instance, from delayed or limited dispersal, are less likely to discriminate between kin and nonkin. On closer inspection this makes sense. If generosity benefits neighbours with which cooperators are anyway related by common descent, recognition and discrimination become less important (Cornwallis et al. 2009).

The ability to discriminate between kin and unrelated conspecifics can be attributed to spatial constellations, familiarity, recognition alleles ('green-beard genes'; Dawkins 1976) or phenotype matching. Nevertheless, as we discussed in Chapter 4, these alternative mechanisms are neither always effective nor mutually exclusive. Testing for a potential effect of kinship and comprehending involved mechanisms therefore requires rigorous experimental scrutiny. It is important to note that the benefits of cooperation among relatives may be offset by the costs of increased competition for resources or reproductive opportunities, hence competition between individuals of a kin group can be similarly strong to that among unrelated group members (Lehmann & Rousset 2010). When in viscous populations competition becomes more local, this involves neighbouring individuals that are relatives, concomitantly reducing selection for cooperation between them. Another context where relatedness may have positive or negative fitness effects regards mating. The inbreeding effects resulting from mating among kin may reduce intersexual conflict and increase lifetime fitness (Kokko & Ots 2006), but the associated reduction in heterozygosity and, hence, lessened genetic diversity typically entails negative fitness effects (Keller & Waller 2002).

As we have illustrated in Chapter 4, a correlation of pay-offs resulting in selection for cooperative behaviour may also result from conditional reciprocation (Trivers 1971). In this scenario, the actor should be able to predict the likelihood and value of the payback (w) that will compensate for the costs involved in the act. If this likelihood exceeds the current cost/benefit ratio, reciprocal cooperation may be selected for ($w > c/b$; Nowak 2006). Various theoretical models identified the conditions under which reciprocal altruism can be evolutionarily stable, and numerous empirical studies suggested that reciprocal cooperation is actually widespread in animals (Table 4.1), which in the past had been often disputed. The decision rules involved in direct and generalized reciprocity are viable, and rigorous experiments with different taxa have recently accumulated convincing evidence that reciprocal exchange of same or different services and commodities does happen in non-human animals (Schweinfurth & Call 2019a). This may be different for indirect reciprocity, which involves higher cognitive demands and may be more important in humans than in other animals.

A helpful act creating net (lifetime) fitness benefits only to the receiver, without any concurrent or future positive feedback to the actor's fitness, will be selected for only if the receiver can force or deceive the potential actor. This means that the fitness balance for the actor is and remains negative ($c > b$), and hence the behaviour is maladaptive. In Chapter 4 we argue that the reasons why such behaviour may still be maintained in a population include (i) rare occurrence and hence negligible fitness consequences, and (ii) high costs of countermeasures against help enforcement in comparison to the costs of the helpful act, i.e. submitting to the coercion is cheaper than resisting it. The occurrence of cooperation based on enforcement or deception may be seen as part of an evolutionary arms race dynamic between the involved parties. This can be plausibly exemplified by the interspecific interaction between brood parasites and their hosts (Davies et al. 1989), as explained in Chapter 5.

We should be aware that, as with any social trait, selection of cooperative behaviour is typically subject to a combination of several evolutionary mechanisms. In interactions among unrelated social partners, cooperation may be selected by a combination of elements of reciprocity and coercion. The outside options for each partner can be particularly important for their choice of strategy. If several options exist, supply and demand in a market-like situation can lead to mutually beneficial exchanges (Hammerstein & Noe 2016). The danger of being exploited may be counteracted by a specialization of roles, which may stabilize cooperation and lead to increased dependence of partners on each other. This is best illustrated by interspecific mutualisms. Biparental care illustrates how individuals interdependent on each other due to their common stakes, in this case shared offspring, may negotiate about their respective contribution, here the investment in brood care. By taking turns in brood-care duties parents can make sure that the partner is also doing their bit, a process reflecting intricate negotiations between mates that may also involve enforcement by the latent threat of desertion (Johnstone & Savage 2019).

In societies containing both related and unrelated members, the evolution of cooperation may be particularly complex, involving several selection mechanisms at the same time. In Chapter 4 we showed that in cooperative breeders, where dominant breeders are supported by subordinate brood-care helpers, the fitness effects of cooperation may depend on an interaction between reciprocal trading of commodities, relatedness between interacting group members, and coercion of help. In cooperatively breeding cichlids, helpers trade brood care against the use of resources in the breeders' territory. At the same time their helping levels are influenced by the dominants' enforcement, administered by aggression and the implicit threat of eviction. On the other hand, brood care of subordinates that are related to the dominants' offspring may be favoured by kin selection. Interestingly, in this interaction between kin selection, reciprocity and coercion, the effect of kin selection on cooperation seems to be smallest (Quinones et al. 2016). Similarly, in vampire bats and Norway rats, where a combination of relatedness, reciprocity and coercion underlies altruistic food donations, relatedness has been shown to be less important for cooperation than reciprocity (Carter & Wilkinson 2013; Schweinfurth & Taborsky 2018a). To obtain quantitative estimates of the relative importance of different evolutionary mechanisms responsible for altruistic cooperation in nature is a major challenge for future studies of sociality, which seems particularly interesting when there are multiple behaviours involved and division of labour among group members (Iserbyt et al. 2017).

6.4 Interspecific Interactions

If members of different species cooperate, selection for concessions between different parties may involve by-product benefits, reciprocal exchange and enforcement; the fourth possible selection mechanism responsible for the evolution of cooperation, the sharing of fitness interests by genetic similarity, is lacking. This is obviously the major difference between evolutionary mechanisms underlying intraspecific and interspecific cooperation. As we show in Chapter 5, cooperative interactions between species contain great potential for conflict. This is not only due to the lack of shared genes, but also because of substantial asymmetries in abilities and pay-offs. Most obvious asymmetries exist if cooperation by one agent is somehow enforced by the other, either by coercion or deceit. Interspecific brood parasitism is a case in point. Such asymmetric, exploitative interactions may result in an arms race between the beneficiary and the inadvertent benefactor, which is well illustrated by the dynamic coevolution between parasites and hosts (Davies et al. 1989).

We have seen in Chapter 5 that transmission mechanisms and assortment may cause pairs of species to cooperate across generations, which might even render indiscriminate cooperation between species (Wyatt et al. 2013), somewhat reminiscent of generalized reciprocity among individuals of the same species. Evolutionarily speaking, the simplest cooperative interaction between different species is commensalism, a one-sided interaction where one partner takes advantage of another without involving a feedback. Think of one species producing 'waste' that can be used by another, such as vertebrate dung used by dung beetles, or which serves a protective function for conspecifics that may be shared by the members of another species, such as by production of alarm calls. Taking advantage of the interspecific relationship may be completely unilateral. The next step in the transition from simple to complex cooperative interactions between species is the two-way interaction characterizing by-product mutualism. Here, both partners of a relationship act in a way benefitting themselves, while at the same time benefitting the partner with no extra costs. Interspecific brood mixing and, in consequence, the shared brood care among parents of different species exemplify this form of interspecific cooperation.

Alternatively, members of different species may reciprocally exchange service and commodities with each other, similarly to reciprocal relationships between conspecifics. The interaction between cleaners and clients demonstrates how such relationships may work. Clients spend time and energy posing for a cleaner, which may also involve increased predation risk, but they benefit from the parasite removal service the cleaner can offer. The latter's benefit from its cleaning service is the nutritional value of the ectoparasites borne by the client. As in any reciprocal relationship, such interaction is prone to cheating, in this case eating of skin and mucus instead of parasites, which can be counteracted through punishment by the mistreated client (Bshary & Grutter 2002). As our examples in Chapter 5 suggested, such interspecific cooperation based on the conditional exchange of service and commodities may involve trading and negotiations just like in many reciprocal interactions among conspecifics. In its most extreme form this may lead to mutual dependency and, finally, cause a transition to a novel unit – an organism combining the previously separate partners (Queller & Strassmann 2009).

When thinking about relationships between different species, we might have adverse effects rather than cooperation in mind. In Chapter 5 we showed that non-interference rivalry for resources can be moderated through character displacement. Alternatively, the coexistence of species in the face of resource competition can be facilitated if specialists meet with generalists. Overlapping resource needs may also cause overt conflict and aggression, with ensuing interspecific territoriality or the exclusion of the competitively inferior party. An interesting facet in the competitive relationship between species is the occurrence of interspecific mating, which is not actually rare in many taxa. To mate with a member of another species involves asymmetric cost/benefit ratios for males and females, as the production of sperm is so much cheaper than the reproductive effort required when playing the female role (Wirtz 1999).

The most extreme adverse relations between species involve the unilateral exploitation of one partner by another, such as in parasite–host and predater–prey relations. Interestingly, the relationship between predators and prey organisms may cause coordination and cooperation among the latter, both among members of the same and of different species. For example, individuals may form aggregations to reduce predation risk, which may consequently facilitate social interactions and, finally, the emergence of cooperation. Mixed-species broods and shared brood care illustrate this point nicely. Even if such interactions may reflect unilateral exploitation, such as when a brood is 'farmed out' to another caregiver, collaborative brood care involving parents of different species may be based on active choice of appropriate 'partners'.

As we have outlined in Chapter 5, interspecific interactions combining more than two species are a particular research challenge as they may involve complex multi-way interactions. We have also stressed that a great many of these interspecific relations, regardless of the degree of conflict or cooperation between the different parties, entail extraordinary ecological significance. Without the cooperation between plants, insects, fungi and other microorganisms, for instance, our current agriculture would be inconceivable (Bronstein 2015).

6.5   General Conclusions

6.5.1   Optimal Responses to Competition

The three alternative ways to cope with competition for resources, *race*, *fight* or *share*, cannot be ranked on a scale from worse to better, and they often occur side by side. Males of the ocellated wrasse, for instance, behave either as bourgeois nest owners, opportunistic sneakers or helpful satellites. They are all selected to fertilize as many eggs as possible, but each male type accomplishes this aim differently: while bourgeois males *fight* for nest ownership among themselves, sneakers *race* into nests to release sperm during spawning and satellites *share* nest defence duties with bourgeois males to increase their fertilization success (Taborsky et al. 1987; Stiver & Alonzo 2013). All three possibilities represent adequate, selected responses to competition in dependence on ecological and social conditions.

As we have seen, certain conditions may cause a change from one optimal response to another. For instance, if cooperation results in the production of resources, the conflict potential is reduced, which may cause a system to switch from *fight* to *share*. Open conflict entails a great damage potential, but cooperation involves the risk of exploitation, so under many circumstances it may be better to scramble or contest than to concede. Conditions that may shift the optimal strategy from conflict to cooperation include the occurrence of outside threats, which may be overcome by combining forces, and the benefits resulting from specializing in certain roles if this goes hand in hand with an exchange of goods and services between parties. The enormous efficiency potential of such division of labour is impressively demonstrated by the performance and productivity of eusocial insects, and the pervasive importance of interspecific mutualisms and symbioses.

We might presume that a change from scramble or contest to cooperation may enhance the complexity involved in social interactions, because of the conflict of interest inherent in any relationship between social partners. This may be true to some extent, as suggested by the varied behaviour of group members in the highly structured societies of cooperative breeders. However, if we develop this thought further, it becomes clear that at the transition to organismality, at the latest, the conflict of interest drops due to the loss of outside options, and the complexity of the interaction concomitantly declines. By this reasoning, the most complex social interactions are probably found at the level of cooperative societies characterized by long-term associations and dynamic group membership. This form of organization provides a playing field for negotiations and trading of goods and services between individuals all trying to optimize their own direct and indirect fitness.

6.5.2   Future Directions

There are obvious and less-apparent challenges worth taking up in future studies of the evolution of social behaviour. We confine ourselves to the issues we find most intriguing.

The ecological and social conditions favouring one or the other response to competition certainly need to be better understood, which should involve measuring fitness consequences of different strategies under varying experimental conditions in nature. This is an enormous challenge. Also, it would be a major advance in our understanding of the evolution of cooperation if we were able to quantify the relative contributions of the alternative selection mechanisms – which include by-product benefits, shared genes, reciprocity and enforcement – for the existence and stability of different forms of cooperative interactions. Perhaps we should not expect very general answers to this question but rather specific explanations for each single case. Nevertheless, as long as we have not worked this out in a certain number of cases and over a range of different systems, we can but speculate. It may also be worth unravelling the continuum apparently existing between bargaining and coercion, in particular in the light of asymmetries between partners regarding their abilities and conditions, including their resource holding potential, alternative options and expected pay-offs.

Another challenge worth taking is the parallel development of theory and empirical/experimental work, which requires close collaboration between theoreticians and empiricists. We tend to be content with a qualitative confirmation of theoretical predictions by a particular system, but this may not be enough, as we cannot expect to have thought of all possible alternative causes responsible for the result. We argue that even in tightly controlled experiments we typically do not fully understand the involved mechanisms well enough to exclude alternative explanations. Biology is inherently complex. Therefore, the more concrete theoretical models describing a system can predict responses to an experimental manipulation, the more confidence we can have that a match between prediction and validation correctly depicts underlying principles. In this endeavour, we should not remain at the rather superficial, functional level scrutinizing fitness correlates, but attempt to also understand the machinery allowing organisms to make adaptive decisions. This again will be a challenge engaging generations to come.

6.5.3   Less Encouraged

We should resist the temptation to expect relatedness and kin selection to explain the majority of social phenomena we wish to understand. In a way, relying all too heavily on the concept of kin selection entails a sort of explanatory laziness, because as long as interactions involve related social partners, we are tempted to think *this is it*. Albeit, this is often unjustified, as the other three selection mechanisms responsible for cooperative behaviour may be involved as well. Recent research in insects, fish and mammals showed that kinship may explain a smaller proportion of variance in social behaviour than, for example, reciprocity and coercion.

Further, we urge that the importance of certain selection mechanisms should not be underestimated simply because we cannot easily imagine how they might work. Reciprocity is a case in point. Due to the scepticism regarding the involved requirements, such as individual recognition and specific social memory, and because of a long-standing lack of suitable experiments testing for the involved decision rules, for quite a while this concept has fallen from favour. Nevertheless, recent research provided evidence that animals do indeed apply the decision rules characterizing reciprocal exchanges of goods and services, and theoretical work has shown that under a wide range of conditions even anonymous generosity can create stable levels of cooperation in a population if it is based on experienced cooperation (i.e. generalized reciprocity).

An unfortunate divide has emerged between theoretical modelling and empirical research. This may be demonstrated with another look at the research on reciprocal cooperation. Literally, thousands of studies have modelled situations theoretically stabilizing direct and indirect reciprocity, but these attempts are typically disregarding the natural conditions prevailing to the target organisms. At the same time, the results of such basic models are often misunderstood by empiricists as generating testable predictions suited to explain animal behaviour. The development of theory for theory's sake is all well and good, but it should not be sold or understood as a recipe for testing the mechanisms underlying animal decisions, and their evolution.

We also caution against the tunnel vision resulting from a narrow focus on particular research traditions. For example, the flourishing field of animal personality has generated a plethora of information that is often bare of astute concepts or a firm theoretical framework. At the same time, a rather comprehensive body of theory has been developed in the field of alternative reproductive and behavioural tactics, which is almost completely ignored by research on behavioural syndromes and animal personality. Working within a certain research tradition should not obfuscate a broader view across imaginary borders.

Last but not least, we would like to discourage defining and applying terms in a highly specific and narrow manner. There will never be full agreement about semantic issues, and it is certainly true that as long as the use of a term is clearly defined, we can communicate, even if we are in disagreement about a particular definition. However, defining terms from everyday language in a way departing from everyday connotations will inevitably cause confusion. This can be illustrated by a look at how a common word such as 'cooperation' has been defined in some literature dealing with its evolution. If the courtship of a male to attract a partner falls within the meaning of this term, but biparental care does not, communication becomes difficult even within a research field, let alone between disciplines. By the same token, if enforcement is defined so that providing incentives to a social partner is included in its meaning, this will cause misunderstandings. It seems that problems of this kind should be easy to avoid.

6.5.4   Final Inference

There is *so* much still to learn about the evolution of social behaviour. To proceed in this direction is our delightful challenge!

Conflict, Cooperation and the Evolution of Menopause

Summary

Humans exhibit a rare life history in which females stop reproducing midway through life. Only a handful of other wild mammals exhibit a similar menopausal life history. The theory of kin selection suggests that post-reproductive survival can be favoured where older females confer fitness benefits on their offspring (the grandmother hypothesis). Numerous studies have shown that older females do help to boost the fitness of their offspring, but such helping benefits are too small to favour reproductive cessation in humans at the observed age of 40–50 years old. Recent models of 'kinship dynamics' suggest that reproductive conflict between generations is a missing factor in the evolution of post-reproductive lifespan. The models further suggest that humans and some cetaceans are predisposed to the evolution of menopause as a consequence of their unusual, and distinct, patterns of mating and dispersal, providing an explanation for the strange taxonomic distribution of this trait. Tests of these models in humans support the predicted effect of demography on patterns of kinship and provide evidence of intergenerational reproductive conflict in some societies. Recent tests of the models in a wild population of another menopausal mammal, the killer whale, have found strong support for the model predictions. Studies of the family conflict in other long-lived mammals can shed new light on how the unusual human life history evolved.

Introduction

As a study animal, humans are the most fascinating and yet most difficult of subjects. Given the power of evolutionary biology to explain the immense diversity of form, function and behaviour that we observe in nature, it is natural that we should wish to apply its methods to ourselves, but doing so is fraught with controversy. Evolutionary studies of human behaviour, in particular, have fuelled fierce debate about the ethics and utility of Darwinian investigations of the more negative aspects of our social lives, such as sexual conflict, racism and war. Less controversial is the use of evolutionary approaches to study our unusual suite of life-history traits. Humans living in 'natural fertility' conditions, without modern medicine or technology, exhibit low adult mortality, a long period of offspring dependency, short female reproductive span, high fertility, and a long period of post-reproductive life. These life-history traits evolved long before the vast cultural, agricultural and technological changes that have occurred in the last 10,000 years. It is therefore reasonable and important to ask how this unusual life history evolved, and apply evolutionary theory and tests to find answers.

For women in natural fertility societies (i.e. societies that lack access to modern medicine or technology) the age at last reproduction averages around 38 years (Cant & Johnstone 2008). Menopause, the permanent cessation of menstruation and loss of fertility, occurs around a decade later. Yet women in these societies who reach the age of 45 can expect to live into their late 60s. In natural fertility human populations, the proportion of the adult female population that is post-reproductive (a measure known as the PrR; Levitis & Lackey 2011) is just less than half, whereas in other wild primate populations this proportion is less than 0.05. The only other wild mammal species that resemble humans in terms of post-reproductive lifespan are resident killer whales ($PrR = 0.22$), short-finned pilot whales ($PrR = 0.28$), beluga whales (*Delphinapterus leucas*: $PrR = 0.27$) and narwhals (*Monodon monocerus*: $PrR = 0.24$; Croft et al. 2015; Ellis et al. 2018; Figure F.1). The prolonged post-reproductive lifespan in these five species (plus semi-captive Asian elephants: Chapman et al. 2019b) represents an outstanding puzzle for evolutionary biology. How can natural selection favour survival so long past the end of reproduction?

For many years the main explanation for the evolution of menopause was the grandmother hypothesis, which suggested that older women survived long past the end of reproduction because of the fitness benefits they could confer on their offspring and grandoffspring. Indeed, numerous studies of humans have found that grandmothers are hardworking helpers, and that having a surviving grandmother boosted the fitness of grandoffspring. But there was a problem. Detailed studies of natural fertility data sets of the Ache (Hill & Hurtado 1996) and a Taiwanese data set from 1906 (Rogers 1993) found that the magnitude of the benefits conferred by grandmothering were too small to favour reproductive cessation around the age of 40–50. Thus the grandmother hypothesis could explain why, in natural fertility populations, older women survived long past the age of reproduction, but this hypothesis couldn't explain the timing of reproductive cessation, or why women gave up reproducing in the first place.

Reproductive Conflict

One important factor missing from early analyses of the grandmother hypotheses is the cost of reproductive conflict. In cooperatively breeding birds and mammals there is intense competition among reproductive females to monopolize reproduction, because each additional offspring produced in a social unit inflicts a fitness cost on other breeders. Younger females typically suppress reproduction to avoid reproductive conflict with older females. Humans are prime candidates to experience reproductive conflict because we share food to a degree unmatched in other primates, and because offspring are reliant upon parents and helpers for a very long period of development. Could the timing of reproductive cessation in older females have to coincide with the onset of reproduction in younger ones, as a mechanism to

avoid intergenerational reproductive conflict? It is certainly the case that humans show an extraordinarily low degree of reproductive overlap between generations. In hunter-gatherers, women have their first baby, on average, at age 19 years, and their last baby, on average, at age 38 years. The average reproductive overlap between generations in human hunter-gatherers is precisely zero (Figure 3.14).

Why, in humans, should older females cease reproduction in the face of reproductive conflict from a younger generation, rather than vice versa? Cant and Johnstone (2008) argued that a major factor is the pattern of sex-specific dispersal, because this determines which females come into reproductive conflict. The pattern of dispersal in ancestral humans has been the subject of considerable debate in the anthropological literature. Early classifications of hunter-gatherer societies suggested that humans were typically 'patrilocal', a social system wherein females disperse from their natal group at reproductive maturity to join their husband's family (Ember 1978). Later studies criticised the strict patrilocal model, mainly on the grounds that there is much variation within and between societies, and that individuals strategically adjust their dispersal behaviour according to their circumstances (Alvarez 2004; Marlowe 2004). This type of flexibility and individual variation is common in other animal populations. However, the evolution of major life-history traits likely depends on the average social environment encountered by genes affecting the schedule of fertility or mortality. Some lines of evidence suggest that mutations affecting the schedule of fertility and mortality are likely to have arisen in an average social environment featuring some degree of female-biased dispersal. First, while dispersal is typically male-biased in mammals (Lawson Handley & Perrin 2007), our closest living relatives, chimpanzees and bonobos, exhibit strongly female-biased dispersal (Eriksson et al. 2006; Langergraber, 2009). Second, genetic evidence suggests that female-biased dispersal was characteristic of *Homo neanderthalensis* (Lalueza-Fox et al. 2011), and isotopic analysis of teeth is consistent with female dispersal in the Pliocene hominins *Australopithecus africanus* and *Paranthropus robustus* (Copeland et al. 2011). Third, analyses of

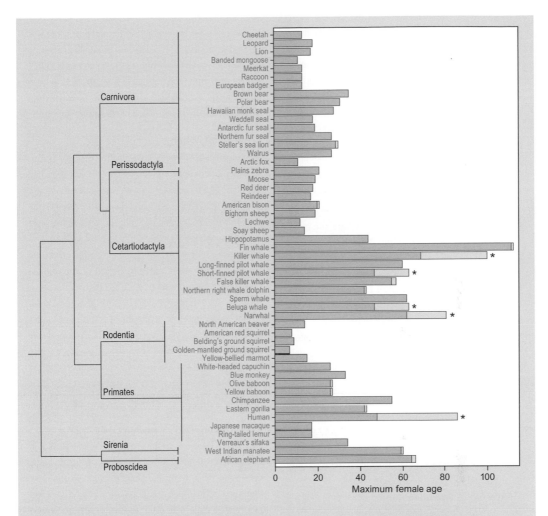

Figure F.1 Extended post-reproductive lifespans are rare in mammals. Bars show the proportion of female years in the population being lived by reproductive (dark grey) and post-reproductive (light grey) females, for 51 species of mammal (compiled from data in Ellis et al. 2018). For five species – humans, killer whales, short-finned pilot whales, narwhals and beluga whales – this proportion is significantly different from zero (marked with an asterisk).

mitochondrial versus Y-chromosome variation are consistent with higher rates of female migration than male migration at the global scale, although there is considerable geographic variation (and inferences are limited by lack of information on human mating systems; Lippold et al. 2014). While not definitive, existing data suggest an ancestral human pattern in which female dispersal and male philopatry was more common than the reverse pattern.

Incorporating an assumption of female-biased dispersal of this kind into a 'tug-of-war' model of reproductive conflict suggests that this demographic pattern has a decisive effect on the predicted outcome of intergenerational reproductive conflict (Cant & Johnstone 2008). The evolutionarily stable solution is for older-generation females to commit irreversibly to zero reproduction and allow younger females to reproduce without hindrance. This is because female-biased dispersal creates a basic relatedness asymmetry in the relatedness of younger and older females to each other's offspring. A young female, newly arrived in a social group, is unrelated to the older female's young and so insensitive to any costs she inflicts on the mother by reproducing. An older female, by contrast, is related to the offspring of the younger female through her son. Given a pattern of female-biased dispersal during the period of lengthening human lifespan, the model predicts that older females should evolve to cease reproduction when females of the younger generation started to reproduce.

In a subsequent paper, Johnstone and Cant (2010) developed a more general model of 'kinship dynamics' to predict how different patterns of mating and dispersal affected the strength of kin selection across the lifespan. Specifically, they investigated how the unusual demography of killer whales and pilot whales, in which neither sex disperses and mating occurs non-locally, influences selection on female helping and harming over the lifespan. As in the human case, this demographic pattern is predicted to result in females becoming more closely related to their local group as they grow older, predisposing them to evolve menopause (Figure F.2A). The model thus provides one explanation for why, of all long-lived mammals, menopause has evolved only in humans and these two toothed whales.

Analysis of patterns of kinship in 19 human societies provides broad support for the predicted effect of sex-biased dispersal on patterns of relatedness across the lifespan (Koster et al. 2019). Lahdenperä et al. (2012) found evidence of severe intergenerational conflict in family groups living in eighteenth- and nineteenth-century Finland. The offspring of mothers-in-law suffered 66 per cent higher mortality when their birth coincided with reproduction by a daughter-in-law in the same household (Lahdenperä et al. 2012). Evidence of fitness costs of intergenerational reproductive conflict has also been found in data from Gambian families collected in the mid-twentieth century (Mace & Alvergne 2012). On the other hand, a study of a historical Norwegian population found no evidence that co-breeding between generations was costly (Skjærvø & Røskaft 2013).

However, in the latter study reproductive conflict was defined to occur when older- and younger-generation females gave birth within 15 years of each other, which may have diluted the power of the study to detect costs of reproductive conflict in the early years of life, when the dependence of offspring is highest.

Enter Killer Whales

A limitation with these tests on human data is that neither modern hunter-gatherers nor historical human populations are perfect windows into our evolutionary past. Patterns of mortality and dispersal in these societies may have changed radically from those that held during the period in which the species-wide trait of menopause evolved in humans. A powerful alternative approach is to study other mammals that exhibit a prolonged post-reproductive life living in the environment in which they evolved. The only other species for which this is possible at present is the resident killer whale, which exhibits a reproductive life history that is very similar to humans. Females become sexually mature around 15 years of age, cease reproduction around the age of 35 or 40, but can survive into their 70s and 80s, perhaps even longer. This information is known thanks to long-term research on two populations of resident killer whales in the Pacific Northwest led by Ken Balcomb of the Center for Whale Research and John Ford of Fisheries and Oceans Canada. Since the 1970s Ken, John and their research teams have identified individuals, monitored births and deaths and recorded social behaviour in the two populations. Subsequent research by Darren Croft, Dan Franks and colleagues at the Universities of Exeter and York has used this long-term data set to test adaptive hypotheses for the evolution of menopause in a non-human mammal. This research has examined (1) whether older females provide mothering and grandmothering benefits; (2) whether killer whale females grow more closely related to the group as they get older, as theoretical models predict; and (3) whether intergenerational conflict is costly.

Foster et al. (2012) found evidence that resident killer whale mothers play a crucial role in the survival of their sons in particular. Indeed, sons become ever more heavily reliant on their mothers for survival as they grow older and larger. This

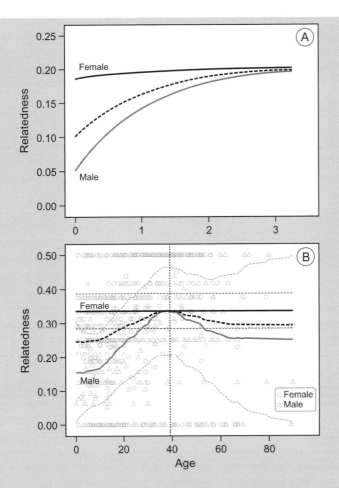

Figure F.2 Age changes in local relatedness in killer whales. (A) Johnstone and Cant's (2010) theoretical prediction of the relationship between female age (scaled relative to mean generation time) and mean relatedness of a female to other females (upper grey line) and males (lower grey line) within the same matriline. Averaged relatedness across both sexes is also shown (black line). (B) Relationship between female age and maternal relatedness in northern and southern resident killer whales, using 43 years of data (200 whales, 846 whale-years). Lines indicate patterns of relatedness as in (A); standard errors are shown as dotted lines. The theoretical model did not predict a drop in relatedness after the end of reproduction because it assumed constant fertility across the lifespan. Redrawn with permission from Croft et al. (2017).

surprising result fits with the prediction of structured population models that take into account the unusual demography of killer whales (Johnstone & Cant 2010). Given a choice over the allocation of investment, mothers do best to invest in sons over daughters because the offspring of sons are born into a different group, the members of whom pay the cost

of rearing. Offspring of daughters, by contrast, remain in the social group and add to levels of local competition. Later work showed that older, post-reproductive females also play a crucial leadership role, using their knowledge to lead the group on foraging trips, particularly when the abundance of salmon (the primary food of resident whales) is low

(Brent et al. 2015). Grandmothers have a measurable impact on the survival of grandoffspring, and this impact is greater if they have stopped reproducing themselves (Nattrass et al. 2019). These studies demonstrate that older, post-reproductive females enhance the fitness of their descendent and non-descendent kin, similar to the demonstrated grand-mothering benefits that post-reproductive females can confer on their offspring in humans (e.g. Lahdenperä et al. 2004; Engelhardt et al. 2019).

Like humans, however, reproductive conflict between generations also plays a critical role in the timing of reproductive cessation. Croft et al. (2017) tested whether patterns of local relatedness in killer whale groups match the patterns predicted by Johnstone and Cant (2010) and tested whether, as predicted, older-generation females suffer dispro-portionate costs in reproductive conflict with younger females (their daughters). The relatedness of females to other members of their social group increases as they age and shows a very close match to theoretical predictions, up to the point at which menopause occurs (Figure F.2B). Interestingly, relatedness drops after females stop reproducing as a grandmother's sons die off – something that is not incorporated in the simple model. Also as predicted, the offspring of older-generation females suffered 1.7 times greater mortality when they competed with the offspring of younger-generation females. Together, the known benefits that older females confer on kin and the costs of competing for repro-duction with younger females can explain the evolu-tion of menopause in killer whales. These findings from killer whales suggest that to explain human life history requires a model incorporating both the inclusive fitness benefits of late-life helping and the inclusive fitness costs of reproductive conflict.

Towards New Frontiers

The kinship dynamics approach aims to predict how features of population demography will shape life history and behaviour in long-lived, family-dwelling animals like ourselves. These models have applica-tion to questions far beyond the topic of the evolution of menopause. How will kinship dynamics shape patterns of investment in offspring during develop-ment, and patterns of conflict and cooperation among group members of different ages? Are cooperative groups subject to evolutionary senescence, in the same way that iteroparous organisms are? Does the pattern of kinship dynamics shape the evolution of early life effects and 'foetal programming' in humans and other mammals? Kinship dynamics models are a first step towards a more general 'social life history theory' capable of tackling these questions.

One promising topic in the study of human life history is to examine how competition within the family unit might shape patterns of growth and devel-opment. For example, another unusual trait of human development is the slow rate of growth from weaning to puberty, followed by an adolescent growth spurt. Chimpanzees grow much more rapidly after weaning, after which growth slows down through to adulthood. Data from hunter-gatherers suggest that the human pattern of slow growth followed by a rapid adolescent growth spurt reduces concurrent demand on parental resources by multiple dependent offspring (Gurven & Walker 2006). Another (speculative) possibility is that offspring suppress their own growth until the age at which (on average) their older sibling has dispersed or become independent, much like the kind of strategic growth adjustment that occurs in fish size hierarchies (Buston 2003a; Wong et al. 2007, 2008; Segers & Taborsky 2012; Reed et al. 2019). The short interbirth interval and consequent high fertility rate of humans may itself be an adaptation to maximize offspring production within the limited time window from age at first reproduction until the onset of inter-generational reproductive conflict. A focus on strat-egies of family conflict as well as cooperation, and a greater appreciation of mammalian comparisons beyond primates, can contribute to a better under-standing of the evolutionary forces that have shaped our own peculiar form and function.

References

Aanen, D.K. & Eggleton, P. 2005. Fungus-growing termites originated in African rain forest. *Current Biology*, 15, 851–855.

Aanen, D.K., Eggleton, P., Rouland-Lefèvre, C., et al. 2002. The evolution of fungus-growing termites and their mutualistic fungal symbionts. *Proceedings of the National Academy of Science of the United States of America*, 99, 14887–14892.

Abbot, P., Withgott, J.H. & Moran, N.A. 2001. Genetic conflict and conditional altruism in social aphid colonies. *Proceedings of the National Academy of Sciences of the United States of America*, 98, 12068–12071.

Abbot, P., Abe, J., Alcock, J., et al. 2011. Inclusive fitness theory and eusociality. *Nature*, 471, E1–E4.

Abrahams, M.V. 1986. Patch choice under perceptual constraints: a cause for departures from an ideal free distribution. *Behavioral Ecology and Sociobiology*, 19, 409–415.

Adami, C. & Hintze, A. 2013. Evolutionary instability of zero-determinant strategies demonstrates that winning is not everything. *Nature Communications*, 4, 2193.

Afshar, M. & Giraldeau, L.A. 2014. A unified modelling approach for producer–scrounger games in complex ecological conditions. *Animal Behaviour*, 96, 167–176.

Akçay, E. & Van Cleve, J. 2016. There is no fitness but fitness, and the lineage is its bearer. *Philosophical Transactions of the Royal Society B: Biological Science*, 371, 20150085.

Alatalo, R.V., Gustafsson, L., Linden, M. & Lundberg, A. 1985. Interspecific competition and niche shifts in tits and the goldcrest: an experiment. *The Journal of Animal Ecology*, 54, 977–984.

Alatalo, R.V., Höglund, J., Lundberg, A. & Sutherland, W.J. 1992. Evolution of black grouse leks: female preferences benefit males in larger leks. *Behavioral Ecology*, 3, 53–59.

Alatalo, R.V., Höglund, J., Lundberg, A., Rintamäki, P.T. & Silverin, B. 1996. Testosterone and male mating success on the black grouse leks. *Proceedings of the Royal Society of London B: Biological Science*, 263, 1697–1702.

Alberts, J.R. 1978. Huddling by rat pups – group behavioral mechanisms of temperature regulation and energy-conservation. *Journal of Comparative and Physiological Psychology*, 92, 231–245.

Alberts, J.R. 2007. Huddling by rat pups: ontogeny of individual and group behavior. *Developmental Psychobiology*, 49, 22–32.

Alerstam, T., Nilsson, S.G. & Ulfstrand, S. 1974. Niche differentiation during winter in woodland birds in southern Sweden and the island of Gotland. *Oikos*, 321–330.

Alexander, R.D. 1974. The evolution of social behavior. *Annual Review of Ecology and Systematics*, 4, 325–383.

Alexander, R.D. 1987. *The Biology of Moral Systems*. New York, NY: Aldine de Gruyter.

Allee, W.C. 1951. *The Social Life of Animals*. New York, NY: Norton & Co.

Allen, B., Nowak, M.A. & Wilson, E.O. 2013. Limitations of inclusive fitness. *Proceedings of the National Academy of Sciences of the United States of America*, 110, 20135–20139.

Allison, S.T. & Kerr, N.L. 1994. Group correspondence biases and the provision of public goods. *Journal of Personality and Social Psychology*, 66, 688.

Almany, G.R., Hamilton, R.J., Bode, M., et al. 2013. Dispersal of grouper larvae drives local resource sharing in a coral reef fishery. *Current Biology*, 23, 626–630.

Alonzo, S.H. 2010. Social and coevolutionary feedbacks between mating and parental investment. *Trends in Ecology & Evolution*, 25, 99–108.

Alonzo, S.H. & Klug, H. 2012. Paternity, maternity, and parental care. In Royle, N.J., Smiseth, P.T. & Kölliker, M. (eds), *The Evolution of Parental Care*. Oxford: Oxford University Press.

Alonzo, S.H., Taborsky, M. & Wirtz, P. 2000. Male alternative reproductive behaviours in a Mediterranean wrasse, *Symphodus ocellatus*: evidence from otoliths for multiple life-history pathways. *Evolutionary Ecology Research*, 2, 997–1007.

Alvard, M.S. & Nolin, D.A. 2002. Rousseau's whale hunt? Coordination among big-game hunters. *Current Anthropology*, 43, 533–559.

Alvarez, H.P. 2004. Residence groups among hunter gatherers: a review of the claims and evidence for patrilocal bands. In Chapais, B. & Berman, C.M. (eds), *Kinship and Behavior in Primates*, pp. 420–442. Oxford: Oxford University Press.

Amos, B., Barrett, J. & Dover, G.A. 1991. Breeding behaviour of pilot whales revealed by DNA fingerprinting. *Heredity*, 67, 49.

Anderholm, S., Waldeck, P., Van der Jeugd, H.P., et al. 2009. Colony kin structure and host–parasite relatedness in the barnacle goose. *Molecular Ecology*, 18, 4955–4963.

Anderson, M.G., Rhymer, J.M. & Rohwer, F.C. 1992. Philopatry, dispersal, and the genetic structure of waterfowl populations. In Batt, B.D.J., Afton, A.D., Anderson, M.G., et al. (eds), *Ecology and Management of Breeding Waterfowl*, pp. 365–395. Minneapolis, MN: University of Minnesota Press.

Andersson, M. 1984. Brood parasitism within species. In Barnard, C.J. (ed.), *Producers and Scroungers: Strategies of Exploitation and Parasitism*, pp. 195–228. London: Croom Helm.

Andersson, M. 1994. *Sexual Selection*. Princeton, NJ: Princeton University Press.

Andersson, M. 2005. Evolution of classical polyandry: three steps to female emancipation. *Ethology*, 111, 1–23.

Andersson, M. & Åhlund, M. 2000. Host–parasite relatedness shown by protein fingerprinting in a brood parasitic bird. *Proceedings of the National Academy of Sciences of the United States of America*, 97, 13188–13193.

Andersson, M. & Simmons, L.W. 2006. Sexual selection and mate choice. *Trends in Ecology & Evolution*, 21, 296–302.

Andersson, M., Ahlund, M. & Waldeck, P. 2019. Brood parasitism, relatedness and sociality: a kinship role in female reproductive tactics. *Biological Reviews*, 94, 307–327.

Andre, J.B. 2015. Contingency in the evolutionary emergence of reciprocal cooperation. *American Naturalist*, 185, 303–316.

Ang, T.Z. & Manica, A. 2010. Aggression, segregation and social stability in a dominance hierarchy. *Proceedings of the Royal Society B: Biological Sciences*, 277, 1337–1343.

Antolin, M.F. 1999. A genetic perspective on mating systems and sex ratios of parasitoid wasps. *Researches on Population Ecology*, 41, 29–37.

Aplin, L.M. & Morand-Ferron, J. 2017. Stable producer–scrounger dynamics in wild birds: sociability and learning speed covary with scrounging behaviour. *Proceedings of the Royal Society B: Biological Sciences*, 284, 20162872.

Archetti, M. & Scheuring, I. 2012. Game theory of public goods in one-shot social dilemmas without assortment. *Journal of Theoretical Biology*, 299, 9–20.

Arnold, C. & Taborsky, B. 2010. Social experience in early ontogeny has lasting effects on social skills in cooperatively breeding cichlids. *Animal Behaviour*, 79, 621–630.

Arnold, K.E. & Owens, I.P.F. 1998. Cooperative breeding in birds: a comparative test of the life history hypothesis. *Proceedings of the Royal Society B: Biological Sciences*, 265, 739–745.

Arnold, K.E. & Owens, I.P. 1999. Cooperative breeding in birds: the role of ecology. *Behavioral Ecology*, 10, 465–471.

Arnold, W. 1988. Social thermoregulation during hibernation in alpine marmots (*Marmota marmota*). *Journal of Comparative Physiology B: Biochemical Systemic and Environmental Physiology*, 158, 151–156.

Arnold, W. 1990a. The evolution of marmot sociality: I. Why disperse late? *Behavioral Ecology and Sociobiology*, 27, 229–237.

Arnold, W. 1990b. The evolution of marmot sociality: II. Costs and benefits of joint hibernation. *Behavioral Ecology and Sociobiology*, 27, 239–246.

Arnott, G. & Elwood, R.W. 2009. Assessment of fighting ability in animal contests. *Animal Behaviour*, 77, 991–1004.

Arnqvist, G. & Rowe, L. 2005. *Sexual Conflict*. Princeton, NJ: Princeton University Press.

Arseneau-Robar, T.J.M., Taucher, A.L., Muller, E., et al. 2016. Female monkeys use both the carrot and the stick to promote male participation in intergroup fights. *Proceedings of the Royal Society B: Biological Sciences*, 283, 20161817.

Ashton, B.J., Ridley, A.R., Edwards, E.K. & Thornton, A. 2018. Cognitive performance is linked to group size and affects fitness in Australian magpies. *Nature*, 554, 364.

Awata, S., Munehara, H. & Kohda, M. 2005. Social system and reproduction of helpers in a cooperatively breeding cichlid fish (*Julidochromis ornatus*) in Lake Tanganyika: field observations and parentage analyses. *Behavioral Ecology and Sociobiology*, 58, 506–516.

Axelrod, R. 1984. *The Evolution of Cooperation*. New York, NY: Basic Books.

Axelrod, R. & Hamilton, W.D. 1981. The evolution of cooperation. *Science*, 211, 1390–1396.

Ågren, J. A. 2014. Evolutionary transitions in individuality: insights from transposable elements. *Trends in Ecology & Evolution*, 29, 90–96.

Ågren, J.A., Davies, N.G. & Foster, K.R. 2019. Enforcement is central to the evolution of cooperation. *Nature Ecology & Evolution*, 3, 1018–1029.

Baba, R. 1990. Brood parasitism and egg robbing among three freshwater fish. *Animal Behaviour*, 40, 776–778.

Babcock, R.C., Bull, G.D., Harrison, P.L., et al. 1986. Synchronous spawnings of 105 scleractinian coral species on the Great Barrier Reef. *Marine Biology*, 90, 379–394.

Babcock, R., Mundy, C., Keesing, J. & Oliver, J. 1992. Predictable and unpredictable spawning events – in-situ behavioral-data from free-spawning coral-reef invertebrates. *Invertebrate Reproduction & Development*, 22, 213–228.

Baglione, V., Canestrari, D., Marcos, J.M., Griesser, M. & Ekman, J. 2002. History, environment and social behaviour: experimentally induced cooperative breeding in the carrion crow. *Proceedings of the Royal Society of London B: Biological Sciences*, 269, 1247–1251.

Baglione, V., Canestrari, D., Marcos, J.M. & Ekman, J. 2003. Kin selection in cooperative alliances of carrion crows. *Science*, 300, 1947–1949.

Baglione, V., Canestrari, D., Marcos, J.M. & Ekman, J. 2006. Experimentally increased food resources in the natal territory promote offspring philopatry and helping in cooperatively breeding carrion crows. *Proceedings of the Royal Society B: Biological Sciences*, 273, 1529–1535.

Baird, T.A., Ryer, C.H. & Olla, B.L. 1991. Social enhancement of foraging on an ephemeral food source in juvenile walleye pollock, *Theragra chalcogramma*. *Environmental Biology of Fishes*, 31, 307–311.

Baker, W.E. & Bulkley, N. 2014. Paying it forward vs. rewarding reputation: mechanisms of generalized reciprocity. *Organization Science*, 25, 1493–1510.

Balasubramaniam, K., Berman, C., Ogawa, H. & Li, J. 2011. Using biological markets principles to examine patterns of grooming exchange in *Macaca thibetana*. *American Journal of Primatology*, 73, 1269–1279.

Balcombe, J.P. 1989. Non-breeder asymmetry in Florida scrub jays. *Evolutionary Ecology*, 3, 77–79.

Baldan, D., Hinde, C.A. & Lessells, C.M. 2019. Turn-taking between provisioning parents: partitioning alternation. *Frontiers in Ecology and Evolution*, 7, 448. doi: 10. 3389/fevo.

Balmford, A. 1992. Social dispersion and lekking in Uganda kob. *Behaviour*, 120, 177–191.

Balmford, A., Deutsch, J.C., Nefdt, R.J.C. & Clutton-Brock, T. 1993. Testing hotspot models of lek evolution: data from three species of ungulates. *Behavioral Ecology and Sociobiology*, 33, 57–65.

Balshine, S. 2012. Patterns of parental care in vertebrates. In Royle, N.J., Smiseth, P.T. & Kölliker, M. (eds), *The Evolution of Parental Care*. Oxford: Oxford University Press.

Balshine, S., Leach, B., Neat, F., et al. 2001. Correlates of group size in a cooperatively breeding cichlid fish. *Behavioral Ecology and Sociobiology*, 50, 134–140.

Balshine-Earn, S. & Lotem, A. 1998. Individual recognition in a cooperatively breeding cichlid: evidence from video playback experiments. *Behaviour*, 135, 369–386.

Balshine-Earn, S., Neat, F.C., Reid, H. & Taborsky, M. 1998. Paying to stay or paying to breed? Field evidence for direct benefits of helping behavior in a cooperatively breeding fish. *Behavioral Ecology*, 9, 432–438.

Balzarini, V., Taborsky, M., Wanner, S., Koch, F. & Frommen, J.G. 2014. Mirror, mirror on the wall: the predictive value of mirror tests for measuring aggression in fish. *Behavioral Ecology and Sociobiology*, 68, 871–878.

Balzarini, V., Taborsky, M., Villa, F. & Frommen, J.G. 2017. Computer animations of color markings reveal the function of visual threat signals in *Neolamprologus pulcher*. *Current Zoology*, 63, 45–54.

Bang, A. & Gadagkar, R. 2012. Reproductive queue without overt conflict in the primitively eusocial wasp *Ropalidia marginata*. *Proceedings of the National Academy of Sciences of the United States of America*, 109, 14494–14499.

Barak, Y. & Yomtov, Y. 1989. The advantage of group hunting in Kuhl's bat *Pipistrellus kuhli* (Microchiroptera). *Journal of Zoology*, 219, 670–675.

Barelli, C., Reichard, U.H. & Mundry, R. 2011. Is grooming used as a commodity in wild white-handed gibbons, *Hylobates lar*? *Animal Behaviour*, 82, 801–809.

Barkan, C.P., Craig, J.L., Strahl, S.D., Stewart, A.M. & Brown, J.L. 1986. Social dominance in communal Mexican jays *Aphelocoma ultramarina*. *Animal Behaviour*, 34, 175–187.

Barker, J.L., Bronstein, J.L., Friesen, M.L., et al. 2017. Synthesizing perspectives on the evolution of cooperation within and between species. *Evolution*, 71, 814–825.

Barlow, G. 2008. *The Cichlid Fishes: Nature's Grand Experiment in Evolution*. New York, NY: Basic Books.

Barlow, G.W. 1974. Contrasts in social behavior between Central American cichlid fishes and coral reef surgeonfishes. *American Zoologist*, 14, 9–34.

Barlow, G.W. 1993. The puzzling paucity of feeding territories among freshwater fishes. *Marine Behaviour & Physiology*, 23, 155–174.

Barnard, C.J. (ed.). 1984. *Producers and Scroungers: Strategies of Exploitation and Parasitism*. London: Croom Helm.

Barnard, C.J. & Sibly, R.M. 1981. Producers and scroungers: a general model and its application to captive flocks of house sparrows. *Animal Behaviour*, 29, 543–550.

Barnett, S.A. 1963. *The Rat – A Study in Behavior*. New Brunswick, NJ: AldineTransaction/Rutgers – The State University.

Barnett, S.A. & Spencer, M.M. 1951. Feeding, social behaviour and interspecific competition in wild rats. *Behaviour*, 3, 229–242.

Barrett, L., Henzi, S.P., Weingrill, T., Lycett, J.E. & Hill, R.A. 1999. Market forces predict grooming reciprocity in female baboons. *Proceedings of the Royal Society B: Biological Sciences*, 266, 665–670.

Barrett, L., Gaynor, D. & Henzi, S.P. 2002. A dynamic interaction between aggression and grooming reciprocity among female chacma baboons. *Animal Behaviour*, 63, 1047–1053.

Barta, Z.N., Houston, A.I., McNamara, J.M. & Szekely, T. 2002. Sexual conflict about parental care: the role of reserves. *American Naturalist*, 159, 687–705.

Barta, Z., McNamara, J.M., Huszar, D.B. & Taborsky, M. 2011. Cooperation among non-relatives evolves by state-dependent generalized reciprocity. *Proceedings of the Royal Society B: Biological Sciences*, 278, 843–848.

Barta, Z., Szekely, T., Liker, A. & Harrison, F. 2014. Social role specialization promotes cooperation between parents. *American Naturalist*, 183, 747–761.

Bartal, I.B., Rodgers, D.A., Sarria, M.S.B., Decety, J. & Mason, P. 2014. Pro-social behavior in rats is modulated by social experience. *Elife*, 3.

Bartlett, M.Y. & DeSteno, D. 2006. Gratitude and prosocial behavior. *Psychological Science*, 17, 319–325.

Basquill, S.P. & Grant, J.W. 1998. An increase in habitat complexity reduces aggression and monopolization of food by zebra fish (*Danio rerio*). *Canadian Journal of Zoology*, 76, 770–772.

Bateman, A.J. 1948. Intra-sexual selection in *Drosophila*. *Heredity*, 2, 349–368.

Bateson, P. 1982. Preferences for cousins in Japanese quail. *Nature*, 295, 236–237.

Bateson, P. & Laland, K.N. 2013. Tinbergen's four questions: an appreciation and an update. *Trends in Ecology & Evolution*, 28, 712–718.

Bateson, P., Gluckman, P. & Hanson, M. 2014. The biology of developmental plasticity and the Predictive Adaptive Response hypothesis. *The Journal of Physiology*, 592, 2357–2368.

Batra, L.R. & Michie, M.D. 1963. Pleomorphism in some ambrosia and related fungi. *Transactions of the Kansas Academy of Science (1903–)*, 66, 470–481.

Bayani, D.M., Taborsky, M. & Frommen, J.G. 2017. To pee or not to pee: urine signals mediate aggressive interactions in the cooperatively breeding cichlid *Neolamprologus pulcher*. *Behavioral Ecology and Sociobiology*, 71, 37.

Bean, D. & Cook, J.M. 2001. Male mating tactics and lethal combat in the nonpollinating fig wasp *Sycoscapter australis*. *Animal Behaviour*, 62, 535–542.

Beani, L. & Turillazzi, S. 1988. Alternative mating tactics in males of *Polistes dominulus* (Hymenoptera: Vespidae). *Behavioral Ecology and Sociobiology*, 22, 257–264.

Beauchamp, G. 2012. Foraging speed in staging flocks of semipalmated sandpipers: evidence for scramble competition. *Oecologia*, 169, 975–980.

Beauchamp, G. & Fernández-Juricic, E. 2004. The group-size paradox: effects of learning and patch departure rules. *Behavioral Ecology*, 16, 352–357.

Beauchamp, G. & Giraldeau, L.A. 1997. Patch exploitation in a producer–scrounger system: test of a hypothesis using flocks of spice finches (*Lonchura punctulata*). *Behavioral Ecology*, 8, 54–59.

Beauplet, G., Barbraud, C., Dabin, W., Küssener, C. & Guinet, C. 2006. Age-specific survival and reproductive performances in fur seals: evidence of senescence and individual quality. *Oikos*, 112, 430–441.

Bebbington, K. & Hatchwell, B.J. 2016. Coordinated parental provisioning is related to feeding rate and reproductive success in a songbird. *Behavioral Ecology*, 27, 652–659.

Bebbington, K., Kingma, S.A., Fairfield, E.A., et al. 2017. Kinship and familiarity mitigate costs of social conflict between Seychelles warbler neighbors. *Proceedings of the National Academy of Sciences of the United States of America*, 114, E9036–E9045.

Beck, N.R., Peakall, R. & Heinsohn, R. 2008. Social constraint and an absence of sex-biased dispersal drive fine-scale genetic structure in white-winged choughs. *Molecular Ecology*, 17, 4346–4358.

Becker, G.S. 1968. Crime and punishment: An economic approach. *Journal of Political Economy*, 76, 169–217.

Beckerman, A.P., Sharp, S.P. & Hatchwell, B.J. 2011. Predation and kin-structured populations: an empirical perspective on the evolution of cooperation. *Behavioral Ecology*, 22, 1294–1303.

Bednarz, J.C. 1988. Cooperative hunting in Harris hawks (*Parabuteo unicinctus*). *Science*, 239, 1525–1527.

Bednekoff, P.A. 1997. Mutualism among safe, selfish sentinels: a dynamic game. *American Naturalist*, 150, 373–392.

Bednekoff, P.A. & Naguib, M. 2015. Sentinel behavior: a review and prospectus. *Advances in the Study of Behavior*, 47, 115–145.

Beekman, M. & Oldroyd, B.P. 2008. When workers disunite: intraspecific parasitism by eusocial bees. *Annual Review of Entomology*, 53, 19–37.

Begon, M., Townsend, C.R. & Harper, J.L. 2006. *Ecology: From Individuals to Ecosystems* (4th ed.). Oxford: Blackwell Publishing.

Bell, G. & Collins, S. 2008. Adaptation, extinction and global change. *Evolutionary Applications*, 1(1), 3–16.

Bell, M.B.V., Nichols, H.J., Gilchrist, J.S., Cant, M.A. & Hodge, S.J. 2012. The cost of dominance: suppressing subordinate reproduction affects the reproductive success of dominant female banded mongooses. *Proceedings of the Royal Society of London B: Biological Sciences*, 279, 619–624.

Bender, N., Heg, D., Hamilton, I.M., et al. 2006. The relationship between social status, behaviour, growth and steroids in male helpers and breeders of a cooperatively breeding cichlid. *Hormones and Behavior*, 50, 173–182.

Bentley, M.G., Olive, P.J.W. & Last, K. 2001. Sexual satellites, moonlight and the nuptial dances of worms: The influence of the Moon on the reproduction of marine animals. *Earth, Moon and Planets*, 85, 67–84.

Bengtsson, B.O. 1978. Avoiding inbreeding: at what cost? *Journal of Theoretical Biology*, 73, 439–444.

Benoit-Bird, K.J. & Au, W.W. 2009. Cooperative prey herding by the pelagic dolphin, *Stenella longirostris*. *Journal of the Acoustical Society of America*, 125, 125–137.

Benson-Amram, S., Dantzer, B., Stricker, G., Swanson, E.M. & Holekamp, K.E. 2016. Brain size predicts problem-solving ability in mammalian carnivores. *Proceedings of the National Academy of Sciences of the United States of America*, 113, 2532–2537.

Benton, T.G. & Foster, W.A. 1992. Altruistic housekeeping in a social aphid. *Proceedings of the Royal Society B: Biological Sciences*, 247, 199–202.

Bercovitch, F.B. 1988. Coalitions, cooperation and reproductive tactics among adult male baboons. *Animal Behaviour*, 36, 1198–1209.

Berec, M. & Bajgar, A. 2011. Choosy outsiders? Satellite males associate with sexy hosts in the European tree frog *Hyla arborea. Acta Zoologica Academiae Scientiarum Hungaricae*, 57, 247–254.

Berg, E.C. 2005. Parentage and reproductive success in the white-throated magpie-jay, *Calocitta formosa*, a cooperative breeder with female helpers. *Animal Behaviour*, 70, 375–385.

Berg, E.C., Eadie, J.M., Langen, T.A. & Russell, A.F. 2009. Reverse sex-biased philopatry in a cooperative bird: genetic consequences and a social cause. *Molecular Ecology*, 18, 3486–3499.

Berger-Tal, R., Lubin, Y., Settepani, V., et al. 2015. Evidence for loss of nepotism in the evolution of permanent sociality. *Scientific Reports*, 5, 13284.

Berghänel, A., Ostner, J., Schröder, U. & Schülke, O. 2011. Social bonds predict future cooperation in male Barbary macaques, *Macaca sylvanus. Animal Behaviour*, 81, 1109–1116.

Bergmüller, R. & Taborsky, M. 2005. Experimental manipulation of helping in a cooperative breeder: helpers 'pay to stay' by pre-emptive appeasement. *Animal Behaviour*, 69, 19–28.

Bergmüller, R. & Taborsky, M. 2007. Adaptive behavioural syndromes due to strategic niche specialization. *BMC Ecology*, 7, 12.

Bergmüller, R. & Taborsky, M. 2010. Animal personality due to social niche specialisation. *Trends in Ecology & Evolution*, 25, 504–511.

Bergmüller, R., Heg, D. & Taborsky, M. 2005a. Helpers in a cooperatively breeding cichlid stay and pay or disperse and breed, depending on ecological constraints. *Proceedings of the Royal Society B: Biological Sciences*, 272, 325–331.

Bergmüller, R., Heg, D., Peer, K. & Taborsky, M. 2005b. Extended safe havens and between-group dispersal of helpers in a cooperatively breeding cichlid. *Behaviour*, 142, 1643–1667.

Bergmüller, R., Johnstone, R.A., Russell, A.F. & Bshary, R. 2007. Integrating cooperative breeding into theoretical concepts of cooperation. *Behavioural Processes*, 76, 61–72.

Bergmüller, R., Schurch, R. & Hamilton, I.M. 2010. Evolutionary causes and consequences of individual variation in cooperative behaviour. *Philosophical Transactions of the Royal Society B: Biological Sciences*, 365, 2751–2764.

Bernasconi, G. & Strassmann, J.E. 1999. Cooperation among unrelated individuals: the ant foundress case. *Trends in Ecology & Evolution*, 14, 477–482.

Bernheim, B.D. & Thomadsen, R. 2005. Memory and anticipation. *The Economic Journal*, 115, 271–304.

Bénabou, R. & Tirole, J. 2009. Over my dead body: bargaining and the price of dignity. *The American Economic Review*, 99, 459–465.

Bhadra, A. & Gadagkar, R. 2008. We know that the wasps 'know': cryptic successors to the queen in *Ropalidia marginata. Biology Letters*, 4, 634–637.

Bhadra, A., Mitra, A., Deshpande, S.A., et al. 2010. Regulation of reproduction in the primitively eusocial wasp *Ropalidia marginata*: on the trail of the queen pheromone. *Journal of Chemical Ecology*, 36, 424–431.

Biedermann, P.H.W. 2010. Observations on sex ratio and behavior of males in *Xyleborinus saxesenii* Ratzeburg (Scolytinae, Coleoptera). *Zookeys*, 56, 253–267.

Biedermann, P.H.W. & Taborsky, M. 2011. Larval helpers and age polyethism in ambrosia beetles. *Proceedings of the National Academy of Sciences of the United States of America*, 108, 17064–17069.

Biedermann, P.H.W. & Taborsky, M. 2021. Experimental social evolution of philopatry and cooperation in fungus-farming beetles. Unpublished data.

Biedermann, P.H.W., Klepzig, K.D. & Taborsky, M. 2009. Fungus cultivation by ambrosia beetles: behavior and laboratory breeding success in three xyleborine species. *Environmental Entomology*, 38, 1096–1105.

Biedermann, P.H.W., Klepzig, K.D. & Taborsky, M. 2011. Costs of delayed dispersal and alloparental care in the fungus-cultivating ambrosia beetle *Xyleborus affinis* Eichhoff (Scolytinae: Curculionidae). *Behavioral Ecology and Sociobiology*, 65, 1753–1761.

Biedermann, P.H.W., Peer, K. & Taborsky, M. 2012. Female dispersal and reproduction in the ambrosia beetle *Xyleborinus saxesenii* Ratzeburg (Coleoptera; Scolytinae). *Mitteilungen der Deutschen Gesellschaft fur Allgemeine und Angewandte Entomologie*, 18, 231–235.

Biedermann, P.H.W., Klepzig, K.D., Taborsky, M. & Six, D.L. 2013. Abundance and dynamics of filamentous fungi in the complex ambrosia gardens of the primitively eusocial beetle *Xyleborinus saxesenii* Ratzeburg (Coleoptera: Curculionidae, Scolytinae). *FEMS Microbiology Ecology*, 83, 711–723.

Bignell, D.E., Roisin, Y. & Lo, N. 2011. *Biology of Termites: A Modern Synthesis*. Heidelberg: Springer.

Bijleveld, A.I., van Gils, J.A., Jouta, J. & Piersma, T. 2015. Benefits of foraging in small groups: an experimental study on public information use in red knots *Calidris canutus. Behavioural Processes*, 117, 74–81.

Binmore, K. 2010. Bargaining in biology? *Journal of Evolutionary Biology*, 23, 1351–1363.

Birch, C.L. 1957. The meanings of competition. *The American Naturalist*, 91, 5–18.

Birch, J. & Okasha, S. 2015. Kin selection and its critics. *Bioscience*, 65, 22–32.

Bird, R.B., Scelza, B., Bird, D.W. & Smith, E.A. 2012. The hierarchy of virtue: mutualism, altruism and signaling in Martu women's cooperative hunting. *Evolution and Human Behavior*, 33, 64–78.

Birkhead, T.R. 1998. Cryptic female choice: criteria for establishing female sperm choice. *Evolution*, 52, 1212–1218.

Bischoff, L.L. 2004. The social structure of the haplodiploid bark beetle, *Xylosandrus germanus*. Diploma thesis, University of Bern, Switzerland.

Bissonnette, A., Franz, M., Schulke, O. & Ostner, J. 2014. Socioecology, but not cognition, predicts male coalitions across primates. *Behavioral Ecology*, 25, 794–801.

Black, J.M. & Owen, M. 1989. Parent–offspring relationships in wintering barnacle geese. *Animal Behaviour*, 37, 187–198.

Blanchard, D.C., Fukunagastinson, C., Takahashi, L.K., Flannelly, K.J. & Blanchard, R.J. 1984. Dominance and aggression in social groups of male and female rats. *Behavioural Processes*, 9, 31–48.

Blanckenhorn, W.U. & Caraco, T. 1992. Social subordinance and a resource queue. *The American Naturalist*, 139, 442–449.

Blanckenhorn, W.U., Morf, C. & Reuter, M. 2000. Are dung flies ideal-free distributed at their oviposition and mating site? *Behaviour*, 137, 233–248.

Blaustein, A.R., Bekoff, M. & Daniels, T.J. 1987. Kin recognition in vertebrates (excluding primates): empirical evidence. In Fletcher, D.J.C. & Michener, C.D. (eds), *Kin Recognition in Animals*, pp. 287–331. London: John Wiley.

Blažek, R., Polačik, M., Smith, C., et al. 2018. Success of cuckoo catfish brood parasitism reflects coevolutionary history and individual experience of their cichlid hosts. *Science Advances*, 4, eaar4380.

Bleay, C., Comendant, T. & Sinervo, B. 2007. An experimental test of frequency-dependent selection on male mating strategy in the field. *Proceedings of the Royal Society B: Biological Sciences*, 274, 2019–2025.

Blumstein, D.T., Ebensperger, L.A., Hayes, L.D., et al. 2010. Toward an integrative understanding of social behavior: new models and new opportunities. *Frontiers in Behavioral Neuroscience*, 4, 34.

Blurton Jones, N.G. 1984. A selfish origin for human food sharing – tolerated theft. *Ethology and Sociobiology*, 5, 1–3.

Blurton Jones, N.G. 1987. Tolerated theft, suggestions about the ecology and evolution of sharing, hoarding and scrounging. *Social Science Information Sur les Sciences Sociales*, 26, 31–54.

Boehm, C. 1999. *Hierarchy in the Forest: The Evolution of Egalitarian Behavior*. Cambridge, MA: Harvard University Press.

Boesch, C. 1994. Cooperative hunting in wild chimpanzees. *Animal Behaviour*, 48, 653–667.

Boesch, C. 2002. Cooperative hunting roles among Tai chimpanzees. *Human Nature – An Interdisciplinary Biosocial Perspective*, 13, 27–46.

Boesch, C. & Boesch, H. 1989. Hunting behavior of wild chimpanzees in the Tai National Park. *American Journal of Physical Anthropology*, 78, 547–573.

Boesch, C., Crockford, C., Herbinger, I., et al. 2008. Intergroup conflicts among chimpanzees in Tai National Park: lethal violence and the female perspective. *American Journal of Primatology: Official Journal of the American Society of Primatologists*, 70, 519–532.

Bogliani, G.I.U.S., Sergio, F.A.B.R. & Tavecchia, G.I.A.C. 1999. Woodpigeons nesting in association with hobby falcons: advantages and choice rules. *Animal Behaviour*, 57, 125–131.

Boland, C.R. 2003. An experimental test of predator detection rates using groups of free-living emus. *Ethology*, 109, 209–222.

Bonduriansky, R. & Chenoweth, S.F. 2009. Intralocus sexual conflict. *Trends in Ecology & Evolution*, 24, 280–288.

Bonneaud, C., Pérez-Tris, J., Federici, P., Chastel, O. & Sorci, G. 2006. Major histocompatibility alleles associated with local resistance to malaria in a passerine. *Evolution*, 60, 383–389.

Bonner, J.T. 1998. The origins of multicellularity. *Integrative Biology: Issues, News, and Reviews*, 1, 27–36.

Boomsma, J.J. 2007. Kin selection versus sexual selection: why the ends do not meet. *Current Biology*, 17, R673–R683.

Boomsma, J.J. 2009. Lifetime monogamy and the evolution of eusociality. *Philosophical Transactions of the Royal Society of London B: Biological Sciences*, 364, 3191–3207.

Boomsma, J.J. 2013. Beyond promiscuity: mate-choice commitments in social breeding. *Philosophical Transactions of the Royal Society B: Biological Sciences*, 368.

Borgeaud, C. & Bshary, R. 2015. Wild vervet monkeys trade tolerance and specific coalitionary support for grooming in experimentally induced conflicts. *Current Biology*, 25, 3011–3016.

Bornbusch, S.L., Lefcheck, J.S. & Duffy, J.E. 2018. Allometry of individual reproduction and defense in eusocial colonies: a comparative approach to trade-offs in social sponge dwelling *Synalpheus* shrimps. *PLoS One*, 13.

Bos, D., van de Koppel, J. & Weissing, F.J. 2004. Dark-bellied Brent geese aggregate to cope with increased levels of primary production. *Oikos*, 107, 485–496.

Böttcher, M.A. & Nagler, J. 2016. Promotion of cooperation by selective group extinction. *New Journal of Physics*, 18.

Bouchard, F. & Huneman, P. 2013. *From Groups to Individuals: Evolution and Emerging Individuality.* Cambridge, MA: MIT Press.

Boucher, D.H. 1985. *The Biology of Mutualism: Ecology and Evolution.* New York, NY: Oxford University Press.

Bourke, A.F. 2005. Genetics, relatedness and social behaviour in insect societies. In Fellowes, M., Holloway, G. & Rolff, J. (eds), *Insect Evolutionary Ecology.* Wallingford: CABI.

Bourke, A.F.G. 1999. Colony size, social complexity and reproductive conflict in social insects. *Journal of Evolutionary Biology*, 12, 245–257.

Bourke, A.F.G. 2009. The kin structure of sexual interactions. *Biology Letters*, 5, 689–692.

Bourke, A.F.G. 2011. *Principles of Social Evolution.* Oxford: Oxford University Press.

Bourke, A.F.G. 2014. Hamilton's rule and the causes of social evolution. *Philosophical Transactions of the Royal Society of London B: Biological Sciences*, 369, 20130362.

Bourke, A.F., Franks, N.R. & Franks, N.R. 1995. *Social Evolution in Ants.* Princeton, NJ: Princeton University Press.

Bowles, S. 2009. Did warfare among ancestral hunter-gatherers affect the evolution of human social behaviors? *Science*, 324, 1293–1298.

Bowles, S. & Gintis, H. 2013. *A Cooperative Species: Human Reciprocity and Its Evolution.* Princeton, NJ: Princeton University Press.

Box, G.E. & Draper, N.R. 1987. *Empirical Model-Building and Response Surfaces.* Oxford: John Wiley & Sons.

Boyd, R. & Richerson, P.J. 1988. The evolution of reciprocity in sizable groups. *Journal of Theoretical Biology*, 132, 337–356.

Boyd, R. & Richerson, P.J. 1989. The evolution of indirect reciprocity. *Social Networks*, 11, 213–236.

Boyd, R. & Richerson, P.J. 1992. Punishment allows the evolution of cooperation (or anything else) in sizable groups. *Ethology and Sociobiology*, 13, 171–195.

Boyd, R., Gintis, H., Bowles, S. & Richerson, P.J. 2003. The evolution of altruistic punishment. *Proceedings of the National Academy of Sciences of the United States of America*, 100, 3531–3535.

Boydston, E.E., Morelli, T.L. & Holekamp, K.E. 2001. Sex differences in territorial behavior exhibited by the spotted hyena (Hyaenidae, *Crocuta crocuta*). *Ethology*, 107, 369–385.

Bradley, B.J., Doran-Sheehy, D.M. & Vigilant, L. 2007. Potential for female kin associations in wild western gorillas despite female dispersal. *Proceedings of the Royal Society of London B: Biological Sciences*, 274, 2179–2185.

Brahma, A., Mandal, S. & Gadagkar, R. 2018. Emergence of cooperation and division of labor in the primitively eusocial wasp *Ropalidia marginata. Proceedings of the National Academy of Sciences of the United States of America*, 115, 756–761.

Brahma, A., Mandal, S. & Gadagkar, R. 2019. To leave or to stay: direct fitness through natural nest foundation in a primitively eusocial wasp. *Insectes Sociaux*, 66, 335–342.

Branconi, R., Baracchi, D., Turillazzi, S. & Cervo, R. 2018. Testing the signal value of clypeal black patterning in an Italian population of the paper wasp *Polistes dominula. Insectes Sociaux*, 65, 161–169.

Brandl, S. & Bellwood, D. 2015. You watch my back and I'll watch yours: coordinated vigilance and reciprocal cooperation in coral reef rabbitfishes. *Scientific Reports*, 5, 14556.

Brandt, H., Ohtsuki, H., Iwasa, Y. & Sigmund, K. 2007. Survey of indirect reciprocity. In Takeuchi, Y., Iwasa, Y. & Sato, K. (eds), *Mathematics for Ecology and Environmental Sciences*, pp. 21–49. Berlin: Springer.

Brandt, M., Foitzik, S., Fischer-Blass, B. & Heinze, J. 2005. The coevolutionary dynamics of obligate ant social parasite system – between prudence and antagonism. *Biological Reviews*, 80, 251–267.

Breder, C.M. & Rosen, D.E. 1966. *Modes of Reproduction in Fishes.* Garden City, NY: Natural History Press.

Breitwisch, R. 1992. Tickling for ticks. *Natural History*, 101, 56–63.

Brent, L.J., Franks, D.W., Foster, E.A., et al. 2015. Ecological knowledge, leadership, and the evolution of menopause in killer whales. *Current Biology*, 25, 746–750.

Bridge, C. & Field, J. 2007. Queuing for dominance: gerontocracy and queue-jumping in the hover wasp *Liostenogaster flavolineata. Behavioral Ecology and Sociobiology*, 61, 1253–1259.

Briffa, M. & Elwood, R.W. 2009. Difficulties remain in distinguishing between mutual and self-assessment in animal contests. *Animal Behaviour*, 77, 759–762.

Briffa, M. & Fortescue, K.J. 2017. Motor pattern during fights in the hermit crab *Pagurus bernhardus*: evidence for the role of skill in animal contests. *Animal Behaviour*, 128, 13–20.

Briffa, M. & Hardy, I.C. 2013. Introduction to animal contests. In Hardy, I.C.W. & Briffa, M. (eds), *Animal Contests*, pp. 1–4. Cambridge: Cambridge University Press.

Briffa, M. & Sneddon, L.U. 2007. Physiological constraints on contest behaviour. *Functional Ecology*, 21, 627–637.

Briffa, M., Hardy, I.C., Gammell, M.P., et al. 2013. Analysis of animal contest data. In Hardy, I.C.W. & Briffa, M. (eds), *Animal Contests*, pp. 47–85. Cambridge: Cambridge University Press.

Bright, M. & Bulgheresi, S. 2010. A complex journey: transmission of microbial symbionts. *Nature Reviews Microbiology*, 8, 218.

Brockmann, H.J. 2001. The evolution of alternative strategies and tactics. *Advances in the Study of Behavior*, 30, 1–51.

Brockmann, H.J. & Taborsky, M. 2008. Alternative reproductive tactics and the evolution of alternative allocation phenotypes. In Oliveira, R.F., Taborsky, M. & Brockmann, H.J. (eds), *Alternative Reproductive Tactics*, pp. 25–51. Cambridge: Cambridge University Press.

Bro-Jørgensen, J. 2003. The significance of hotspots to lekking topi antelopes (*Damaliscus lunatus*). *Behavioral Ecology and Sociobiology*, 53, 324–331.

Bronstein, J.L. 1994a. Conditional outcomes in mutualistic interactions. *Trends in Ecology & Evolution*, 9, 214–217.

Bronstein, J.L. 1994b. Our current understanding of mutualism. *Quarterly Review of Biology*, 69, 31–51.

Bronstein, J.L. 2015. *Mutualism*. Oxford: Oxford University Press.

Bronstein, J.L., Alarcon, R. & Geber, M. 2006. The evolution of plant–insect mutualisms. *New Phytologist*, 172, 412–428.

Brooker, M.G., Rowley, I., Adams, M. & Baverstock, P.R. 1990. Promiscuity: an inbreeding avoidance mechanism in a socially monogamous species? *Behavioral Ecology and Sociobiology*, 26, 191–199.

Broom, M., Johanis, M. & Rychtá, J. 2015. The effect of fight cost structure on fighting behaviour. *Journal of Mathematical Biology*, 71, 979–996.

Brosnan, S.F., Salwiczek, L. & Bshary, R. 2010. The interplay of cognition and cooperation. *Philosophical Transactions of the Royal Society of London B: Biological Sciences*, 365, 2699–2710.

Brouwer, L., Heg, D. & Taborsky, M. 2005. Experimental evidence for helper effects in a cooperatively breeding cichlid. *Behavioral Ecology*, 16, 667–673.

Brouwer, L., Richardson, D.S., Eikenaar, C. & Komdeur, J. 2006. The role of group size and environmental factors on survival in a cooperatively breeding tropical passerine. *Journal of Animal Ecology*, 75, 1321–1329.

Brouwer, L., Tinbergen, J.M., Both, C., et al. 2009. Experimental evidence for density-dependent reproduction in a cooperatively breeding passerine. *Ecology*, 90, 729–741.

Brouwer, L., Van De Pol, M., Atema, E.L.S. & Cockburn, A. 2011. Strategic promiscuity helps avoid inbreeding at multiple levels in a cooperative breeder where both sexes are philopatric. *Molecular Ecology*, 20, 4796–4807.

Brouwer, L., Richardson, D.S. & Komdeur, J. 2012. Helpers at the nest improve late-life offspring performance: evidence from a long-term study and a cross-foster experiment. *Plos One*, 7, e33167.

Brouwer, L., van de Pol, M. & Cockburn, A. 2014. The role of social environment on parental care: offspring benefit more from the presence of female than male helpers. *Journal of Animal Ecology*, 83, 491–503.

Brown, C., Garwood, M.P. & Williamson, J.E. 2012. It pays to cheat: tactical deception in a cephalopod social signalling system. *Biology Letters*, 8, 729–732.

Brown, C.R. 1986. Cliff swallow colonies as information centers. *Science*, 234, 83–85.

Brown, C.R., Brown, M.B. & Shaffer, M.L. 1991. Food-sharing signals among socially foraging cliff swallows. *Animal Behaviour*, 42, 551–564.

Brown, J.L. 1964. The evolution of diversity in avian territorial systems. *The Wilson Bulletin*, 76, 160–169.

Brown, J.L. 1980. Fitness in complex avian social systems. In Markl, H. (ed.), *Evolution of Social Behavior: Hypotheses and Empirical Tests*, pp. 115–128. Weinheim: Verlag Chemie.

Brown, J.L. 1983. Cooperation – a biologists dilemma. *Advances in the Study of Behavior*, 13, 1–37.

Brown, J.L. 1987. *Helping and Communal Breeding in Birds: Ecology and Evolution*. Princeton, NJ: Princeton University Press.

Brown, J.L. & Brown, E.R. 1980. Reciprocal aid-giving in a communal bird. *Zeitschrift für Tierpsychologie – Journal of Comparative Ethology*, 53, 313–324.

Brown, J.L. & Brown, E.R. 1984. Parental facilitation: parent–offspring relations in communally breeding birds. *Behavioral Ecology and Sociobiology*, 14, 203–209.

Brown, J.L. & Brown, E.R. 1990. Mexican jays: uncooperative breeding. In Stacey, P.B. & Koenig, W.D. (eds), *Cooperative Breeding in Birds*, pp. 267–288. Cambridge: Cambridge University Press.

Brown, J.L. & Orians, G.H. 1970. Spacing patterns in mobile animals. *Annual Review of Ecology and Systematics*, 1, 239–262.

Brown, W.L. & Wilson, E.O. 1956. Character displacement. *Systematic Zoology*, 5, 49–64.

Browne, F.G. 1961. The biology of Malayan Scolytidae and Platypodidae. *Malayan Forest Records*, 22, 1–255.

Browne, F.G. 1965. Types of ambrosia beetle attack on living trees. *Proceedings of the International Congress of Entomology*, 12, 680.

Brucks, D. & von Bayern, A.M.P. 2020. Parrots voluntarily help each other to obtain food rewards. *Current Biology*, 30, 292–297.

Bruintjes, R. & Taborsky, M. 2008. Helpers in a cooperative breeder pay a high price to stay: effects of demand, helper size and sex. *Animal Behaviour*, 75, 1843–1850.

Bruintjes, R. & Taborsky, M. 2011. Size-dependent task specialization in a cooperative cichlid in response to experimental variation of demand. *Animal Behaviour*, 81, 387–394.

Bruintjes, R., Hekman, R. & Taborsky, M. 2010. Experimental global food reduction raises resource acquisition costs of brood care helpers and reduces their helping effort. *Functional Ecology*, 24, 1054–1063.

Bruintjes, R., Bonfils, D., Heg, D. & Taborsky, M. 2011. Paternity of subordinates raises cooperative effort in cichlids. *PLoS One*, 6, e25673.

Bruintjes, R., Heg-Bachar, Z. & Heg, D. 2013. Subordinate removal affects parental investment, but not offspring survival in a cooperative cichlid. *Functional Ecology*, 27, 730–738.

Bruintjes, R., Lynton-Jenkins, J., Jones, J.W., et al. 2016. Out-group threat promotes within-group affiliation in a cooperative fish. *The American Naturalist*, 187, 274–282.

Brunner, E. & Heinze, J. 2009. Worker dominance and policing in the ant *Temnothorax unifasciatus*. *Insectes Sociaux*, 56, 397–404.

Bshary, R. 2002. Biting cleaner fish use altruism to deceive image-scoring client reef fish. *Proceedings of the Royal Society B: Biological Sciences*, 269, 2087–2093.

Bshary, R. & Bergmüller, R. 2008. Distinguishing four fundamental approaches to the evolution of helping. *Journal of Evolutionary Biology*, 21, 405–420.

Bshary, R. & Grutter, A.S. 2002. Asymmetric cheating opportunities and partner control in a cleaner fish mutualism. *Animal Behaviour*, 63, 547–555.

Bshary, R. & Grutter, A.S. 2005. Punishment and partner switching cause cooperative behaviour in a cleaning mutualism. *Biology Letters*, 1, 396–399.

Bshary, R. & Grutter, A.S. 2006. Image scoring and cooperation in a cleaner fish mutualism. *Nature*, 441, 975–978.

Bshary, R. & Schäffer, D. 2002. Choosy reef fish select cleaner fish that provide high-quality service. *Animal Behaviour*, 63, 557–564.

Bshary, R., Hohner, A., Ait-el-Djoudi, K. & Fricke, H. 2006. Interspecific communicative and coordinated hunting between groupers and giant moray eels in the Red Sea. *PLoS Biology*, 4, e431.

Bshary, R., Zuberbuhler, K. & van Schaik, C.P. 2016. Why mutual helping in most natural systems is neither conflict-free nor based on maximal conflict. *Philosophical Transactions of the Royal Society B: Biological Sciences*, 371, 20150091.

Buckley, N.J. 1996. Food finding and the influence of information, local enhancement, and communal roosting on foraging success of North American vultures. *The Auk*, 113, 473–488.

Buckley, N.J. 1997. Experimental tests of the information-center hypothesis with black vultures (*Coragypsatratus*) and turkey vultures (*Cathartesaura*). *Behavioral Ecology and Sociobiology*, 41, 267–279.

Bugnyar, T. & Kotrschal, K. 2002. Observational learning and the raiding of food caches in ravens, *Corvus corax*: is it 'tactical' deception? *Animal Behaviour*, 64, 185–195.

Bugnyar, T. & Kotrschal, K. 2004. Leading a conspecific away from food in ravens (*Corvus corax*)? *Animal Cognition*, 7, 69–76.

Burgerhout, E., Tudorache, C., Brittijn, S.A., et al. 2013. Schooling reduces energy consumption in swimming male European eels, *Anguilla anguilla* L. *Journal of Experimental Marine Biology and Ecology*, 448, 66–71.

Burke, T., Davies, N.B., Bruford, M.W. & Hatchwell, B.J. 1989. Parental care and mating behaviour of polyandrous dunnocks *Prunella modularis* related to paternity by DNA fingerprinting. *Nature*, 338, 249–251.

Burnet, F.M. 1970. The concept of immunological surveillance. *Immunological Aspects of Neoplasia*, 13, 1–27.

Burnovski, M. & Safra, Z. 1994. Deterrence effects of sequential punishment policies: should repeat offenders be more severely punished? *International Review of Law and Economics*, 14, 341–350.

Burt, A. & Trivers, R. 2006. *Genes in Conflict: the Biology of Selfish Genetic Elements*. Cambridge, MA: Harvard University Press.

Burt, D.B. & Peterson, A.T. 1993. Biology of cooperative-breeding scrub jays (*Aphelocoma coerulescens*) of Oaxaca, Mexico. *The Auk*, 110, 207–214.

Buss, L.W. 1987. *The Evolution of Individuality*. Princeton, NJ: Princeton University Press.

Buston, P. 2003a. Forcible eviction and prevention of recruitment in the clown anemonefish. *Behavioral Ecology*, 14, 576–582.

Buston, P. 2003b. Social hierarchies: size and growth modification in clownfish. *Nature*, 424, 145–146.

Buston, P.M. & Cant, M.A. 2006. A new perspective on size hierarchies in nature: patterns, causes, and consequences. *Oecologia*, 149, 362–372.

Buston, P.M., Fauvelot, C., Wong, M.Y. & Planes, S. 2009. Genetic relatedness in groups of the humbug damselfish *Dascyllus aruanus*: small, similar-sized individuals may be close kin. *Molecular Ecology*, 18, 4707–4715.

Buzatto, B.A., Tomkins, J.L. & Simmons, L.W. 2014. Alternative phenotypes within mating systems. In Shuker, D. & Simmons, L. (eds), *The Evolution of Insect Mating Systems*, pp. 106–128. Oxford: Oxford University Press.

Byrne, R.W. 2007. Ape society: trading favours. *Current Biology*, 17, R775–R776.

Cade, W.H. & Cade, S. 1992. Male mating success, calling and searching behaviour at high and low densities in the field cricket, *Gryllus integer*. *Animal Behaviour*, 43, 49–56.

Caine, N.G., Addington, R.L. & Windfelder, T.L. 1995. Factors affecting the rates of food calls given by red-bellied tamarins. *Animal Behaviour*, 50, 53–60.

Cam, E., Link, W.A., Cooch, E.G., Monnat, J.Y. & Danchin, E. 2002. Individual covariation in life-history traits: seeing the trees despite the forest. *The American Naturalist*, 159, 96–105.

Cam, E., Monnat, J. & Royle, A. 2004. Dispersal and individual quality in a long lived species. *Oikos*, 106, 386–398.

Campbell, L.A., Tkaczynski, P.J., Lehmann, J., Mouna, M. & Majolo, B. 2018. Social thermoregulation as a potential mechanism linking sociality and fitness: Barbary macaques with more social partners form larger huddles. *Scientific Reports*, 8, 6074.

Campenni, M., Manciocco, A., Vitale, A. & Schino, G. 2015. Exchanging grooming, but not tolerance and aggression in common marmosets (*Callithrix jacchus*). *American Journal of Primatology*, 77, 222–228.

Canestrari, D., Marcos, J.M. & Baglione, V. 2005. Effect of parentage and relatedness on the individual contribution to cooperative chick care in carrion crows *Corvus corone corone*. *Behavioral Ecology and Sociobiology*, 57, 422–428.

Canestrari, D., Marcos, J.M. & Baglione, V. 2011. Helpers at the nest compensate for reduced maternal investment in egg size in carrion crows. *Journal of Evolutionay Biology*, 24, 1870–1878.

Caniglia, G. 2015. Understanding societies from inside the organisms. Leo Pardi's work on social dominance in *Polistes* wasps (1937–1952). *Journal of the History of Biology*, 48, 455–486.

Canonge, S., Deneubourg, J.L. & Sempo, G. 2011. Group living enhances individual resources discrimination: the use of public information by cockroaches to assess shelter quality. *PLoS One*, 6.

Cant, M.A. 1998. A model for the evolution of reproductive skew without reproductive suppression. *Animal Behaviour*, 55, 163–169.

Cant, M.A. 2000. Social control of reproduction in banded mongooses. *Animal Behaviour*, 59, 147–158.

Cant, M.A. 2003. Patterns of helping effort in cooperatively breeding banded mongooses (*Mungos mungo*). *Journal of Zoology*, 259, 115–121.

Cant, M.A. 2006. A tale of two theories: parent–offspring conflict and reproductive skew. *Animal Behaviour*, 71, 255–263.

Cant, M.A. 2011. The role of threats in animal cooperation. *Proceedings of the Royal Society B: Biological Sciences*, 278, 170–178.

Cant, M.A. 2012. Suppression of social conflict and evolutionary transitions to cooperation. *American Naturalist*, 179, 293–301.

Cant, M.A. & Croft, D.P. 2019. Life-history evolution: grandmothering in space and time. *Current Biology*, 29 (6), R215–R218.

Cant, M.A. & Field, J. 2001. Helping effort and future fitness in cooperative animal societies. *Proceedings of the Royal Society of London B: Biological Sciences*, 268, 1959–1964.

Cant, M.A. & Johnstone, R.A. 1999. Costly young and reproductive skew in animal societies. *Behavioral Ecology*, 10, 178–184.

Cant, M.A. & Johnstone, R.A. 2006. Self-serving punishment and the evolution of cooperation. *Journal of Evolutionary Biology*, 19, 1383–1385.

Cant, M.A. & Johnstone, R.A. 2008. Reproductive conflict and the separation of reproductive generations in humans. *Proceedings of the National Academy of Sciences of the United States of America*, 105, 5332–5336.

Cant, M.A. & Johnstone, R.A. 2009. How threats influence the evolutionary resolution of within-group conflict. *American Naturalist*, 173, 759–771.

Cant, M.A. & Reeve, H.K. 2002. Female control of the distribution of paternity in cooperative breeders. *American Naturalist*, 160, 602–611.

Cant, M.A. & Shen, S.F. 2006. Endogenous timing in competitive interactions among relatives. *Proceedings of the Royal Society of London B: Biological Sciences*, 273, 171–178.

Cant, M.A. & Young, A.J. 2013. Resolving social conflict among females without overt aggression. *Philosophical Transactions of the Royal Society of London B: Biological Sciences*, 368, 20130076.

Cant, M.A., English, S., Reeve, H.K. & Field, J. 2006a. Escalated conflict in a social hierachy. *Proceedings of the Royal Society B: Biological Sciences*, 273, 1471–2954.

Cant, M.A., Llop, J.B. & Field, J. 2006b. Individual variation in social aggression and the probability of inheritance: theory and a field test. *American Naturalist*, 167, 837–852.

Cant, M.A., Hodge, S.J., Gilchrist, J.S., Bell, M.B.V. & Nichols, H.J. 2010. Reproductive control via eviction (but not the threat of eviction) in banded mongooses. *Proceedings of the Royal Society of London B: Biological Sciences*, 277, 2219–2226.

Cant, M.A., Vitikainen, E. & Nichols, H.J. 2013. Demography and social evolution of banded mongooses. *Advances in the Study of Behavior*, 45, 407–445.

Cant, M.A., Nichols, H.J., Johnstone, R.A. & Hodge, S.J. 2014. Policing of reproduction by hidden threats in a cooperative mammal. *Proceedings of the National Academy of Sciences of the United States of America*, 111, 326–330.

Cant, M.A., Nichols, H.J., Thompson, F.J. & Vitikainen, E.I. 2016. Banded mongooses: demography, life history, and social behavior. In Koenig, W.D. & Dickinson, J.L. (eds), *Cooperative Breeding in Vertebrates: studies of ecology, evolution and behavior*, pp. 318–337. Cambridge: Cambridge University Press.

Carayon, J. 1966. *Traumatic insemination and the paragenital system. Monograph of Cimicidae (Hemiptera, Heteroptera)*, pp. 81–166. College Park, MD: Entomological Society of America.

Carazo, P., Tan, C.K., Allen, F., Wigby, S. & Pizzari, T. 2014. Within-group male relatedness reduces harm to females in *Drosophila*. *Nature*, 505, 672.

Carbone, C. & Taborsky, M. 1996. Mate choice or harassment avoidance? A question of female control at the lek. *Behavioral Ecology*, 7, 370–378.

Carey, H.V. & Moore, P. 1986. Foraging and predation risk in yellow-bellied marmots. *American Midland Naturalist*, 267–275.

Carlstead, K. 1986. Predictability of feeding: its effect on agonistic behaviour and growth in grower pigs. *Applied Animal Behaviour Science*, 16, 25–38.

Carne, C., Wiper, S. & Semple, S. 2011. Reciprocation and interchange of grooming, agonistic support, feeding tolerance, and aggression in semi-free-ranging Barbary macaques. *American Journal of Primatology*, 73, 1127–1133.

Carpenter, F.L. 1987. Food abundance and territoriality – to defend or not to defend. *American Zoologist*, 27, 387–399.

Carpenter, F.L. & Macmillen, R.E. 1976. Threshold model of feeding territoriality and test with a Hawaiian honeycreeper. *Science*, 194, 639–642.

Carter, G. 2014. The reciprocity controversy. *Animal Behavior and Cognition*, 1, 368–386.

Carter, G.G. & Wilkinson, G.S. 2013. Food sharing in vampire bats: reciprocal help predicts donations more than relatedness or harassment. *Proceedings of the Royal Society B: Biological Sciences*, 280, 20122573.

Carter, G.G. & Wilkinson, G.S. 2015. Social benefits of non-kin food sharing by female vampire bats. *Proceedings of the Royal Society B: Biological Sciences*, 282, 20152524.

Carter, G.G. & Wilkinson, G.S. 2016. Common vampire bat contact calls attract past food-sharing partners. *Animal Behaviour*, 116, 45–51.

Carter, G.G., Farine, D.R. & Wilkinson, G.S. 2017. Social bet-hedging in vampire bats. *Biology Letters*, 13.

Carter, G.G., Schino, G. & Farine, D. 2019. Challenges in assessing the roles of nepotism and reciprocity in cooperation networks. *Animal Behaviour*, 150, 255–271.

Carter, G.G., Farine, D.R., Crisp, R.J., et al. 2020. Development of new food-sharing relationships in vampire bats. *Current Biology*, 30, 1275–1279.

Case, T.J. & Gilpin, M.E. 1974. Interference competition and niche theory. *Proceedings of the National Academy of Sciences of the United States of America*, 71, 3073–3077.

Cervo, R., Dapporto, L., Beani, L., Strassmann, J.E. & Turillazzi, S. 2008. On status badges and quality signals in the paper wasp *Polistes dominulus*: body size, facial colour patterns and hierarchical rank. *Proceedings of the Royal Society B: Biological Sciences*, 275, 1189–1196.

Chakrabarti, S. & Jhala, Y.V. 2017. Selfish partners: resource partitioning in male coalitions of Asiatic lions. *Behavioral Ecology*, 28, 1532–1539.

Chancellor, R.L. & Isbell, L.A. 2009. Female grooming markets in a population of gray-cheeked mangabeys (*Lophocebus albigena*). *Behavioral Ecology*, 20, 79–86.

Chandrashekara, K. & Gadagkar, R. 1992. Queen succession in the primitively eusocial tropical wasp *Ropalidia marginata* (Lep.) (Hymenoptera: Vespidae). *Journal of Insect Behaviour*, 5, 193–209.

Chapman, S.N., Pettay, J.E., Lummaa, V. & Lahdenperä, M. 2019a. Limits to fitness benefits of prolonged post-reproductive lifespan in women. *Current Biology*, 29, 645–650.

Chapman, S.N., Jackson, J., Htut, W., Lummaa, V. & Lahdenperä, M. 2019b. Asian elephants exhibit post-reproductive lifespans. *BMC Evolutionary Biology*, 19, 193.

Chapman, T. 2006. Evolutionary conflicts of interest between males and females. *Current Biology*, 16, R744–R754.

Chapuisat, M. & Keller, L. 1999. Testing kin selection with sex allocation data in eusocial Hymenoptera. *Heredity*, 82, 473.

Charlesworth, D. & Charlesworth, B. 1987. Inbreeding depression and its evolutionary consequences. *Annual Review of Ecology and Systematics*, 18, 237–268.

Charnov, E.L. 1978a. Evolution of eusocial behavior: offspring choice or parental parasitism? *Journal of Theoretical Biology*, 75, 451–465.

Charnov, E.L. 1978b. Sex-ratio selection in eusocial Hymenoptera. *The American Naturalist*, 112, 317–326.

Charnov, E.L. 1982. *The Theory of Sex Allocation* (18th ed.). Princeton, NJ: Princeton University Press.

Chase, I. 1980. Cooperative and non-cooperative behavior in animals. *American Naturalist*, 115, 827–857.

Chellappa, S. & Huntingford, F.A. 1989. Depletion of energy reserves during reproductive aggression in male three-spined stickleback, *Gasterostem aculeatus* L. *Journal of Fish Biology*, 35, 315-316.

Chen, M.K. & Hauser, M. 2005. Modeling reciprocation and cooperation in primates: evidence for a punishing strategy. *Journal of Theoretical Biology*, 235, 5–12.

Chen, S.H., Fan, Z.Y., Chen, C.S. & Lu, Y.W. 2011. The breeding biology of Chinese crested terns in mixed species colonies in eastern China. *Bird Conservation International*, 21, 266–273.

Cheney, D.L. 2011. Extent and limits of cooperation in animals. *Proceedings of the National Academy of Sciences of the United States of America*, 108, 10902–10909.

Cheney, D.L., Moscovice, L.R., Heesen, M., Mundry, R. & Seyfarth, R.M. 2010. Contingent cooperation between wild female baboons. *Proceedings of the National Academy of Sciences of the United States of America*, 107, 9562–9566.

Chervet, N., Zöttl, M., Schürch, R., Taborsky, M. & Heg, D. 2011. Repeatability and heritability of behavioural types in a social cichlid. *International Journal of Evolutionary Biology*, 2011, 321729.

Chiang, Y.S. & Takahashi, N. 2011. Network homophily and the evolution of the pay-it-forward reciprocity. *PLoS One*, 6, e29188.

Chiba, S. & Leong, K. 2015. An example of conflicts of interest as pandering disincentives. *Economics Letters*, 131, 20–23.

Chiong, R. & Kirley, M. 2015. Promotion of cooperation in social dilemma games via generalised indirect reciprocity. *Connection Science*, 27, 417–433.

Choi, J.K. & Bowles, S. 2007. The coevolution of parochial altruism and war. *Science*, 318, 636–640.

Christe, P., Richner, H. & Oppliger, A. 1996. Of great tits and fleas: sleep baby sleep. *Animal Behaviour*, 52, 1087–1092.

Christensen, C. & Radford, A.N. 2018. Dear enemies or nasty neighbors? Causes and consequences of variation in the responses of group-living species to territorial intrusions. *Behavioral Ecology*, 29, 1004–1013.

Claidiere, N., Whiten, A., Mareno, M.C., et al. 2015. Selective and contagious prosocial resource donation in capuchin monkeys, chimpanzees and humans. *Scientific Reports*, 5, 7631.

Clark, C.W. & Mangel, M. 1986. The evolutionary advantages of group foraging. *Theoretical Population Biology*, 30, 45–75.

Clarke, F.M. & Faulkes, C.G. 1997. Dominance and queen succession in captive colonies of the eusocial naked mole-rat, *Heterocephalus glaber*. *Proceedings of the Royal Society of London B: Biological Sciences*, 264, 993–1000.

Clarke, F.M. & Faulkes, C.C. 2001. Intracolony aggression in the eusocial naked mole-rat, *Heterocephalus glaber*. *Animal Behaviour*, 61, 311–324.

Clarke, F.M., Miethe, G.H. & Bennett, N.C. 2001. Reproductive suppression in female Damaraland mole-rats *Cryptomys damarensis*: dominant control or self-restraint? *Proceedings of the Royal Society of London B: Biological Sciences*, 268, 899–909.

Clarke, M.F. 1984. Co-operative breeding by the Australian bell miner *Manorina melanophrys* Latham: a test of kin selection theory. *Behavioral Ecology* and Sociobiology, 14, 137–146.

Clarke, M.F. 1989. The pattern of helping in the bell miner (*Manorina melanophrys*). *Ethology*, 80, 292–306.

Clarke, M.F. & Heathcote, C.F. 1990. Dispersal, survivorship and demography in the co-operatively-breeding bell miner *Manorina melanophrys*. *Emu*, 90, 15–23.

Clobert, J., Danchin, E., Dhondt, A.A. & Nichols, J. 2001. *Dispersal*. Oxford: Oxford University Press.

Clutton-Brock, T.H. 1985. Size, sexual dimorphism, and polygyny in primates. In Jungers, W.L. (ed.), *Size and Scaling in Primate Biology*. Advances in Primatology, pp. 51–60. Boston, MA: Springer.

Clutton-Brock, T.H. 1991. *The Evolution of Parental Care*. Princeton, NJ: Princeton University Press.

Clutton-Brock, T. 2002. Breeding together: kin selection and mutualism in cooperative vertebrates. *Science*, 296 (5565), 69–72.

Clutton-Brock, T. 2009. Cooperation between non-kin in animal societies. *Nature*, 462, 51–57.

Clutton-Brock, T. & Huchard, E. 2013a. Social competition and its consequences in female mammals. *Journal of Zoology*, 289, 151–171.

Clutton-Brock, T.H. & Huchard, E. 2013b. Social competition and selection in males and females. *Philosophical Transactions of the Royal Society B: Biological Sciences*, 368, 20130074.

Clutton-Brock, T.H. & Lukas, D. 2012. The evolution of social philopatry and dispersal in female mammals. *Molecular Ecology*, 21, 472–492.

Clutton-Brock, T.H. & Manser, M. 2016. Meerkats: cooperative breeding in the Kalahari. In Koenig, W.D. & Dickinson, J.L. (eds), *Cooperative Breeding in Vertebrates*, pp. 294–317. Cambridge: Cambridge University Press.

Clutton-Brock, T.H. & Parker, G.A. 1995a. Punishment in animal societies. *Nature*, 373, 209–216.

Clutton-Brock, T.H. & Parker, G.A. 1995b. Sexual coercion in animal societies. *Animal Behaviour*, 49, 1345–1365.

Clutton-Brock, T. & Sheldon, B.C. 2010. Individuals and populations: the role of long-term, individual-based studies of animals in ecology and evolutionary biology. *Trends in Ecology & Evolution*, 25, 562–573.

Clutton-Brock, T.H., Albon, S.D. & Guinness, F.E. 1989. Fitness costs of gestation and lactation in wild mammals. *Nature*, 337, 260.

Clutton-Brock, T.H., Deutsch, J.C. & Nefdt, R.J.C. 1993. The evolution of ungulate leks. *Animal Behaviour*, 46, 1121–1138.

Clutton-Brock, T.H., Brotherton, P.N.M., Smith, R., et al. 1998. Infanticide and expulsion of females in a cooperative mammal. *Proceedings of the Royal Society of London B: Biological Sciences*, 265, 2291–2295.

Clutton-Brock, T.H., Gaynor, D., McIlrath, G.M., et al. 1999a. Predation, group size and mortality in a cooperative mongoose, *Suricata suricatta*. *Journal of Animal Ecology*, 68, 672–683.

Clutton-Brock, T.H., O'Riain, M.J., Brotherton, P.N., et al. 1999b. Selfish sentinels in cooperative mammals. *Science*, 284, 1640–1644.

Clutton-Brock, T.H., Brotherton, P.N.M., O'Riain, M.J., et al. 2000. Individual contributions to babysitting in a cooperative mongoose, *Suricata suricatta*. *Proceedings of the Royal Society of London B: Biological Sciences*, 267, 301–305.

Clutton-Brock, T.H., Brotherton, P.N.M., O'Riain, M.J., et al. 2001a. Contributions to cooperative rearing in meerkats. *Animal Behaviour*, 61, 705–710.

Clutton-Brock, T.H., Brotherton, P.N., Russell, A.F., et al. 2001b. Cooperation, control, and concession in meerkat groups. *Science*, 291, 478–481.

Clutton-Brock, T.H., Russell, A.F., Sharpe, L.L. & Jordan, N.R. 2005. 'False feeding' and aggression in meerkat societies. *Animal Behaviour*, 69, 1273–1284.

Clutton-Brock, T.H., Hodge, S.J. & Flower, T.P. 2008. Group size and the suppression of subordinate reproduction in Kalahari meerkats. *Animal Behaviour*, 76, 689–700.

Clutton-Brock, T.H., Hodge, S.J., Flower, T.P., Spong, G.F. & Young, A.J. 2010. Adaptive suppression of subordinate reproduction in cooperative mammals. *The American Naturalist*, 176, 664–673.

Cockburn, A. 1998. Evolution of helping behavior in cooperatively breeding birds. *Annual Review of Ecology and Systematics*, 29, 141–177.

Cockburn, A. 2004. Mating systems and sexual conflict in birds. In Koenig, W. & Dickinson, J. (eds), *Ecology and Evolution of Cooperative Breeding in Birds*, pp. 81–101. Cambridge: Cambridge University Press.

Cockburn, A. 2006. Prevalence of different modes of parental care in birds. *Proceedings of the Royal Society of London B: Biological Sciences*, 273, 1375–1383.

Cockburn, A., Osmond, H.L., Mulder, R.A., Double, M.C. & Green, D.J. 2008. Demography of male reproductive queues in cooperatively breeding superb fairy-wrens *Malurus cyaneus*. *Journal of Animal Ecology*, 77, 297–304.

Coffie, P.A. 1998. Status of the spinynose sculpin, *Asemichthys taylori*, in Canada. *Canadian Field Naturalist*, 112, 130–132.

Cohen, L.B. & Dearborn, D.C. 2004. Great frigatebirds, *Fregata minor*, choose mates that are genetically similar. *Animal Behaviour*, 68, 1229–1236.

Collar, N.J. & Stuart, S.N. 1985. *Threatened Birds of Africa and Related Islands: The ICBP/IUCN Red Data Book*. (Third Edition, Part 1). Cambridge: International Council for Bird Preservation, and International Union for Conservation of Nature and Natural Resources.

Concannon, M.R., Stein, A.C. & Uy, J.A. 2012. Kin selection may contribute to lek evolution and trait introgression across an avian hybrid zone. *Molecular Ecology*, 21, 1477–1486.

Connor, R.C. 1986. Pseudo-reciprocity – investing in mutualism. *Animal Behaviour*, 34, 1562–1566.

Connor, R.C. 1995a. The benefits of mutualism – a conceptual framework. *Biological Reviews of the Cambridge Philosophical Society*, 70, 427–457.

Connor, R.C. 1995b. Impala allogrooming and the parceling model of reciprocity. *Animal Behaviour*, 49, 528–530.

Connor, R.C. 1995c. Altruism among non-relatives – alternatives to the prisoners-dilemma. *Trends in Ecology & Evolution*, 10, 84–86.

Connor, R.C. & Curry, R.L. 1995. Helping non-relatives – a role for deceit. *Animal Behaviour*, 49, 389–393.

Connor, R.C., Cioffi, W.R., Randic, S., et al. 2017. Male alliance behaviour and mating access varies with habitat in a dolphin social network. *Scientific Reports*, 7, 46354.

Conrad, K.F., Robertson, R.J. & Boag, P.T. 1998. Frequency of extrapair young increases in second broods of eastern phoebes. *The Auk*, 115, 497–502.

Conradt, L., Krause, J., Couzin, I.D. & Roper, T.J. 2009. 'Leading according to need' in self-organizing groups. *The American Naturalist*, 173, 304–312.

Cook, D.F. 1990. Differences in courtship, mating and postcopulatory behaviour between male morphs of the dung beetle *Onthophagus binodis* Thunberg (Coleoptera: Scarabaeidae). *Animal Behaviour*, 40, 428–436.

Cook, J.M., Compton, S.G., Herre, E.A. & West, S.A. 1997. Alternative mating tactics and extreme male dimorphism in fig wasps. *Proceedings of the Royal Society of London B: Biological Sciences*, 264, 747–754.

Cooke, S.J., Schreer, J.F., Wahl, D.H. & Philipp, D.P. 2010. Cardiovascular performance of six species of field-acclimatized centrarchid sunfish during the parental care period. *Journal of Experimental Biology*, 213, 2332–2342.

Coolen, I., van Bergen, Y., Day, R.L. & Laland, K.N. 2003. Species difference in adaptive use of public information in sticklebacks. *Proceedings of the Royal Society of London B: Biological Sciences*, 270, 2413–2419.

Cooney, R. & Bennett, N.C. 2000. Inbreeding avoidance and reproductive skew in a cooperative mammal. *Proceedings of the Royal Society of London B: Biological Sciences*, 267, 801–806.

Cooper, G.A., Levin, S.R., Wild, G. & West, S.A. 2018. Modeling relatedness and demography in social evolution. *Evolution Letters*, 2, 260–271.

Cooper, M.A., Aureli, F. & Singh, M. 2004. Between-group encounters among bonnet macaques (*Macaca radiata*). *Behavioral Ecology and Sociobiology*, 56, 217–227.

Copeland, S.R., Sponheimer, M., de Ruiter, D.J., et al. 2011. Strontium isotope evidence for landscape use by early hominins. *Nature*, 474, 76–78.

Cordero, O.X., Ventouras, L.A., DeLong, E.F. & Polz, M.F. 2012. Public good dynamics drive evolution of iron acquisition strategies in natural bacterioplankton populations. *Proceedings of the National Academy of Sciences of the United States of America*, 109, 20059–20064.

Cords, M. 2002. Friendship among adult female blue monkeys (*Cercopithecus mitis*). *Behaviour*, 139, 291–314.

Cornelissen, T., Cintra, F. & Santos, J.C. 2016. Shelter-building insects and their role as ecosystem engineers. *Neotropical entomology*, 45, 1–12.

Cornforth, D.M., Sumpter, D.J., Brown, S.P. & Brannstrom, A. 2012. Synergy and group size in microbial cooperation. *American Naturalist*, 180, 296–305.

Corning, P.A. & Szathmary, E. 2015. 'Synergistic selection': a Darwinian frame for the evolution of complexity. *Journal of Theoretical Biology*, 371, 45–58.

Cornwallis, C.K., West, S.A. & Griffin, A.S. 2009. Routes to indirect fitness in cooperatively breeding vertebrates: kin discrimination and limited dispersal. *Journal of Evolutionary Biology*, 22, 2445–2457.

Cornwallis, C.K., West, S.A., Davis, K.E. & Griffin, A.S. 2010. Promiscuity and the evolutionary transition to complex societies. *Nature*, 466, 969–972.

Cornwallis, C.K., Botero, C.A., Rubenstein, D.R., et al. 2017. Cooperation facilitates the colonization of harsh environments. *Nature Ecology & Evolution*, 1, 0057.

Courchamp, F., Grenfell, B. & Clutton-Brock, T. 1999. Population dynamics of obligate cooperators. *Proceedings of the Royal Society of London B: Biological Sciences*, 266, 557–563.

Courtene-Jones, W. & Briffa, M. 2014. Boldness and asymmetric contests: role-and outcome-dependent effects of fighting in hermit crabs. *Behavioral Ecology*, 25, 1073–1082.

Couzin, I.D. & Krause, J. 2003. Self-organization and collective behavior in vertebrates. *Advances in the Study of Behavior*, 32, 1–75.

Couzin, I.D., Krause, J., James, R., Ruxton, G.D. & Franks, N.R. 2002. Collective memory and spatial sorting in animal groups. *Journal of Theoretical Biology*, 218, 1–11.

Covas, R. & Griesser, M. 2007. Life history and the evolution of family living in birds. *Proceedings of the Royal Society of London B: Biological Sciences*, 274, 1349–1357.

Covas, R., Doutrelant, C. & du Plessis, M.A. 2004. Experimental evidence of a link between breeding conditions and the decision to breed or to help in a colonial cooperative bird. *Proceedings of the Royal Society of London. Series B: Biological Sciences*, 271, 827–832.

Covas, R., Dalecky, A., Caizergues, A. & Doutrelant, C. 2006. Kin associations and direct vs indirect fitness benefits in colonial cooperatively breeding sociable weavers *Philetairus socius*. *Behavioral Ecology and Sociobiology*, 60, 323–331.

Cox, J.A. 2012. Social grooming in the brown-headed nuthatch may have expanded functions. *Southeastern Naturalist*, 11, 771–774.

Coyne, J.A. & Sohn, J.J. 1978. Interspecific brood care in fishes: reciprocal altruism or mistaken identity? *The American Naturalist*, 112, 447–450.

Craig, D.M. 1982. Group selection versus individual selection – an experimental analysis. *Evolution*, 36, 271–282.

Crawford, J.C., Liu, Z., Nelson, T.A., Nielsen, C.K. & Bloomquist, C.K. 2009. Genetic population structure within and between beaver (*Castor canadensis*) populations in Illinois. *Journal of Mammalogy*, 90, 373–379.

Creel, S. & Creel, N.M. 1995. Communal hunting and pack size in African wild dogs, *Lycaon pictus*. *Animal Behaviour*, 50, 1325–1339.

Creel, S. & Creel, N.M. 2002. *The African Wild Dog: Behavior, Ecology, and Conservation*. Princeton, NJ: Princeton University Press.

Creel, S.R., Monfort, S.L., Wildt, D.E. & Waser, P.M. 1991. Spontaneous lactation is an adaptive result of pseudopregnancy. *Nature*, 351, 660.

Creel, S., Schuette, P. & Christianson, D. 2014. Effects of predation risk on group size, vigilance, and foraging behavior in an African ungulate community. *Behavioral Ecology*, 25, 773–784.

Cremer, S., Armitage, S.A.O. & Schmid-Hempel, P. 2007. Social immunity. *Current Biology*, 17, R693–R702.

Crespi, B.J. 1992. Eusociality in Australian gall thrips. *Nature*, 359, 724–726.

Crespi, B.J. & Ragsdale, J.E. 2000. A skew model for the evolution of sociality via manipulation: why it is better to be feared than loved. *Proceedings of the Royal Society B: Biological Sciences*, 267, 821–828.

Crick, H.Q.P. 1992. Load-lightening in cooperatively breeding birds and the cost of reproduction. *Ibis*, 134, 56–61.

Crick, J., Suchak, M., Eppley, T.M., Campbell, M.W. & de Waal, F.B. 2013. The roles of food quality and sex in chimpanzee sharing behavior (*Pan troglodytes*). *Behaviour*, 150, 1203–1224.

Crimaldi, J.P. 2012. The role of structured stirring and mixing on gamete dispersal and aggregation in broadcast spawning. *Journal of Experimental Biology*, 215, 1031–1039.

Crimaldi, J.P. & Zimmer, R.K. 2014. The physics of broadcast spawning in benthic invertebrates. *Annual Review of Marine Science*, 6(6), 141–165.

Croft, D.P., James, R., Thomas, P.O.R., et al. 2006. Social structure and co-operative interactions in a wild population of guppies (*Poecilia reticulata*). *Behavioral Ecology and Sociobiology*, 59, 644–650.

Croft, D.P., Krause, J., Darden, S.K., et al. 2009. Behavioural trait assortment in a social network: patterns and implications. *Behavioral Ecology and Sociobiology*, 63, 1495–1503.

Croft, D.P., Brent, L.J., Franks, D.W. & Cant, M.A. 2015. The evolution of prolonged life after reproduction. *Trends in Ecology & Evolution*, 30, 407–416.

Croft, D.P., Johnstone, R.A., Ellis, S., et al. 2017. Reproductive conflict and the evolution of menopause in killer whales. *Current Biology*, 27, 298–304.

Crompton, B., Thomason, J.C. & McLachlan, A. 2003. Mating in a viscous universe: the race is to the agile, not to the swift. *Proceedings of the Royal Society of London B: Biological Sciences*, 270, 1991–1995.

Cronin, K.A., Schroeder, K.K.E. & Snowdon, C.T. 2010. Prosocial behaviour emerges independent of reciprocity in cottontop tamarins. *Proceedings of the Royal Society B: Biological Sciences*, 277, 3845–3851.

Crook, J.H. 1972. Sexual selection, dimorphism and social organization in the primates. In Campbell, B.G. (ed.), *Sexual Selection and the Descent of Man*. Chicago, IL: Aldine.

Crozier, R.G. & Giese, R.L. 1967a. The Columbian timber beetle, *Corthylus columbianus* (Coleoptera: Scolytidae). III. Definition of epiphytotics. *Journal of Economic Entomology*, 60, 55–58.

Crozier, R.G. & Giese, R.L. 1967b. The Columbian timber beetle, *Corthylus columbianus* (Coleoptera: Scolytidae). IV. Intrastand population distribution. *The Canadian Entomologist*, 99, 1203–1214.

Crozier, R.H. & Pamilo, P. 1996. *Evolution of Social Insect Colonies*. Oxford: Oxford University Press.

Cubaynes, S., MacNulty, D.R., Stahler, D.R., et al. 2014. Density-dependent intraspecific aggression regulates survival in northern Yellowstone wolves (*Canis lupus*). *Journal of Animal Ecology*, 83, 1344–1356.

Curry, R.L. 1988. Influence of kinship on helping behavior in Galapagos mockingbirds. *Behavioral Ecology and Sociobiology*, 22, 141–152.

Curry, R.L. & Grant, P.R. 1990. Galapagos mockingbirds: territorial cooperative breeding in a climatically variable environment. In Stacey, P.B. & Koenig, W.D. (eds), *Cooperative Breeding in Birds: Long-Term Studies of Ecology and Behavior*, pp. 291–331. Cambridge: Cambridge University Press.

Dandekar, A.A., Chugani, S. & Greenberg, E.P. 2012. Bacterial quorum sensing and metabolic incentives to cooperate. *Science*, 338, 264–266.

Daniels, R.A. 1978. Nesting behaviour of *Harpagifer bispinis* in Arthur Harbour, Antarctic Peninsula. *Journal of Fish Biology*, 12, 465–474.

Daniels, R.A. 1979. Nest guard replacement in the Antarctic fish *Harpagifer bispinis*: possible altruistic behavior. *Science*, 205, 831–833.

Darch, S.E., West, S.A., Winzer, K. & Diggle, S.P. 2012. Density-dependent fitness benefits in quorum-sensing bacterial populations. *Proceedings of the National Academy of Sciences of the United States of America*, 109, 8259–8263.

Darwin, C. 1859. *On the Origin of Species By Means of Natural Selection, or the Preservation of Favoured Races in the Struggle for Life*. London: John Murray.

Darwin, C. 1871. *The Descent of Man, and Selection in Relation to Sex*. London: John Murray.

Dausmann, K.H., Glos, J., Ganzhorn, J.U. & Heldmaier, G. 2004. Physiology: hibernation in a tropical primate – even in the wound-down hibernating state, this lemur can warm up without waking up. *Nature*, 429, 825–826.

David, M., Gillingham, M.A.F., Salignon, M., Laskowski, K.L. & Giraldeau, L.A. 2014. Speed–accuracy trade-off and its consequences in a scramble competition context. *Animal Behaviour*, 90, 255–262.

Davies, N.B. 1986. Reproductive success of dunnocks, *Prunella modularis*, in a variable mating system. I. Factors influencing provisioning rate, nestling weight and fledging success. *The Journal of Animal Ecology*, 55, 123–138.

Davies, N.B. 1992. *Dunnock Behaviour and Social Evolution*. Oxford: Oxford University Press.

Davies, N.B. 2000. *Cuckoos, Cowbirds and Other Cheats*. London: T & AD Poyser Ltd.

Davies, N.B. 2015. *Cuckoo: Cheating by Nature*. London: Bloomsbury Publishing.

Davies, N.B. & Brooke, M. de L. 1988. Cuckoos versus reed warblers: adaptations and counteradaptations. *Animal Behaviour*, 36, 262–284.

Davies, N.B. & Brooke, M. de L. 1989a. An experimental study of co-evolution between the cuckoo, *Cuculus canorus*, and its hosts. I. Host egg discrimination. *Journal of Animal Ecology*, 58, 207–214.

Davies, N.B. & Brooke, M. de L. 1989b. An experimental study of co-evolution between the cuckoo, *Cuculus canorus* and its hosts. II. Host egg markings, chick discrimination and general discussion. *Journal of Animal Ecology*, 58, 225–236.

Davies, N.B. & Houston, A.I. 1981. Owners and satellites: the economics of territory defence in the pied wagtail, *Motacilla alba*. *The Journal of Animal Ecology*, 157–180.

Davies, N.B. & Lundberg, A. 1984. Food distribution and a variable mating system in the dunnock, *Prunella modularis*. *The Journal of Animal Ecology*, 895–912.

Davies, N.B., Bourke, A.F.G. & Brooke, M. de L. 1989. Cuckoos and parasitic ants – interspecific brood parasitism as an evolutionary arms-race. *Trends in Ecology & Evolution*, 4, 274–278.

Davies, N.B., Kilner, R.M. & Noble, D.G. 1998. Nestling cuckoos, *Cuculus canorus*, exploit hosts with begging calls that mimic a brood. *Proceedings of the Royal Society of London B: Biological Sciences*, 265, 673–678.

Davis, D.E. 1953. The characteristics of rat populations. *Quarterly Review of Biology*, 28, 373–401.

Dawkins, R. 1976 [2016]. *The Selfish Gene*. Oxford: Oxford University Press.

Dawkins, R., Krebs, J.R., Maynard, S.J. & Holliday, R. 1979. Arms races between and within species. *Proceedings of the Royal Society of London B: Biological Sciences*, 205, 489–511.

De Boer, B.A. 1981. Influence of population density on the territorial, courting and spawning behaviour of male *Chromis cyanea* (Pomacentridae). *Behaviour*, 77, 99–120.

De Fine Licht, H. & Biedermann, P.H. 2012. Patterns of functional enzyme activity in fungus farming ambrosia beetles. *Frontiers in Zoology*, 9, 13.

de Kort, S.R., Emery, N.J. & Clayton, N.S. 2006. Food sharing in jackdaws, *Corvus monedula*: what, why and with whom? *Animal Behaviour*, 72, 297–304.

De Leon, L.F., Podos, J., Gardezi, T., Herrel, A. & Hendry, A.P. 2014. Darwin's finches and their diet niches: the sympatric coexistence of imperfect generalists. *Journal of Evolutionary Biology*, 27, 1093–1104.

de Luca, D.W. & Ginsberg, J.R. 2001. Dominance, reproduction and survival in banded mongooses: towards an egalitarian social system? *Animal Behaviour*, 61, 17–30.

de Ruiter, J.R. & Geffen, E. 1998. Relatedness of matrilines, dispersing males and social groups in long-tailed macaques (*Macaca fascicularis*). *Proceedings of the Royal Society of London B: Biological Sciences*, 265, 79–87.

De Souza, A.R. & Prezoto, F. 2012. Aggressive interactions for a decentralized regulation of foraging activity in the social wasp *Polistes versicolor*. *Insectes Sociaux*, 59, 463–467.

de Waal, F.B.M. 1989. Food sharing and reciprocal obligations among chimpanzees. *Journal of Human Evolution*, 18, 433–459.

de Waal, F.B.M. 1997a. Food transfers through mesh in brown capuchins. *Journal of Comparative Psychology*, 111, 370–378.

de Waal, F.B.M. 1997b. The chimpanzee's service economy: food for grooming. *Evolution and Human Behavior*, 18, 375–386.

de Waal, F.B.M. 2000. Attitudinal reciprocity in food sharing among brown capuchin monkeys. *Animal Behaviour*, 60, 253–261.

de Waal, F.B. & Brosnan, S.F. 2006. Simple and complex reciprocity in primates. In Kappeler, P.M. & van Schaik, C.P. (eds), *Cooperation in Primates and Humans*, pp. 85–105. Berlin: Springer.

de Waal, F.B. & Luttrell, L.M. 1988. Mechanisms of social reciprocity in three primate species: symmetrical relationship characteristics or cognition? *Ethology and Sociobiology*, 9, 101–118.

de Waal, F.B.M. & Berger, M.L. 2000. Payment for labour in monkeys. *Nature*, 404, 563.

Dechmann, D.K., Kranstauber, B., Gibbs, D. & Wikelski, M. 2010. Group hunting – a reason for sociality in molossid bats? *PLoS One*, 5.

Delattre, O., Blatrix, R., Châline, N., et al. 2012. Do host species evolve a specific response to slave-making ants? *Frontiers in Zoology*, 9, 38.

DeLay, L.S., Faaborg, J., Naranjo, J., et al. 1996. Paternal care in the cooperatively polyandrous Galapagos hawk. *Condor*, 98, 300–311.

Delgado, M.M., Nicholas, M., Petrie, D.J. & Jacobs, L.F. 2014. Fox squirrels match food assessment and cache effort to value and scarcity. *PLoS One*, 9.

Delmas, G.E., Lew, S.E. & Zanutto, B.S. 2019. High mutual cooperation rates in rats learning reciprocal altruism: the role of pay-off matrix. *PLoS One*, 14.

Demsar, J. & Bajec, I.L. 2013. Family bird: a heterogeneous simulated flock. In *Advances in Artificial Life*, ECAL 12, pp. 1114–1115.

Denault, L.K. & Mcfarlane, D.A. 1995. Reciprocal altruism between male vampire bats, *Desmodus rotundus*. *Animal Behaviour*, 49, 855–856.

Desjardins, J.K., Stiver, K.A., Fitzpatrick, J.L. & Balshine, S. 2008a. Differential responses to territory intrusions in cooperatively breeding fish. *Animal Behaviour*, 75, 595–604.

Desjardins, J.K., Stiver, K.A., Fitzpatrick, J.L., et al. 2008b. Sex and status in a cooperative breeding fish: behavior and androgens. *Behavioral Ecology and Sociobiology*, 62, 785–794.

DeWoody, J.A., Fletcher, D.E., Wilkins, S.D. & Avise, J.C. 2001. Genetic documentation of filial cannibalism in nature. *Proceedings of the National Academy of Sciences of the United States of America*, 98, 5090–5092.

Dey, C.J., Reddon, A.R., O'Connor, C.M. & Balshine, S. 2013. Network structure is related to social conflict in a cooperatively breeding fish. *Animal Behaviour*, 85, 395–402.

Dey, C.J., O'Connor, C.M., Wilkinson, H., et al. 2017. Direct benefits and evolutionary transitions to complex societies. *Nature Ecology & Evolution*, 1(5), 137.

Díaz-Muñoz, S.L., DuVal, E.H., Krakauer, A.H. & Lacey, E.A. 2014. Cooperating to compete: altruism, sexual selection and causes of male reproductive cooperation. *Animal Behaviour*, 88, 67–78.

DiBitetti, M.S. 1997. Evidence for an important social role of allogrooming in a platyrrhine primate. *Animal Behaviour*, 54, 199–211.

Dickinson, J.L. 2004. A test of the importance of direct and indirect fitness benefits for helping decisions in western bluebirds. *Behavioral Ecology*, 15, 233–238.

Dickinson, J.L. & Akre, J.J. 1998. Extrapair paternity, inclusive fitness, and within-group benefits of helping in western bluebirds. *Molecular Ecology*, 7, 95–105.

Dickinson, J.L. & Hatchwell, B.J. 2004. Fitness consequences of helping. In Koenig, W.D. & Dickinson, J.L. (eds), *Ecology and Evolution of Cooperative Breeding in Birds*, pp. 48–66. Cambridge: Cambridge University Press.

Dickinson, J.L. & McGowan, A. 2005. Winter resource wealth drives delayed dispersal and family-group living in western bluebirds. *Proceedings of the Royal Society of London B: Biological Sciences*, 272, 2423–2428.

Dickinson, J.L., Koenig, W.D. & Pitelka, F.A. 1996. Fitness consequences of helping behavior in the western bluebird. *Behavioral Ecology*, 7, 168–177.

Dickinson, J.L., Ferree, E.D., Stern, C.A., Swift, R. & Zuckerberg, B. 2014. Delayed dispersal in western bluebirds: teasing apart the importance of resources and parents. *Behavioral Ecology*, 25, 843–851.

Dierkes, P., Taborsky, M. & Kohler, U. 1999. Reproductive parasitism of broodcare helpers in a cooperatively breeding fish. *Behavioral Ecology*, 10, 510–515.

Dierkes, P., Heg, D., Taborsky, M., Skubic, E. & Achmann, R. 2005. Genetic relatedness in groups is sex-specific and declines with age of helpers in a cooperatively breeding cichlid. *Ecology Letters*, 8, 968–975.

Dierkes, P., Taborsky, M. & Achmann, R. 2008. Multiple paternity in the cooperatively breeding fish *Neolamprologus pulcher*. *Behavioral Ecology and Sociobiology*, 62, 1581–1589.

Diggle, S.P., Griffin, A.S., Campbell, G.S. & West, S.A. 2007. Cooperation and conflict in quorum-sensing bacterial populations. *Nature*, 450, 411–414.

Dijk, R.E., Kaden, J.C., Ticó, A., et al. 2014. Cooperative investment in public goods is kin directed in communal nests of social birds. *Ecology Letters*, 17, 1141–1148.

Dill, L.M. 1978. Energy-based model of optimal feeding-territory size. *Theoretical Population Biology*, 14, 396–429.

Dill, L.M., Ydenberg, R.C. & Fraser, A.H.G. 1981. Food abundance and territory size in juvenile Coho salmon (*Oncorhynchus kisutch*). *Canadian Journal of Zoology–Revue Canadienne de Zoologie*, 59, 1801–1809.

Dloniak, S.M., French, J.A. & Holekamp, K.E. 2006. Rank-related maternal effects of androgens on behaviour in wild spotted hyaenas. *Nature*, 440, 1190.

Dobson, F.S. 1982. Competition for mates and predominant juvenile male dispersal in mammals. *Animal Behaviour*, 30, 1183–1192.

Dobson, F.S., Viblanc, V.A., Arnaud, C.M. & Murie, J.O. 2012. Kin selection in Columbian ground squirrels: direct and indirect fitness benefits. *Molecular Ecology*, 21, 524–531.

Doebeli, M. & Hauert, C. 2005. Models of cooperation based on the Prisoner's Dilemma and the Snowdrift game. *Ecology Letters*, 8, 748–766.

Doebeli, M. & Knowlton, N. 1998. The evolution of inter-specific mutualisms. *Proceedings of the National Academy of Sciences of the United States of America*, 95, 8676–8680.

Doerr, E.D. & Doerr, V.A. 2006. Comparative demography of treecreepers: evaluating hypotheses for the evolution and maintenance of cooperative breeding. *Animal Behaviour*, 72, 147–159.

Dolivo, V. & Taborsky, M. 2015a. Norway rats reciprocate help according to the quality of help they received. *Biology Letters*, 11, 20140959.

Dolivo, V. & Taborsky, M. 2015b. Cooperation among Norway rats: the importance of visual cues for reciprocal cooperation, and the role of coercion. *Ethology*, 121, 1071–1080.

Dolivo, V. & Taborsky, M. 2017. Environmental enrichment of young adult rats (*Rattus norvegicus*) in different sensory modalities has long-lasting effects on their ability to learn via specific sensory channels. *Journal of Comparative Psychology*, 131, 79–88.

Dolivo, V., Rutte, C. & Taborsky, M. 2016. Ultimate and proximate mechanisms of reciprocal altruism in rats. *Learning & Behavior*, 44, 223–226.

Domeier, M.L. & Colin, P.L. 1997. Tropical reef fish spawning aggregations: defined and reviewed. *Bulletin of Marine Science*, 60, 698–726.

Donaldson, L., Thompson, F.J., Field, J. & Cant, M.A. 2013. Do paper wasps negotiate over helping effort? *Behavioral Ecology*, 25, 88–94.

Double, M.C. & Cockburn, A. 2003. Subordinate superb fairy-wrens (*Malurus cyaneus*) parasitize the reproductive success of attractive dominant males. *Proceedings of the Royal Society of London B: Biological Sciences*, 270, 379–384.

Double, M.C., Peakall, R., Beck, N.R. & Cockburn, A. 2005. Dispersal, philopatry, and infidelity: dissecting local genetic structure in superb fairy-wrens (*Malurus cyaneus*). *Evolution*, 59, 625–635.

Douglas, A.E. 2010. *The Symbiotic Habit*. Princeton, NJ: Princeton University Press.

Dowds, B.M. & Elwood, R.W. 1985. Shell wars II: the influence of relative size on decisions made during hermit crab shell fights. *Animal Behaviour*, 33, 649–656.

Dowling, D.K., Richardson, D.S., Blaakmeer, K. & Komdeur, J. 2001. Feather mite loads influenced by salt exposure, age and reproductive stage in the Seychelles warbler *Acrocephalus sechellensis*. *Journal of Avian Biology*, 32, 364–369.

Downing, P.A., Griffin, A.S. & Cornwallis, C.K. 2018. Sex differences in helping effort reveal the effect of future reproduction on cooperative behaviour in birds. *Proceedings of the Royal Society of London B: Biological Sciences*, 285, 20181164.

Doyle, R.W. & Talbot, A.J. 1986. Artificial selection on growth and correlated selection on competitive behaviour in fish. *Canadian Journal of Fisheries and Aquatic Sciences*, 43, 1059–1064.

Drea, C.M. & Carter, A.N. 2009. Cooperative problem solving in a social carnivore. *Animal Behaviour*, 78, 967–977.

Drury, D.W., Siniard, A.L. & Wade, M.J. 2009. Genetic differentiation among wild populations of *Tribolium castaneum* estimated using microsatellite markers. *Journal of Heredity*, 100, 732–741.

Drury, J.P., Okamoto, K.W., Anderson, C.N. & Grether, G.F. 2015. Reproductive interference explains persistence of aggression between species. *Proceedings of the Royal Society B: Biological Sciences*, 282, 20142256.

Du Plessis, M.A. 1993. Helping behaviour in cooperatively-breeding green woodhoopoes: selected or unselected trait? *Behaviour*, 127, 49–65.

Du Plessis, M.A. & Williams, J.B. 1994. Communal cavity roosting in green woodhoopoes – consequences for energy-expenditure and the seasonal pattern of mortality. *Auk*, 111, 292–299.

Dubois, F. & Giraldeau, L.A. 2003. The forager's dilemma: food sharing and food defense as risk-sensitive foraging options. *The American Naturalist*, 162, 768–779.

Duckworth, R.A. & Badyaev, A.V. 2007. Coupling of dispersal and aggression facilitates the rapid range expansion of a passerine bird. *Proceedings of the National Academy of Sciences of the United States of America*, 104, 15017–15022.

Dufour, V., Pele, M., Neumann, M., Thierry, B. & Call, J. 2009. Calculated reciprocity after all: computation behind token transfers in orang-utans. *Biology Letters*, 5, 172–175.

Duftner, N., Sefc, K.M., Koblmuller, S., et al. 2007. Parallel evolution of facial stripe patterns in the *Neolamprologus brichardi/pulcher* species complex endemic to Lake Tanganyika. *Molecular Phylogenetics and Evolution*, 45, 706–715.

Dugatkin, L.A. 1997. *Cooperation Among Animals: an Evolutionary Perspective*. New York, NY: Oxford University Press.

Dugatkin, L.A. 2002. Animal cooperation among unrelated individuals. *Naturwissenschaften*, 89, 533–541.

Dugatkin, L.A. & Alfieri, M. 1991. Guppies and the TIT FOR TAT strategy: preference based on past interaction. *Behavioral Ecology and Sociobiology*, 28, 243–246.

Dugatkin, L.A. & Biederman, L. 1991. Balancing asymmetries in resource holding power and resource value in the pumpkinseed sunfish. *Animal Behaviour*, 42, 691–692.

Dumke, M., Herberstein, M.E. & Schneider, J.M. 2018. Advantages of social foraging in crab spiders: groups capture more and larger prey despite the absence of a web. *Ethology*, 124, 695–705.

Dunbar, R.I.M. & Dunbar, P. 1988. Maternal time budgets of gelada baboons. *Animal Behaviour*, 36, 970–980.

Dunbar, R.I.M. & Sharman, M. 1984. Is social grooming altruistic? *Zeitschrift für Tierpsychologie – Journal of Comparative Ethology*, 64, 163–173.

Duncan, C., Gaynor, D., Clutton-Brock, T. & Dyble, M. 2019. The evolution of indiscriminate altruism in a cooperatively breeding mammal. *The American Naturalist*, 193, 841–851.

Duncan, F.D. & Crewe, R.M. 1994. Group hunting in a ponerine ant, *Leptogenys nitida* Smith. *Oecologia*, 97, 118–123.

Dunford, C. 1977. Behavioral limitation of round-tailed ground squirrel density. *Ecology*, 58, 1254–1268.

Dunn, J., Dunn, D.W., Strand, M.R. & Hardy, I.C.W. 2014. Higher aggression towards closer relatives by soldier larvae in a polyembryonic wasp. *Biology Letters*, 10, 20140229.

Dunn, P.O., Cockburn, A. & Mulder, R.A. 1995. Fairy-wren helpers often care for young to which they are unrelated. *Proceedings of the Royal Society of London B: Biological Sciences*, 259, 339–343.

Durrant, R. 2011. Collective violence: an evolutionary perspective. *Aggression and Violent Behavior*, 16, 428–436.

DuVal, E.H. 2007a. Social organization and variation in cooperative alliances among male lance-tailed manakins. *Animal Behaviour*, 73, 391–401.

DuVal, E.H. 2007b. Cooperative display and lekking behavior of the lance-tailed manakin (*Chiroxiphia lanceolata*). *Auk*, 124, 1168–1185.

DuVal, E.H. 2007c. Adaptive advantages of cooperative courtship for subordinate male lance-tailed manakins. *American Naturalist*, 169, 423–432.

Earley, R.L. & Dugatkin, L.A. 2002. Eavesdropping on visual cues in green swordtail (*Xiphophorus helleri*) fights: a case for networking. *Proceedings of the Royal Society of London B: Biological Sciences*, 269, 943–952.

Ebensperger, L.A., Hurtado, M.J. & Valdivia, I. 2006. Lactating females do not discriminate between their own young and unrelated pups in the communally breeding rodent, *Octodon degus*. *Ethology*, 112, 921–929.

Eberhard, W.G. 1996. *Female Control: Sexual Selection by Cryptic Female Choice*. Princeton, NJ: Princeton University Press.

Ebersole, J.P. 1977. The adaptive significance of interspecific territoriality in the reef fish *Eupomacentrus leucostictus*. *Ecology*, 58, 914–920.

Eccard, J.A. & Ylönen, H. 2002. Direct interference or indirect exploitation? An experimental study of fitness costs of interspecific competition in voles. *Oikos*, 99, 580–590.

Edenbrow, M., Bleakley, B.H., Darden, S.K., et al. 2017. The evolution of cooperation: interacting phenotypes among social partners. *American Naturalist*, 189, 630–643.

Edvardsson, M. & Tregenza, T. 2005. Why do male *Callosobruchus maculatus* harm their mates? *Behavioral Ecology*, 16, 788–793.

Edwards, S.V. 1993. Mitochondrial gene genealogy and gene flow among island and mainland populations of a sedentary songbird, the grey-crowned babbler (*Pomatostomus temporalis*). *Evolution*, 47, 1118–1137.

Eichhoff, W. 1881. *Die Europäischen Borkenkäfer*. Berlin: Julius Springer.

Eikenaar, C., Richardson, D.S., Brouwer, L. & Komdeur, J. 2007. Parent presence, delayed dispersal, and territory acquisition in the Seychelles warbler. *Behavioral Ecology*, 18, 874–879.

Eikenaar, C., Richardson, D.S., Brouwer, L. & Komdeur, J. 2008a. Sex biased natal dispersal in a closed, saturated population of Seychelles warblers *Acrocephalus sechellensis*. *Journal of Avian Biology*, 39, 73–80.

Eikenaar, C., Richardson, D.S., Brouwer, L., Bristol, R. & Komdeur, J. 2008b. Experimental evaluation of sex differences in territory acquisition in a cooperatively breeding bird. *Behavioral Ecology*, 20, 207–214.

Eisenberg, J.F., Muckenhirn, N.A. & Rudran, R. 1972. The relation between ecology and social structure in primates. *Science*, 176, 863–874.

Ekman, J. 2004. Delayed dispersal. In Koenig, W.D. & Dickinson, J.L. (eds), *Ecology and Evolution of Cooperative Breeding in Birds*, pp. 35–47. Cambridge, MA: Cambridge University Press.

Ekman, J. 2006. Family living among birds. *Journal of Avian Biology*, 37, 289–298.

Ekman, J. & Griesser, M. 2002. Why offspring delay dispersal: experimental evidence for a role of parental tolerance. *Proceedings of the Royal Society of London B: Biological Sciences*, 269, 1709–1713.

Ekman, J., Sklepkovych, B. & Tegelstrom, H. 1994. Offspring retention in the Siberian jay (*Perisoreus infaustus*): the prolonged brood care hypothesis. *Behavioral Ecology*, 5, 245–253.

Ekman, J., Baglione, V., Eggers, S. & Griesser, M. 2001. Delayed dispersal: living under the reign of nepotistic parents. *The Auk*, 118, 1–10.

Ekvall, K. 1998. Effects of social organization, age and aggressive behaviour on allosuckling in wild fallow deer. *Animal Behaviour*, 56, 695–703.

El Mouden, C. & Gardner, A. 2008. Nice natives and mean migrants: the evolution of dispersal-dependent social behaviour in viscous populations. *Journal of Evolutionary Biology*, 21, 1480–1491.

El Mouden, C., West, S.A. & Gardner, A. 2010. The enforcement of cooperation by policing. *Evolution*, 64, 2139–2152.

Eldakar, O.T., Dlugos, M.J., Pepper, J.W. & Wilson, D.S. 2009. Population structure mediates sexual conflict in water striders. *Science*, 326, 816.

Elgar, M.A. 1986. House sparrows establish foraging flocks by giving chirrup calls if the resources are divisible. *Animal Behaviour*, 34, 169–174.

Ellis, S., Franks, D.W., Nattrass, S., et al. 2018. Analyses of ovarian activity reveal repeated evolution of post-reproductive lifespans in toothed whales. *Scientific Reports*, 8, 1–10.

Elwood, R.W. 1991. Ethical implications of studies on infanticide and maternal aggression in rodents. *Animal Behaviour*, 42, 841–849.

Ember, C.R. 1978. Myths about hunter gatherers. *Ethnology*, 17, 439–448.

Emlen, D.J. 1997. Alternative reproductive tactics and male-dimorphism in the horned beetle *Onthophagus acuminatus* (Coleoptera: Scarabaeidae). *Behavioral Ecology and Sociobiology*, 41, 335–341.

Emlen, S.T. 1982. The evolution of helping. I. An ecological constraints model. *The American Naturalist*, 119, 29–39.

Emlen, S.T. 1991. Evolution of cooperative breeding in birds and mammals. In Krebs, J.R. & Davies, N.B. (eds), *Behavioural Ecology: An Evolutionary Approach* (3rd ed.), pp. 301–337. Oxford: Blackwell.

Emlen, S.T. 1995. An evolutionary theory of the family. *Proceedings of the National Academy of Sciences of the United States of America*, 92, 8092–8099.

Emlen, S.T. 1997. Predicting family dynamics in social vertebrates. In Krebs, J.R. & Davies, N.B. (eds), *Behavioural Ecology: An Evolutionary Approach* (4th ed.), pp. 228–253. Cambridge, MA: Blackwell.

Emlen, S.T. & Oring, L.W. 1977. Ecology, sexual selection, and the evolution of mating systems. *Science*, 197, 215–223.

Emlen, S.T. & Wrege, P.H. 1988. The role of kinship in helping decisions among white-fronted bee-eaters. *Behavioral Ecology and Sociobiology*, 23, 305–315.

Emlen, S.T. & Wrege, P.H. 1991. Breeding biology of white-fronted bee-eaters at Nakuru – the influence of helpers on breeder fitness. *Journal of Animal Ecology*, 60, 309–326.

Emlen, S.T., Reeve, H.K., Sherman, P.W., et al. 1991. Adaptive versus nonadaptive explanations of behavior: the case of alloparental helping. *The American Naturalist*, 138, 259–270.

Emonds, G., Declerck, C.H., Boone, C., Vandervliet, E.J. & Parizel, P.M. 2012. The cognitive demands on cooperation in social dilemmas: an fMRI study. *Social Neuroscience*, 7, 494–509.

Endler, A., Hölldobler, B. & Liebig, J. 2007. Lack of physical policing and fertility cues in egg-laying workers of the ant *Camponotus floridanus*. *Animal Behaviour*, 74, 1171–1180.

Engelhardt, S.C. & Taborsky, M. 2020. Broad definitions of enforcement are unhelpful for understanding evolutionary mechanisms of cooperation. *Nature Ecology & Evolution*, 4, 323.

Engelhardt, S.C., Weladji, R.B., Holand, O., Roed, K.H. & Nieminen, M. 2015. Evidence of reciprocal allonursing in reindeer, *Rangifer tarandus*. *Ethology*, 121, 245–259.

Engelhardt, S.C., Bergeron, P., Gagnon, A., Dillon, L. & Pelletier, F. 2019. Using geographical distance as a potential proxy for help in the assessment of the grandmother hypothesis. *Current Biology*, 29, 651–656.

Engelmann, J.M., Herrmann, E. & Tomasello, M. 2015. Chimpanzees trust conspecifics to engage in low-cost reciprocity. *Proceedings of the Royal Society of London B: Biological Sciences*, 282, 20142083.

Enquist, M. & Leimar, O. 1983. Evolution of fighting behaviour: decision rules and assessment of relative strength. *Journal of Theoretical Biology*, 102, 387–410.

Enquist, M. & Leimar, O. 1987. Evolution of fighting behaviour: the effect of variation in resource value. *Journal of Theoretical Biology*, 127, 187–205.

Engqvist, L. & Taborsky, M. 2016. The evolution of genetic and conditional alternative reproductive tactics. *Proceedings of the Royal Society of London B: Biological Sciences*, 283, 20152945.

Eppley, T.M., Watzek, J., Dausmann, K.H., Ganzhorn, J.U. & Donati, G. 2017. Huddling is more important than rest site selection for thermoregulation in southern bamboo lemurs. *Animal Behaviour*, 127, 153–161.

Eriksson, J., Siedel, H., Lukas, D., et al. 2006. Y-chromosome analysis confirms highly sex-biased dispersal and suggests a low male effective population size in bonobos (*Pan paniscus*). *Molecular Ecology*, 15, 939–949.

Ermeidou, C. 2016. The influence of kinship on helper acceptance and reproductive behaviour in the cooperatively breeding fish *Neolamrologus pulcher*. MSc thesis, University of Bern, Switzerland.

Ermeidou, C., Taborsky, M. & Frommen, J.G. 2021. Inbreeding depression, but no inbreeding avoidance in the cichlid fish *Neolamprologus pulcher*. Unpublished manuscript.

Eshel, I. & Shaked, A. 2001. Partnership. *Journal of Theoretical Biology*, 208, 457–474.

Espmark, Y. & Knudsen, T. 2001. Intraspecific brood adoption in the convict cichlid with respect to fry of two colour morphs. *Journal of Fish Biology*, 59, 504–514.

Estrela, S., Libby, E., Van Cleve, J., et al. 2019. Environmentally mediated social dilemmas. *Trends in Ecology & Evolution*, 34, 6–18.

Ewald, P.W. & Carpenter, F.L. 1978. Territorial responses to energy manipulations in the Anna hummingbird. *Oecologia*, 31, 277–292.

Faber, D.B. & Baylis, J.R. 1993. Effects of body size on agonistic encounters between male jumping spiders (Araneae: Salticidae). *Animal Behaviour*, 45, 289–299.

Fagan, J. & Meares, T.L. 2008. Punishment, deterrence and social control: the paradox of punishment in minority communities. *Ohio State Journal of Criminal Law*, 6, 173.

Fairbanks, B.M. & Dobson, F.S. 2010. Kinship does not affect vigilance in Columbian ground squirrels (*Urocitellus columbianus*). *Canadian Journal of Zoology*, 88, 266–270.

Faria, G.S. & Gardner, A. 2020. Does kin discrimination promote cooperation? *Biology Letters*, 16(3), 20190742.

Farine, D.R., Garroway, C.J. & Sheldon, B.C. 2012. Social network analysis of mixed-species flocks: exploring the structure and evolution of interspecific social behaviour. *Animal Behaviour*, 84, 1271–1277.

Farmer, M.B. & Alonzo, S.H. 2008. Competition for territories does not explain allopaternal care in the tessellated darter. *Environmental Biology of Fishes*, 83, 391–395.

Farrell, B.D., Sequeira, A.S., O'Meara, B.C., et al. 2001. The evolution of agriculture in beetles (Curculionidae: Scolytinae and Platypodinae). *Evolution*, 55, 2011–2027.

Faulkes, C.G., Arruda, M.F. & Monteiro da Cruz, M.A.O. 2003. Matrilineal genetic structure within and among populations of the cooperatively breeding common marmoset, *Callithrix jacchus*. *Molecular Ecology*, 12, 1101–1108.

Fawcett, T.W., Hamblin, S. & Giraldeau, L.A. 2013. Exposing the behavioral gambit: the evolution of learning and decision rules. *Behavioral Ecology*, 24, 2–11.

Feeney, W.E., Welbergen, J.A. & Langmore, N.E. 2014. Advances in the study of coevolution between avian brood parasites and their hosts. *Annual Review of Ecology, Evolution, and Systematics*, 45, 227–246.

Feh, C. 1999. Alliances and reproductive success in Camargue stallions. *Animal Behaviour*, 57, 705–713.

Feh, C. & Demazieres, J. 1993. Grooming at a preferred site reduces heart-rate in horses. *Animal Behaviour*, 46, 1191–1194.

Fehr, E. & Gachter, S. 2002. Altruistic punishment in humans. *Nature*, 415, 137–140.

Feldblum, J.T., Wroblewski, E.E., Rudicell, R.S., et al. 2014. Sexually coercive male chimpanzees sire more offspring. *Current Biology*, 24, 2855–2860.

Ferreira, C.E.L., Goncalves, J.E.A., Coutinho, R. & Peret, A.C. 1998. Herbivory by the dusky damselfish *Stegastes fuscus* (Cuvier, 1830) in a tropical rocky shore: effects on the benthic community. *Journal of Experimental Marine Biology and Ecology*, 229, 241–264.

Field, J. 1992. Intraspecific parasitism as an alternative reproductive tactic in nest-building wasps and bees. *Biological Reviews*, 67, 79–126.

Field, J. & Cant, M.A. 2009. Reproductive skew in primitively eusocial wasps: how useful are current models? In Hager, R. & Jones, C.B. (eds), *Reproductive Skew in Vertebrates: Proximate and Ultimate Causes*, pp. 305–333. Cambridge: Cambridge University Press.

Field, J. & Leadbeater, E. 2016. Cooperation between non-relatives in a primitively eusocial paper wasp, *Polistes dominula*. *Philosophical Transactions of the Royal Society B: Biological Sciences*, 371, 20150093.

Field, J., Solís, C.R., Queller, D.C. & Strassmann, J.E. 1998. Social and genetic structure of paper wasp cofoundress associations: tests of reproductive skew models. *The American Naturalist*, 151, 545–563.

Field, J., Cronin, A. & Bridge, C. 2006. Future fitness and helping in social queues. *Nature*, 441, 214–217.

Firman, R.C., Gasparini, C., Manier, M.K. & Pizzari, T. 2017. Postmating female control: 20 years of cryptic female choice. *Trends in Ecology & Evolution*, 32, 368–382.

Fischer, E.A. 1980. The relationship between mating system and simultaneous hermaphroditism in the coral-reef fish, *Hypoplectrus nigricans* (Serranidae). *Animal Behaviour*, 28, 620–633.

Fischer, E.A. 1984. Egg trading in the chalk bass, *Serranus torgurarum*, a simultaneous hermaphrodite. *Zeitschrift für Tierpsychologie*, 66, 143–151.

Fischer, S., Zöttl, M., Groenewoud, F. & Taborsky, B. 2014. Group-size-dependent punishment of idle subordinates in a cooperative breeder where helpers pay to stay. *Proceedings of the Royal Society of London B: Biological Sciences*, 281, 20140184.

Fischer, S., Bessert-Nettelbeck, M., Kotrschal, A. & Taborsky, B. 2015. Rearing-group size determines social competence and brain structure in a cooperatively breeding cichlid. *American Naturalist*, 186, 123–140.

Fitzpatrick, J.L., Desjardins, J.K., Stiver, K.A., Montgomerie, R. & Balshine, S. 2006. Male reproductive suppression in the cooperatively breeding fish *Neolamprologus pulcher*. *Behavioral Ecology*, 17, 25–33.

Fitzpatrick, J.W. & Bowman, R. 2016. Florida scrub-jays: oversized territories and group defense in a fire-maintained habitat. In Koenig, W.D. & Dickinson, J.L. (eds), *Cooperative Breeding in Vertebrates: Studies of Ecology, Evolution, and Behavior*, pp. 77–96. New York, NY: Cambridge University Press.

Fletcher, D.J.C. & Ross, K.G. 1985. Regulation of reproduction in eusocial Hymenoptera. *Annual Review of Entomology*, 30, 319–343.

Fletcher, J.A. & Doebeli, M. 2009. A simple and general explanation for the evolution of altruism. *Proceedings of the Royal Society of London B: Biological Sciences*, 276, 13–19.

Flower, T. 2011. Fork-tailed drongos use deceptive mimicked alarm calls to steal food. *Proceedings of the Royal Society of London B: Biological Sciences*, 278, 1548–1555.

Flower, T.P., Gribble, M. & Ridley, A.R. 2014. Deception by flexible alarm mimicry in an African bird. *Science*, 344, 513–516.

Foley, A.M., Hewitt, D.G., DeYoung, R.W., et al. 2018. Reproductive effort and success of males in scramble-competition polygyny: evidence for trade-offs between foraging and mate search. *Journal of Animal Ecology*, 87, 1600–1614.

Folse III, H.J. & Roughgarden, J. 2010. What is an individual organism? A multilevel selection perspective. *The Quarterly Review of Biology*, 85, 447–472.

Forsgren, E., Karlsson, A. & Kvarnemo, C. 1996. Female sand gobies gain direct benefits by choosing males with eggs in their nests. *Behavioral Ecology and Sociobiology*, 39, 91–96.

Forstmeier, W., Nakagawa, S., Griffith, S.C. & Kempenaers, B. 2014. Female extra-pair mating: adaptation or genetic constraint? *Trends in Ecology & Evolution*, 29, 456–464.

Forsyth, A. & Alcock, J. 1990. Female mimicry and resource defense polygyny by males of a tropical rove beetle, *Leistotrophus versicolor* (Coleoptera: Staphylinidae). *Behavioral Ecology and Sociobiology*, 26, 325–330.

Foster, E.A., Franks, D.W., Mazzi, S., et al. 2012. Adaptive prolonged postreproductive life span in killer whales. *Science*, 337, 1313.

Foster, E.G., Ritz, D.A., Osborn, J.E. & Swadling, K.M. 2001. Schooling affects the feeding success of Australian salmon (*Arripis trutta*) when preying on mysid swarms (*Paramesopodopsis rufa*). *Journal of Experimental Marine Biology and Ecology*, 261, 93–106.

Foster, K.R. 2004. Diminishing returns in social evolution: the not-so-tragic commons. *Journal of Evolutionary Biology*, 17, 1058–1072.

Foster, K.R. & Wenseleers, T. 2006. A general model for the evolution of mutualisms. *Journal of Evolutionary Biology*, 19, 1283–1293.

Foster, K.R., Wenseleers, T. & Ratnieks, F.L. 2006. Kin selection is the key to altruism. *Trends in Ecology & Evolution*, 21, 57-60.

Foster, M.S. 1977. Odd couples in manakins: a study of social organization and cooperative breeding in *Chiroxiphia linearis*. *The American Naturalist*, 111.

Foster, M.S. 1981. Cooperative behavior and social organization of the swallow-tailed manakin (*Chiroxiphia caudata*). *Behavioral Ecology and Sociobiology*, 9, 167–177.

Foster, N.L. & Briffa, M. 2014. Familial strife on the seashore: aggression increases with relatedness in the sea anemone *Actinia equina*. *Behavioural Processes*, 103, 243–245.

Foster, W.A. & Treherne, J.E. 1981. Evidence for the dilution effect in the selfish herd from fish predation on a marine insect. *Nature*, 293, 466–467.

Fowler, A.C. 2005. Fine-scale spatial structuring in cackling Canada geese related to reproductive performance and breeding philopatry. *Animal Behaviour*, 69, 973–981.

Fowler, J.H. 2005. Altruistic punishment and the origin of cooperation. *Proceedings of the National Academy of Sciences of the United States of America*, 102, 7047–7049.

Fowler, J.H. & Christakis, N.A. 2010. Cooperative behavior cascades in human social networks. *Proceedings of the National Academy of Sciences of the United States of America*, 107, 5334–5338.

Francisco, M.R., Gibbs, H.L. & Galetti, P.M. Jr. 2009. Patterns of individual relatedness at blue manakin (*Chiroxiphia caudata*) leks. *Auk*, 126, 47–53.

Francke-Grosmann, H. 1967. Ectosymbiosis in wood-inhabiting insects. In Henry, M.S. (ed.), *Symbiosis: Associations of Invertebrates, Birds, Ruminants, and Other Biota*, pp. 141–205. New York, NY: Academic Press.

Frank, R.E. & Silk, J.B. 2009a. Grooming exchange between mothers and non-mothers: the price of natal attraction in wild baboons (*Papio anubis*). *Behaviour*, 146, 889–906.

Frank, R.E. & Silk, J.B. 2009b. Impatient traders or contingent reciprocators? Evidence for the extended time-course of grooming exchanges in baboons. *Behaviour*, 146, 1123–1135.

Frank, S.A. 1993. Coevolutionary genetics of plants and pathogens. *Evolutionary Ecology*, 7, 45–75.

Frank, S.A. 1994. Genetics of mutualism: the evolution of altruism between species. *Journal of Theoretical Biology*, 170, 393–400.

Frank, S.A. 1995. Mutual policing and repression of competition in the evolution of cooperative groups. *Nature*, 377, 520–522.

Frank, S.A. 1998. *Foundations of Social Evolution*. Princeton, NJ: Princeton University Press.

Frank, S.A. 2003. Repression of competition and the evolution of cooperation. *Evolution*, 57, 693–705.

Frank, S.A. 2013. Natural selection. VII. History and interpretation of kin selection theory. *Journal of Evolutionary Biology*, 26, 1151–1184.

Franks, N.R. 1986. Teams in social insects – group retrieval of prey by army ants (*Eciton burchelli*, Hymenoptera, Formicidae). *Behavioral Ecology and Sociobiology*, 18, 425–429.

Fraser, O.N. & Bugnyar, T. 2012. Reciprocity of agonistic support in ravens. *Animal Behaviour*, 83, 171–177.

Fraser, S.A., Wisenden, B.D. & Keenleyside, M.H.A. 1993. Aggressive behaviour among convict cichlid (*Cichlasoma nigrofasciatum*) fry of different sizes and its importance to brood adoption. *Canadian Journal of Zoology*, 71, 2358–2362.

Freidin, E., Carballo, F. & Bentosela, M. 2017. Direct reciprocity in animals: the roles of bonding and affective processes. *International Journal of Psychology*, 52, 163–170.

French, B.W. & Cade, W.H. 1989. Sexual selection at varying population densities in male field crickets, *Gryllus veletis* and *G. pennsylvanicus. Journal of Insect Behavior*, 2, 105–121.

Fretwell, S.D. 1972[2020]. *Populations in a Seasonal Environment*. Princeton, NJ: Princeton University Press.

Fretwell, S.D. & Lucas, H.L. 1970. On territorial behaviour and other factors influencing habitat distribution in birds. *Acta Biotheoretica*, 19, 16–36.

Frommen, J.G. & Bakker, T.C. 2006. Inbreeding avoidance through non-random mating in sticklebacks. *Biology Letters*, 2, 232–235.

Frommen, J.G., Luz, C. & Bakker, T.C. 2007. Kin discrimination in sticklebacks is mediated by social learning rather than innate recognition. *Ethology*, 113, 276–282.

Fruteau, C., Voelkl, B., van Damme, E. & Noe, R. 2009. Supply and demand determine the market value of food providers in wild vervet monkeys. *Proceedings of the National Academy of Sciences of the United States of America*, 106, 12007–12012.

Fruteau, C., Lemoine, S., Hellard, E., van Damme, E. & Noe, R. 2011a. When females trade grooming for grooming: testing partner control and partner choice models of cooperation in two primate species. *Animal Behaviour*, 81, 1223–1230.

Fruteau, C., van de Waal, E., van Damme, E. & Noe, R. 2011b. Infant access and handling in sooty mangabeys and vervet monkeys. *Animal Behaviour*, 81, 153–161.

Fu, F., Nowak, M.A. & Hauert, C. 2010. Invasion and expansion of cooperators in lattice populations: prisoner's dilemma vs. snowdrift games. *Journal of Theoretical Biology*, 266, 358–366.

Furrer, R.D. & Manser, M.B. 2009. The evolution of urgency-based and functionally referential alarm calls in ground-dwelling species. *The American Naturalist*, 173, 400–410.

Gadagkar, R. 1997. *Survival Strategies: Cooperation and Conflict in Animal Societies*. Cambridge, MA: Harvard University Press.

Gadagkar, R. 2001. *The Social Biology of Ropalidia marginata: Toward Understanding the Evolution of Eusociality*. Cambridge, MA: Harvard University Press.

Gadagkar, R. 2016. Evolution of social behaviour in the primitively eusocial wasp *Ropalidia marginata*: do we need to look beyond kin selection? *Philosophical Transactions of the Royal Society of London B: Biological Sciences*, 371, 20150094.

Gadgil, M. 1975. Evolution of social-behavior through interpopulation selection. *Proceedings of the National Academy of Sciences of the United States of America*, 72, 1199–1201.

Galliard, J.L., Ferrière, & Clobert, J. 2003. Mother–offspring interactions affect natal dispersal in a lizard. *Proceedings of the Royal Society of London. Series B: Biological Sciences*, 270, 1163–1169.

Gaillard, J.M., Festa-Bianchet, M., Delorme, D. & Jorgenson, J. 2000. Body mass and individual fitness in female ungulates: bigger is not always better. *Proceedings of the Royal Society of London B: Biological Sciences*, 267, 471–477.

Galef Jr, B.G. & Giraldeau, L.A. 2001. Social influences on foraging in vertebrates: causal mechanisms and adaptive functions. *Animal Behaviour*, 61, 3–15.

Gamboa, G.J., Wacker, T.L., Scope, J.A., Cornell, T.J. & Shellmanreeve, J. 1990. The mechanism of queen regulation of foraging by workers in paper wasps (*Polistes fuscatus*, Hymenoptera, Vespidae). *Ethology*, 85, 335–343.

Gandon, S. & Rousset, F. 1999. Evolution of stepping-stone dispersal rates. *Proceedings of the Royal Society of London B: Biological Sciences*, 266, 2507–2513.

Garay, J. 2009. Cooperation in defence against a predator. *Journal of Theoretical Biology*, 257, 45–51.

Garcia, R.A., Cabeza, M., Rahbek, C. & Araújo, M.B. 2014. Multiple dimensions of climate change and their implications for biodiversity. *Science*, 344, 1247579.

Gardner, A. 2010. Sex-biased dispersal of adults mediates the evolution of altruism among juveniles. *Journal of Theoretical Biology*, 262, 339–345.

Gardner, A. & Grafen, A. 2009. Capturing the superorganism: a formal theory of group adaptation. *Journal of Evolutionary Biology*, 22, 659–671.

Gardner, A. & West, S.A. 2004. Cooperation and punishment, especially in humans. *The American Naturalist*, 164, 753–764.

Gardner, A. & West, S.A. 2006. Demography, altruism, and the benefits of budding. *Journal of Evolutionary Biology*, 19, 1707–1716.

Gardner, A. & West, S.A. 2010. Greenbeards. *Evolution*, 64, 25–38.

Gardner, A., West, S.A. & Buckling, A. 2004. Bacteriocins, spite and virulence. *Proceedings of the Royal Society of London B: Biological Sciences*, 271, 1529–1535.

Gardner, A., West, S. & Barton, N. 2007. The relation between multilocus population genetics and social evolution theory. *The American Naturalist*, 169, 207–226.

Gardner, A., West, S. & Wild, G. 2011. The genetical theory of kin selection. *Journal of Evolutionary Biology*, 24, 1020–1043.

Garfinkel, M.R. & Skaperdas, S. 2007. Economics of conflict: an overview. *Handbook of Defense Economics*, 2, 649–709.

Garroway, C.J., Radersma, R., Sepil, I., et al. 2013. Fine-scale genetic structure in a wild bird population: the role of limited dispersal and environmentally based selection as causal factors. *Evolution*, 67, 3488–3500.

Garza, J.C., Dallas, J., Duryadi, D., et al. 1997. Social structure of the mound-building mouse *Mus spicilegus* revealed by genetic analysis with microsatellites. *Molecular Ecology*, 6, 1009–1017.

Gaspari, S., Azzellino, A., Airoldi, S. & Hoelzel, A.R. 2007. Social kin associations and genetic structuring of striped dolphin populations (*Stenella coeruleoalba*) in the Mediterranean Sea. *Molecular Ecology*, 16, 2922–2933.

Gasparini, C. & Pilastro, A. 2011. Cryptic female preference for genetically unrelated males is mediated by ovarian fluid in the guppy. *Proceedings of the Royal Society of London B: Biological Sciences*, 278, 2495–2501.

Gaston, A.J. 1978. The evolution of group territorial behavior and cooperative breeding. *The American Naturalist*, 112, 1091–1100.

Gautrais, J., Jost, C., Soria, M., et al. 2009. Analyzing fish movement as a persistent turning walker. *Journal of Mathematical Biology*, 58, 429–445.

Gavrilets, S. 2012. On the evolutionary origins of the egalitarian syndrome. *Proceedings of the National Academy of Sciences of the United States of America*, 109, 14069–14074.

Gavrilets, S. & Fortunato, L. 2014. A solution to the collective action problem in between-group conflict with within-group inequality. *Nature Communications*, 5, 3526.

Gazda, S.K., Connor, R.C., Edgar, R.K. & Cox, F. 2005. A division of labour with role specialization in group-hunting bottlenose dolphins (*Tursiops truncatus*) off Cedar Key, Florida. *Proceedings of the Royal Society of London B: Biological Sciences*, 272, 135–140.

Gerber, N., Schweinfurth, M.K. & Taborsky, M. 2020. The smell of cooperation: rats increase helpful behaviour when receiving odour cues of a conspecific performing a cooperative task. *Proceedings of the Royal Society of London B: Biological Sciences*, 287, 20202327.

Gerlach, G. & Lysiak, N. 2006. Kin recognition and inbreeding avoidance in zebrafish, *Danio rerio*, is based on phenotype matching. *Animal Behaviour*, 71, 1371–1377.

Gfrerer, N. 2017. Cooperation, social competence and working ability in Swiss military dogs. PhD thesis, University of Bern, Switzerland.

Gfrerer, N. & Taborsky, M. 2017. Working dogs cooperate among one another by generalised reciprocity. *Scientific Reports*, 7, 43867.

Gfrerer, N. & Taborsky, M. 2018. Working dogs transfer different tasks in reciprocal cooperation. *Biology Letters*, 14, 20170460.

Ghoul, M., Griffin, A.S. & West, S.A. 2014. Toward an evolutionary definition of cheating. *Evolution*, 68, 318–331.

Gibbs, H.L., Goldizen, A.W., Bullough, C. & Goldizen, A.R. 1994. Parentage analysis of multi-male social groups of Tasmanian native hens (*Tribonyx mortierii*): genetic evidence for monogamy and polyandry. *Behavioral Ecology and Sociobiology*, 35, 363–371.

Gibson, R.M., Pires, D., Delaney, K.S. & Wayne, R.K. 2005. Microsatellite DNA analysis shows that greater sage grouse leks are not kin groups. *Molecular Ecology*, 14, 4453–4459.

Gilbert, C., McCafferty, D., Le Maho, Y., et al. 2010. One for all and all for one: the energetic benefits of huddling in endotherms. *Biological Reviews*, 85, 545–569.

Gilbert, W.M., Nolan, P.M., Stoehr, A.M. & Hill, G.E. 2005. Filial cannibalism at a house finch nest. *The Wilson Bulletin*, 117, 413–415.

Gilby, I.C. 2006. Meat sharing among the Gombe chimpanzees: harassment and reciprocal exchange. *Animal Behaviour*, 71, 953–963.

Gilchrist, J.S. 2004. Pup escorting in the communal breeding banded mongoose: behavior, benefits, and maintenance. *Behavioral Ecology*, 15, 952–960.

Gilchrist, J.S. 2008. Aggressive monopolization of mobile carers by young of a cooperative breeder. *Proceedings of the Royal Society of London B: Biological Sciences*, 275, 2491–2498.

Gill, F.B. & Wolf, L.L. 1975. Economics of feeding territoriality in golden-winged sunbird. *Ecology*, 56, 333–345.

Gill, S.A. 2012. Strategic use of allopreening in family-living wrens. *Behavioral Ecology and Sociobiology*, 66, 757–763.

Gillespie, J.H. 1977. Natural selection for variances in offspring numbers: a new evolutionary principle. *The American Naturalist*, 111, 1010–1014.

Ginther, A.J. & Snowdon, C.T. 2009. Expectant parents groom adult sons according to previous alloparenting in a biparental cooperatively breeding primate. *Animal Behaviour*, 78, 287–297.

Giorgi, M.S., Arlettaz, R., Christe, P. & Vogel, P. 2001. The energetic grooming costs imposed by a parasitic mite (*Spinturnix myoti*) upon its bat host (*Myotis myotis*). *Proceedings of the Royal Society of London B: Biological Sciences*, 268, 2071–2075.

Giraldeau, L.A. 1988. The stable group and the determinants of foraging group size. In Slobodchikoff, C.N. (ed.), *The Ecology of Social Behavior*, pp. 33–53. San Diego, CA: Academic Press.

Girman, D.J., Mills, M.G.L., Geffen, E. & Wayne, R.K. 1997. A molecular genetic analysis of social structure, dispersal, and interpack relationships of the African wild dog (*Lycaon pictus*). *Behavioral Ecology and Sociobiology*, 40, 187–198.

Giron, D., Dunn, D.W., Hardy, I.C. & Strand, M.R. 2004. Aggression by polyembryonic wasp soldiers correlates with kinship but not resource competition. *Nature*, 430, 676.

Glonekova, M., Brandlova, K. & Pluhacek, J. 2016. Stealing milk by young and reciprocal mothers: high incidence of allonursing in giraffes, *Giraffa camelopardalis*. *Animal Behaviour*, 113, 113–123.

Godfray, H.C. 1995. Evolutionary theory of parent–offspring conflict. *Nature*, 376, 133.

Godin, J.G. & Keenleyside, M.H. 1984. Foraging on patchily distributed prey by a cichlid fish (Teleostei, Cichlidae): a test of the ideal free distribution theory. *Animal Behaviour*, 32, 120–131.

Goldberg, J.L., Grant, J.W. & Lefebvre, L. 2001. Effects of the temporal predictability and spatial clumping of food on the intensity of competitive aggression in the Zenaida dove. *Behavioral Ecology*, 12, 490–495.

Goldizen, A.W., Putland, D.A. & Goldizen, A.R. 1998a. Variable mating patterns in Tasmanian native hens (*Gallinula mortierii*): correlates of reproductive success. *Journal of Animal Ecology*, 67, 307–317.

Goldizen, A.W., Goldizen, A.R., Putland, D.A., et al. 1998b. 'Wife-sharing' in the Tasmanian native hen (*Gallinula mortierii*): is it caused by a male-biased sex ratio? *The Auk*, 115, 528–532.

Goldizen, A.W., Buchan, J.C., Putland, D.A., Goldizen, A.R. & Krebs, E.A. 2000. Patterns of mate-sharing in a population of Tasmanian native hens *Gallinula mortierii*. *Ibis*, 142, 40–47.

Goldschmidt, T.G., Bakker, T.C. & Feuth-de Bruijn, E. 1993. Selective copying in mate choice of female sticklebacks. *Animal Behaviour*, 45, 547.

Gomes, C.M. & Boesch, C. 2009. Wild chimpanzees exchange meat for sex on a long-term basis. *PLoS One*, 4(4), e5116.

Gomes, C.M. & Boesch, C. 2011. Reciprocity and trades in wild West African chimpanzees. *Behavioral Ecology and Sociobiology*, 65, 2183–2196.

Gomes, C.M., Mundry, R. & Boesch, C. 2009. Long-term reciprocation of grooming in wild West African chimpanzees. *Proceedings of the Royal Society B: Biological Sciences*, 276, 699–706.

Gomez-Gardenes, J., Campillo, M., Floria, L. & Moreno, Y. 2007. Dynamical organization of cooperation in complex topologies. *Physical Review Letters*, 98, 108103.

Goodale, E., Beauchamp, G., Magrath, R.D., Nieh, J.C. & Ruxton, G.D. 2010. Interspecific information transfer influences animal community structure. *Trends in Ecology & Evolution*, 25, 354–361.

Goodall, J. 1986. *The Chimpanzees of Gombe: Patterns of Behavior*. Cambridge, MA: Belknap Press.

Goodall, J. 2000. *In the Shadow of Man*. Boston, MA: Houghton Mifflin Harcourt.

Goodnight, C. 2013a. On multilevel selection and kin selection: contextual analysis meets direct fitness. *Evolution*, 67, 1539–1548.

Goodnight, C.J. 2013b. Defining the individual. In Bouchad, F. & Huneman, P. (eds), *From Groups to Individuals – Evolution and Emerging Individuality*, pp. 37–53. Cambridge, MA: MIT Press.

Goodnight, C.J. & Stevens, L. 1997. Experimental studies of group selection: what do they tell us about group selection in nature? *American Naturalist*, 150, S59–S79.

Gore, J., Youk, H. & van Oudenaarden, A. 2009. Snowdrift game dynamics and facultative cheating in yeast. *Nature*, 459, 253–256.

Gorrell, J.C., McAdam, A.G., Coltman, D.W., Humphries, M.M. & Boutin, S. 2010. Adopting kin enhances inclusive fitness in asocial red squirrels. *Nature Communications*, 1, 22.

Grafen, A. 1979. The hawk–dove game played between relatives. *Animal Behaviour*, 27(Part 3), 905–907.

Grafen, A. 1984. Natural selection, kin selection and group selection. *Behavioural Ecology: An Evolutionary Approach*, 2, 62–84.

Grafen, A. 2007. The formal Darwinism project: a mid-term report. *Journal of Evolutionary Biology*, 20, 1243–1254.

Grafen, A. 2009. Formalizing Darwinism and inclusive fitness theory. *Philosophical Transactions of the Royal Society of London B: Biological Sciences*, 364, 3135–3141.

Grafen, A. 2014. The formal Darwinism project in outline. *Biology & Philosophy*, 29, 155–174.

Grant, J.W. 1993. Whether or not to defend? The influence of resource distribution. *Marine & Freshwater Behaviour & Physiology*, 23, 137–153.

Grant, J.W. & Kramer, D.L. 1992. Temporal clumping of food arrival reduces its monopolization and defence by zebrafish, *Brachydanio rerio*. *Animal Behaviour*, 44, 101–110.

Grant, J.W. & Noakes, D.L. 1988. Aggressiveness and foraging mode of young-of-the-year brook charr, *Salvelinus fontinalis* (Pisces, Salmonidae). *Behavioral Ecology and Sociobiology*, 22, 435–445.

Grant, J.W.A., Girard, I.L., Breau, C. & Weir, L.K. 2002. Influence of food abundance on competitive aggression in juvenile convict cichlids. *Animal Behaviour*, 63, 323–330.

Grantner, A. & Taborsky, M. 1998. The metabolic rates associated with resting, and with the performance of agonistic, submissive and digging behaviours in the cichlid fish *Neolamprologus pulcher* (Pisces: Cichlidae). *Journal of Comparative Physiology B*, 168, 427–433.

Grasmuck, V. & Desor, D. 2002. Behavioural differentiation of rats confronted to a complex diving-for-food situation. *Behavioural Processes*, 58, 67–77.

Gray, K., Ward, A.F. & Norton, M.I. 2014. Paying it forward: generalized reciprocity and the limits of generosity. *Journal of Experimental Psychology – General*, 143, 247–254.

Green, J.P. & Hatchwell, B. 2018. Inclusive fitness consequences of dispersal decisions in a cooperatively breeding bird, the long-tailed tit (*Aegithalos caudatus*). *Proceedings of the National Academy of Sciences of the United States of America*, 115, 12011–12016.

Green, J.P., Cant, M.A. & Field, J. 2014. Using social parasitism to test reproductive skew models in a primitively eusocial wasp. *Proceedings of the Royal Society of London B: Biological Sciences*, 281, 20141206.

Green, J.P., Freckleton, R.P. & Hatchwell, B.J. 2016. Variation in helper effort among cooperatively breeding bird species is consistent with Hamilton's Rule. *Nature Communications*, 7, 12663.

Green, P.A. & Patek, S.N. 2018. Mutual assessment during ritualized fighting in mantis shrimp (Stomatopoda). *Proceedings of the Royal Society of London B: Biological Sciences*, 285, 20172542.

Green, P.A., McHenry, M.J. and Patek, S.N., 2019. Context-dependent scaling of kinematics and energetics during contests and feeding in mantis shrimp. *Journal of Experimental Biology*, 222(7).

Greenwood, P.J. 1980. Mating systems, philopatry and dispersal in birds and mammals. *Animal Behaviour*, 28, 1140–1162.

Greiner, B. & Levati, M.V. 2005. Indirect reciprocity in cyclical networks – an experimental study. *Journal of Economic Psychology*, 26, 711–731.

Grether, G.F., Losin, N., Anderson, C.N. & Okamoto, K. 2009. The role of interspecific interference competition in character displacement and the evolution of competitor recognition. *Biological Reviews*, 84, 617–635.

Grether, G.F., Anderson, C.N., Drury, J.P., et al. 2013. The evolutionary consequences of interspecific aggression. *Annals of the New York Academy of Sciences*, 1289, 48–68.

Griesser, M. 2003. Nepotistic vigilance behavior in Siberian jay parents. *Behavioral Ecology*, 14, 246–250.

Griesser, M. & Ekman, J. 2004. Nepotistic alarm calling in the Siberian jay, *Perisoreus infaustus*. *Animal Behaviour*, 67, 933–939.

Griesser, M. & Ekman, J. 2005. Nepotistic mobbing behaviour in the Siberian jay, *Perisoreus infaustus*. *Animal Behaviour*, 69, 345–352.

Griesser, M., Nystrand, M. & Ekman, J. 2006. Reduced mortality selects for family cohesion in a social species. *Proceedings of the Royal Society of London B: Biological Sciences*, 273, 1881–1886.

Griesser, M., Drobniak, S.M., Nakagawa, S. & Botero, C.A. 2017. Family living sets the stage for cooperative breeding and ecological resilience in birds. *PLoS Biology*, 15, e2000483.

Griffin, A.S. & West, S.A. 2002. Kin selection: fact and fiction. *Trends in Ecology & Evolution*, 17, 15–21.

Griffin, A.S. & West, S.A. 2003. Kin discrimination and the benefit of helping in cooperatively breeding vertebrates. *Science*, 302, 634–636.

Griffin, A.S., West, S.A. & Buckling, A. 2004. Cooperation and competition in pathogenic bacteria. *Nature*, 430, 1024–1027.

Griffith, S.C., Owens, I.P. & Thuman, K.A. 2002. Extra pair paternity in birds: a review of interspecific variation and adaptive function. *Molecular Ecology*, 11, 2195–2212.

Grinsted, L. & Field, J. 2017. Market forces influence helping behaviour in cooperatively breeding paper wasps. *Nature Communications*, 8.

Grinsted, L. & Field, J. 2018. Predictors of nest growth: diminishing returns for subordinates in the paper wasp *Polistes dominula*. *Behavioral Ecology and Sociobiology*, 72, 88.

Groenewoud, F., Frommen, J.G., Josi, D., et al. 2016. Predation risk drives social complexity in cooperative breeders. *Proceedings of the National Academy of Sciences of the United States of America*, 113, 4104–4109.

Groenewoud, F., Kingma, S.A., Hammers, M., et al. 2018. Subordinate females in the cooperatively breeding Seychelles warbler obtain direct benefits by joining unrelated groups. *Journal of Animal Ecology*, 87, 1251–1263.

Groom, M.J. 1992. Sand-colored nighthawks parasitize the antipredator behavior of three nesting bird species. *Ecology*, 73, 785–793.

Groothuis, T.G. & Kraak, S.B. 1994. Female preference for nests with eggs is based on the presence of the eggs themselves. *Behaviour*, 131, 189–206.

Gross, M.R. 1996. Alternative reproductive strategies and tactics: diversity within sexes. *Trends in Ecology & Evolution*, 11, 92–98.

Gröning, J. & Hochkirch, A. 2008. Reproductive interference between animal species. *The Quarterly Review of Biology*, 83, 257–282.

Gruber-Vodicka, H.R., Dirks, U., Leisch, N., et al. 2011. *Paracatenula*, an ancient symbiosis between thiotrophic *Alphaproteobacteria* and catenulid flatworms. *Proceedings of the National Academy of Sciences*, 108, 12078–12083.

Grüter, C. & Taborsky, B. 2005. Sex ratio and the sexual conflict about brood care in a biparental mouthbrooder. *Behavioral Ecology and Sociobiology*, 58, 44–52.

Gumert, M.D. 2007. Payment for sex in a macaque mating market. *Animal Behaviour*, 74, 1655–1667.

Gumert, M.D. & Ho, M.H. 2008. The trade balance of grooming and its coordination of reciprocation and tolerance in Indonesian long-tailed macaques (*Macaca fascicularis*). *Primates*, 49, 176–185.

Gunnarsson, G.S. & Steingrimsson, S.O. 2011. Contrasting patterns of territoriality and foraging mode in two stream-dwelling salmonids, Arctic char (*Salvelinus alpinus*) and brown trout (*Salmo trutta*). *Canadian Journal of Fisheries and Aquatic Sciences*, 68, 2090–2100.

Gurven, M. & Kaplan, H. 2007. Longevity among hunter-gatherers: a cross-cultural examination. *Population and Development Review*, 33, 321–365.

Gurven, M. & Walker, R. 2006. Energetic demand of multiple dependents and the evolution of slow human growth. *Proceedings of the Royal Society of London B: Biological Sciences*, 273, 835–841.

Hack, M.A. 1997. Assessment strategies in the contests of male crickets, *Acheta domesticus* (L.). *Animal Behaviour*, 53, 733–747.

Hadfield, J.D., Richardson, D.S. & Burke, T. 2006. Towards unbiased parentage assignment: combining genetic, behavioural and spatial data in a Bayesian framework. *Molecular Ecology*, 15, 3715–3730.

Haemig, P.D. 2001. Symbiotic nesting of birds with formidable animals: a review with applications to biodiversity conservation. *Biodiversity & Conservation*, 10, 527–540.

Hager, R. & Jones, C.B. 2009. *Reproductive Skew in Vertebrates. Proximate and Ultimate Causes.* Cambridge: Cambridge University Press.

Haig, D. 1993. Genetic conflicts in human pregnancy. *Quarterly Review of Biology*, 68, 495–532.

Haig, D. 2014. Genetic dissent and individual compromise. *Biology & Philosophy*, 29, 233-239.

Haig, D. 2015. Maternal–fetal conflict, genomic imprinting and mammalian vulnerabilities to cancer. *Philosophical Transactions of the Royal Society of London B: Biological Sciences*, 370, 20140178.

Haig, D. & Grafen, A. 1991. Genetic scrambling as a defence against meiotic drive. *Journal of Theoretical Biology*, 153, 531–558.

Haig, D. & Wilkins, J.F. 2000. Genomic imprinting, sibling solidarity and the logic of collective action. *Philosophical Transactions of the Royal Society of London B: Biological Sciences*, 355, 1593–1597.

Halling, L.A., Oldroyd, B.P., Wattanachaiyingcharoen, W., et al. 2001. Worker policing in the bee *Apis florea*. *Behavioral Ecology and Sociobiology*, 49, 509–513.

Halliwell, B., Uller, T., Wapstra, E. & While, G.M. 2017. Resource distribution mediates social and mating behavior in a family living lizard. *Behavioral Ecology*, 28, 145–153.

Halpin, Z.T. 1991. Kin recognition cues of vertebrates. In Hepper, P.G. (ed.), *Kin Recognition*, pp. 220–258. Cambridge: Cambridge University Press.

Hamel, S., Gaillard, J.M., Festa-Bianchet, M. & Côté, S.D. 2009a. Individual quality, early-life conditions, and reproductive success in contrasted populations of large herbivores. *Ecology*, 90, 1981–1995.

Hamel, S., Côté, S.D., Gaillard, J.M. & Festa-Bianchet, M. 2009b. Individual variation in reproductive costs of reproduction: high-quality females always do better. *Journal of Animal Ecology*, 78, 143–151.

Hamilton, I.M. & Dill, L.M. 2002. Monopolization of food by zebrafish (*Danio rerio*) increases in risky habitats. *Canadian Journal of Zoology*, 80, 2164–2169.

Hamilton, I. & Heg, D. 2008. Sex differences in the effect of social status on the growth of subordinates in a cooperatively breeding cichlid. *Journal of Fish Biology*, 72, 1079–1088.

Hamilton, I.M. & Ligocki, I.Y. 2012. The extended personality: indirect effects of behavioural syndromes on the behaviour of others in a group-living cichlid. *Animal Behaviour*, 84, 659–664.

Hamilton, I.M. & Taborsky, M. 2005a. Contingent movement and cooperation evolve under generalized reciprocity. *Proceedings of the Royal Society of London B: Biological Sciences*, 272, 2259–2267.

Hamilton, I.M. & Taborsky, M. 2005b. Unrelated helpers will not fully compensate for costs imposed on breeders when they pay to stay. *Proceedings of the Royal Society of London B: Biological Sciences*, 272, 445–454.

Hamilton, I.M., Heg, D. & Bender, N. 2005. Size differences within a dominance hierarchy influence conflict and help in a cooperatively breeding cichlid. *Behaviour*, 142, 1591–1613.

Hamilton, W.D. 1963. The evolution of altruistic behavior. *The American Naturalist*, 97, 354–356.

Hamilton, W.D. 1964. The genetical evolution of social behaviour I and II. *Journal of Theoretical Biology*, 7, 17–52.

Hamilton, W.D. 1967. Extraordinary sex ratios. *Science*, 156, 477–488.

Hamilton, W.D. 1970. Selfish and spiteful behaviour in an evolutionary model. *Nature*, 228, 1218–1220.

Hamilton, W.D. 1971. Geometry for the selfish herd. *Journal of Theoretical Biology*, 31, 295–311.

Hamilton, W.D. 1972. Altruism and related phenomena, mainly in social insects. *Annual Review of Ecology and Systematics*, 3, 193–232.

Hamilton, W.D. 1975. Innate social aptitudes of man: an approach from evolutionary genetics. *Biosocial Anthropology*, 53, 133–155.

Hamilton, W.D. 1979. Wingless and fighting males in fig wasps and other insects. In Blum, M.S. & Blum, N.A. (eds), *Reproductive Competition, Mate Choice, and Sexual Selection in Insects*, pp. 167–220. New York, NY: Plenum.

Hamilton, W.D. 1996. *Narrow Roads of Gene Land*. New York, NY: W.H. Freeman.

Hamilton, W.D. & May, R.M. 1977. Dispersal in stable habitats. *Nature*, 269, 578.

Hammers, M., Kingma, S.A., Spurgin, L.G., et al. 2019. Breeders that receive help age more slowly in a cooperatively breeding bird. *Nature Communications*, 10, 1301.

Hammerstein, P. 1981. The role of asymmetries in animal contests. *Animal Behaviour*, 29, 193–205.

Hammerstein, P. 2003. Why is reciprocity so rare in social animals? A protestant appeal. In Hammerstein, P. (ed.), *Dahlem Workshop Report. Genetic and Cultural Evolution of Cooperation*, pp. 83–93. Cambridge, MA: MIT Press.

Hammerstein, P. & Noe, R. 2016. Biological trade and markets. *Philosophical Transactions of the Royal Society of London B: Biological Sciences*, 371.

Hammerstein, P. & Parker, G.A. 1982. The asymmetric war of attrition. *Journal of Theoretical Biology*, 96, 647–682.

Handegard, N.O., Boswell, K.M., Ioannou, C.C., et al. 2012. The dynamics of coordinated group hunting and collective information transfer among schooling prey. *Current Biology*, 22, 1213–1217.

Hankinson, T.L. 1920. Report on investigations of the fish of the Galien River, Berrien County, Michigan. *Occasional Papers of the Museum of Zoology, University of Michigan*, 89, 1–14.

Hannon, S.J., Mumme, R.L., Koenig, W.D. & Pitelka, F.A. 1985. Replacement of breeders and within-group conflict in the cooperatively breeding acorn woodpecker. *Behavioral Ecology and Sociobiology*, 17, 303–312.

Hanwell, A. & Peaker, M. 1977. Physiological effects of lactation on the mother. In *Comparative Aspects of Lactation, Symposia of the Zoological Society of London*, 41, 297–312. London: Academic Press.

Harcourt, J.L., Sweetman, G., Manica, A. & Johnstone, R.A. 2010. Pairs of fish resolve conflicts over coordinated movement by taking turns. *Current Biology*, 20, 156–160.

Hardin, G. 1968. The tragedy of the commons. *Science*, 162, 1243–1248.

Hardy, I.C., Goubault, M. & Batchelor, T.P. 2013. Hymenopteran contests and agonistic behaviour. In Hardy, I.C.W. & Briffa, M. (eds), *Animal Contests*, p. 147. Cambridge: Cambridge University Press.

Hario, M., Koljonen, M.L. & Rintala, J. 2012. Kin structure and choice of brood care in a common cider (*Somateria m. mollissima*) population. *Journal of Ornithology*, 153, 963–973.

Harris, A.C. & Madden, G.J. 2002. Delay discounting and performance on the prisoner's dilemma game. *Psychological Record*, 52, 429–40.

Harris, J.A., Campbell, K.G. & Wright, G.M. 1976. Ecological studies on the horizontal borer '*Austroplatypus incompertus*' (Schedl) (Coleoptera: Platypodidae). *Journal of the Entomological Society of Australia (NSW)*, 9, 11–21.

Harrison, F., Barta, Z., Cuthill, I. & Szekely, T. 2009. How is sexual conflict over parental care resolved? A meta analysis. *Journal of Evolutionary Biology*, 22, 1800–1812.

Harrisson, K.A., Pavlova, A., Amos, J.N., et al. 2013. Disrupted fine-scale population processes in fragmented landscapes despite large-scale genetic connectivity for a widespread and common cooperative breeder: the superb fairy-wren (*Malurus cyaneus*). *Journal of Animal Ecology*, 82, 322–333.

Hart, B.L. & Hart, L.A. 1992. Reciprocal allogrooming in impala, *Aepyceros melampus*. *Animal Behaviour*, 44, 1073–1083.

Hart, B.L., Hart, L.A., Mooring, M.S. & Olubayo, R. 1992. Biological basis of grooming behavior in antelope – the body-size, vigilance and habitat principles. *Animal Behaviour*, 44, 615–631.

Hart, D.D. 1987. Feeding territoriality in aquatic insects – cost–benefit models and experimental tests. *American Zoologist*, 27, 371–386.

Hart, M.K., Kratter, A.W. & Crowley, P.H. 2016. Partner fidelity and reciprocal investments in the mating system of a simultaneous hermaphrodite. *Behavioral Ecology*, 27, 1471–1479.

Harten, L., Prat, Y., Ben Cohen, S., Dor, R. & Yovel, Y. 2019. Food for sex in bats revealed as producer males reproduce with scrounging females. *Current Biology*, 29, 1895–1900.

Hartley, I.R., Davies, N.B., Hatchwell, B.J., et al. 1995. The polygynandrous mating system of the alpine accentor, *Prunella collaris*. II. Multiple paternity and parental effort. *Animal Behaviour*, 49, 789–803.

Harts, A.M. & Kokko, H. 2013. Understanding promiscuity: when is seeking additional mates better than guarding an already found one? *Evolution*, 67, 2838–2848.

Hasson, O. 1994. Cheating signals. *Journal of Theoretical Biology*, 167, 223–238.

Hatchwell, B.J. 1999. Investment strategies of breeders in avian cooperative breeding systems. *American Naturalist*, 154, 205–219.

Hatchwell, B.J. 2009. The evolution of cooperative breeding in birds: kinship, dispersal and life history. *Philosophical Transactions of the Royal Society of London B: Biological Sciences*, 364, 3217–3227.

Hatchwell, B.J. & Komdeur, J. 2000. Ecological constraints, life history traits and the evolution of cooperative breeding. *Animal Behaviour*, 59, 1079–1086.

Hatchwell, B.J., Ross, D.J., Fowlie, M.K. & McGowan, A. 2001. Kin discrimination in cooperatively breeding long-tailed tits. *Proceedings of the Royal Society of London B: Biological Sciences*, 268, 885–890.

Hatchwell, B.J., Ross, D.J., Chaline, N., Fowlie, M.K. & Burke, T. 2002. Parentage in the cooperative breeding system of long-tailed tits, *Aegithalos caudatus*. *Animal Behaviour*, 64, 55–63.

Hatchwell, B.J., Russell, A.F., MacColl, A.D., et al. 2004. Helpers increase long-term but not short-term productivity in cooperatively breeding long-tailed tits. *Behavioral Ecology*, 15, 1–10.

Hattori, Y., Kuroshima, H. & Fujita, K. 2005. Cooperative problem solving by tufted capuchin monkeys (*Cebus apella*): spontaneous division of labor, communication, and reciprocal altruism. *Journal of Comparative Psychology*, 119, 335–342.

Hauert, C., Michor, F., Nowak, M.A. & Doebeli, M. 2006. Synergy and discounting of cooperation in social dilemmas. *Journal of Theoretical Biology*, 239, 195–202.

Haunhorst, C.B., Schülke, O. & Ostner, J. 2016. Opposite-sex social bonding in wild Assamese macaques. *American Journal of Primatology*, 78, 872–882.

Hauser, M.D., Teixidor, P., Field, L. & Flaherty, R. 1993. Food-elicited cells in chimpanzees: effects of food quantity and divisibility. *Animal Behaviour*, 45, 817–819.

Hauser, M.D., Chen, M.K., Chen, F., Chuang, E. & Chuang, E. 2003. Give unto others: genetically unrelated cotton-top tamarin monkeys preferentially give food to those who altruistically give food back. *Proceedings of the Royal Society of London B: Biological Sciences*, 270, 2363–2370.

Hawlena, H., Bashary, D., Abramsky, Z. & Krasnov, B.R. 2007. Benefits, costs and constraints of anti-parasitic grooming in adult and juvenile rodents. *Ethology*, 113, 394–402.

Hayden, B.Y. 2016. Time discounting and time preference in animals: a critical review. *Psychonomic Bulletin & Review*, 23, 39–53.

Haydock, J., Koenig, W.D. & Stanback, M.T. 2001. Shared parentage and incest avoidance in the cooperatively breeding acorn woodpecker. *Molecular Ecology*, 10, 1515–1525.

Healy, W.M. 1992. *Behavior*, pp. 46–65. Mechanicsburg, PA: Stackpole Books.

Hector, D.P. 1986. Cooperative hunting and its relationship to foraging success and prey size in an avian predator. *Ethology*, 73, 247–257.

Heg, D. 2008. Reproductive suppression in female cooperatively breeding cichlids. *Biology Letters*, 4, 606–609.

Heg, D. 2010. Status-dependent and strategic growth adjustments in female cooperative cichlids. *Behavioral Ecology and Sociobiology*, 64, 1309–1316.

Heg, D. & Hamilton, I.M. 2008. Tug-of-war over reproduction in a cooperatively breeding cichlid. *Behavioral Ecology and Sociobiology*, 62, 1249–1257.

Heg, D. & Taborsky, M. 2010. Helper response to experimentally manipulated predation risk in the cooperatively breeding cichlid *Neolamprologus pulcher*. *PLoS One*, 5, e10784.

Heg, D., Bachar, Z., Brouwer, L. & Taborsky, M. 2004a. Predation risk is an ecological constraint for helper dispersal in a cooperatively breeding cichlid. *Proceedings of the Royal Society of London B: Biological Sciences*, 271, 2367–2374.

Heg, D., Bender, N. & Hamilton, I. 2004b. Strategic growth decisions in helper cichlids. *Proceedings of the Royal Society of London B: Biological Sciences*, 271, S505–S508.

Heg, D., Brouwer, L., Bachar, Z. & Taborsky, M. 2005a. Large group size yields group stability in the cooperatively breeding cichlid *Neolamprologus pulcher*. *Behaviour*, 142, 1615–1641.

Heg, D., Bachar, Z. & Taborsky, M. 2005b. Cooperative breeding and group structure in the Lake Tanganyika cichlid *Neolamprologus savoryi*. *Ethology*, 111, 1017–1043.

Heg, D., Bergmuller, R., Bonfils, D., et al. 2006. Cichlids do not adjust reproductive skew to the availability of independent breeding options. *Behavioral Ecology*, 17, 419–429.

Heg, D., Heg-Bachar, Z., Brouwer, L. & Taborsky, M. 2008a. Experimentally induced helper dispersal in colonially breeding cooperative cichlids. *Environmental Biology of Fishes*, 83, 191–206.

Heg, D., Jutzeler, E., Bonfils, D. & Mitchell, J.S. 2008b. Group composition affects male reproductive partitioning in a cooperatively breeding cichlid. *Molecular Ecology*, 17, 4359–4370.

Heg, D., Jutzeler, E., Mitchell, J.S. & Hamilton, I.M. 2009. Helpful female subordinate cichlids are more likely to reproduce. *PLoS One*, 4, e5458.

Heg, D., Rothenberger, S. & Schuerch, R. 2011. Habitat saturation, benefits of philopatry, relatedness, and the extent of co-operative breeding in a cichlid. *Behavioral Ecology*, 22, 82–92.

Heg, D., Josi, D., Takeyama, T., et al. (submitted). Age- and sex-dependent relatedness explains reproductive skew, territory inheritance and workload in highly social cichlids.

Heinrich, B. 1988. Winter foraging at carcasses by three sympatric corvids, with emphasis on recruitment by the raven, *Corvus corax*. *Behavioral Ecology and Sociobiology*, 23, 141–156.

Heinsohn, R.G. 1991. Kidnapping and reciprocity in cooperatively breeding white-winged choughs. *Animal Behaviour*, 41, 1097–1100.

Heinsohn, R.G. 2004. Parental care, load-lightening, and costs. In Koenig, W.D. & Dickinson, J.L. (eds), *Ecology and Evolution of Cooperative Breeding in Birds*, pp. 67–80. Cambridge: Cambridge University Press.

Heinsohn, R. & Legge, S. 1999. The cost of helping. *Trends in Ecology & Evolution*, 14, 53–57.

Heinsohn, R., Dunn, P., Legge, S. & Double, M. 2000. Coalitions of relatives and reproductive skew in cooperatively breeding white-winged choughs. *Proceedings of the Royal Society of London B: Biological Sciences*, 267, 243–249.

Heitman, T.L., Koski, K.G. & Scott, M.E. 2003. Energy deficiency alters behaviours involved in transmission of *Heligmosomoides polygyrus* (Nematoda) in mice. *Canadian Journal of Zoology – Revue Canadienne de Zoologie*, 81, 1767–1773.

Hellmann, J.K. & Hamilton, I.M. 2018. Dominant and subordinate outside options alter help and eviction in a pay-to-stay negotiation model. *Behavioral Ecology*, 29, 553–562.

Hellmann, J.K., Ligocki, I.Y., O'Connor, C.M., et al. 2015. Reproductive sharing in relation to group and colony-level attributes in a cooperative breeding fish. *Proceedings of the Royal Society of London B: Biological Sciences*, 282, 20150954.

Hemelrijk, C.K. 1990. Models of, and tests for, reciprocity, unidirectionality and other social-interaction patterns at a group level. *Animal Behaviour*, 39, 1013–1029.

Hemelrijk, C.K. 1994. Support for being groomed in long-tailed macaques, *Macaca fascicularis*. *Animal Behaviour*, 48, 479–481.

Hemelrijk, C.K. & Ek, A. 1991. Reciprocity and interchange of grooming and support in captive chimpanzees. *Animal Behaviour*, 41, 923–935.

Hemelrijk, C.K. & Luteijn, M. 1998. Philopatry, male presence and grooming reciprocation among female primates: a comparative perspective. *Behavioral Ecology and Sociobiology*, 42, 207–215.

Henter, H.J. 2003. Inbreeding depression and haplodiploidy: experimental measures in a parasitoid and comparisons across diploid and haplodiploid insect taxa. *Evolution*, 57, 1793–1803.

Henzi, S.P. & Barrett, L. 2002. Infants as a commodity in a baboon market. *Animal Behaviour*, 63, 915–921.

Henzi, S.P., Lycett, J.E. & Weingrill, T. 1997. Cohort size and the allocation of social effort by female mountain baboons. *Animal Behaviour*, 54, 1235–1243.

Hepper, P.G. 1991. *Recognizing Kin: Ontogeny and Classification*. Cambridge: Cambridge University Press.

Herberstein, M.E., Painting, C.J. & Holwell, G.I. 2017. Scramble competition polygyny in terrestrial arthropods. *Advances in the Study of Behavior*, 49, 237–295.

Herbert-Read, J.E., Romanczuk, P., Krause, S., et al. 2016. Proto-cooperation: group hunting sailfish improve hunting success by alternating attacks on grouping prey. *Proceedings of the Royal Society of London B: Biological Sciences*, 283, 20161671.

Herbert-Read, J.E., Rosén, E., Szorkovszky, A., et al. 2017. How predation shapes the social interaction rules of shoaling fish. *Proceedings of the Royal Society of London B: Biological Sciences*, 284, 20171126.

Herne, K., Lappalainen, O. & Kestila-Kekkonen, E. 2013. Experimental comparison of direct, general, and indirect reciprocity. *Journal of Socio-Economics*, 45, 38–46.

Herre, E.A., Knowlton, N., Mueller, U.G. & Rehner, S.A. 1999. The evolution of mutualisms: exploring the paths between conflict and cooperation. *Trends in Ecology & Evolution*, 14, 49–53.

Herrmann, E., Call, J., Hernández-Lloreda, M.V., Hare, B. & Tomasello, M. 2007. Humans have evolved specialized skills of social cognition: the cultural intelligence hypothesis. *Science*, 317, 1360–1366.

Hershey, A.E. 1987. Tubes and foraging behavior in larval Chironomidae – implications for predator avoidance. *Oecologia*, 73, 236–241.

Hert, E. 1985. Individual recognition of helpers by the breeders in the cichlid fish *Lamprologus brichardi* (Poll, 1974). *Zeitschrift für Tierpsychologie*, 68, 313–325.

Heymann, E.W. & Hsia, S.S. 2015. Unlike fellows – a review of primate–non-primate associations. *Biological Reviews*, 90, 142–156.

Higashi, M. & Yamamura, N. 1993. What determines animal group size? Insider–outsider conflict and its resolution. *The American Naturalist*, 142, 553–563.

Higginson, D.M., Miller, K.B., Segraves, K.A. & Pitnick, S. 2012. Female reproductive tract form drives the evolution of complex sperm morphology. *Proceedings of the National Academy of Sciences of the United States of America*, 109, 4538–4543.

Hilbe, C., Nowak, M.A. & Sigmund, K. 2013. Evolution of extortion in Iterated Prisoner's Dilemma games. *Proceedings of the National Academy of Sciences of the United States of America*, 110, 6913–6918.

Hilbe, C., Rohl, T. & Milinski, M. 2014. Extortion subdues human players but is finally punished in the prisoner's dilemma. *Nature Communications*, 5, 3976.

Hilbe, C., Hagel, K. & Milinski, M. 2016. Asymmetric power boosts extortion in an economic experiment. *PLoS One*, 11, e0163867.

Hill, K. & Hurtado, A.M. 1996. *Ache Life History: the Ecology and Demography of a Foraging People*. New York, NY: de Gruyter.

Hinde, C.A. & Kilner, R.M. 2007. Negotiations within the family over the supply of parental care. *Proceedings of the Royal Society of London B: Biological Sciences*, 274, 53–60.

Hinsch, M. & Komdeur, J. 2010. Defence, intrusion and the evolutionary stability of territoriality. *Journal of Theoretical Biology*, 266, 606–613.

Hinsch, M. & Komdeur, J. 2017. What do territory owners defend against? *Proceedings of the Royal Society of London B: Biological Sciences*, 284, 20162356.

Hinsch, M., Pen, I. & Komdeur, J. 2013. Evolution of defense against depletion of local food resources in a mechanistic foraging model. *Behavioral Ecology*, 24, 245–252.

Hintz, W.D. & Lonzarich, D.G. 2018. Maximizing foraging success: the roles of group size, predation risk, competition, and ontogeny. *Ecosphere*, 9, e02456.

Hirschenhauser, K., Canario, A.V., Ros, A.F., Taborsky, M. & Oliveira, R.F. 2008. Social context may affect urinary excretion of 11-ketotestosterone in African cichlids. *Behaviour*, 145, 1367–1388.

Hirshleifer, J. 1989. Conflict and rent-seeking success functions: ratio versus difference models of relative success. *Public Choice*, 63, 101–112.

Hirshleifer, J. 2001. *The Dark Side of the Force: Economic Foundations of Conflict Theory*. Cambridge: Cambridge University Press.

Hoare, D.J., Couzin, I.D., Godin, J.G. & Krause, J. 2004. Context-dependent group size choice in fish. *Animal Behaviour*, 67, 155–164.

Hochberg, M.E., Rankin, D.J. & Taborsky, M. 2008. The coevolution of cooperation and dispersal in social groups and its implications for the emergence of multicellularity. *BMC Evolutionary Biology*, 8, 238.

Hochkirch, A., Groning, J. & Bucker, A. 2007. Sympatry with the devil: reproductive interference could hamper species coexistence. *Journal of Animal Ecology*, 76, 633–642.

Hodge, S.J. 2005. Helpers benefit offspring in both the short and long-term in the cooperatively breeding banded mongoose. *Proceedings of the Royal Society of London B: Biological Sciences*, 272, 2479–2484.

Hodge, S.J., Bell, M.B.V., Mwanghuya, F., et al. 2009. Maternal weight, offspring competition and the evolution of communal breeding. *Behavioral Ecology*, 20, 729–735.

Hodge, S.J., Bell, M.B. & Cant, M.A. 2011. Reproductive competition and the evolution of extreme birth synchrony in a cooperative mammal. *Biology Letters*, 7, 54–56.

Hoeksema, J.D. & Bruna, E.M. 2000. Pursuing the big questions about interspecific mutualism: a review of theoretical approaches. *Oecologia*, 125, 321–330.

Hof, C., Levinsky, I., Araújo, M.B. & Rahbek, C. 2011. Rethinking species' ability to cope with rapid climate change. *Global Change Biology*, 17, 2987–2990.

Hoffmann, A.A. & Sgrò, C.M. 2011. Climate change and evolutionary adaptation. *Nature*, 470, 479.

Hofmann, H.A., Beery, A.K., Blumstein, D.T., et al. 2014. An evolutionary framework for studying mechanisms of social behavior. *Trends in Ecology & Evolution*, 29, 581–589.

Holbrook, C.T., Barden, P.M. & Fewell, J.H. 2011. Division of labor increases with colony size in the harvester ant *Pogonomyrmex californicus*. *Behavioral Ecology*, 22, 960–966.

Holman, L., Jorgensen, C.G., Nielsen, J. & d'Ettorre, P. 2010. Identification of an ant queen pheromone regulating worker sterility. *Proceedings of the Royal Society of London B: Biological Sciences*, 277, 3793–3800.

Holmes, W.G. & Sherman, P.W. 1983. Kin recognition in animals: the prevalence of nepotism among animals raises basic questions about how and why they distinguish relatives from unrelated individuals. *The American Scientist*, 71, 46–55.

Holt, R.D. 1977. Predation, apparent competition, and the structure of prey communities. *Theoretical Population Biology*, 12, 197–229.

Honza, M., Taborsky, B., Taborsky, M., et al. 2002. Behaviour of female common cuckoos, *Cuculus canorus*, in the vicinity of host nests before and during egg laying: a radiotelemetry study. *Animal Behaviour*, 64, 861–868.

Hoppitt, W. & Laland, K.N. 2013. *Social Learning: an Introduction to Mechanisms, Methods, and Models*. Princeton, NJ: Princeton University Press.

Horak, P., Tegelmann, L., Ots, I. & Möller, A.P. 1999. Immune function and survival of great tit nestlings in relation to growth conditions. *Oecologia*, 121, 316–322.

Horner, V., Carter, J., Suchak, M. & de Waal, F.B. 2011. Spontaneous prosocial choice by chimpanzees. *Proceedings of the National Academy of Sciences of the United States of America*, 108, 13847–13851.

Houston, A.I. & Davies, N.B. 1985. The evolution of cooperation and life history in the dunnock *Prunella modularis*. In Sibley, R.M. & Smith, R.H. (eds), *Behavioural Ecology*, pp. 471–487. Oxford: Blackwell Scientific.

Houston, A.I. & McNamara, J.M. 1991. Evolutionarily stable strategies in the repeated hawk–dove game. *Behavioral Ecology*, 2, 219–227.

Houston, A.I., McCleery, R.H. & Davies, N.B. 1985. Territory size, prey renewal and feeding rates – interpretation of observations on the pied wagtail (*Motacilla alba*) by simulation. *Journal of Animal Ecology*, 54, 227–239.

Houston, A.I., Szekely, T. & McNamara, J.M. 2005. Conflict between parents over care. *Trends in Ecology & Evolution*, 20, 33–38.

Höglund, J. 2003. Lek-kin in birds – provoking theory and surprising new results. *Annales Zoologici Fennici*, 40, 249–253.

Höglund, J. & Alatalo, R.V. 1995. *Leks*. Princeton, NJ: Princeton University Press.

Höglund, J., Alatalo, R.V., Lundberg, A., Rintamäki, P.T. & Lindell, J. 1999. Microsatellite markers reveal the potential for kin selection on black grouse leks. *Proceedings of the Royal Society of London B: Biological Sciences*, 266, 813–816.

Hölldobler, B. & Wilson, E.O. 1990. *The Ants*. New York, NY: Belknap Press.

Hölldobler, B. & Wilson, E.O. 2009. *The Superorganism: The Beauty, Elegance and Strangeness of Insect Societies*. New York, NY: W.W. Norton & Company.

Hsu, Y.Y., Earley, R.L. & Wolf, L.L. 2006. Modulation of aggressive behaviour by fighting experience: mechanisms and contest outcomes. *Biological Reviews*, 81, 33–74.

Hughes, J.M., Mather, P.B., Toon, A., et al. 2003. High levels of extra-group paternity in a population of Australian magpies *Gymnorhina tibicen*: evidence from microsatellite analysis. *Molecular Ecology*, 12, 3441–3450.

Hughes, W.O.H., Oldroyd, B.P., Beekman, M. & Ratnieks, F.L.W. 2008. Ancestral monogamy shows kin selection is key to the evolution of eusociality. *Science*, 320, 1213–1216.

Hulcr, J. & Dunn, R.R. 2011. The sudden emergence of pathogenicity in insect–fungus symbioses threatens naive forest ecosystems. *Proceedings of the Royal Society of London B: Biological Sciences*, 278, 2866–2873.

Huntingford, F.A. & Turner, A.K. 1987. *Animal Conflict*. London: Chapman and Hall.

Huntingford, F.A., Lazarus, J., Barrie, B.D. & Webb, S. 1994. A dynamic analysis of cooperative predator inspection in sticklebacks. *Animal Behaviour*, 47, 413–423.

Huth, A. & Wissel, C. 1994. The simulation of fish schools in comparison with experimental data. *Ecological Modelling*, 75, 135–146.

Iguchi, K. & Abe, S. 2002. Territorial defense of an excess food supply by an algal grazing fish, ayu. *Ecological Research*, 17, 373–380.

Ilmonen, P., Stundner, G., Thoss, M. & Penn, D.J. 2009. Females prefer the scent of outbred males: good-genes-as-heterozygosity? *BMC Evolutionary Biology*, 9, 104.

Inglis, R.F., Garfjeld Roberts, P., Gardner, A. & Buckling, A. 2011. Spite and the scale of competition in *Pseudomonas aeruginosa*. *The American Naturalist*, 178, 276–285.

Inglis, R.F., West, S. & Buckling, A. 2014. An experimental study of strong reciprocity in bacteria. *Biology Letters*, 10, 20131069.

Ingvarsson, P.K. 1998. Kin-structured colonization in *Phalacrus substriatus*. *Heredity*, 80, 456.

Innes, R.J., McEachern, M.B., Van Vuren, D.H., et al. 2012. Genetic relatedness and spatial associations of dusky-footed woodrats (*Neotoma fuscipes*). *Journal of Mammalogy*, 93, 439–446.

Inzani, E.L., Marshall, H.H., Sanderson, J.L., et al. 2016. Female reproductive competition explains variation in prenatal investment in wild banded mongooses. *Scientific Reports*, 6, 20013.

Ioannou, C.C., Guttal, V. & Couzin, I.D. 2012. Predatory fish select for coordinated collective motion in virtual prey. *Science*, 337, 1212–1215.

Irwin, A.J. & Taylor, P.D. 2001. Evolution of altruism in stepping-stone populations with overlapping generations. *Theoretical Population Biology*, 60, 315–325.

Isack, H.A. & Reyer, H.U. 1989. Honeyguides and honey gatherers: interspecific communication in a symbiotic relationship. *Science*, 243, 1343–1346.

Iserbyt, A., Farrell, S., Eens, M. & Muller, W. 2015. Sex-specific negotiation rules in a costly conflict over parental care. *Animal Behaviour*, 100, 52–58.

Iserbyt, A., Fresneau, N., Kortenhoff, T., Eens, M. & Muller, W. 2017. Decreasing parental task specialization promotes conditional cooperation. *Scientific Reports*, 7, 6565.

Isvaran, K. & Ponkshe, A. 2013. How general is a female mating preference for clustered males in lekking species? A meta-analysis. *Animal Behaviour*, 86, 417–425.

Ito, K., McNamara, J.M., Yamauchi, A. & Higginson, A.D. 2017. The evolution of cooperation by negotiation in a noisy world. *Journal of Evolutionary Biology*, 30, 603–615.

IUCN. 2013. The IUCN Red List of Threatened Species. www.iucnredlist.org.

Iwagami, A. & Masuda, N. 2010. Upstream reciprocity in heterogeneous networks. *Journal of Theoretical Biology*, 265, 297–305.

Izawa, K. 1980. Social behavior of the wild black-capped capuchin (*Cebus apella*). *Primates*, 21, 443–467.

Jaafar, Z. & Zeng, Y. 2012. Visual acuity of the goby-associated shrimp, *Alpheus rapax* Fabricius, 1798 (Decapoda, Alpheidae). *Crustaceana*, 85, 1487–1497.

Jaatinen, K., Jaari, S., O'Hara, R.B., Jöst, M. & Merilä, J. 2009. Relatedness and spatial proximity as determinants of host–parasite interactions in the brood parasitic Barrow's goldeneye (*Bucephala islandica*). *Molecular Ecology*, 18, 2713–2721.

Jacobs, D.S. & Jarvis, J.U.M. 1996. No evidence for the work-conflict hypothesis in the eusocial naked mole-rat (*Heterocephalus glaber*). *Behavioral Ecology and Sociobiology*, 39, 401–409.

Jaeggi, A.V. & Gurven, M. 2013. Natural cooperators: food sharing in humans and other primates. *Evolutionary Anthropology*, 22, 186–195.

Jaeggi, A.V. & van Schaik, C.P. 2011. The evolution of food sharing in primates. *Behavioral Ecology and Sociobiology*, 65, 2125–2140.

Jaeggi, A.V., Stevens, J.M. & Van Schaik, C.P. 2010. Tolerant food sharing and reciprocity is precluded by despotism among bonobos but not chimpanzees. *American Journal of Physical Anthropology*, 143, 41–51.

Jaeggi, A.V., De Groot, E., Stevens, J.M. & Van Schaik, C.P. 2013. Mechanisms of reciprocity in primates: testing for short-term contingency of grooming and food sharing in bonobos and chimpanzees. *Evolution and Human Behavior*, 34, 69–77.

Jamieson, I.G., Quinn, J.S., Rose, P.A. & White, B.N. 1994. Shared paternity among non-relatives is a result of an egalitarian mating system in a communally breeding bird, the pukeko. *Proceedings of the Royal Society of London B: Biological Sciences*, 257, 271–277.

Jandt, J.M., Tibbetts, E.A. & Toth, A.L. 2014. *Polistes* paper wasps: a model genus for the study of social dominance hierarchies. *Insectes Sociaux*, 61, 11–27.

Jaramillo, J.L., Ospina, C.M., Gil, Z.N., Montoya, E.C. & Benavides, P. 2011. Advances on the biology of *Corthylus zulmae* (Coleoptera: Curculionidae) in *Alnus acuminata* (Betulaceae). *Revista Colombiana de Entomologia*, 37, 48–55.

Jeanne, R.L. 1991. The swarm-founding Polistinae. In Ross, K.G. & Matthews, R.W. (eds), *The Social Biology of Wasps*, pp. 191–231. Ithaca, NY: Cornell University Press.

Jennions, M.D. & Macdonald, D.W. 1994. Cooperative breeding in mammals. *Trends in Ecology & Evolution*, 9, 89–93.

Jetz, W. & Rubenstein, D.R. 2011. Environmental uncertainty and the global biogeography of cooperative breeding in birds. *Current Biology*, 21, 72–78.

Jirotkul, M. 1999. Population density influences male–male competition in guppies. *Animal Behaviour*, 58, 1169–1175.

Johansen, J.L., Vaknin, R., Steffensen, J.F. & Domenici, P. 2010. Kinematics and energetic benefits of schooling in the labriform fish, striped surfperch *Embiotoca lateralis*. *Marine Ecology Progress Series*, 420, 221–229.

Johns, P.M., Howard, K.J., Breisch, N.L., Rivera, A. & Thorne, B.L. 2009. Nonrelatives inherit colony resources in a primitive termite. *Proceedings of the National Academy of Sciences of the United States of America*, 106, 17452–17456.

Johnston, C.E. 1994. Nest association in fishes: evidence for mutualism. *Behavioral Ecology and Sociobiology*, 35, 379–383.

Johnstone, R.A. 2000. Models of reproductive skew: a review and synthesis. *Ethology*, 106, 5–26.

Johnstone, R.A. 2001. Eavesdropping and animal conflict. *Proceedings of the National Academy of Sciences of the United States of America*, 98, 9177–9180.

Johnstone, R.A. 2008. Kin selection, local competition, and reproductive skew. *Evolution*, 62, 2592–2599.

Johnstone, R.A. 2011. Load lightening and negotiation over offspring care in cooperative breeders. *Behavioral Ecology*, 22, 436–444.

Johnstone, R.A. & Cant, M.A. 1999. Reproductive skew and the threat of eviction: a new perspective. *Proceedings of the Royal Society of London B: Biological Sciences*, 266, 275–279.

Johnstone, R.A. & Cant, M.A. 2008. Sex differences in dispersal and the evolution of helping and harming. *American Naturalist*, 172, 318–330.

Johnstone, R. & Cant, M.A. 2009. Models of reproductive skew: outside options and the resolution of reproductive conflict. In Hager, R. & Jones, C.B. (eds), *Reproductive Skew in Vertebrates: Proximate and Ultimate Causes*, pp. 3–23. Cambridge: Cambridge University Press.

Johnstone, R.A. & Cant, M.A. 2010. The evolution of menopause in cetaceans and humans: the role of demography. *Proceedings of the Royal Society of London B: Biological Sciences*, 277, 3765–3771.

Johnstone, R.A. & Hinde, C. 2006. Negotiation over offspring care – how should parents respond to each other's efforts? *Behavioral Ecology*, 17, 818–827.

Johnstone, R.A. & Keller, L. 2000. How males can gain by harming their mates: sexual conflict, seminal toxins, and the cost of mating. *The American Naturalist*, 156, 368–377.

Johnstone, R.A. & Roulin, A. 2003. Sibling negotiation. *Behavioral Ecology*, 14, 780–786.

Johnstone, R.A. & Savage, J.L. 2019. Conditional cooperation and turn-taking in parental care. *Frontiers in Ecology and Evolution*, 7, 335.

Johnstone, R.A., Cant, M.A. & Field, J. 2012. Sex-biased dispersal, haplodiploidy and the evolution of helping in social insects. *Proceedings of the Royal Society of London B: Biological Sciences*, 279, 787–793.

Johnstone, R.A., Manica, A., Fayet, A.L., et al. 2014. Reciprocity and conditional cooperation between great tit parents. *Behavioral Ecology*, 25, 216–222.

Johnstone, R.A., Cant, M.A., Cram, D. & Thompson, F.J. 2020. Exploitative leaders incite violent intergroup conflict in a social mammal. *Proceedings of the National Academy of Sciences of the United States of America*, 117, 29759–29766.

Jolles, J.W., King, A.J., Manica, A. & Thornton, A. 2013. Heterogeneous structure in mixed-species corvid flocks in flight. *Animal Behaviour*, 85, 743–750.

Jolles, J.W., Boogert, N.J., Sridhar, V.H., Couzin, I.D. & Manica, A. 2017. Consistent individual differences drive collective behavior and group functioning of schooling fish. *Current Biology*, 27, 2862–2868.

Jolles, J.W., King, A.J. & Killen, S.S. 2020. The role of individual heterogeneity in collective animal behaviour. *Trends in Ecology & Evolution*, 35, 278–291.

Jones, E.I., Bronstein, J.L. & Ferriere, R. 2012. The fundamental role of competition in the ecology and evolution of mutualisms. *Year in Evolutionary Biology*, 1256, 66–88.

Jones, H.A.C., Noble, C., Damsgård, B. & Pearce, G.P. 2012. Investigating the influence of predictable and unpredictable feed delivery schedules upon the behaviour and welfare of Atlantic salmon parr (*Salmo salar*) using social network analysis and fin damage. *Applied Animal Behaviour Science*, 138, 132–140.

Jordal, B.H. & Cognato, A.I. 2012. Molecular phylogeny of bark and ambrosia beetles reveals multiple origins of fungus farming during periods of global warming. *BMC Evolutionary Biology*, 12, 133.

Jordan, L.A., Wong, M.Y. & Balshine, S.S. 2010. The effects of familiarity and social hierarchy on group membership decisions in a social fish. *Biology Letters*, 6, 301–303.

Jordan, N.R., Buse, C., Wilson, A.M., et al. 2017. Dynamics of direct inter-pack encounters in endangered African wild dogs. *Behavioral Ecology and Sociobiology*, 71, 115.

Josi, D., Taborsky, M. & Frommen, J.G. 2020a. Investment of group members is contingent on helper number and the presence of young in a cooperative breeder. *Animal Behaviour*, 160, 35–42.

Josi, D., Freudiger, A., Taborsky, M. & Frommen, J.G. 2020b. Experimental predator intrusions in a cooperative breeder reveal task partitioning of group members. *Behavioral Ecology*, 31, 1369–1378.

Jungwirth, A. & Taborsky, M. 2015. First- and second-order sociality determine survival and reproduction in cooperative cichlids. *Proceedings of the Royal Society of London B: Biological Sciences*, 282, 20151971.

Jungwirth, A., Walker, J. & Taborsky, M. 2015a. Prospecting precedes dispersal and increases survival chances in cooperatively breeding cichlids. *Animal Behaviour*, 106, 107–114.

Jungwirth, A., Josi, D., Walker, J. & Taborsky, M. 2015b. Benefits of coloniality: communal defence saves antipredator effort in cooperative breeders. *Functional Ecology*, 29, 1218–1224.

Kaburu, S.S. & Newton-Fisher, N.E. 2015. Egalitarian despots: hierarchy steepness, reciprocity and the grooming-trade model in wild chimpanzees, *Pan troglodytes*. *Animal Behaviour*, 99, 61–71.

Kagel, J.H., Green, L. & Caraco, T. 1986. When foragers discount the future – constraint or adaptation. *Animal Behaviour*, 34, 271–283.

Kaniewska, P., Alon, S., Karako-Lampert, S., Hoegh-Guldberg, O. & Levy, O. 2015. Signaling cascades and the importance of moonlight in coral broadcast mass spawning. *Elife*, 4, e09991.

Kappeler, P.M. 2013. Why male mammals are monogamous. *Science*, 341, 469–470.

Kappeler, P.M. 2017. Sex roles and adult sex ratios: insights from mammalian biology and consequences for primate behaviour. *Philosophical Transactions of the Royal Society of London B: Biological Sciences*, 372, 20160321.

Kappeler, P.M. & Fichtel, C. 2012. Female reproductive competition in *Eulemur rufifrons*: eviction and reproductive restraint in a plurally breeding Malagasy primate. *Molecular Ecology*, 21, 685–698.

Kappeler, P.M. & van Schaik, C.P. 2002. Evolution of primate social systems. *International Journal of Primatology*, 23, 707–740.

Kardile, S.P. & Gadagkar, R. 2002. Docile sitters and active fighters in paper wasps: a tale of two queens. *Naturwissenschaften*, 89, 176–179.

Karplus, I. & Thompson, A. 2011. The partnership between gobiid fishes and burrowing alpheid shrimps. In Patzner, R.A., Van Tassell, J.L., Kovačić, M. & Kapoor, B.G. (eds), *The Biology of Gobies*, pp. 559–607. New York, NY: Science Publishers.

Kasper, C., Colombo, M., Aubin-Horth, N. & Taborsky, B. 2018. Brain activation patterns following a cooperation opportunity in a highly social cichlid fish. *Physiology & Behavior*, 195, 37–47.

Katula, R.S. & Page, L.M. 1998. Nest association between a large predator, the bowfin (*Amia calva*), and its prey, the golden shiner (*Notemigonus crysoleucas*). *Copeia*, 220–221.

Katz, L., Levitt, S.D. & Shustorovich, E. 2003. Prison conditions, capital punishment, and deterrence. *American Law and Economics Review*, 5, 318–343.

Katz, Y., Tunström, K., Ioannou, C.C., Huepe, C. & Couzin, I.D. 2011. Inferring the structure and dynamics of interactions in schooling fish. *Proceedings of the National Academy of Sciences of the United States of America*, 108, 18720–18725.

Kawasaki, Y., Ito, M., Miura, K. & Kajimura, H. 2010. Superinfection of five *Wolbachia* in the alnus ambrosia beetle, *Xylosandrus germanus* (Blandford) (Coleoptera: Curuculionidae). *Bulletin of Entomological Research*, 100, 231–239.

Keane, B., Waser, P.M., Creel, S.R., et al. 1994. Subordinate reproduction in dwarf mongooses. *Animal Behaviour*, 47, 65–75.

Keen, W.H. & Reed, R.W. 1985. Territorial defense of space and feeding sites by a plethodontid salamander. *Animal Behaviour*, 33, 1119–1123.

Keenleyside, M.H.A. 1991. Parental care. In Keenleyside, M.H.A. (ed.), *Cichlid Fishes: Behaviour, Ecology and Evolution*, pp. 191–208. London: Chapman and Hall.

Keller, L. 1997. Indiscriminate altruism: unduly nice parents and siblings. *Trends in Ecology & Evolution*, 12, 99–103.

Keller, L. & Reeve, H.K. 1994. Partitioning of reproduction in animal societies. *Trends in Ecology & Evolution*, 9, 98–102.

Keller, L. & Ross, K.G. 1998. Selfish genes: a green beard in the red fire ant. *Nature*, 394, 573.

Keller, L.F. & Waller, D.M. 2002. Inbreeding effects in wild populations. *Trends in Ecology & Evolution*, 17, 230–241.

Keller, L., Peer, K., Bernasconi, C., Taborsky, M. & Shuker, D.M. 2011. Inbreeding and selection on sex ratio in the bark beetle *Xylosandrus germanus*. *BMC Evolutionary Biology*, 11, 359.

Kellogg, K.A., Markert, J.A., Stuaffer, J.R. Jr & Kocher, T.D. 1995. Microsatellite variation demonstrates multiple paternity in lekking cichlid fishes from Lake Malawi, Africa. *Proceedings of the Royal Society of London B: Biological Sciences*, 260, 79–84.

Kellogg, K.A., Markert, J.A., Stauffer, J.R. & Kocher, T.D. 1998. Intraspecific brood mixing and reduced polyandry in a maternal mouth-brooding cichlid. *Behavioral Ecology*, 9, 309–312.

Kemp, A.C. & Woodcock, M. 1995. *The Hornbills*. Oxford: Oxford University Press.

Kempenaers, B.A.R.T. & Dhondt, A.A. 1993. Why do females engage in extra-pair copulations? A review of hypotheses and their predictions. *Belgian Journal of Zoology*, 123, 93.

Kempenaers, B.A.R.T. & Sheldon, B.C. 1997. Studying paternity and paternal care: pitfalls and problems. *Animal Behaviour*, 53, 423–427.

Kennedy, P., Higginson, A.D., Radford, A.N. & Sumner, S. 2018. Altruism in a volatile world. *Nature*, 555, 359–362.

Kent, D.I., Fisher, J.D. & Marliave, J.B. 2011. Interspecific nesting in marine fishes: spawning of the spinynose sculpin, *Asemichthys taylori*, on the eggs of the buffalo sculpin, *Enophrys bison*. *Ichthyological Research*, 58, 355–359.

Kent, D.S. & Simpson, J.A. 1992. Eusociality in the beetle *Austroplatypus incompertus* (Coleoptera, Curculionidae). *Naturwissenschaften*, 79, 86–87.

Kern, J.M. & Radford, A.N. 2018. Experimental evidence for delayed contingent cooperation among wild dwarf mongooses. *Proceedings of the National Academy of Sciences of the United States of America*, 115, 6255–6260.

Kerth, G. 2008. Causes and consequences of sociality in bats. *Bioscience*, 58, 737–746.

Kerth, G. & Reckardt, K. 2003. Information transfer about roosts in female Bechstein's bats: an experimental field study. *Proceedings of the Royal Society of London B: Biological Sciences*, 270, 511–515.

Kettler, N., Schweinfurth, M.K. & Taborsky, M. 2021. Rats show direct reciprocity when interacting with multiple partners. *Scientific Reports*, 11, 3228.

Keynan, O., Ridley, A.R. & Lotem, A. 2015. Social foraging strategies and acquisition of novel foraging skills in cooperatively breeding Arabian babblers. *Behavioral Ecology*, 26, 207–214.

Kiers, E.T. & West, S.A. 2015. Evolving new organisms via symbiosis. *Science*, 348, 392–394.

Kiers, E.T., Duhamel, M., Beesetty, Y., et al. 2011. Reciprocal rewards stabilize cooperation in the mycorrhizal symbiosis. *Science*, 333, 880–882.

Killingback, T. & Doebeli, M. 2002. The continuous prisoner's dilemma and the evolution of cooperation through reciprocal altruism with variable investment. *American Naturalist*, 160, 421–438.

Kilner, R.M. & Hinde, C.A. 2008. Information warfare and parent–offspring conflict. *Advances in the Study of Behavior*, 38, 283–336.

Kilner, R.M. & Hinde, C.A. 2012. Parent–offspring conflict. In Royle, N.J., Smiseth, P.T. & Kölliker, M. (eds), *The Evolution of Parental Care*, pp. 119–132. Oxford: Oxford University Press.

Kilner, R.M. & Langmore, N.E. 2011. Cuckoos versus hosts in insects and birds: adaptations, counter-adaptations and outcomes. *Biological Reviews*, 86, 836–852.

Kim, J.-W., Wood, J.L.A., Grant, J.W.A. & Brown, G.E. 2011. Acute and chronic increases in predation risk affect the territorial behaviour of juvenile Atlantic salmon in the wild. *Animal Behaviour*, 81, 93–99.

King, W.J. 1989a. Spacing of female kin in Columbian ground squirrels (*Spermophilus columbianus*). *Canadian Journal of Zoology*, 67, 91–95.

King, W.J. 1989b. Kin-differential behaviour of adult female Columbian ground squirrels. *Animal Behaviour*, 38, 354–356.

Kingma, S.A. 2017. Direct benefits explain interspecific variation in helping behaviour among cooperatively breeding birds. *Nature Communications*, 8, 1–7.

Kingma, S.A., Santema, P., Taborsky, M. & Komdeur, J. 2014. Group augmentation and the evolution of cooperation. *Trends in Ecology & Evolution*, 29, 476–484.

Kingma, S.A., Bebbington, K., Hammers, M., Richardson, D.S. & Komdeur, J. 2016a. Delayed dispersal and the costs and benefits of different routes to independent breeding in a cooperatively breeding bird. *Evolution*, 70, 2595–2610.

Kingma, S.A., Komdeur, J., Hammers, M. & Richardson, D.S. 2016b. The cost of prospecting for dispersal opportunities in a social bird. *Biology Letters*, 12, 20160316.

Kingma, S.A., Komdeur, J., Burke, T. & Richardson, D.S. 2017. Differential dispersal costs and sex-biased dispersal distance in a cooperatively breeding bird. *Behavioral Ecology*, 28, 1113–1121.

Kirkendall, L.R. 1993. Ecology and evolution of biased sex ratios in bark and ambrosia beetles. In Wrensch, D.L. & Ebbert, M.A. (eds), *Evolution and Diversity of Sex Ratio in Insects and Mites*, pp. 235–345. New York, NY: Chapman & Hall.

Kirkendall, L.R. 2006. A new host-specific, *Xyleborus vochysiae* (Curculionidae: Scolytinae), from Central America breeding in live trees. *Annals of the Entomological Society of America*, 99, 211–217.

Kirkendall, L.R., Kent, D.S. & Raffa, K.F. 1997. Interactions among males, females and offspring in bark and ambrosia beetles: the significance of living in tunnels for the evolution of social behavior. In Choe, J.C. & Crespi, B.J. (eds), *The Evolution of Social Behavior in Insects and Arachnids*, pp. 181–215. Cambridge: Cambridge University Press.

Kirkendall, L.R., Biedermann, P.H. & Jordal, B.H. 2015. Evolution and diversity of bark and ambrosia beetles. In Vega, F.E. & Hofstetter, R.W. (eds), *Bark Beetles. Biology and Ecology of Native and Invasive Species*, pp. 85–156. Amsterdam: Academic Press.

Klaassen, M., Brenninkmeijer, A., Boix-Hinzen, C. & Mendelsohn, J. 2003. Fathers with highly demanding partners and offspring in a semidesert environment: energetic aspects of the breeding system of Monteiro's hornbills (*Tockus monteiri*) in Namibia. *Auk*, 120, 866–873.

Klug, H. 2018. Why monogamy? A review of potential ultimate drivers. *Frontiers in Ecology and Evolution*, 6, 30.

Klug, H. & Bonsall, M.B. 2007. When to care for, abandon, or eat your offspring: the evolution of parental care and filial cannibalism. *The American Naturalist*, 170, 88–901.

Knapp, R.A. & Sargent, R.C. 1989. Egg-mimicry as a mating strategy in the fantail darter, *Etheostoma flabellare*: females prefer males with eggs. *Behavioural Ecology and Sociobiology*, 25, 321–326.

Knapp, R., Wingfield, J.C. & Bass, A.H. 1999. Steroid hormones and paternal care in the plainfin midshipman fish (*Porichthys notatus*). *Hormones and Behavior*, 35, 81–89.

Knell, R.J. 2009. Population density and the evolution of male aggression. *Journal of Zoology*, 278, 83–90.

Knopp, T., Heimovirta, M., Kokko, H. & Merilä, J. 2008. Do male moor frogs (*Rana arvalis*) lek with kin? *Molecular Ecology*, 17, 2522–2530.

Koblmüller, S., Odhiambo, E.A., Sinyinza, D., Sturmbauer, C. & Sefc, K.M. 2015. Big fish, little divergence: phylogeography of Lake Tanganyika's giant cichlid, *Boulengerochromis microlepis*. *Hydrobiologia*, 748, 29–38.

Koenig, W.D. & Dickinson, J.L. 2004. *Ecology and Evolution of Cooperative Breeding in Birds.* Cambridge: Cambridge University Press.

Koenig, W.D. & Dickinson, J.L. 2016. *Cooperative Breeding in Vertebrates.* Cambridge: Cambridge University Press.

Koenig, W. & Haydock, J. 2004. Incest and incest avoidance. In Koenig, W. & Dickinson, J. (eds), *Ecology and Evolution of Cooperative Breeding in Birds,* pp. 142–156. Cambridge: Cambridge University Press.

Koenig, W.D. & Walters, E.L. 2011. Age-related provisioning behaviour in the cooperatively breeding acorn woodpecker: testing the skills and the pay-to-stay hypotheses. *Animal Behaviour,* 82, 437–444.

Koenig, W.D., Pitelka, F.A., Carmen, W.J., Mumme, R.L. & Stanback, M.T. 1992. The evolution of delayed dispersal in cooperative breeders. *The Quarterly Review of Biology,* 67, 111–150.

Koenig, W.D., Haydock, J. & Stanback, M.T. 1998. Reproductive roles in the cooperatively breeding acorn woodpecker: incest avoidance versus reproductive competition. *The American Naturalist,* 151, 243–255.

Koenig, W.D., Hooge, P.N., Stanback, M.T. & Haydock, J. 2000. Natal dispersal in the cooperatively breeding acorn woodpecker. *The Condor,* 102, 492–502.

Koenig, W.D., Walters, E.L. & Haydock, J. 2009. Helpers and egg investment in the cooperatively breeding acorn woodpecker: testing the concealed helper effects hypothesis. *Behavioral Ecology and Sociobiology,* 63, 1659–1665.

Koenig, W.D., Dickinson, J.L. & Emlen, S.T. 2016. Synthesis: cooperative breeding in the twenty-first century. In Koenig, W.D. & Dickinson, J.L. (eds), *Cooperative Breeding in Vertebrates: Studies of Ecology, Evolution, and Behavior,* pp. 353–374. New York, NY: Cambridge University Press.

Koenig, W.D., Walters, E.L. & Barve, S. 2019. Does helping-at-the-nest help? The case of the acorn woodpecker. *Frontiers in Ecology and Evolution,* 7, 272.

Koga, T. & Ikeda, S. 2010. Perceived predation risk and mate defense jointly alter the outcome of territorial fights. *Behavioral Ecology and Sociobiology,* 64, 827–833.

Kohda, M. 1997. Interspecific society among herbivorous cichlid fishes. In Kawanabe, H., Hori, M. & Nagoshi, M. (eds), *Fish Communities of Lake Tanganyika,* pp. 107–120. Kyoto: Kyoto University Press.

Kohda, M., Heg, D., Makino, Y., et al. 2009. Living on the wedge: female control of paternity in a cooperatively polyandrous cichlid. *Proceedings of the Royal Society of London B: Biological Sciences,* 276, 4207–4214.

Kohda, M., Jordan, L.A., Hotta, T., et al. 2015. Facial recognition in a group-living cichlid fish. *PLoS One,* 10, e0142552.

Kokko, H. 2013. Dyadic contests: modelling flights between two individuals. In Hardy, I.C.W. & Briffa,

M. (eds), *Animal Contests.* Cambridge: Cambridge University Press

Kokko, H. & Lindström, J. 1996. Kin selection and the evolution of leks: whose success do young males maximize? *Proceedings of the Royal Society of London B: Biological Sciences,* 263, 919–923.

Kokko, H. & Ots, I. 2006. When not to avoid inbreeding. *Evolution,* 60, 467–475.

Kokko, H., Johnstone, R.A. & Clutton-Brock, T.H. 2001. The evolution of cooperative breeding through group augmentation. *Proceedings of the Royal Society of London B: Biological Sciences,* 268, 187–196.

Kokko, H., Johnstone, R.A. & Wright, J. 2002. The evolution of parental and alloparental effort in cooperatively breeding groups: when should helpers pay to stay? *Behavioral Ecology,* 13, 291–300.

Komdeur, J. 1992. Importance of habitat saturation and territory quality for evolution of cooperative breeding in the Seychelles warbler. *Nature,* 358, 493–495.

Komdeur, J. 1993. Fitness-related dispersal. *Nature,* 366, 23.

Komdeur, J. 1994a. Experimental evidence for helping and hindering by previous offspring in the cooperative-breeding Seychelles warbler *Acrocephalus sechellensis.* *Behavioral Ecology and Sociobiology,* 34, 175–186.

Komdeur, J. 1994b. The effect of kinship on helping in the cooperative breeding Seychelles warbler (*Acrocephalus sechellensis*). *Proceedings of the Royal Society of London B: Biological Sciences,* 256, 47–52.

Komdeur, J. 1994c. Conserving the Seychelles warbler *Acrocephalus sechellensis* by translocation from Cousin Island to the islands of Aride and Cousine. *Biological Conservation,* 67, 143–152.

Komdeur, J. 1996a. Influence of age on reproductive performance in the Seychelles warbler. *Behavioral Ecology,* 7, 417–425.

Komdeur, J. 1996b. Seasonal timing of reproduction in a tropical bird, the Seychelles warbler: a field experiment using translocation. *Journal of Biological Rhythms,* 11, 333–346.

Komdeur, J. 1996c. Influence of helping and breeding experience on reproductive performance in the Seychelles warbler: a translocation experiment. *Behavioral Ecology,* 7, 326–333.

Komdeur, J. & Daan, S. 2005. Breeding in the monsoon: semi-annual reproduction in the Seychelles warbler (*Acrocephalus sechellensis*). *Journal of Ornithology,* 146, 305–313.

Komdeur, J. & Edelaar, P. 2001a. Male Seychelles warblers use territory budding to maximize lifetime fitness in a saturated environment. *Behavioral Ecology,* 12, 706–715.

Komdeur, J. & Edelaar, P. 2001b. Evidence that helping at the nest does not result in territory inheritance in the Seychelles warbler. *Proceedings of the Royal Society of London B: Biological Sciences,* 268, 2007–2012.

Komdeur, J. & Ekman, J. 2010. Adaptations and constraints in the evolution of delayed dispersal: implications for cooperation. In Szekely, T., Moore, A.J. & Komdeur, J. (eds), *Social Behaviour. Genes, Ecology and Evolution*, pp. 306–327. Cambridge: Cambridge University Press.

Komdeur, J. & Hatchwell, B.J. 1999. Kin recognition: function and mechanism in avian societies. *Trends in Ecology & Evolution*, 14, 237–241.

Komdeur, J. & Kats, R.K. 1999. Predation risk affects trade-off between nest guarding and foraging in Seychelles warblers. *Behavioral Ecology*, 10, 648–658.

Komdeur, J. & Pels, M.t.D. 2005. Rescue of the Seychelles warbler on Cousin Island, Seychelles: the role of habitat restoration. *Biological Conservation*, 124, 15–26.

Komdeur, J., Huffstadt, A., Prast, et al. 1995. Transfer experiments of Seychelles warblers to new islands: changes in dispersal and helping behaviour. *Animal Behaviour*, 49, 695–708.

Komdeur, J., Daan, S., Tinbergen, J. & Mateman, C. 1997. Extreme adaptive modification in sex ratio of the Seychelles warbler's eggs. *Nature*, 385, 522–525.

Komdeur, J., Richardson, D.S., Hammers, M., et al. 2001. The evolution of cooperative breeding in vertebrates. *eLS*, 1–11.

Komdeur, J., Piersma, T., Kraaijeveld, K., Kraaijeveld-Smit, F. & Richardson, D.S. 2004a. Why Seychelles warblers fail to recolonize nearby islands: unwilling or unable to fly there? *Ibis*, 146, 298–302.

Komdeur, J., Richardson, D.S. & Burke, T. 2004b. Experimental evidence that kin discrimination in the Seychelles warbler is based on association and not on genetic relatedness. *Proceedings of the Royal Society of London B: Biological Sciences*, 271, 963.

Komdeur, J., Eikenaar, C., Brouwer, L. & Richardson, D.S. 2008. The evolution and ecology of cooperative breeding in vertebrates. *eLS*.

Komdeur, J., Burke, T., Dugdale, H.L. & Richardson, D.S. 2016. Seychelles warblers: Complexities of the helping paradox. In Koenig, W.D. & Dickinson, J.L. (eds), *Cooperative Breeding in Vertebrates. Studies of Ecology, Evolution and Behaviour*, pp. 197–216. New York, NY: Cambridge University Press.

Komdeur, J., Richardson, D.S., Hammers, M., et al. 2017. The evolution of cooperative breeding in vertebrates. *eLS*. https://doi.org/10.1002/9780470015902.a0021218 .pub2

Kondoh, M. & Higashi, M. 2000. Reproductive isolation mechanism resulting from resolution of intragenomic conflict. *American Naturalist*, 156, 511–518.

Korb, J. & Heinze, J. 2004. Multilevel selection and social evolution of insect societies. *Naturwissenschaften*, 91, 291–304.

Korolev, K.S., Xavier, J.B. & Gore, J. 2014. Turning ecology and evolution against cancer. *Nature Reviews Cancer*, 14, 371.

Korpimäki, E., Norrdahl, K. & Rinta-Jaskari, T. 1991. Responses of stoats and least weasels to fluctuating food abundances: is the low phase of the vole cycle due to mustelid predation? *Oecologia*, 88, 552–561.

Korpimäki, E., Oksanen, L., Oksanen, T., et al. 2005. Vole cycles and predation in temperate and boreal zones of Europe. *Journal of Animal Ecology*, 74, 1150–1159.

Koster, J., Lukas, D., Nolin, D., et al. 2019. Kinship ties across the lifespan in human communities. *Philosophical Transactions of the Royal Society of London B: Biological Sciences*, 374.

Kotiaho, J.S., Simmons, L.W., Hunt, J. & Tomkins, J.L. 2003. Males influence maternal effects that promote sexual selection: a quantitative genetic experiment with dung beetles *Onthophagus taurus*. *The American Naturalist*, 161, 852–859.

Kotrschal, A. & Taborsky, B. 2010. Resource defence or exploded lek? – A question of perspective. *Ethology*, 116, 1189–1198.

Kotrschal, K., Hemetsberger, J. & Dittami, J. 1993. Food exploitation by a winter flock of greylag geese – behavioral dynamics, competition and social status. *Behavioral Ecology and Sociobiology*, 33, 289–295.

Koyama, N. 1973. Dominance, grooming, and clasped-sleeping relationships among bonnet monkeys in India. *Primates*, 14, 225–244.

Koyama, N., Caws, C. & Aureli, F. 2006. Interchange of grooming and agonistic support in chimpanzees. *International Journal of Primatology*, 27, 1293–1309.

Koykka, C. & Wild, G. 2015. The evolution of group dispersal with leaders and followers. *Journal of Theoretical Biology*, 371, 117–126.

Kölliker, M., Boos, S., Wong, J.W.Y., et al. 2015. Parent–offspring conflict and the genetic trade-offs shaping parental investment. *Nature Communications*, 6, 6850.

König, B. 1989. Kin recognition and maternal care under restricted feeding in house mice (*Mus domesticus*). *Ethology*, 82, 328–343.

König, B. 1994. Components of lifetime reproductive success in communally and solitarily nursing house mice – a laboratory study. *Behavioral Ecology and Sociobiology*, 34, 275–283.

Kraak, S.B. 1996. Female preference and filial cannibalism in *Aidablennius sphynx* (Teleostei, Blenniidae); a combined field and laboratory study. *Behavioural Processes*, 36, 85–97.

Kraak, S.B.M. & Groothuis, T.G.G. 1994. Female preference for nests with eggs is based on the presence of the eggs themselves. *Behaviour*, 131, 189–206.

Kraak, S.B.M., Bakker, T.C.M. & Mundwiler, B. 1999. Correlates of the duration of the egg collecting phase in the three-spined stickleback. *Journal of Fish Biology*, 54, 1038–1049.

Krafft, B., Colin, C. & Peignot, P. 1994. Diving for food – a new model to assess social roles in a group of laboratory rats. *Ethology*, 96, 11–23.

Krakauer, A.H. 2005. Kin selection and cooperative court-ship in wild turkeys. *Nature*, 434, 69–72.

Krakauer, A.H. & DuVal, E.H. 2011. Kin selection and cooperative courtship in birds. In Salmon, C.A. & Shackelford, T.K. (eds), *The Oxford Handbook of Evolutionary Family Psychology*. New York, NY: Oxford University Press.

Krama, T., Vrublevska, J., Freeberg, T.M., et al. 2012. You mob my owl, I'll mob yours: birds play tit-for-tat game. *Scientific Reports*, 2, 800.

Kramer, J., Klauke, N., Bauer, M. & Schaefer, H.M. 2016. No evidence for enforced alloparental care in a coopera-tively breeding parrot. *Ethology*, 122, 389–398.

Krams, I., Krama, T., Igaune, K. & Maend, R. 2008. Experimental evidence of reciprocal altruism in the pied flycatcher. *Behavioral Ecology and Sociobiology*, 62, 599–605.

Krams, I., Berzins, A., Krama, T., et al. 2010. The increased risk of predation enhances cooperation. *Proceedings of the Royal Society of London B: Biological Sciences*, 277, 513–518.

Krams, I., Kokko, H., Vrublevska, J., et al. 2013. The excuse principle can maintain cooperation through for-givable defection in the Prisoner's Dilemma game. *Proceedings of the Royal Society of London B: Biological Sciences*, 280, 20131475.

Krasheninnikova, A., Brucks, D., Blanc, S. & von Bayern, A.M.P. 2019. Assessing African grey parrots' prosocial tendencies in a token choice paradigm. *Royal Society Open Science*, 6, 190696.

Krause, J. & Godin, J.G. 1994. Shoal choice in the banded killifish (*Fundulus diaphanus*, Teleostei, Cyprinodontidae): effects of predation risk, fish size, species composition and size of shoals. *Ethology*, 98, 128–136.

Krause, J. & Ruxton, G.D. 2002. *Living in Groups*. Oxford: Oxford University Press.

Krebs, J.R. 1974. Colonial nesting and social feeding as strategies for exploiting food resources in the great blue heron (*Ardea herodias*). *Behaviour*, 51, 99–134.

Kruuk, H. 1972. *The Spotted Hyena: a Study of Predation and Social Behavior*. Chicago, IL: University of Chicago Press.

Kuijper, B. & Johnstone, R.A. 2018. Maternal effects and parent–offspring conflict. *Evolution*, 72, 220–233.

Kunz, T.H. (ed.). 1982. Roosting ecology of bats. In *Ecology of Bats*, pp. 1–55. Boston, MA: Springer.

Kutsukake, N. & Clutton-Brock, T.H. 2006a. Aggression and submission reflect reproductive conflict between females in cooperatively breeding meerkats *Suricata suricatta*. *Behavioral Ecology and Sociobiology*, 59, 541–548.

Kutsukake, N. & Clutton-Brock, T.H. 2006b. Social func-tions of allogrooming in cooperatively breeding meer-kats. *Animal Behaviour*, 72, 1059–1068.

Kutsukake, N. & Clutton-Brock, T.H. 2010. Grooming and the value of social relationships in cooperatively breed-ing meerkats. *Animal Behaviour*, 79, 271–279.

Kutsukake, N., Inada, M., Sakamoto, S.H. & Okanoya, K. 2012. A distinct role of the queen in coordinated work-load and soil distribution in eusocial naked mole-rats. *PLoS One*, 7, e44584.

Kümmerli, R., Gardner, A., West, S.A. & Griffin, A.S. 2009a. Limited dispersal, budding dispersal, and cooper-ation: an experimental study. *Evolution*, 63, 939–949.

Kümmerli, R., Griffin, A.S., West, S.A., Buckling, A. & Harrison, F. 2009b. Viscous medium promotes cooper-ation in the pathogenic bacterium *Pseudomonas aerugi-nosa*. *Proceedings of the Royal Society of London B: Biological Sciences*, 276, 3531–3538.

Kvarnemo, C. 2018. Why do some animals mate with one partner rather than many? A review of causes and conse-quences of monogamy. *Biological Reviews*, 93, 1795–1812.

Lacey, E.A. & Sherman, P.W. 1991. Social organization of naked mole-rat colonies: evidence for divisions of labor. In Sherman, P.W., Jarvis, J.U.M. & Alexander, R.D. (eds), *The Biology of the Naked Mole-Rat*, pp. 275–336. Princeton, NJ: Princeton University Press.

Lacey, E.A., Braude, S.H. & Wieczorek, J.R. 1998. Solitary burrow use by adult Patagonian tuco-tucos (*Ctenomys haigi*). *Journal of Mammalogy*, 79, 986–991.

Lacey, E., O'Brien, S.L., Sobrero, R. & Ebensperger, L.A. 2019. Spatial relationships among free-living cururos (*Spalacopus cyanus*) demonstrate burrow sharing and communal nesting. *Journal of Mammalogy*, 100, 1918–1927.

Lahdenperä, M., Lummaa, V., Helle, S., Tremblay, M. & Russell, A.F. 2004. Fitness benefits of prolonged post-reproductive lifespan in women. *Nature*, 428, 178–181.

Lahdenperä, M., Gillespie, D.O., Lummaa, V. & Russell, A.F. 2012. Severe intergenerational reproductive conflict and the evolution of menopause. *Ecology Letters*, 15, 1283–1290.

Laidre, M.E. 2011. Ecological relations between hermit crabs and their shell-supplying gastropods: constrained consumers. *Journal of Experimental Marine Biology and Ecology*, 397, 65–70.

Laidre, M.E. 2013. Eavesdropping foragers use level of collective commotion as public information to target high quality patches. *Oikos*, 122, 1505–1511.

Laland, K.N., Sterelny, K., Odling-Smee, J., Hoppitt, W. & Uller, T. 2011. Cause and effect in biology revisited: is Mayr's proximate–ultimate dichotomy still useful? *Science*, 334, 1512–1516.

Lalueza-Fox, C., Rosas, A., Estalrrich, A., et al. 2011. Genetic evidence for patrilocal mating behavior among Neandertal groups. *Proceedings of the National Academy of Sciences of the United States of America*, 108, 250–253.

Lamba, S., Kazi, Y.C., Deshpande, S., et al. 2007. A possible novel function of dominance behaviour in queen-less colonies of the primitively eusocial wasp *Ropalidia marginata*. *Behavioural Processes*, 74, 351–356.

Lambert, D.M., Millar, C.D., Jack, K., Anderson, S. & Craig, J.L. 1994. Single and multilocus DNA fingerprinting of communally breeding pukeko: do copulations or dominance ensure reproductive success? *Proceedings of the National Academy of Sciences of the United States of America*, 91, 9641–9645.

Landa, J.T. 1998. Bioeconomics of schooling fishes: selfish fish, quasi-free riders, and other fishy tales. *Environmental Biology of Fishes*, 53, 353–364.

Langen, K., Schwarzer, J., Kullmann, H., Bakker, T.C. & Thünken, T. 2011. Microsatellite support for active inbreeding in a cichlid fish. *PLoS One*, 6, e24689.

Langer, P., Hogendoorn, K. & Keller, L. 2004. Tug-of-war over reproduction in a social bee. *Nature*, 428, 844–847.

Langergraber, K., Mitani, J. & Vigilant, L. 2009. Kinship and social bonds in female chimpanzees (*Pan troglodytes*). *American Journal of Primatology*, 71, 840–851.

Lank, D.B. & Smith, C.M. 1992. Females prefer larger leks: field experiments with ruffs (*Philomachus pugnax*). *Behavioral Ecology and Sociobiology*, 30, 323–329.

Lank, D.B., Smith, C.M., Hanotte, O., Burke, T. & Cooke, F. 1995. Genetic polymorphism for alternative mating-behavior in lekking male ruff *Philomachus pugnax*. *Nature*, 378, 59–62.

Lank, D.B., Smith, C.M., Hanotte, O., et al. 2002. High frequency of polyandry in a lek mating system. *Behavioral Ecology*, 13, 209–215.

Larose, K. & Dubois, F. 2011. Constraints on the evolution of reciprocity: an experimental test with zebra finches. *Ethology*, 117, 115–123.

Laundré, J.W., Hernández, L. & Altendorf, K.B. 2001. Wolves, elk, and bison: reestablishing the 'landscape of fear' in Yellowstone National Park, USA. *Canadian Journal of Zoology*, 79, 1401–1409.

Lawler, R.R., Richard, A.F. & Riley, M.A. 2003. Genetic population structure of the white sifaka (*Propithecus verreauxi verreauxi*) at Beza Mahafaly Special Reserve, southwest Madagascar (1992–2001). *Molecular Ecology*, 12, 2307–2317.

Lawson Handley, L.L. & Perrin, N. 2007. Advances in our understanding of mammalian sex-biased dispersal. *Molecular Ecology*, 16, 1559–1578.

Lazaro-Perea, C. 2001. Intergroup interactions in wild common marmosets, *Callithrix jacchus*: territorial defence and assessment of neighbours. *Animal Behaviour*, 62, 11–21.

Le Comber, S.C., Faulkes, C.G., Formosinho, J. & Smith, C. 2003. Response of territorial males to the threat of sneaking in the three-spined stickleback (*Gasterosteus aculeatus*): a field study. *Journal of Zoology*, 261, 15–20.

Le Roux, A., Cherry, M.I., Gygax, L. & Manser, M.B. 2009. Vigilance behaviour and fitness consequences: comparing a solitary foraging and an obligate group-foraging mammal. *Behavioral Ecology and Sociobiology*, 63, 1097–1107.

Le Roux, A., Snyder-Mackler, N., Roberts, E.K., Beehner, J.C. & Bergman, T.J. 2013. Evidence for tactical concealment in a wild primate. *Nature Communications*, 4, 1–6.

Le Vin, A., Mable, B. & Arnold, K. 2010. Kin recognition via phenotype matching in a cooperatively breeding cichlid, *Neolamprologus pulcher*. *Animal Behaviour*, 79, 1109–1114.

Le Vin, A., Mable, B., Taborsky, M., Heg, D. & Arnold, K. 2011. Individual variation in helping in a cooperative breeder: relatedness versus behavioural type. *Animal Behaviour*, 82, 467–477.

Leadbeater, E., Carruthers, J.M., Green, J.P., van Heusden, J. & Field, J. 2010. Unrelated helpers in a primitively eusocial wasp: is helping tailored toward direct fitness? *PLoS One*, 5, e11997.

Leadbeater, E., Carruthers, J.M., Green, J.P., Rosser, N.S. & Field, J. 2011. Nest inheritance is the missing source of direct fitness in a primitively eusocial insect. *Science*, 333, 874–876.

Lebigre, C., Alatalo, R.V., Forss, H.E. & Siitari, H. 2008. Low levels of relatedness on black grouse leks despite male philopatry. *Molecular Ecology*, 17, 4512–4521.

Leclaire, S., Nielsen, J.F., Thavarajah, N.K., Manser, M. & Clutton-Brock, T.H. 2013. Odour-based kin discrimination in the cooperatively breeding meerkat. *Biology Letters*, 9, 20121054.

Lee, J.W., Jang, B.S., Dawson, D.A., Burke, T. & Hatchwell, B.J. 2009. Fine-scale genetic structure and its consequence in breeding aggregations of a passerine bird. *Molecular Ecology*, 18, 2728–2739.

Lee, J.W., Lee, Y.K. & Hatchwell, B.J. 2010. Natal dispersal and philopatry in a group-living but noncooperative passerine bird, the vinous-throated parrotbill. *Animal Behaviour*, 79, 1017–1023.

Leggett, H.C., El Mouden, C., Wild, G. & West, S. 2011. Promiscuity and the evolution of cooperative breeding. *Proceedings of the Royal Society of London B: Biological Sciences*, 279, 1405–1411.

Leggett, H.C., Wild, G., West, S.A. & Buckling, A. 2017. Fast-killing parasites can be favoured in spatially structured populations. *Philosophical Transactions of the Royal Society of London B: Biological Sciences*, 372, 20160096.

Lehmann, L. 2007. The evolution of trans-generational altruism: kin selection meets niche construction. *Journal of Evolutionary Biology*, 20, 181–189.

Lehmann, L. & Balloux, F. 2007. Natural selection on fecundity variance in subdivided populations: kin selection meets bet hedging. *Genetics*, 176, 361–377.

Lehmann, L. & Feldman, M.W. 2008. War and the evolution of belligerence and bravery. *Proceedings of the Royal Society of London B: Biological Sciences*, 275, 2877–2885.

Lehmann, L. & Keller, L. 2006a. The evolution of cooperation and altruism – a general framework and a classification of models. *Journal of Evolutionary Biology*, 19, 1365–1376.

Lehmann, L. & Keller, L. 2006b. Synergy, partner choice and frequency dependence: their integration into inclusive fitness theory and their interpretation in terms of direct and indirect fitness effects. *Journal of Evolutionary Biology*, 19, 1426–1436.

Lehmann, L. & Perrin, N. 2003. Inbreeding avoidance through kin recognition: choosy females boost male dispersal. *The American Naturalist*, 162, 638–652.

Lehmann, L. & Rousset, F. 2010. How life history and demography promote or inhibit the evolution of helping behaviours. *Philosophical Transactions of the Royal Society of London B: Biological Sciences*, 365, 2599–2617.

Lehmann, L., Bargum, K. & Reuter, M. 2006. An evolutionary analysis of the relationship between spite and altruism. *Journal of Evolutionary Biology*, 19, 1507–1516.

Lehmann, L., Keller, L., West, S. & Roze, D. 2007. Group selection and kin selection: two concepts but one process. *Proceedings of the National Academy of Sciences of the United States of America*, 104, 6736–6739.

Lehner, S.R., Rutte, C. & Taborsky, M. 2011. Rats benefit from winner and loser effects. *Ethology*, 117, 949–960.

Lehtonen, J. 2016. Multilevel selection in kin selection language. *Trends in Ecology & Evolution*, 31, 752–762.

Leigh, E.G.J. 2010. The evolution of mutualism. *Journal of Evolutionary Biology*, 23, 2507–2528.

Leighton, G.M. & Vander Meiden, L. 2016. Sociable weavers increase cooperative nest construction after suffering aggression. *PLoS One*, 11, e0150953.

Leimar, O. & Hammerstein, P. 2001. Evolution of cooperation through indirect reciprocity. *Proceedings of the Royal Society of London B: Biological Sciences*, 268, 745–753.

Leimar, O. & Hammerstein, P. 2010. Cooperation for direct fitness benefits. *Philosophical Transactions of the Royal Society of London B: Biological Sciences*, 365, 2619–2626.

Leimar, O., Austad, S. & Enquist, M. 1991. A test of the sequential assessment game: fighting in the bowl and doily spider *Frontinella pyramitela*. *Evolution*, 45, 862–874.

Leimgruber, K.L. 2018. The developmental emergence of direct reciprocity and its influence on prosocial behavior. *Current Opinion in Psychology*, 20, 122–126.

Leimgruber, K.L., Ward, A.F., Widness, J., et al. 2014. Give what you get: capuchin monkeys (*Cebus apella*) and 4-year-old children pay forward positive and negative outcomes to conspecifics. *PLoS One*, 9, e87035.

Leinfelder, I., De Vries, H., Deleu, R. & Nelissen, M. 2001. Rank and grooming reciprocity among females in a mixed-sex group of captive hamadryas baboons. *American Journal of Primatology*, 55, 25–42.

Lenormand, T., Engelstädter, J., Johnston, S.E., Wijnker, E. & Haag, C.R. 2016. Evolutionary mysteries in meiosis. *Philosophical Transactions of the Royal Society of London B*, 371, 20160001.

Lessells, C.M. 1991. The evolution of life histories. In Krebs, J.R. & Davies, N.B. (eds), *Behavioural Ecology: An Evolutionary Approach*, pp. 32–68. Oxford: Blackwell Scientific.

Lessells, C.M. 2006. The evolutionary outcome of sexual conflict. *Philosophical Transactions of the Royal Society of London B*, 361, 301–317.

Lessells, C.M. 2012. Sexual conflict. In Royle, N.J., Smiseth, P.T. & Kölliker, M. (eds), *The Evolution of Parental Care*, pp. 150–170. Oxford: Oxford University Press.

Lessells, C. & McNamara, J.M. 2012. Sexual conflict over parental investment in repeated bouts: negotiation reduces overall care. *Proceedings of the Royal Society of London B: Biological Sciences*, 279, 1506–1514.

Levin, S.R., Gandon, S. & West, S.A. 2020. The social coevolution hypothesis for the origin of enzymatic cooperation. *Nature Ecology & Evolution*, 4, 132–137.

Levitan, D.R. 1995. The ecology of fertilization in free-spawning invertebrates. In McEdward, L. (ed.), *Ecology of Marine Invertebrate Larvae*, pp. 123–156. Marine Science Series. Boca Raton, FL: CRC Press.

Levitan, D.R., Sewell, M.A. & Chia, F.S. 1991. Kinetics of fertilization in the sea urchin *Strongylocentrotus franciscanus*: interaction of gamete dilution, age, and contact time. *The Biological Bulletin*, 181, 371–378.

Levitis, D.A. & Lackey, L.B. 2011. A measure for describing and comparing postreproductive life span as a population trait. *Methods in Ecology and Evolution*, 2, 446–453.

Lewis, D.S.C. 1980. Mixed species broods in Lake Malawi cichlids: an alternative to the cuckoo theory. *Copeia*, 4, 874–875.

Lewis, S., Roberts, G., Harris, M.P., Prigmore, C. & Wanless, S. 2007. Fitness increases with partner and neighbour allopreening. *Biology Letters*, 3, 386–389.

Liao, X.Y., Rong, S. & Queller, D.C. 2015. Relatedness, conflict, and the evolution of eusociality. *PLoS Biology*, 13, e1002098.

Liebl, A.L., Nomano, F.Y., Browning, L.E. & Russell, A.F. 2016. Experimental evidence for fully additive care among male carers in the cooperatively breeding chestnut-crowned babbler. *Animal Behaviour*, 115, 47–53.

Lievin-Bazin, A., Pineaux, M., Le Covec, M., et al. 2019. Food sharing and affiliation: an experimental and longitudinal study in cockatiels (*Nymphicus hollandicus*). *Ethology*, 125, 276–288.

Ligon, J.D. 1983. Cooperation and reciprocity in avian social systems. *American Naturalist*, 121, 366–384.

Ligon, J.D. & Burt, D.B. 2004. Evolutionary origins. In Koenig, W.D. & Dickinson, J.L. (eds), *Ecology and Evolution of Cooperative Breeding in Birds*, pp. 5–34. Cambridge: Cambridge University Press.

Ligon, J.D. & Ligon, S.H. 1978a. Communal breeding in green woodhoopoes as a case for reciprocity. *Nature*, 276, 496–498.

Ligon, J.D. & Ligon, S.H. 1978b. The communal social system of the green woodhoopoe in Kenya. *Living Bird*, 17, 159–197.

Ligon, J.D. & Ligon, S.H. 1983. Reciprocity in the green woodhoopoe (*Phoeniculus purpureus*). *Animal Behaviour*, 31, 480–489.

Ligon, J.D., Ligon, S.H. & Ford, H.A. 1991. An experimental study of the bases of male philopatry in the cooperatively breeding superb fairy-wren *Malurus cyaneus*. *Ethology*, 87, 134–148.

Lill, J.T. & Marquis, R.J. 2007. Microhabitat manipulation: ecosystem engineering by shelter-building insects. In Cuddington, K., Byers, J.E., Wilson, W.G. & Hastings, A. (eds), *Ecosystem Engineers: Plants to Protists*, pp. 107–138. New York, NY: Elsevier.

Lima, M.R., Macedo, R.H., Muniz, L., Pacheco, A. & Graves, J.A. 2011. Group composition, mating system, and relatedness in the communally breeding guira cuckoo (*Guira guira*) in Central Brazil. *The Auk*, 128, 475–486.

Lima, S.L. & Dill, L.M. 1990. Behavioral decisions made under the risk of predation: a review and prospectus. *Canadian Journal of Zoology*, 68, 619–640.

Limberger, D. 1983. Pairs and harems in a cichlid fish, *Lamprologus brichardi*. *Zeitschrift für Tierpsychologie*, 62, 115–144.

Lion, S. & Boots, M. 2010. Are parasites 'prudent' in space? *Ecology Letters*, 13, 1245–1255.

Lippold, S., Xu, H., Ko, A., et al. 2014. Human paternal and maternal demographic histories: insights from high-resolution Y chromosome and mtDNA sequences. *Investigative Genetics*, 5, 13.

Little, A.E.F. & Currie, C.R. 2007. Symbiotic complexity: discovery of a fifth symbiont in the attine ant–microbe symbiosis. *Biology Letters*, 3, 501–504.

Loiselle, B.A., Blake, J.G., Durães, R., Ryder, T.B. & Tori, W. 2007. Environmental and spatial segregation of leks among six co-occurring species of manakins (Pipridae) in eastern Ecuador. *The Auk*, 124, 420–431.

Loke, L.H.L., Ladle, R.J., Bouma, T.J. & Todd, P.A. 2015. Creating complex habitats for restoration and reconciliation. *Ecological Engineering*, 77, 307–313.

LoPresti, E.F. & Morse, D.H. 2013. Costly leaf shelters protect moth pupae from parasitoids. *Arthropod–Plant Interactions*, 7, 445–453.

Lopuch, S. & Popik, P. 2011. Cooperative behavior of laboratory rats (*Rattus norvegicus*) in an instrumental task. *Journal of Comparative Psychology*, 125, 250–253.

Lorenz, K. 1963. *Das Sogenannte Böse. Zur Naturgeschichte Der Aggression*. Vienna: Borotha-Schoeler.

Losin, N., Drury, J.P., Peiman, K.S., Storch, C. & Grether, G.F. 2016. The ecological and evolutionary stability of interspecific territoriality. *Ecology Letters*, 19, 260–267.

Lott, D.F. 1991. *Intraspecific Variation in the Social Systems of Wild Vertebrates* (2nd ed.). Cambridge: Cambridge University Press.

Loukola, O.J., Perry, C.J., Coscos, L. & Chittka, L. 2017. Bumblebees show cognitive flexibility by improving on an observed complex behavior. *Science*, 355, 833–836.

Løvlie, H., Gillingham, M.A., Worley, K., Pizzari, T. & Richardson, D.S. 2013. Cryptic female choice favours sperm from major histocompatibility complex-dissimilar males. *Proceedings of the Royal Society of London B: Biological Sciences*, 280, 20131296.

Lubin, Y. & Bilde, T. 2007. The evolution of sociality in spiders. *Advances in the Study of Behavior*, 37, 83–145.

Lucherini, M. & Birochio, D.E. 1997. Lack of aggression and avoidance between vicuna and guanaco herds grazing in the same Andean habitat. *Studies on Neotropical Fauna and Environment*, 32, 72–75.

Lukas, D. & Clutton-Brock, T.H. 2012a. The evolution of mammalian societies: cooperative breeding monogamy and polytocy. *Proceeding of the Royal Society of London B: Biological Sciences*, 279, 4065–4070.

Lukas, D. & Clutton-Brock, T. 2012b. Cooperative breeding and monogamy in mammalian societies. *Proceedings of the Royal Society of London B: Biological Sciences*, 279, 2151–2156.

Lukas, D. & Clutton-Brock, T.H. 2013. The evolution of social monogamy in mammals. *Science*, 341, 526–530.

Lukas, D. & Clutton-Brock, T. 2017. Climate and the distribution of cooperative breeding in mammals. *Royal Society Open Science*, 4, 160897.

Lutermann, H., Verburgt, L. & Rendigs, A. 2010. Resting and nesting in a small mammal: sleeping sites as a limiting resource for female grey mouse lemurs. *Animal Behaviour*, 79, 1211–1219.

Lüscher, M. 1961. Social control of polymorphism in termites. In Kennedy, J.S. (ed.), *Insect Polymorphism*, pp. 57–67. London: Royal Entomological Society.

Lynch, M. & Walsh, B. 1998. *Genetics and Analysis of Quantitative Traits*. Sunderland, MA: Sinauer.

Maan, M.E. & Taborsky, M. 2007. Sexual conflict over breeding substrate causes female expulsion and offspring loss in a cichlid fish. *Behavioral Ecology*, 19, 302–308.

MacColl, A.D. & Hatchwell, B.J. 2004. Determinants of lifetime fitness in a cooperative breeder, the long-tailed tit *Aegithalos caudatus*. *Journal of Animal Ecology*, 73, 1137–1148.

MacDougall-Shackleton, S.A. 2011. The levels of analysis revisited. *Philosophical Transactions of the Royal Society of London B: Biological Sciences*, 366, 2076–2085.

Mace, R. & Alvergne, A. 2012. Female reproductive competition within families in rural Gambia. *Proceedings of the Royal Society of London B: Biological Sciences*, 279, 2219–2227.

Macedo, R.H. & Bianchi, C.A. 1997. Communal breeding in tropical Guira cuckoos *Guira guira*: sociality in the absence of a saturated habitat. *Journal of Avian Biology*, 28, 207–215.

Machanda, Z.P., Gilby, I.C. & Wrangham, R.W. 2014. Mutual grooming among adult male chimpanzees: the immediate investment hypothesis. *Animal Behaviour*, 87, 165–174.

Mackenzie, A., Reynolds, J.D., Brown, V.J. & Sutherland, W.J. 1995. Variation in male mating success on leks. *The American Naturalist*, 145, 633–652.

MacLeod, K. & Clutton-Brock, T. 2015. Low costs of allonursing in meerkats: mitigation by behavioral change? *Behavioral Ecology*, 26, 697–705.

MacLeod, K.J. & Lukas, D. 2014. Revisiting non-offspring nursing: allonursing evolves when the costs are low. *Biology Letters*, 10, 20140378.

MacLeod, K.J., Nielsen, J.F. & Clutton-Brock, T.H. 2013. Factors predicting the frequency, likelihood and duration of allonursing in the cooperatively breeding meerkat. *Animal Behaviour*, 86, 1059–1067.

Madden, J.R., Lowe, T.J., Fuller, H.V., et al. 2004. Neighbouring male spotted bowerbirds are not related, but do maraud each other. *Animal Behaviour*, 68, 751–758.

Madden, J.R. & Clutton-Brock, T.H. 2009. Manipulating grooming by decreasing ectoparasite load causes unpredicted changes in antagonism. *Proceedings of the Royal Society of London B: Biological Sciences*, 276, 1263–1268.

Madgwick, P.G., Belcher, L.J. & Wolf, J.B. 2019. Greenbeard genes: theory and reality. *Trends in Ecology & Evolution*, 34, 1092–1103.

Magnus, D.B.E. 1967. Zur Ökologie sedimentbewohnender *Alpheus garnelen* (Decapoda, Natantia) des Roten Meeres. *Helgoländer Wissenschaftliche Meeresuntersuchungen*, 15, 506.

Magrath, R.D. & Whittingham, L.A. 1997. Subordinate males are more likely to help if unrelated to the breeding female in cooperatively breeding white-browed scrubwrens. *Behavioral Ecology and Sociobiology*, 41, 185–192.

Magurran, A.E. 1990. The adaptive significance of schooling as an anti-predator defence in fish. *Annales Zoologici Fennici*, 27, 51–66.

Maher, C.R. & Lott, D.F. 2000. A review of ecological determinants of territoriality within vertebrate species. *American Midland Naturalist*, 143, 1–29.

Mainwaring, M.C. 2011. The use of nestboxes by roosting birds during the non-breeding season: a review of the costs and benefits. *Ardea*, 99, 167–176.

Majolo, B., Schino, G. & Aureli, F. 2012. The relative prevalence of direct, indirect and generalized reciprocity in macaque grooming exchanges. *Animal Behaviour*, 83, 763–771.

Manica, A. 2002. Filial cannibalism in teleost fish. *Biological Reviews*, 77, 261–277.

Manica, A., Fayet, A.L., Hinde, C.A., et al. 2013. Reciprocity and conditional cooperation between great tit parents. *Behavioral Ecology*, 25, 216–222.

Manser, M.B. 2001. The acoustic structure of suricates' alarm calls varies with predator type and the level of response urgency. *Proceedings of the Royal Society of London B: Biological Sciences*, 268, 2315–2324.

Manson, J.H., Navarrete, C.D., Silk, J.B. & Perry, S. 2004. Time-matched grooming in female primates? New analyses from two species. *Animal Behaviour*, 67, 493–500.

Marconato, A. & Bisazza, A. 1986. Males whose nests contain eggs are preferred by female *Cottus gobio* L. (Pisces, Cottidae). *Animal Behaviour*, 34, 1580–1582.

Marler, P., Dufty, A. & Pickert, R. 1986a. Vocal communication in the domestic chicken: I. Does a sender communicate information about the quality of a food referent to a receiver? *Animal Behaviour*, 34, 188–193.

Marler, P., Dufty, A. & Pickert, R. 1986b. Vocal communication in the domestic chicken: II. Is a sender sensitive to the presence and nature of a receiver? *Animal Behaviour*, 34, 194–198.

Marlowe, F.W. 2004. Marital residence among foragers. *Current Anthropology*, 45, 277–284.

Marshall, H.H., Sanderson, J.L., Mwanghuya, F., et al. 2016. Variable ecological conditions promote male helping by changing banded mongoose group composition. *Behavioral Ecology*, 27, 978–987.

Marshall, J.A.R. 2011. Group selection and kin selection: formally equivalent approaches. *Trends in Ecology & Evolution*, 26, 325–332.

Martel, G. 1996. Growth rate and influence of predation risk on territoriality in juvenile coho salmon (*Oncorhynchus kisutch*). *Canadian Journal of Fisheries and Aquatic Sciences*, 53, 660–669.

Martel, G. & Dill, L.M. 1993. Feeding and aggressive behaviours in juvenile coho salmon (*Oncorhynchus kisutch*) under chemically-mediated risk of predation. *Behavioral Ecology and Sociobiology*, 32, 365–370.

Martin, E. & Taborsky, M. 1997. Alternative male mating tactics in a cichlid, *Pelvicachromis pulcher*: a comparison of reproductive effort and success. *Behavioral Ecology and Sociobiology*, 41, 311–319.

Martin, S.J., Beekman, M., Wossler, T.C. & Ratnieks, F.L.W. 2002. Parasitic Cape honeybee workers, *Apis mellifera capensis*, evade policing. *Nature*, 415, 163–165.

Marzluff, J.M. & Balda, R.P. 1990. Pinyon jays: making the best of a bad situation by helping. In Koenig, W.D. & Dickinson, J.L. (eds), *Cooperative Breeding in Vertebrates: Studies of Ecology, Evolution, and Behavior*, pp. 199–237. New York, NY: Cambridge University Press.

Marzluff, J.M. & Heinrich, B. 1991. Foraging by common ravens in the presence and absence of territory holders: an experimental analysis of social foraging. *Animal Behaviour*, 42, 755–770.

Marzluff, J.M., Heinrich, B. & Marzluff, C.S. 1996. Raven roosts are mobile information centres. *Animal Behaviour*, 51, 89–103.

Maslow, A.H. 1936. The rôle of dominance in the social and sexual behavior of infra-human primates: I. observations at vilas park zoo. *Pedagogical Seminary and Journal of Genetic Psychology*, 48, 261–277.

Masse, A. & Cote, S.D. 2013. Spatiotemporal variations in resources affect activity and movement patterns of white-tailed deer (*Odocoileus virginianus*) at high density. *Canadian Journal of Zoology*, 91, 252–263.

Massen, J.J.M., Ritter, C. & Bugnyar, T. 2015. Tolerance and reward equity predict cooperation in ravens (*Corvus corax*). *Scientific Reports*, 5, 15021.

Masuda, N. 2007. Participation costs dismiss the advantage of heterogeneous networks in evolution of cooperation. *Proceedings of the Royal Society of London B: Biological Sciences*, 274, 1815–1821.

Masuda, N. 2011. Clustering in large networks does not promote upstream reciprocity. *PLoS One*, 6, e25190.

Masuda, N. 2012. Evolution of cooperation driven by zealots. *Scientific Reports*, 2, 646.

Matsumoto, K. & Kohda, M. 2004. Territorial defense against various food competitors in the Tanganyikan benthophagous cichlid *Neolamprologus tetracanthus*. *Ichthyological Research*, 51, 354–359.

Matsuura, K. 2012. Multifunctional queen pheromone and maintenance of reproductive harmony in termite colonies. *Journal of Chemical Ecology*, 38, 746–754.

Mattey, S.N. & Smiseth, P.T. 2015. No inbreeding avoidance by female burying beetles regardless of whether they encounter males simultaneously or sequentially. *Ethology*, 121, 1031–1038.

May, R.M., Conway, G.R., Hassell, M.P. & Southwood, T.R.E. 1974. Time delays, density-dependence and single-species oscillations. *The Journal of Animal Ecology*, 747–770.

May, R.M. 1981. The evolution of cooperation. *Nature*, 292, 291–292.

Maynard Smith, J. 1964. Group selection and kin selection. *Nature*, 201, 1145–1147.

Maynard Smith, J. 1974. The theory of games and the evolution of animal conflicts. *Journal of Theoretical Biology*, 47, 209–221.

Maynard Smith, J. 1977. Parental investment: a prospective analysis. *Animal Behaviour*, 25, 1–9.

Maynard Smith, J. 1982a. *Evolution and the Theory of Games*. Cambridge: Cambridge University Press.

Maynard Smith, J. 1982b. The evolution of social behaviour – a classification of models. In *Current Problems in Sociobiology*, pp. 29–44. Cambridge: Cambridge University Press.

Maynard Smith, J. 1988. Evolutionary progress and levels of selection. In Nitecki, M.H. (ed.), *Evolutionary Progress*, pp. 219–230. Chicago, IL: University of Chicago Press.

Maynard Smith, J. & Harper, D. 2003. *Animal Signals*. New York, NY: Oxford University Press.

Maynard Smith, J. & Parker, G.A. 1976. The logic of asymmetric contests. *Animal Behaviour*, 24, 159–175.

Maynard Smith, J. & Price, G.R. 1973. The logic of animal conflict. *Nature*, 246, 15–18.

Maynard Smith, J. & Ridpath, M.G. 1972. Wife sharing in the Tasmaninan native hen, *Tribonyx mortierii* – a case of kin selection? *American Naturalist*, 106, 447–452.

Maynard Smith, J. & Szathmary, E. 1995. *The Major Transitions in Evolution*. Oxford: Oxford University Press.

Mayr, E. 1961. Cause and effect in biology. *Science*, 134, 1501–1506.

McDonald, D.B. 1993a. Delayed plumage maturation and orderly queues for status: a manakin mannequin experiment. *Ethology*, 94, 31–45.

McDonald, D.B. 1993b. Demographic consequences of sexual selection in the long-tailed manakin. *Behavioral Ecology*, 4, 297–309.

McDonald, D.B. 2009. Young-boy networks without kin clusters in a lek-mating manakin. *Behavioral Ecology and Sociobiology*, 63, 1029–1034.

McDonald, D.B. & Potts, W.K. 1994. Cooperative display and relatedness among males in a lek-mating bird. *Science*, 266, 1030–1032.

McDonald, P.G. 2014. Cooperative breeding beyond kinship: why else do helpers help? *Emu*, 114, 91–96.

McDonald, P.G. & Wright, J. 2011. Bell miner provisioning calls are more similar among relatives and are used by helpers at the nest to bias their effort towards kin. *Proceedings of the Royal Society of London B: Biological Sciences*, 278, 3403–3411.

McDonald, P.G., Kazem, A.J.N., Clarke, M.F. & Wright, J. 2008a. Helping as a signal: does removal of potential audiences alter helper behavior in the bell miner? *Behav. Ecol.*, 19, 1047–1055.

McDonald, P.G., Te Marvelde, L., Kazem, A.J. & Wright, J. 2008b. Helping as a signal and the effect of a potential audience during provisioning visits in a cooperative bird. *Animal Behaviour*, 75, 1319–1330.

McEachern, M.B., Eadie, J.M. & Van Vuren, D.H. 2007. Local genetic structure and relatedness in a solitary mammal, *Neotoma fuscipes*. *Behavioral Ecology and Sociobiology*, 61, 1459–1469.

McFall-Ngai, M. 2014. Divining the essence of symbiosis: insights from the squid–*Vibrio* model. *PLoS Biology*, 12, e1001783.

McGregor, P.K. 2005. *Animal Communication Networks*. Cambridge: Cambridge University Press.

McInnes, A.M., McGeorge, C., Ginsberg, S., Pichegru, L. & Pistorius, P.A. 2017. Group foraging increases foraging efficiency in a piscivorous diver, the African penguin. *Royal Society Open Science*, 4.

McKaye, K.R. 1977. Defense of a predator's young by a herbivorous fish: an unusual strategy. *The American Naturalist*, 111, 301–315.

McKaye, K.R. 1979. Defense of a predator's young revisited. *The American Naturalist*, 114, 595–601.

McKaye, K.R. 1985. Cichlid–catfish mutualistic defense of young in Lake Malawi, Africa. *Oecologia*, 66, 358–363.

McKaye, K.R. & McKaye, N.M. 1977. Communal care and kidnapping of young by parental cichlids. *Evolution*, 31, 674–681.

McKaye, K.R. & Oliver, M.K. 1980. Geometry of a selfish school: defence of cichlid young by bagrid catfish in Lake Malawi, Africa. *Animal Behaviour*, 28, 1287.

McKaye, K.R., Mughogho, D.E. & Lovullo, T.J. 1992. Formation of the selfish school. *Environmental Biology of Fishes*, 35, 213–218.

McKinnon, L., Gilchrist, H.G. & Scribner, K.T. 2006. Genetic evidence for kin-based female social structure in common eiders (*Somateria mollissima*). *Behavioral Ecology*, 17, 614–621.

McMahon, B.F. & Evans, R.M. 1992. Foraging strategies of American white pelicans. *Behaviour*, 120, 69–89.

McNamara, J.M. 2013. Towards a richer evolutionary game theory. *Journal of the Royal Society Interface*, 10, 20130544.

McNamara, J.M. & Houston, A.I. 2002. Credible threats and promises. *Philosophical Transactions of the Royal Society of London B: Biological Sciences*, 357, 1607–1616.

McNamara, J.M. & Houston, A.I. 2009. Integrating function and mechanism. *Trends in Ecology & Evolution*, 24, 670–675.

McNamara, J.M., Gasson, C.E. & Houston, A.I. 1999. Incorporating rules for responding into evolutionary games. *Nature*, 401, 368–371.

McNamara, J.M., Houston, A.I., Barta, Z. & Osorno, J.L. 2003. Should young ever be better off with one parent than with two? *Behavioral Ecology*, 14, 301–310.

McNamara, J.M., Barta, Z., Fromhage, L. & Houston, A.I. 2008. The coevolution of choosiness and cooperation. *Nature*, 451, 189–192.

McPherson, M., Smith-Lovin, L. & Cook, J.M. 2001. Birds of a feather: homophily in social networks. *Annual Review of Sociology*, 27, 415–444.

McRae, S.B. 1996. Family values: costs and benefits of communal nesting in the moorhen. *Animal Behaviour*, 52, 225–245.

Mech, L.D. 2003. *The Wolves of Denali*. Minneapolis, MN: University of Minnesota Press.

Medawar, P.B. 1957. *Uniqueness of the Individual*. London: Methuen.

Mehlis, M., Bakker, T.C. & Frommen, J.G. 2008. Smells like sib spirit: kin recognition in three-spined sticklebacks (*Gasterosteus aculeatus*) is mediated by olfactory cues. *Animal Cognition*, 11, 643–650.

Mehlis, M., Bakker, T.C., Engqvist, L. & Frommen, J.G. 2010. To eat or not to eat: egg-based assessment of paternity triggers fine-tuned decisions about filial cannibalism. *Proceedings of the Royal Society of London B: Biological Sciences*, 277, 2627–2635.

Mehlis, M., Thunken, T., Bakker, T. & Frommen, J. 2015. Quantification acuity in spontaneous shoaling decisions of three-spined sticklebacks. *Animal Cognition*, 18, 1125–1131.

Meise, K., von Engelhardt, N., Forcada, J. & Hoffman, J.I. 2016. Offspring hormones reflect the maternal prenatal social environment: potential for foetal programming? *PLoS One*, 11, e0145352.

Melis, A.P., Hare, B. & Tomasello, M. 2008. Do chimpanzees reciprocate received favours? *Animal Behaviour*, 76, 951–962.

Melis, A.P., Hare, B. & Tomasello, M. 2009. Chimpanzees coordinate in a negotiation game. *Evolution and Human Behavior*, 30, 381–392.

Mendres, K.A. & de Waal, F.B.M. 2000. Capuchins do cooperate: the advantage of an intuitive task. *Animal Behaviour*, 60, 523–529.

Mennella, J.A., Blumberg, M.S., McClintock, M.K. & Moltz, H. 1990. Inter-litter competition and communal nursing among Norway rats: advantages of birth synchrony. *Behavioral Ecology and Sociobiology*, 27, 183–190.

Mesterton-Gibbons, M. & Dugatkin, L.A. 1992. Cooperation among unrelated individuals – evolutionary factors. *Quarterly Review of Biology*, 67, 267–281.

Metheny, J.D., Kalcounis-Rueppell, M.C., Bondo, K.J. & Brigham, R.M. 2008. A genetic analysis of group movement in an isolated population of tree-roosting bats. *Proceedings of the Royal Society of London B: Biological Sciences*, 275, 2265–2272.

Meunier, J. 2015. Social immunity and the evolution of group living in insects. *Philosophical Transactions of the Royal Society of London B: Biological Sciences*, 370, 20140102.

Meunier, J., West, S.A. & Chapuisat, M. 2008. Split sex ratios in the social Hymenoptera: a meta-analysis. *Behavioral Ecology*, 19, 382–390.

Meunier, J., Delaplace, L. & Chapuisat, M. 2010. Reproductive conflicts and egg discrimination in a socially polymorphic ant. *Behavioral Ecology and Sociobiology*, 64, 1655–1663.

Michael, R.P. & Zumpe, D. 1993. A review of hormonal factors influencing the sexual and aggressive behavior of macaques. *American Journal of Primatology*, 30, 213–241.

Michod, R.E. 2000. *Darwinian Dynamics: Evolutionary Transitions in Fitness and Individuality*. Princeton, NJ: Princeton University Press.

Mielke, A., Crockford, C. & Wittig, R.M. 2019. Snake alarm calls as a public good in sooty mangabeys. *Animal Behaviour*, 158, 201–209.

Milinski, M. 1977. Experiments on the selection by predators against spatial oddity of their prey. *Zeitschrift für Tierpsychologie*, 43, 311–325.

Milinski, M. 1979. An evolutionarily stable feeding strategy in sticklebacks 1. *Zeitschrift für Tierpsychologie*, 51, 36–40.

Milinski, M. 2016. Reputation, a universal currency for human social interactions. *Philosophical Transactions of the Royal Society of London B: Biological Sciences*, 371, 20150100.

Milinski, M. & Wedekind, C. 1998. Working memory constrains human cooperation in the Prisoner's Dilemma. *Proceedings of the National Academy of Sciences of the United States of America*, 95, 13755–13758.

Milinski, M., Pfluger, D., Kulling, D. & Kettler, R. 1990. Do sticklebacks cooperate repeatedly in reciprocal pairs? *Behavioral Ecology and Sociobiology*, 27, 17–21.

Milinski, M., Semmann, D. & Krambeck, H.J. 2002. Reputation helps solve the 'tragedy of the commons'. *Nature*, 415, 424–426.

Mills, A.D., Crawford, L.L., Domjan, M. & Faure, J.M. 1997. The behavior of the Japanese or domestic quail *Coturnix japonica*. *Neuroscience & Biobehavioral Reviews*, 21, 261–281.

Miramontes, O. 1993. Complexity and behaviour in *Leptothorax* ants. *CopIt ArXives*.

Mitani, J.C. 2006. Reciprocal exchange in chimpanzees and other primates. In Kappeler, P.M. & van Schaik, C.P. (eds), *Cooperation in Primates: Mechanisms and Evolution*, pp. 101–113. Heidelberg: Springer-Verlag.

Mitani, J.C. & Watts, D.P. 1999. Demographic influences on the hunting behavior of chimpanzees. *American Journal of Physical Anthropology*, 109, 439–454.

Mitani, J.C. & Watts, D.P. 2001. Why do chimpanzees hunt and share meat? *Animal Behaviour*, 61, 915–924.

Mitani, J.C., Watts, D.P. & Amsler, S.J. 2010. Lethal intergroup aggression leads to territorial expansion in wild chimpanzees. *Current Biology*, 20, R507–R508.

Mitchell, J.S., Jutzeler, E., Heg, D. & Taborsky, M. 2009a. Dominant members of cooperatively-breeding groups adjust their behaviour in response to the sexes of their subordinates. *Behaviour*, 146, 1665–1686.

Mitchell, J.S., Jutzeler, E., Heg, D. & Taborsky, M. 2009b. Gender differences in the costs that subordinate group members impose on dominant males in a cooperative breeder. *Ethology*, 115, 1162–1174.

Mitchell, J.S., Ocana, S.W. & Taborsky, M. 2014. Male and female shell-brooding cichlids prefer different shell characteristics. *Animal Behaviour*, 98, 131–137.

Mitri, S., Floreano, D. & Keller, L. 2009. The evolution of information suppression in communicating robots with conflicting interests. *Proceedings of the National Academy of Sciences of the United States of America*, 106, 15786–15790.

Mitteldorf, J. & Wilson, D.S. 2000. Population viscosity and the evolution of altruism. *Journal of Theoretical Biology*, 204, 481–496.

Miyazawa, E., Seguchi, A., Takahashi, N., Motai, A. & Izawa, E.I. 2020. Different patterns of allopreening in the same-sex and opposite-sex interactions of juvenile large-billed crows (*Corvus macrorhynchos*). *Ethology*, 126, 195–206.

Mock, D.W. & Parker, G.A. 1997. *The Evolution of Sibling Rivalry*. Oxford: Oxford University Press.

Mock, D.W., Dugas, M.B. & Strickler, S.A. 2011. Honest begging: expanding from signal of need. *Behavioral Ecology*, 22, 909–917.

Moczek, A.P. & Emlen, D.J. 2000. Male horn dimorphism in the scarab beetle, *Onthophagus taurus*: do alternative reproductive tactics favour alternative phenotypes? *Animal Behaviour*, 59, 459–466.

Moffett, M.W. 2012. Supercolonies of billions in an invasive ant: What is a society? *Behavioral Ecology*, 23, 925–933.

Molbo, D., Machado, C.A., Herre, E.A. & Keller, L. 2004. Inbreeding and population structure in two pairs of cryptic fig wasp species. *Molecular Ecology*, 13, 1613–1623.

Molesti, S. & Majolo, B. 2017. Evidence of direct reciprocity, but not of indirect and generalized reciprocity, in the grooming exchanges of wild Barbary macaques (*Macaca sylvanus*). *American Journal of Primatology*, 79.

Monaghan, P. & Metcalfe, N.B. 1985. Group foraging in wild brown hares: effects of resource distribution and social status. *Animal Behaviour*, 33, 993–999.

Monnin, T. & Peeters, C. 1999. Dominance hierarchy and reproductive conflicts among subordinates in a monogynous queenless ant. *Behavioral Ecology*, 10, 323–332.

Moody, M. 2008. Serial reciprocity: a preliminary statement. *Sociological Theory*, 26, 130–151.

Moore, J.C., Loggenberg, A. & Greeff, J.M. 2005. Kin competition promotes dispersal in a male pollinating fig wasp. *Biology Letters*, 2, 17–19.

Mooring, M.S. 1995. The effect of tick challenge on grooming rate by impala. *Animal Behaviour*, 50, 377–392.

Mooring, M.S. & Hart, B.L. 1995. Costs of allogrooming in impala – distraction from vigilance. *Animal Behaviour*, 49, 1414–1416.

Mooring, M.S. & Hart, B.L. 1997. Reciprocal allogrooming in wild impala lambs. *Ethology*, 103, 665–680.

Mooring, M.S. & Samuel, W.M. 1999. Premature loss of winter hair in free-ranging moose (*Alces alces*) infested with winter ticks (*Dermacentor albipictus*) is correlated with grooming rate. *Canadian Journal of Zoology – Revue Canadienne de Zoologie*, 77, 148–156.

Morand-Ferron, J. & Quinn, J.L. 2011. Larger groups of passerines are more efficient problem solvers in the wild. *Proceedings of the National Academy of Sciences of the United States of America*, 108, 15898–15903.

Moreira, J., Vukov, J., Sousa, C., et al. 2013. Individual memory and the emergence of cooperation. *Animal Behaviour*, 85, 233–239.

Morgan, L.D. & Fine, M.L. 2020. Agonistic behavior in juvenile blue catfish *Ictalurus furcatus*. *Journal of Ethology*, 38, 29–40.

Mori, S. 1995. Factors associated with and fitness effects of nest-raiding in the three-spined stickleback, *Gasterosteus aculeatus*, in a natural situation. *Behaviour*, 132, 1011–1023.

Morris, B.E.L., Henneberger, R., Hube, H. & Moissl-Eichinger, C. 2013. Microbial syntrophy: interaction for the common good. *FEMS Microbiology Reviews*, 37, 384–406.

Morris, D.W. 1996. Coexistence of specialist and generalist rodents via habitat selection. *Ecology*, 77, 2352–2364.

Morrow, E.H. & Arnqvist, G. 2003. Costly traumatic insemination and a female counter-adaptation in bed bugs. *Proceedings of the Royal Society of London B: Biological Sciences*, 270, 2377–2381.

Morse, D.H. 1978. Structure and foraging patterns of flocks of tits and associated species in an English woodland during the winter. *Ibis*, 120, 298–312.

Mottley, K. & Giraldeau, L.A. 2000. Experimental evidence that group foragers can converge on predicted producer–scrounger equilibria. *Animal Behaviour*, 60, 341–350.

Mueller, C.A. & Cant, M.A. 2010. Imitation and traditions in wild banded mongooses. *Current Biology*, 20, 1171–1175.

Mueller, U.G., Rehner, S.A. & Schultz, T.R. 1998. The evolution of agriculture in ants. *Science*, 281, 2034–2038.

Mueller, U.G., Gerardo, N.M., Aanen, D.K., Six, D.L. & Schultz, T.R. 2005. The evolution of agriculture in insects. *Annual Review of Ecology, Evolution, and Systematics*, 36, 563–595.

Mulder, R.A. & Langmore, N.E. 1993. Dominant males punish helpers for temporary defection in the superb fairy wren. *Animal Behaviour*, 45, 830–833.

Mulder, R.A., Dunn, P.O., Cockburn, A., Cohen, K.A.L. & Howell, M.J. 1994. Helpers liberate female fairy-wrens from constraints on extra-pair mate choice. *Proceedings of the Royal Society of London B: Biological Sciences*, 255, 223–229.

Muller, C.A. & Manser, M.B. 2007. 'Nasty neighbours' rather than 'dear enemies' in a social carnivore. *Proceedings of the Royal Society of London B: Biological Sciences*, 274, 959–965.

Muller, C.A. & Bell, M.B.V. 2009. Kidnapping and infanticide between groups of banded mongooses. *Mammalian Biology*, 74, 315–318.

Mumme, R.L. 1992. Do helpers increase reproductive success? *Behavioral Ecology and Sociobiology*, 31, 319–328.

Mumme, R.L., Koenig, W.D. & Pitelka, F.A. 1983. Reproductive competition in the communal acorn woodpecker – sisters destroy each other's eggs. *Nature*, 306, 583–584.

Mumme, R.L., Koenig, W.D. & Ratnieks, F.L. 1989. Helping behaviour, reproductive value, and the future component of indirect fitness. *Animal Behaviour*, 38, 331–343.

Myrberg, A.A. Jr & Thresher, R.E. 1974. Interspecific aggression and its relevance to the concept of territoriality in reef fishes. *American Zoologist*, 14, 81–96.

Naef, J. & Taborsky, M. 2020a. Commodity-specific punishment for experimentally induced defection in cooperatively breeding fish. *Royal Society Open Science*, 7, 191808.

Naef, J. & Taborsky, M. 2020b. Punishment controls helper defence against egg predators but not against predators of adults in cooperatively breeding cichlids. *Animal Behaviour*, 168, 137–147.

Nagoshi, M. & Gashagaza, M.M. 1988. Growth of the larvae of a Tanganyikan cichlid, *Lamprologus attenuatus*, under parental care. *Japanese Journal of Ichthyology*, 35, 392–395.

Nakamaru, M., Matsuda, H. & Iwasa, Y. 1997. The evolution of cooperation in a lattice-structured population. *Journal of Theoretical Biology*, 184, 65–81.

Nakazawa, T. & Yamamura, N. 2009. Theoretical considerations for the maintenance of interspecific brood care by a Nicaraguan cichlid fish: behavioral plasticity and spatial structure. *Journal of Ethology*, 27, 67–73.

Nam, K.B., Simeoni, M., Sharp, S.P. & Hatchwell, B.J. 2010. Kinship affects investment by helpers in a cooperatively breeding bird. *Proceedings of the Royal Society of London B: Biological Sciences*, 277, 3299–3306.

Nattrass, S., Croft, D.P., Ellis, S., et al. 2019. Postreproductive killer whale grandmothers improve the survival of their grandoffspring. *Proceedings of the National Academy of Sciences of the United States of America*, 116, 26669–26673.

Neems, R.M., Lazarus, J. & Mclachlan, A.J. 1992. Swarming behavior in male chironomid midges: a cost–benefit analysis. *Behavioral Ecology*, 3, 285–290.

Neff, B.D. 2003. Decisions about parental care in response to perceived paternity. *Nature*, 422, 716.

Neff, B.D. & Sherman, P.W. 2003. Nestling recognition via direct cues by parental male bluegill sunfish (*Lepomis macrochirus*). *Animal Cognition*, 6, 87–92.

Neff, B.D. & Svensson, E.I. 2013. Polyandry and alternative mating tactics. *Philosophical Transactions of the Royal Society of London B*, 368, 20120045.

Nelson, R.M. & Greeff, J.M. 2009. Evolution of the scale and manner of brother competition in pollinating fig wasps. *Animal Behaviour*, 77, 693–700.

Neukom, R., Barboza, L.A., Erb, M.P., et al. 2019. Consistent multi-decadal variability in global temperature reconstructions and simulations over the Common Era. *Nature Geoscience*, 12, 643–649.

Nevo, E. 1979. Adaptive convergence and divergence of subterranean mammals. *Annual Review of Ecology and Systematics*, 10, 269–308.

Newby, J., Darden, T., Bassos-Hull, K. & Shedlock, A.M. 2014. Kin structure and social organization in the spotted eagle ray, *Aetobatus narinari*, off coastal Sarasota, FL. *Environmental Biology of Fishes*, 97, 1057–1065.

Newton-Fisher, N.E. & Lee, P.C. 2011. Grooming reciprocity in wild male chimpanzees. *Animal Behaviour*, 81, 439–446.

Nichols, H.J., Jordan, N.R., Jamie, G.A., Cant, M.A. & Hoffman, J.I. 2012a. Fine-scale spatiotemporal patterns of genetic variation reflect budding dispersal coupled with strong natal philopatry in a cooperatively breeding mammal. *Molecular Ecology*, 21, 5348–5362.

Nichols, H.J., Amos, W., Bell, M.B., et al. 2012b. Food availability shapes patterns of helping effort in a cooperative mongoose. *Animal Behaviour*, 83, 1377–1385.

Nichols, H.J., Cant, M.A. & Sanderson, J.L. 2015. Adjustment of costly extra-group paternity according to inbreeding risk in a cooperative mammal. *Behavioral Ecology*, 26, 1486–1494.

Nicholson, A.J. 1954. An outline of the dynamics of animal populations. *Australian Journal of Zoology*, 2, 9–65.

Nicola, G.G., Ayllon, D., Elvira, B. & Almodovar, A. 2016. Territorial and foraging behaviour of juvenile Mediterranean trout under changing conditions of food and competitors. *Canadian Journal of Fisheries and Aquatic Sciences*, 73, 990–998.

Nielsen, C.L.R., Gates, R.J. & Parker, P.G. 2006. Intraspecific nest parasitism of wood ducks in natural cavities: comparisons with nest boxes. *The Journal of Wildlife Management*, 70, 835–843.

Nielsen, J.F., English, S., Goodall-Copestake, W.P., et al. 2012. Inbreeding and inbreeding depression of early life traits in a cooperative mammal. *Molecular Ecology*, 21, 2788–2804.

Niklas, K.J., Cobb, E.D. & Kutschera, U. 2014. Did meiosis evolve before sex and the evolution of eukaryotic life cycles? *Bioessays*, 36, 1091–1101.

Noë, R. 1990. A veto game played by baboons: a challenge to the use of the prisoner's dilemma as a paradigm for reciprocity and cooperation. *Animal Behavior*, 39, 78–90.

Noë, R. 2006. Cooperation experiments: coordination through communication versus acting apart together. *Animal Behaviour*, 71, 1–18.

Noë, R. & Hammerstein, P. 1994. Biological markets – supply-and-demand determine the effect of partner choice in cooperation, mutualism and mating. *Behavioral Ecology and Sociobiology*, 35, 1–11.

Noë, R. & Hammerstein, P. 1995. Biological markets. *Trends in Ecology & Evolution*, 10, 336–339.

Noë, R., Vanschaik, C.P. & Vanhooff, J.A.R.A. 1991. The market effect – an explanation for pay-off asymmetries among collaborating animals. *Ethology*, 87, 97–118.

Noël, M.V., Grant, J.W. & Carrigan, J.G. 2005. Effects of competitor-to-resource ratio on aggression and size variation within groups of convict cichlids. *Animal Behaviour*, 69, 1157–1163.

Nomano, F.Y., Browning, L.E., Savage, J.L., et al. 2015. Unrelated helpers neither signal contributions nor suffer retribution in chestnut-crowned babblers. *Behavioral Ecology*, 26, 986–995.

Nonacs, P. 2011. Kinship, greenbeards, and runaway social selection in the evolution of social insect cooperation. *Proceedings of the National Academy of Sciences of the United States of America*, 108, 10808–10815.

Normark, B.B., Jordal, B.H. & Farrell, B.D. 1999. Origin of a haplodiploid beetle lineage. *Proceedings of the Royal Society of London B: Biological Sciences*, 266, 2253–2259.

Norris, D.M. & Chu, H.-M. 1985. *Xyleborus ferrugineus*. In Singh, P. & Moore, R.F. (eds), *Handbook of Insect Rearing*, Vol. I, pp. 303–315. Amsterdam: Elsevier.

Nowak, M.A. 2006. Five rules for the evolution of cooperation. *Science*, 314, 1560–1563.

Nowak, M.A. & May, R.M. 1992. Evolutionary games and spatial chaos. *Nature*, 359, 826–829.

Nowak, M.A. & Roch, S. 2007. Upstream reciprocity and the evolution of gratitude. *Proceedings of the Royal Society of London B: Biological Sciences*, 274, 605–610.

Nowak, M.A. & Sigmund, K. 1992. Tit-for-tat in heterogeneous populations. *Nature*, 355, 250–253.

Nowak, M. & Sigmund, K. 1993. A strategy of win stay, lose shift that outperforms tit-for-tat in the prisoners-dilemma game. *Nature*, 364, 56–58.

Nowak, M.A. & Sigmund, K. 1998a. The dynamics of indirect reciprocity. *Journal of Theoretical Biology*, 194, 561–574.

Nowak, M.A. & Sigmund, K. 1998b. Evolution of indirect reciprocity by image scoring. *Nature*, 393, 573–577.

Nowak, M.A. & Sigmund, K. 2005. Evolution of indirect reciprocity. *Nature*, 437, 1291–1298.

Nowak, M.A., Tarnita, C.E. & Wilson, E.O. 2010a. The evolution of eusociality. *Nature*, 466, 1057–1062.

Nowak, M.A., Tarnita, C.E. & Antal, T. 2010b. Evolutionary dynamics in structured populations.

Philosophical Transactions of the Royal Society of London B: Biological Sciences, 365, 19–30.

Nuotcla, J.A., Taborsky, M. & Biedermann, P.H.W. 2014. The importance of blocking the gallery entrance in the ambrosia beetle *Xyleborinus saxesenii* ratzeburg (Coleoptera; Scolytinae). *Mitteilungen der Deutschen Gesellschaft fur Allgemeine und Angewandte Entomologie*, 19, 203–207.

Nuotclá, J.A., Biedermann, P.H. & Taborsky, M. 2019. Pathogen defence is a potential driver of social evolution in ambrosia beetles. *Proceedings of the Royal Society of London B: Biological Sciences*, 286, 20192332.

Nuotclá, J.A., Diehl, J.M.C. & Taborsky, M. 2021. Habitat quality determines dispersal decisions and fitness in a beetle–fungus mutualism. *Frontiers in Ecology and Evolution*, 9, 242.

Nutt, K.J. 2008. A comparison of techniques for assessing dispersal behaviour in gundis: revealing dispersal patterns in the absence of observed dispersal behaviour. *Molecular Ecology*, 17, 3541–3556.

O'Brien, S., Luján, A.M., Paterson, S., Cant, M.A. & Buckling, A. 2017. Adaptation to public goods cheats in *Pseudomonas aeruginosa*. *Proceedings of the Royal Society of London B: Biological Sciences*, 284, 20171089.

O'Connor, C.M., Reddon, A.R., Ligocki, I.Y., et al. 2015. Motivation but not body size influences territorial contest dynamics in a wild cichlid fish. *Animal Behaviour*, 107, 19–29.

O'Donnell, S. 2001. Worker biting interactions and task performance in a swarm-founding eusocial wasp (*Polybia occidentalis*, Hymenoptera: Vespidae). *Behavioral Ecology*, 12, 353–359.

Ochi, H. & Yanagisawa, Y. 1996. Interspecific brood-mixing in Tanganyikan cichlids. *Environmental Biology of Fishes*, 45, 141–149.

Ochi, H. & Yanagisawa, Y. 2005. Farming-out of offspring is a predominantly male tactic in a biparental mouth-brooding cichlid *Perrisodus mircolepis*. *Environmental Biology of Fishes*, 73, 335–340.

Ochi, H., Yanagisawa, Y. & Omori, K. 1995. Intraspecific brood-mixing of the cichlid fish *Perissodus microlepis* in Lake Tanganyika. *Environmental Biology of Fishes*, 43, 201–206.

Ochi, H., Onchiand, T. & Yanagisawa, Y. 2001. Alloparental care between catfishes in Lake Tanganyika. *Journal of Fish Biology*, 59, 1279–1286.

Ohtsuki, H. 2018. Evolutionary dynamics of coordinated cooperation. *Frontiers in Ecology and Evolution*, 6, 62.

Ohtsuki, H. & Iwasa, Y. 2004. How should we define goodness? Reputation dynamics in indirect reciprocity. *Journal of Theoretical Biology*, 231, 107–120.

Ohtsuki, H. & Iwasa, Y. 2006. The leading eight: social norms that can maintain cooperation by indirect reciprocity. *Journal of Theoretical Biology*, 239, 435–444.

Ohtsuki, H., Hauert, C., Lieberman, E. & Nowak, M.A. 2006. A simple rule for the evolution of cooperation on graphs and social networks. *Nature*, 441, 502–505.

Oi, C.A., Van Oystaeyen, A., Oliveira, R.C., et al. 2015a. Dual effect of wasp queen pheromone in regulating insect sociality. *Current Biology*, 25, 1638–1640.

Oi, C.A., van Zweden, J.S., Oliveira, R.C., et al. 2015b. The origin and evolution of social insect queen pheromones: novel hypotheses and outstanding problems. *Bioessays*, 37, 808–821.

Oka, R. & Kusimba, C.M. 2008. The archaeology of trading systems, part 1: towards a new trade synthesis. *Journal of Archaeological Research*, 16, 339–395.

Okasha, S. 2005. Altruism, group selection and correlated interaction. *British Journal for the Philosophy of Science*, 56, 703–725.

Okasha, S. 2006. *Evolution and Levels of Selection*. Oxford: Oxford University Press.

Okasha, S. 2012. Social justice, genomic justice and the veil of ignorance: Harsanyi meets Mendel. *Economics & Philosophy*, 28, 43–71.

Okasha, S. 2016. The relation between kin and multilevel selection: an approach using causal graphs. *British Journal for the Philosophy of Science*, 67, 435–470.

Okasha, S. & Paternotte, C. 2012. Group adaptation, formal Darwinism and contextual analysis. *Journal of Evolutionary Biology*, 25, 1127–1139.

Oksanen, T. & Henttonen, H. 1996. Dynamics of voles and small mustelids in the taiga landscape of northern Fennoscandia in relation to habitat quality. *Ecography*, 19, 432–443.

Okuda, N. 2001. The costs of reproduction to males and females of a paternal mouthbrooding cardinalfish *Apogon notatus*. *Journal of Fish Biology*, 58, 776–787.

Oldroyd, B.P., Halling, L.A., Good, G., et al. 2001. Worker policing and worker reproduction in *Apis cerana*. *Behavioral Ecology and Sociobiology*, 50, 371–377.

Olendorf, R., Getty, T. & Scribner, K. 2004. Cooperative nest defence in red-winged blackbirds: reciprocal altruism, kinship or by-product mutualism? *Proceedings of the Royal Society of London B: Biological Sciences*, 271, 177–182.

Oli, M.K. 2003. Hamilton goes empirical: estimation of inclusive fitness from life-history data. *Proceedings of the Royal Society of London B: Biological Sciences*, 270, 307–311.

Oliveira, R.F., McGregor, P.K. & Latruffe, C. 1998. Know thine enemy: fighting fish gather information from observing conspecific interactions. *Proceedings of the Royal Society of London B: Biological Sciences*, 265, 1045–1049.

Oliveira, R.F., Taborsky, M. & Brockmann, H.J. 2008. *Alternative Reproductive Tactics: an Integrative Approach*. Cambridge: Cambridge University Press.

Oliver, A.S. 1997. Size and density dependent mating tactics in the simultaneously hermaphroditic seabass *Serranus subligarius* (Cope, 1870). *Behaviour*, 134, 563–594.

Olson, L.E. & Blumstein, D.T. 2009. A trait-based approach to understand the evolution of complex coalitions in male mammals. *Behavioral Ecology*, 20, 624–632.

Oosthuizen, M.K., Bennett, N.C., Lutermann, H. & Coen, C.W. 2008. Reproductive suppression and the seasonality of reproduction in the social Natal mole-rat (*Cryptomys hottentotus natalensis*). *General and Comparative Endocrinology*, 159, 236–240.

Orians, G.H. & Willson, M.F. 1964. Interspecific territories of birds. *Ecology*, 45, 736–745.

Ortega, J. & Arita, H.T. 2000. Defence of females by dominant males of *Artibeus jamaicensis* (Chiroptera: Phyllostomidae). *Ethology*, 106, 395–407.

Ortega, J. & Arita, H.T. 2002. Subordinate males in harem groups of Jamaican fruit-eating bats (*Artibeus jamaicensis*): Satellites or sneaks? *Ethology*, 108, 1077–1091.

Ortego, J., Calabuig, G., Aparicio, J.M. & Cordero, P.J. 2008. Genetic consequences of natal dispersal in the colonial lesser kestrel. *Molecular Ecology*, 17, 2051–2059.

Ostner, J., Schülke, O. & Nunn, C.L. 2008. Female reproductive synchrony predicts skewed paternity across primates. *Behavioral Ecology*, 19, 1150–1158.

Owen-Smith, N., Martin, J. & Yoganand, K. 2015. Spatially nested niche partitioning between syntopic grazers at foraging arena scale within overlapping home ranges. *Ecosphere*, 6(9), 1–17.

Öst, M. & Tierala, T. 2011. Synchronized vigilance while feeding in common eider brood-rearing coalitions. *Behavioral Ecology*, 22, 378–384.

Öst, M., Jaatinen, K. & Steele, B. 2007. Aggressive females seize central positions and show increased vigilance in brood-rearing coalitions of eiders. *Animal Behaviour*, 73, 239–247.

Öst, M., Smith, B.D. & Kilpi, M. 2008. Social and maternal factors affecting duckling survival in eiders *Somateria mollissima*. *Journal of Animal Ecology*, 77, 315–325.

Östlund-Nilsson, S. 2002. Does paternity or paternal investment determine the level of paternal care and does female choice explain egg stealing in the fifteen-spined stickleback? *Behavioral Ecology*, 13, 188–192.

Packer, C. 1977. Reciprocal altruism in *Papio anubis*. *Nature*, 265, 441–443.

Packer, C. & Pusey, A.E. 1982. Cooperation and competition within coalitions of male lions – kin selection or game theory. *Nature*, 296, 740–742.

Packer, C. & Pusey, A.E. 1983. Adaptations of female lions to infanticide by incoming males. *The American Naturalist*, 121, 716–728.

Packer, C. & Pusey, A.E. 1993. Dispersal, kinship, and inbreeding in African lions. In Thornhill, N.W. (ed.), *The Natural History of Inbreeding and Outbreeding: Theoretical and Impirical Perspectives*, pp. 375–391. Chicago, IL: University of Chicago Press.

Packer, C. & Ruttan, L. 1988. The evolution of cooperative hunting. *American Naturalist*, 132, 159–198.

Packer, C., Scheel, D. & Pusey, A.E. 1990. Why lions form groups: food is not enough. *The American Naturalist*, 136, 1–19.

Packer, C., Gilbert, D.A., Pusey, A.E. & Obrien, S.J. 1991. A molecular genetic-analysis of kinship and cooperation in African lions. *Nature*, 351, 562–565.

Packer, C., Lewis, S. & Pusey, A. 1992. A comparative analysis of non-offspring nursing. *Animal Behaviour*, 43, 265–281.

Packer, C., Pusey, A.E. & Eberly, L.E. 2001. Egalitarianism in female African lions. *Science*, 293, 690–693.

Painter, J.N., Crozier, R.H., Poiani, A., Robertson, R.J. & Clarke, M.F. 2000. Complex social organization reflects genetic structure and relatedness in the cooperatively breeding bell miner, *Manorina melanophrys*. *Molecular Ecology*, 9, 1339–1347.

Pamilo, P. 1990. Sex allocation and queen–worker conflict in polygynous ants. *Behavioral Ecology and Sociobiology*, 27, 31–36.

Pamilo, P. & Rosengren, R. 1984. Evolution of nesting strategies of ants: genetic evidence from different population types of *Formica* ants. *Biological Journal of the Linnean Society*, 21, 331–348.

Pande, S., Shitut, S., Freund, L., et al. 2015. Metabolic cross-feeding via intercellular nanotubes among bacteria. *Nature Communications*, 6, 6238.

Paquet, M., Doutrelant, C., Loubon, M., et al. 2016. Communal roosting, thermoregulatory benefits and breeding group size predictability in cooperatively breeding sociable weavers. *Journal of Avian Biology*, 47, 749–755.

Park, T. 1954. Experimental studies of interspecies competition II. Temperature, humidity, and competition in two species of *Tribolium*. *Physiological Zoology*, 27, 177–238.

Parker, A.K., Parker, C.H. & Codding, B.F. 2019. When to defend? Optimal territoriality across the Numic homeland. *Quaternary International*, 518, 3–10.

Parker, G.A. 1970. The reproductive behaviour and the nature of sexual selection in *Scatophaga stercoraria* L. (Diptera: Scatophagidae): II. The fertilization rate and the spatial and temporal relationships of each sex around the site of mating and oviposition. *The Journal of Animal Ecology*, 39, 205–228.

Parker, G.A. 1974. Assessment strategy and evolution of fighting behavior. *Journal of Theoretical Biology*, 47, 223–243.

Parker, G.A. 1979. Sexual selection and sexual conflict. In Blum, M.S. & Blum, N.A. (eds), *Sexual Selection and Reproductive Competition in Insects*, pp. 123–166. New York, NY: Academic Press.

Parker, G.A. 1984. Evolutionarily stable strategies. In Krebs, J.R. & Davies, N.B. (eds), *Behavioural Ecology. An Evolutionary Approach*, pp. 30–61. Oxford: Blackwell Scientific.

Parker, G.A. 1985. Models of parent–offspring conflict V: effects of the behaviour of two parents. *Animal Behaviour*, 33, 519–533.

Parker, G.A. 2000. Scramble in behaviour and ecology. *Philosophical Transactions of the Royal Society of London B: Biological Sciences*, 355, 1637–1645.

Parker, G.A. 2006. Sexual conflict over mating and fertilization: an overview. *Philosophical Transactions of the Royal Society of London B: Biological Sciences*, 361, 235–259.

Parker, G.A. & Sutherland, W.J. 1986. Ideal free distributions when individuals differ in competitive ability: phenotype-limited ideal free models. *Animal Behaviour*, 34, 1222–1242.

Parker, G.A., Ramm, S.A., Lehtonen, J. & Henshaw, J.M. 2018. The evolution of gonad expenditure and gonadosomatic index (GSI) in male and female broadcast-spawning invertebrates. *Biological Reviews*, 93, 693–753.

Parmentier, T., Dekoninck, W. & Wenseleers, T. 2015. Context-dependent specialization in colony defence in the red wood ant *Formica rufa*. *Animal Behaviour*, 103, 161–167.

Parrish, A.E., Brosnan, S.F. & Beran, M.J. 2015. Capuchin monkeys alternate play and reward in a dual computerized task. *Animal Behavior and Cognition*, 2, 334–347.

Partridge, B.L., Johansson, J. & Kalish, J. 1983. The structure of schools of giant bluefin tuna in Cape Cod Bay. *Environmental Biology of Fishes*, 9, 253–262.

Patricelli, G.L., Krakauer, A.H. & McElreath, R. 2011. Assets and tactics in a mating market: economic models of negotiation offer insights into animal courtship dynamics on the lek. *Current Zoology*, 57, 225–236.

Payne, R.J. 1998. Gradually escalating fights and displays: the cumulative assessment model. *Animal Behaviour*, 56, 651–662.

Payne, R.J. & Pagel, M. 1997. Why do animals repeat displays? *Animal Behaviour*, 54, 109–119.

Peake, T.M. 2005. Eavesdropping in communication networks. In McGregor, P.K. (ed.), *Animal Communication Networks*, pp. 13–37. Cambridge: Cambridge University Press.

Peake, T.M., Terry, A.M.R., McGregor, P.K. & Dabelsteen, T. 2001. Male great tits eavesdrop on simulated male-to-male vocal interactions. *Proceedings of the Royal Society of London B: Biological Sciences*, 268, 1183–1187.

Peer, K. & Taborsky, M. 2004. Female ambrosia beetles adjust their offspring sex ratio according to outbreeding opportunities for their sons. *Journal of Evolutionary Biology*, 17, 257–264.

Peer, K. & Taborsky, M. 2005. Outbreeding depression, but no inbreeding depression in haplodiploid ambrosia beetles with regular sibling mating. *Evolution*, 59, 317–323.

Peer, K. & Taborsky, M. 2007. Delayed dispersal as a potential route to cooperative breeding in ambrosia beetles. *Behavioral Ecology and Sociobiology*, 61, 729–739.

Peeters, C. & Ito, F. 2001. Colony dispersal and the evolution of queen morphology in social Hymenoptera. *Annual Review of Entomology*, 46, 601–630.

Pena, J. & Rochat, Y. 2012. Bipartite graphs as models of population structures in evolutionary multiplayer games. *PLoS One*, 7, e44514.

Pena, J., Pestelacci, E., Berchtold, A. & Tomassini, M. 2011. Participation costs can suppress the evolution of upstream reciprocity. *Journal of Theoretical Biology*, 273, 197–206.

Pepper, J.W. & Smuts, B.B. 2002. A mechanism for the evolution of altruism among nonkin: positive assortment through environmental feedback. *American Naturalist*, 160, 205–213.

Perc, M., Gomez-Gardenes, J., Szolnoki, A., Floria, L.M. & Moreno, Y. 2013. Evolutionary dynamics of group interactions on structured populations: a review. *Journal of the Royal Society Interface*, 10, 20120997.

Petersen, C.W. 1995. Reproductive behavior, egg trading, and correlates of male mating success in the simultaneous hemaphrodite, *Serranus tabacarius*. *Environmental Biology of Fishes*, 43, 351–361.

Petit, O. & Bon, R. 2010. Decision-making processes: the case of collective movements. *Behavioural Processes*, 84, 635–647.

Petrie, M. & Moller, A.P. 1991. Laying eggs in other's nests: intraspecific brood parasitism in birds. *TREE*, 6, 315–320.

Petrie, M., Krupa, A. & Burke, T. 1999. Peacocks lek with relatives even in the absence of social and environmental cues. *Nature*, 401, 155.

Peyton, K.A., Valentino, L.M. & Maruska, K.P. 2014. Dual roles of an algal farming damselfish as a cultivator and opportunistic browser of an invasive seaweed. *PLoS One*, 9, e109007.

Pfeiffer, T., Rutte, C., Killingback, T., Taborsky, M. & Bonhoeffer, S. 2005. Evolution of cooperation by generalized reciprocity. *Proceedings of the Royal Society of London B: Biological Sciences*, 272, 1115–1120.

Pfennig, D.W. 1992. Polyphenism in spadefoot toad tadpoles as a locally adjusted evolutionarily stable strategy. *Evolution*, 46, 1408–1420.

Pfennig K.S. 2007. Facultative mate choice drives adaptive hybridization. *Science*, 318, 965–967

Pfennig, K.S. & Simovich, M.A. 2002. Differential selection to avoid hybridization in two toad species. *Evolution*, 56, 1840–1848.

Phillips, T. 2018. The concepts of asymmetric and symmetric power can help resolve the puzzle of altruistic and cooperative behaviour. *Biological Reviews*, 93, 457–468.

Picchi, L., Cabanes, G., Ricci-Bonot, C. & Lorenzi, M.C. 2018. Quantitative matching of clutch size in reciprocating hermaphroditic worms. *Current Biology*, 28, 3254–3259.

Pietsch, T.W. 2005. Dimorphism, parasitism, and sex revisited: modes of reproduction among deep-sea ceratioid anglerfishes (Teleostei: Lophiiformes). *Ichthyological Research*, 52, 207–236.

Piper, W.H. 1994. Courtship, copulation, nesting behavior and brood parasitism in the Venezuelan stripe-backed wren. *Condor*, 96, 654–671.

Pitcher, T.J. 1986. Functions of shoaling behaviour in teleosts. In Pitcher, T.J. (ed.), *The Behaviour of Teleost Fishes*, pp. 294–337. London: Croom Helm.

Pitcher, T.J. 1992. Who dares, wins: the function and evolution of predator inspection behaviour in shoaling fish. *Netherlands Journal of Zoology*, 42, 371–391.

Piyapong, C., Butlin, R.K., Faria, J.J., et al. 2011. Kin assortment in juvenile shoals in wild guppy populations. *Heredity*, 106, 749.

Pizzari, T. & Birkhead, T.R. 2000. Female feral fowl eject sperm of subdominant males. *Nature*, 405, 787–789.

Pizzari, T. & Gardner, A. 2012. The sociobiology of sex: inclusive fitness consequences of inter-sexual interactions. *Philosophical Transactions of the Royal Society of London B: Biological Sciences*, 367, 2314–2323.

Plantan, T., Howitt, M., Kotzé, A. & Gaines, M. 2013. Feeding preferences of the red-billed oxpecker, *Buphagus erythrorhynchus*: a parasitic mutualist? *African Journal of Ecology*, 51, 325–336.

Platt, T.G. & Bever, J.D. 2009. Kin competition and the evolution of cooperation. *Trends in Ecology & Evolution*, 24, 370–377.

Poethke, H.J. & Kaiser, H. 1987. The territoriality threshold – a model for mutual avoidance in dragonfly mating systems. *Behavioral Ecology and Sociobiology*, 20, 11–19.

Pope, T.R. 1998. Effects of demographic change on group kin structure and gene dynamics of populations of red howling monkeys. *Journal of Mammalogy*, 79, 692–712.

Port, M., Clough, D. & Kappeler, P.M. 2009. Market effects offset the reciprocation of grooming in free-ranging redfronted lemurs, *Eulemur fulvus rufus*. *Animal Behaviour*, 77, 29–36.

Port, M., Schulke, O. & Ostner, J. 2017. From individual to group territoriality: competitive environments promote the evolution of sociality. *American Naturalist*, 189, E46–E57.

Power, M.E. 1983. Grazing responses of tropical freshwater fishes to different scales of variation in their food. *Environmental Biology of Fishes*, 9, 103–115.

Powers, D.R. 1987. Effects of variation in food quality on the breeding territoriality of the male Anna's hummingbird. *Condor*, 89, 103–111.

Pradeu, T. 2010. What is an organism? An immunological answer. *History and Philosophy of the Life Sciences*, 32, 247–267.

Pradeu, T. 2013. Immunity and the emergence of individuality. In Bouchard, F. & Huneman, P. (eds), *From Groups to Individuals: Evolution and Emerging*

Individuality, pp. 77–96. Cambridge, MA: The MIT Press.

Pravosudova, E.V. & Grubb Jr, T.C. 2000. An experimental test of the prolonged brood care model in the tufted titmouse (*Baeolophus bicolor*). *Behavioral Ecology*, 11, 309–314.

Premnath, S., Sinha, A. & Gadagkar, R. 1996. Dominance relationship in the establishment of reproductive division of labour in a primitively eusocial wasp (*Ropalidia marginata*). *Behavioral Ecology and Sociobiology*, 39, 125–132.

Premoli, M.C. & Sella, G. 1995. Alloparental egg care in the polychaete worm *Ophryotrocha diadema*. *Ethology*, 101, 177–186.

Press, W.H. & Dyson, F.J. 2012. Iterated prisoner's dilemma contains strategies that dominate any evolutionary opponent. *Proceedings of the National Academy of Sciences of the United States of America*, 109, 10409–10413.

Pressley, P.H. 1981. Pair formation and joint territoriality in a simultaneous hermaphrodite: the coral reef fish *Serranus tigrinus*. *Zeitschrift für Tierpsychologie*, 56, 33–46.

Pruett-Jones, S.G. & Lewis, M.J. 1990. Sex ratio and habitat limitation promote delayed dispersal in superb fairy-wrens. *Nature*, 348, 541.

Pruitt, J.N. & Riechert, S.E. 2011. Within-group behavioral variation promotes biased task performance and the emergence of a defensive caste in a social spider. *Behavioral Ecology and Sociobiology*, 65, 1055–1060.

Pusey, A.E. & Packer, C. 1987. The evolution of sex-biased dispersal in lions. *Behaviour*, 101, 275–310.

Pusey, A.E. & Packer, C. 1994. Non-offspring nursing in social carnivores: minimizing the costs. *Behavioral Ecology*, 5, 362–374.

Pusey, A. & Wolf, M. 1996. Inbreeding avoidance in animals. *Trends in Ecology & Evolution*, 11, 201–206.

Queller, D.C. 1984. Kin selection and frequency dependence: a game theoretic approach. *Biological Journal of the Linnean Society*, 23, 133–143.

Queller, D.C. 1985. Kinship, reciprocity and synergism in the evolution of social-behavior. *Nature*, 318, 366–367.

Queller, D.C. 1992. Does population viscosity promote kin selection? *Trends in Ecology & Evolution*, 7, 322–324.

Queller, D.C. 1994a. Genetic relatedness in viscous populations. *Evolutionary Ecology*, 8, 70–73.

Queller, D.C. 1994b. Male–female conflict and parent–offspring conflict. *The American Naturalist*, 144, S84–S99.

Queller, D.C. & Goodnight, K.F. 1989. Estimating relatedness using genetic markers. *Evolution*, 43, 258–275.

Queller, D.C. & Strassmann, J.E. 1998. Kin selection and social insects. *Bioscience*, 48, 165–175.

Queller, D.C. & Strassmann, J.E. 2009. Beyond society: the evolution of organismality. *Philosophical Transactions* of the Royal Society of London B: Biological Sciences, 364, 3143–3155.

Queller, D.C., Zacchi, F., Cervo, R., et al. 2000. Unrelated helpers in a social insect. Nature, 405, 784–787.

Queller, D.C., Ponte, E., Bozzaro, S. & Strassmann, J.E. 2003. Single-gene greenbeard effects in the social amoeba Dictyostelium discoideum. Science, 299, 105–106.

Quilichini, A., Debussche, M. & Thompson, J.D. 2001. Evidence for local outbreeding depression in the Mediterranean island endemic Anchusa crispa Viv. (Boraginaceae). Heredity, 87, 190.

Quinn, J.L. & Kokorev, Y. 2002. Trading-off risks from predators and from aggressive hosts. Behavioral Ecology and Sociobiology, 51, 455–460.

Quinn, J.L. & Ueta, M. 2008. Protective nesting associations in birds. Ibis, 150, 146–167.

Quinn, J.L., Prop, J., Kokorev, Y. & Black, J.M. 2003. Predator protection or similar habitat selection in red-breasted goose nesting associations: extremes along a continuum. Animal Behaviour, 65, 297–307.

Quinn, J.S., Woolfenden, G.E., Fitzpatrick, J.W. & White, B.N. 1999. Multi-locus DNA fingerprinting supports genetic monogamy in Florida scrub-jays. Behavioral Ecology and Sociobiology, 45(1), 1–10.

Quinones, A.E., van Doorn, G.S., Pen, I., Weissing, F.J. & Taborsky, M. 2016. Negotiation and appeasement can be more effective drivers of sociality than kin selection. Philosophical Transactions of the Royal Society of London B: Biological Sciences, 371, 20150089.

Quirici, V., Palma, M., Sobrero, R.I., Faugeron, S. & Ebensperger, L.A. 2013. Relatedness does not predict vigilance in a population of the social rodent Octodon degus. Acta Ethologica, 16, 1–8.

Rabenold, K.N. 1985. Cooperation in breeding by nonreproductive wrens: kinship, reciprocity, and demography. Behavioral Ecology and Sociobiology, 17, 1–17.

Radford, A.N. 2008a. Type of threat influences postconflict allopreening in a social bird. Current Biology, 18, R114–R115.

Radford, A.N. 2008b. Duration and outcome of intergroup conflict influences intragroup affiliative behaviour. Proceedings of the Royal Society of London B: Biological Sciences, 275, 2787–2791.

Radford, A.N. & Du Plessis, M.A. 2006. Dual function of allopreening in the cooperatively breeding green woodhoopoe, Phoeniculus purpureus. Behavioral Ecology and Sociobiology, 61, 221–230.

Radford, A.N. & Ridley, A.R. 2006. Recruitment calling: a novel form of extended parental care in an altricial species. Current Biology, 16, 1700–1704.

Radford, A.N., Bell, M.B.V., Hollén, L.I. & Ridley, A.R. 2011. Singing for your supper: sentinel calling by kleptoparasites can mitigate the cost to victims. Evolution, 65, 900–906.

Radford, A.N., Majolo, B. & Aureli, F. 2016. Within-group behavioural consequences of between-group conflict: a prospective review. Proceedings of the Royal Society of London B: Biological Sciences, 283, 20161567.

Raignier, A. & Van Boven, J. 1955. Étude taxonomique, biologique at biometrique des Dorylus du sous-genre Annoma (Hymenoptera: Formicidae). Annales de la Museum Royale de Congo Belgique, 2, 1–359.

Raihani, N.J. & Bshary, R. 2015. Third-party punishers are rewarded, but third-party helpers even more so. Evolution, 69, 993–1003.

Raihani, N.J., Grutter, A.S. & Bshary, R. 2010. Punishers benefit from third-party punishment in fish. Science, 327, 171.

Raihani, N.J., Thornton, A. & Bshary, R. 2012. Punishment and cooperation in nature. Trends in Ecology & Evolution, 27, 288–295.

Ramos, A., Fonseca, P.J., Modesto, T., Almada, V.C. & Amorim, M.C. 2012. Alloparental behavior in the highly vocal Lusitanian toadfish. Journal of Experimental Marine Biology and Ecology, 434, 58–62.

Rand, D.G., Tarnita, C.E., Ohtsuki, H. & Nowak, M.A. 2013. Evolution of fairness in the one-shot anonymous Ultimatum Game. Proceedings of the National Academy of Sciences of the United States of America, 110, 2581–2586.

Randall, J.A., McCowan, B., Collins, K.C., Hooper, S.L. & Rogovin, K. 2005. Alarm signals of the great gerbil: acoustic variation by predator context, sex, age, individual, and family group. The Journal of the Acoustical Society of America, 118, 2706–2714.

Rangel-Negrín, A., Flores-Escobar, E., Coyohua-Fuentes, A., et al. 2015. Behavioural and glucocorticoid responses of a captive group of spider monkeys to short-term variation in food presentation. Folia Primatologica, 86, 433–445.

Rankin, D.J. 2011. Kin selection and the evolution of sexual conflict. Journal of Evolutionary Biology, 24, 71–81.

Rankin, D.J. & Taborsky, M. 2009. Assortment and the evolution of generalized reciprocity. Evolution, 63, 1913–1922.

Rankin, D.J., Bargum, K. & Kokko, H. 2007. The tragedy of the commons in evolutionary biology. Trends in Ecology & Evolution, 22, 643–651.

Rasa, O.A. 1977. The ethology and sociology of the dwarf mongoose (Helogale undulata rufula). Zeitschrift für Tierpsychologie, 43, 337–406.

Rasa, O.A. 1986. Coordinated vigilance in dwarf mongoose family groups: the 'watchman's song' hypothesis and the costs of guarding. Ethology, 71, 340–344.

Rasa, O.A.E. 1989. The costs and effectiveness of vigilance behavior in the dwarf mongoose – implications for fitness and optimal group-size. Ethology Ecology & Evolution, 1, 265–282.

Rasmussen, G.S.A., Gusset, M., Courchamp, F. & Macdonald, D.W. 2008. Achilles' heel of sociality revealed by energetic poverty trap in cursorial hunters. *The American Naturalist*, 172, 508–518.

Ratcliffe, J.M. & ter Hofstede, H.M. 2005. Roosts as information centres: social learning of food preferences in bats. *Biology Letters*, 1, 72–74.

Ratledge, C. & Dover, L.G. 2000. Iron metabolism in pathogenic bacteria. *Annual Reviews in Microbiology*, 54, 881–941.

Ratnieks, F.L.W. 1988. Reproductive harmony via mutual policing by workers in eusocial Hymenoptera. *The American Naturalist*, 132, 217–236.

Ratnieks, F.L.W. & Visscher, K.P. 1989. Worker policing in the honeybee. *Nature*, 342, 796–797.

Ratnieks, F.L.W. & Wenseleers, T. 2005. Policing insect societies. *Science*, 307, 54–56.

Ratnieks, F.L. & Wenseleers, T. 2008. Altruism in insect societies and beyond: voluntary or enforced? *Trends in Ecology & Evolution*, 23, 45–52.

Ratnieks, F.L.W., Foster, K.R. & Wenseleers, T. 2006. Conflict resolution in insect societies. *Annual Review of Entomology*, 51, 581–608.

Ratzeburg, J.T.C. 1839. *Die Forst-Insecten*. Berlin: Nicolaische Buchhandlung.

Rautiala, P., Helantera, H. & Puurtinen, M. 2019. Extended haplodiploidy hypothesis. *Evolution Letters*, 3, 263–270.

Raveh, A., Kotler, B.P., Abramsky, Z. & Krasnov, B.R. 2011. Driven to distraction: detecting the hidden costs of flea parasitism through foraging behaviour in gerbils. *Ecology Letters*, 14, 47–51.

Reader, S.M., Hager, Y. & Laland, K.N. 2011. The evolution of primate general and cultural intelligence. *Philosophical Transactions of the Royal Society B: Biological Sciences*, 366, 1017–1027.

Recer, G.M., Blanckenhorn, W.U., Newman, J.A., et al. 1987. Temporal resource variability and the habitat-matching rule. *Evolutionary Ecology*, 1, 363–378.

Reddon, A.R., Voisin, M.R., Menon, N., et al. 2011a. Rules of engagement for resource contests in a social fish. *Animal Behaviour*, 82, 93–99.

Reddon, A.R., Balk, D. & Balshine, S. 2011b. Sex differences in group-joining decisions in social fish. *Animal Behaviour*, 82, 229–234.

Reed, C., Branconi, R., Majoris, J., Johnson, C. & Buston, P. 2019. Competitive growth in a social fish. *Biology Letters*, 15, 20180737.

Reed, T.M. 1982. Interspecific territoriality in the chaffinch and great tit on islands and the mainland of Scotland: playback and removal experiments. *Animal Behaviour*, 30, 171–181.

Reeve, H.K. 1989. The evolution of conspecific acceptance thresholds. *The American Naturalist*, 133, 407–435.

Reeve, H.K. 1991. *Polistes*. In Ross, K.R. & Matthews, R.W. (eds), *The Social Biology of Wasps*, pp. 99–148. Ithaca, NY: Cornell University Press.

Reeve, H.K. 1992. Queen activation of lazy workers in colonies of the eusocial naked mole-rat. *Nature*, 358, 147–149.

Reeve, H.K. 2000. A transactional theory of within-group conflict. *The American Naturalist*, 155, 365–382.

Reeve, H.K. & Gamboa, G.J. 1983. Colony activity integration in primitively eusocial wasps – the role of the queen (*Polistes fuscatus*, Hymenoptera, Vespidae). *Behavioral Ecology and Sociobiology*, 13, 63–74.

Reeve, H.K. & Gamboa, G.J. 1987. Queen regulation of worker foraging in paper wasps – a social feedback-control system (*Polistes fuscatus*, Hymenoptera, Vespidae). *Behaviour*, 102, 147–167.

Reeve, H.K. & Hölldobler, B. 2007. The emergence of a superorganism through intergroup competition. *Proceedings of the National Academy of Sciences of the United States of America*, 104, 9736–9740.

Reeve, H.K. & Keller, L. 1995. Partitioning of reproduction in mother-daughter versus sibling associations – a test of optimal skew theory. *The American Naturalist*, 145, 119–132.

Reeve, H.K. & Nonacs, P. 1997. Within-group aggression and the value of group members: theory and a field test with social wasps. *Behavioral Ecology*, 8, 75–82.

Reeve, H.K. & Ratnieks, F.L.W. 1993. Queen–queen conflicts in polygynous societies: mutual tolerance and reproductive skew. In Keller, L. (ed.), *Queen Number and Sociality in Insects*, pp. 45–85. Oxford: Oxford University Press.

Reeve, H.K. & Sherman, P.W. 1991. Intracolonial aggression and nepotism by the breeding female naked mole-rat. In Sherman, P.W., Jarvis, J.U.M. & Alexander, R.D. (eds), *The Biology of the Naked Mole-Rat*. Princeton, NJ: Princeton University Press.

Reeve, H.K., Westneat, D.F., Noon, W.A., Sherman, P.W. & Aquadro, C.F. 1990. DNA 'fingerprinting' reveals high levels of inbreeding in colonies of the eusocial naked mole-rat. *Proceedings of the National Academy of Sciences of the United States of America*, 87, 2496–2500.

Reeve, H.K., Emlen, S.T. & Keller, L. 1998a. Reproductive sharing in animal societies: reproductive incentives or incomplete control by dominant breeders? *Behavioral Ecology*, 9, 267–278.

Reeve, H.K., Peters, J.M., Nonacs, P. & Starks, P.T. 1998b. Dispersal of first 'workers' in social wasps: causes and implications of an alternative reproductive strategy. *Proceedings of the National Academy of Sciences of the United States of America*, 95, 13737–13742.

Refardt, D., Bergmiller, T. & Kümmerli, R. 2013. Altruism can evolve when relatedness is low: evidence from bacteria committing suicide upon phage infection. *Proceedings of the Royal Society of London B: Biological Sciences*, 280, 20123035.

Regnaut, S., Christe, P., Chapuisat, M. & Fumagalli, L. 2006. Genotyping faeces reveals facultative kin association on capercaillie's leks. *Conservation Genetics*, 7, 665–674.

Reuter, M., Ward, P.I. & Blanckenhorn, W.U. 1998. An ESS treatment of the pattern of female arrival at the mating site in the yellow dung fly *Scathophaga stercoraria* (L.). *Journal of Theoretical Biology*, 195, 363–370.

Reyer, H.U. 1980. Flexible helper structure as an ecological adaptation in the pied kingfisher (*Ceryle rudis rudis* L.). *Behavioral Ecology and Sociobiology*, 6, 219–227.

Reyer, H.U. 1984. Investment and relatedness: a cost/benefit analysis of breeding and helping in the pied kingfisher (*Ceryle rudis*). *Animal Behaviour*, 32, 1163–1178.

Reyer, H.U. 1986. Breeder–helper interactions in the pied kingfisher reflect the costs and benefits of cooperative breeding. *Behaviour*, 96, 277–303.

Reynolds, S.M., Dryer, K., Bollback, J., et al. 2007. Behavioral paternity predicts genetic paternity in satin bowerbirds (*Ptilonorhynchus violaceus*), a species with a non-resource-based mating system. *The Auk*, 124, 857–867.

Ribbink, A.J. 1977. Cuckoo among Lake Malawi cichlid fish. *Nature*, 267, 243.

Ribbink, A.J., Marsh, A.C., Marsh, B. & Sharp, B.J. 1980. Parental behaviour and mixed broods among cichlid fish of Lake Malawi. *African Zoology*, 15, 1–6.

Ribeiro, A.M., Lloyd, P., Feldheim, K.A. & Bowie, R.C. 2012. Microgeographic socio-genetic structure of an African cooperative breeding passerine revealed: integrating behavioural and genetic data. *Molecular Ecology*, 21, 662–672.

Richardson, D.S. & Bolen, G.M 1999. A nesting association between semi-colonial Bullock's orioles and yellow-billed magpies: evidence for the predator protection hypothesis. *Behavioral Ecology and Sociobiology*, 46, 373–380.

Richardson, D.S. & Burke, T. 2001. Extrapair paternity and variance in reproductive success related to breeding density in Bullock's orioles. *Animal Behaviour*, 62, 519–525.

Richardson, D.S., Jury, F.L., Blaakmeer, K., Komdeur, J. & Burke, T. 2001. Parentage assignment and extra-group paternity in a cooperative breeder: the Seychelles warbler (*Acrocephalus sechellensis*). *Molecular Ecology*, 10, 2263–2273.

Richardson, D.S., Burke, T. & Komdeur, J. 2002. Direct benefits and the evolution of female-biased cooperative breeding in Seychelles warblers. *Evolution*, 56, 2313–2321.

Richardson, D.S., Burke, T. & Komdeur, J. 2003a. Sex-specific associative learning cues and inclusive fitness benefits in the Seychelles warbler. *Journal of Evolutionary Biology*, 16, 854–861.

Richardson, D.S., Komdeur, J. & Burke, T. 2003b. Avian behaviour: altruism and infidelity among warblers. *Nature*, 422, 580.

Richardson, D.S., Komdeur, J., Burke, T. & Von Schantz, T. 2005. MHC-based patterns of social and extra-pair

mate choice in the Seychelles warbler. *Proceedings of the Royal Society of London B: Biological Sciences*, 272, 759–767.

Richardson, D.S., Burke, T. & Komdeur, J. 2007. Grandparent helpers: the adaptive significance of older, postdominant helpers in the Seychelles warbler. *Evolution*, 61, 2790–2800.

Rickard, I.J. & Lummaa, V. 2007. The predictive adaptive response and metabolic syndrome: challenges for the hypothesis. *Trends in Endocrinology & Metabolism*, 18, 94–99.

Ridley, A.R. 2016. Southern pied babblers: the dynamics of conflict and cooperation in a group living society. In Koenig, W.D. & Dickinson, J.L. (eds), *Cooperative Breeding in Vertebrates: Studies of Ecology, Evolution, and Behavior*, pp. 115–132. New York, NY: Cambridge University Press.

Ridley, A.R. & Raihani, N.J. 2007. Facultative response to a kleptoparasite by the cooperatively breeding pied babbler. *Behavioral Ecology*, 18, 324–330.

Ridley, A.R., Nelson-Flower, M.J. & Thompson, A.M. 2013. Is sentinel behaviour safe? An experimental investigation. *Animal Behaviour*, 85, 137–142.

Ridley, J., Komdeur, J. & Sutherland, W.J. 2003. Population regulation in group-living birds: predictive models of the Seychelles warbler. *Journal of Animal Ecology*, 72, 588–598.

Ridley, M. & Rechten, C. 1981. Female sticklebacks prefer to spawn with males whose nests contain eggs. *Behaviour*, 76, 152–161.

Riebli, T., Avgan, B., Bottini, A.M., et al. 2011. Behavioural type affects dominance and growth in staged encounters of cooperatively breeding cichlids. *Animal Behaviour*, 81, 313–323.

Riebli, T., Taborsky, M., Chervet, N., et al. 2012. Behavioural type, status and social context affect behaviour and resource allocation in cooperatively breeding cichlids. *Animal Behaviour*, 84, 925–936.

Riedman, M.L. 1982. The evolution of alloparental care and adoption in mammals and birds. *The Quarterly Review of Biology*, 57, 405–435.

Riehl, C. 2011a. Living with strangers: direct benefits favour non-kin cooperation in a communally nesting bird. *Proceedings of the Royal Society of London B: Biological Sciences*, 278, 1728–1735.

Riehl, C. 2011b. Paternal investment and the 'sexually selected hypothesis' for the evolution of eggshell coloration: revisiting the assumptions. *The Auk*, 128, 175–179.

Riehl, C. 2013. Evolutionary routes to non-kin cooperative breeding in birds. *Proceedings of the Royal Society of London B: Biological Sciences*, 280, 20132245.

Riehl, C. 2016. Infanticide and within-clutch competition select for reproductive synchrony in a cooperative bird. *Evolution*, 70, 1760–1769.

Riehl, C. & Frederickson, M.E. 2016. Cheating and punishment in cooperative animal societies. *Philosophical Transactions of the Royal Society of London B: Biological Sciences*, 371, 20150090.

Riehl, C. & Strong, M.J. 2019. Social parasitism as an alternative reproductive tactic in a cooperatively breeding cuckoo. *Nature*, 567, 96–99.

Rieucau, G. & Giraldeau, L.A. 2009. Group size effect caused by food competition in nutmeg mannikins (*Lonchura punctulata*). *Behavioral Ecology*, 20, 421–425.

Ritz, D.A., Hobday, A.J., Montgomery, J.C. & Ward, A.J. 2011. Social aggregation in the pelagic zone with special reference to fish and invertebrates. In Lesser, M. (ed.), *Advances in Marine Biology*, Volume 60, pp. 161–227. Oxford: Elsevier.

Roberts, G. 1998. Competitive altruism: from reciprocity to the handicap principle. *Proceedings of the Royal Society of London B: Biological Sciences*, 265, 427–431.

Roberts, G. 2005. Cooperation through interdependence. *Animal Behaviour*, 70, 901–908.

Roberts, H. 1960. *Trachyostus ghanaensis* Schedl (Col., Platypodidae), an ambrosia beetle attacking wawa, *Triplochiton scleroxylon* K. Schum. Technical Bulletin, West African Timber Borer Research Unit.

Robertson, D.R. 1984. Cohabitation of competing territorial damselfishes on a caribbean coral-reef. *Ecology*, 65, 1121–1135.

Robertson, D.R. & Warner, R.R. 1978. *Sexual patterns in the labroid fishes of the Western Caribbean, II, the parrotfishes (Scaridae)*. Smithsonian Contributions to Zoology No. 255. Washington, DC: Smithsonian Institution Press.

Robertson, D.R., Sweatman, H.P.A., Fletcher, E.A. & Cleland, M.G. 1976. Schooling as a mechanism for circumventing the territoriality of competitors. *Ecology*, 57, 1208–1220.

Robinson, E.J.H. 2014. Polydomy: the organisation and adaptive function of complex nest systems in ants. *Current Opinion in Insect Science*, 5, 37–43.

Robinson, E.J. & Barker, J.L. 2017. Inter-group cooperation in humans and other animals. *Biology Letters*, 13, 20160793.

Rodrigues, A.M. & Gardner, A. 2012. Evolution of helping and harming in heterogeneous populations. *Evolution: International Journal of Organic Evolution*, 66, 2065–2079.

Rodrigues, A.M. & Gardner, A. 2013. Evolution of helping and harming in viscous populations when group size varies. *The American Naturalist*, 181, 609–622.

Rogers, A.R. 1993. Why menopause? *Evolutionary Ecology*, 7, 406–426.

Rohwer, S. 1978. Parent cannibalism of offspring and egg raiding as a courtship strategy. *The American Naturalist*, 112, 429–440.

Romero, T. & Aureli, F. 2008. Reciprocity of support in coatis (*Nasua nasua*). *Journal of Comparative Psychology*, 122, 19–25.

Ronce, O., Gandon, S. & Rousset, F. 2000. Kin selection and natal dispersal in an age-structured population. *Theoretical Population Biology*, 58, 143–159.

Rood, J.P. 1990. Group size, survival, reproduction, and routes to breeding in dwarf mongooses. *Animal Behaviour*, 39, 566–572.

Rose, L.M. 1997. Vertebrate predation and food-sharing in *Cebus* and *Pan*. *International Journal of Primatology*, 18, 727–765.

Rosenbaum, S. & Gettler, L.T. 2018. With a little help from her friends (and family) part I: the ecology and evolution of non-maternal care in mammals. *Physiology & Behavior*, 193, 1–11.

Rosenbaum, S., Vecellio, V. & Stoinski, T. 2016. Observations of severe and lethal coalitionary attacks in wild mountain gorillas. *Scientific Reports*, 6, 37018.

Rosengrave, P., Montgomerie, R. & Gemmell, N. 2016. Cryptic female choice enhances fertilization success and embryo survival in chinook salmon. *Proceedings of the Royal Society of London B: Biological Sciences*, 283, 20160001.

Ross, L., Gardner, A., Hardy, N. & West, S. 2013. Ecology, not the genetics of sex determination, determines who helps in eusocial populations. *Current Biology*, 23, 2383–2387.

Ross, R.M. 1978. Territorial behavior and ecology of the anemonefish *Amphiprion melanopus* on Guam 1. *Zeitschrift für Tierpsychologie*, 46, 71–83.

Rothstein, S.I. & Pierotti, R. 1988. Distinctions among reciprocal altruism, kin selection, and cooperation and a model for the initial evolution of beneficent behavior. *Ethology and Sociobiology*, 9, 189–209.

Roulin, A., Des Monstiers, B., Ifrid, E., et al. 2016. Reciprocal preening and food sharing in colour-polymorphic nestling barn owls. *Journal of Evolutionary Biology*, 29, 380–394.

Roulin, A. 2002. The sibling negotiation hypothesis. In Wright, J. & Leonard, M.L. (eds), *The Evolution of Begging*, pp. 107–126. Dordrecht: Kluwer Academic.

Rousset, F. & Gandon, S. 2002. Evolution of the distribution of dispersal distance under distance-dependent cost of dispersal. *Journal of Evolutionary Biology*, 15, 515–523.

Rousseu, F., Charette, Y. & Belisle, M. 2014. Resource defense and monopolization in a marked population of ruby-throated hummingbirds (*Archilochus colubris*). *Ecology and Evolution*, 4, 776–793.

Rowell, T.E., Wilson, C. & Cords, M. 1991. Reciprocity and partner preference in grooming of female blue monkeys. *International Journal of Primatology*, 12, 319–336.

Roy Nielsen, C.L., Parker, P.G. & Gates, R.J. 2008. Partial clutch predation, dilution of predation risk, and the evolution of intraspecific nest parasitism. *The Auk*, 125, 679–686.

Royle, N.J., Smiseth, P.T. & Kölliker, M. 2012. *The Evolution of Parental Care*. Oxford: Oxford University Press.

Royle, N.J., Alonzo, S.H. & Moore, A.J. 2016. Co-evolution, conflict and complexity: what have we learned about the evolution of parental care behaviours? *Current Opinion in Behavioral Sciences*, 12, 30–36.

Rubenstein, D.I. 1981. Population density, resource patterning, and territoriality in the Everglades pygmy sunfish. *Animal Behaviour*, 29, 155–172.

Rubenstein, D.I. & Nuñez, C.M. 2009. Sociality and reproductive skew in horses and zebras. In Hager, R. & Jones, C.B. (eds), *Reproductive Skew in Vertebrates: Proximate and Ultimate Causes*, pp. 196–226. Cambridge: Cambridge University Press.

Rubenstein, D.R. 2007. Female extrapair mate choice in a cooperative breeder: trading sex for help and increasing offspring heterozygosity. *Proceedings of the Royal Society of London B: Biological Sciences*, 274, 1895–1903.

Rubenstein, D.R. 2011. Spatiotemporal environmental variation, risk aversion, and the evolution of cooperative breeding as a bet-hedging strategy. *Proceedings of the National Academy of Sciences of the United States of America*, 108, 10816–10822.

Rubenstein, D.R. & Abbot, P. 2017. *Comparative Social Evolution*. Cambridge: Cambridge University Press.

Rubenstein, D.R. & Lovette, I.J. 2007. Temporal environmental variability drives the evolution of cooperative breeding in birds. *Current Biology*, 17, 1414–1419.

Rubinstein, A. 1979. An optimal conviction policy for offenses that may have been committed by accident. In Brams, S.J., Schotter, A. & Schwödiauer, G. (eds), *Applied Game Theory*, pp. 406–413. Heidelberg: Physica.

Rubinstein, A. 1980. On an anomaly of the deterrent effect of punishment. *Economics Letters*, 6, 89–94.

Rueger, T., Barbasch, T.A., Wong, M.Y., et al. 2018. Reproductive control via the threat of eviction in the clown anemonefish. *Proceedings of the Royal Society of London B: Biological Sciences*, 285, 20181295.

Rumbaugh, K.P., Diggle, S.P., Watters, C.M., et al. 2009. Quorum sensing and the social evolution of bacterial virulence. *Current Biology*, 19, 341–345.

Rusch, H. & Gavrilets, S. 2017. The logic of animal intergroup conflict: a review. *Journal of Economic Behavior & Organization*, 178, 1014–1030.

Russell, A.F. 2000. Ecological constraints and the cooperative breeding system of the long-tailed tit *Aegithalos caudatus*. PhD thesis, University of Sheffield, UK.

Russell, A.F. 2004. Mammals: comparisons and contrasts. In Koenig, W.D. & Dickinson, J.L. (eds), *Ecology and Evolution of Cooperative Breeding in Birds*, pp. 210–227. Cambridge: Cambridge University Press.

Russell, A.F. & Hatchwell, B.J. 2001. Experimental evidence for kin-biased helping in a cooperatively breeding vertebrate. *Proceedings of the Royal Society of London B: Biological Sciences*, 268, 2169–2174.

Russell, A.F., Sharpe, L.L., Brotherton, P.N.M. & Clutton-Brock, T.H. 2003. Cost minimization by helpers in cooperative vertebrates. *Proceedings of the National Academy of Sciences*, 100, 3333-3338.

Russell, A., Langmore, N., Cockburn, A., Astheimer, L. & Kilner, R. 2007a. Reduced egg investment can conceal helper effects in cooperatively breeding birds. *Science*, 317, 941–944.

Russell, A.F., Young, A.J., Spong, G., Jordan, N.R. & Clutton-Brock, T.H. 2007b. Helpers increase the reproductive potential of offspring in cooperative meerkats. *Proceedings of the Royal Society B: Biological Sciences*, 274, 513–524.

Russell, E.M., Yom-Tov, Y. & Geffen, E. 2004. Extended parental care and delayed dispersal: northern, tropical, and southern passerines compared. *Behavioral Ecology*, 15, 831–838.

Rusu, A.S. & Krackow, S. 2004. Kin-preferential cooperation, dominance-dependent reproductive skew, and competition for mates in communally nesting female house mice. *Behavioral Ecology and Sociobiology*, 56, 298–305.

Rutte, C. & Taborsky, M. 2007. Generalized reciprocity in rats. *PLoS Biology*, 5, 1421–1425.

Rutte, C. & Taborsky, M. 2008. The influence of social experience on cooperative behaviour of rats (*Rattus norvegicus*): direct vs generalised reciprocity. *Behavioral Ecology and Sociobiology*, 62, 499–505.

Rutte, C., Taborsky, M. & Brinkhof, M.W.G. 2006. What sets the odds of winning and losing? *Trends in Ecology & Evolution*, 21, 16–21.

Ryder, T.B., Parker, P.G., Blake, J.G. & Loiselle, B.A. 2009. It takes two to tango: reproductive skew and social correlates of male mating success in a lek-breeding bird. *Proceedings of the Royal Society of London B: Biological Sciences*, 276, 2377–2384.

Sabbatini, G., Vizioli, A.D., Visalberghi, E. & Schino, G. 2012. Food transfers in capuchin monkeys: an experiment on partner choice. *Biology Letters*, 8, 757–759.

Sachs, J., Mueller, U., Wilcox, T. & Bull, J. 2004. The evolution of cooperation. *The Quarterly Review of Biology*, 79, 135–160.

Saha, P., Balasubramaniam, K., Kalyani, J., et al. 2012. Clinging to royalty: *Ropalidia marginata* queens can employ both pheromone and aggression. *Insectes Sociaux*, 59, 41–44.

Sakai, M., Hishii, T., Takeda, S. & Kohshima, S. 2006. Flipper rubbing behaviors in wild bottlenose dolphins (*Tursiops aduncus*). *Marine Mammal Science*, 22, 966–978.

Salles, O.C., Pujol, B., Maynard, J.A., et al. 2016. First genealogy for a wild marine fish population reveals multigenerational philopatry. *Proceedings of the National Academy of Sciences of the United States of America*, 113, 13245–13250.

Sandell, M. & Liberg, O. 1992. Roamers and stayers – a model on male mating tactics and mating systems. *American Naturalist*, 139, 177–189.

Sanderson, J.L., Wang, J.L., Vitikainen, E.I.K., Cant, M.A. & Nichols, H.J. 2015a. Banded mongooses avoid inbreeding when mating with members of the same natal group. *Molecular Ecology*, 24, 3738–3751.

Sanderson, J.L., Nichols, H.J., Marshall, H.H., et al. 2015b. Elevated glucocorticoid concentrations during gestation predict reduced reproductive success in subordinate female banded mongooses. *Biology Letters*, 11, 20150620.

Sankey, D.W., Shepard, E.L., Biro, D. & Portugal, S.J. 2019. Speed consensus and the 'Goldilocks principle' in flocking birds (*Columba livia*). *Animal Behaviour*, 157, 105–119.

Santema, P. & Clutton-Brock, T. 2012. Dominant female meerkats do not use aggression to elevate work rates of helpers in response to increased brood demand. *Animal Behaviour*, 83, 827–832.

Santoro, F.H. 1963. Bioecología de *Platypus sulcatus* Chapuis (Coeloptera, Platypodidae). *Revista de Investigaciones Forestales*, 4, 47–79.

Santos, F.C. & Pacheco, J.M. 2005. Scale-free networks provide a unifying framework for the emergence of cooperation. *Physical Review Letters*, 95, 098104.

Santos, F.C. & Pacheco, J.M. 2006. A new route to the evolution of cooperation. *Journal of Evolutionary Biology*, 19, 726–733.

Santos, F.C., Pacheco, J.M. & Lenaerts, T. 2006. Evolutionary dynamics of social dilemmas in structured heterogeneous populations. *Proceedings of the National Academy of Sciences of the United States of America*, 103, 3490–3494.

Santos, J. & Lacey, E. 2011. Burrow sharing in the desert-adapted torch-tail spiny rat, *Trinomys yonenagae*. *Journal of Mammalogy*, 92, 3–11.

Sato, N., Tan, L., Tate, K. & Okada, M. 2015. Rats demonstrate helping behavior toward a soaked conspecific. *Animal Cognition*, 18, 1039–1047.

Sato, T. 1987. A brood parasitic catfish of the mouthbrooding cichlid fishes in Lake Tanganyika. In Kawanabe, H. (ed.), *Ecological and Limnological Studies on Lake Tanganyika and Its Adjacent Areas*, pp. 43–44. Kyoto: Kyoto University Press.

Sato, T., Hirose, M., Taborsky, M. & Kimura, S. 2004. Size-dependent male alternative reproductive tactics in the shell-brooding cichlid fish *Lamprologus callipterus* in Lake Tanganyika. *Ethology*, 110, 49–62.

Saunders, J.L. & Knoke, J.K. 1967. Diets for rearing the ambrosia beetle *Xyleborus ferrugineus* (Fabricius) in vitro. *Science*, 157, 460–463.

Savage, J.L., Russell, A.F. & Johnstone, R.A. 2013. Intra-group relatedness affects parental and helper investment rules in offspring care. *Behavioral Ecology and Sociobiology*, 67, 1855–1865.

Savage, J.L., Russell, A.F. & Johnstone, R.A. 2015. Maternal allocation in cooperative breeders: should mothers match or compensate for expected helper contributions? *Animal Behaviour*, 102, 189–197.

Savage, J.L., Browning, L.E., Manica, A., Russell, A.F. & Johnstone, R.A. 2017. Turn-taking in cooperative offspring care: by-product of individual provisioning behavior or active response rule? *Behavioral Ecology and Sociobiology*, 71, 162.

Sæther, B.E. & Engen, S. 2015. The concept of fitness in fluctuating environments. *Trends in Ecology & Evolution*, 30, 273–281.

Schacht, R. & Bell, A.V. 2016. The evolution of monogamy in response to partner scarcity. *Scientific Reports*, 6, 32472.

Schaedelin, F.C., van Dongen, W.F.D. & Wagner, R.H. 2013. Nonrandom brood mixing suggests adoption in a colonial cichlid. *Behavioral Ecology*, 24, 540–546.

Scheel, D. & Packer, C. 1991. Group hunting behavior of lions – a search for cooperation. *Animal Behaviour*, 41, 697–709.

Scheid, C., Schmidt, J. & Noe, R. 2008. Distinct patterns of food offering and co-feeding in rooks. *Animal Behaviour*, 76, 1701–1707.

Schel, A.M., Machanda, Z., Townsend, S.W., Zuberbühler, K. & Slocombe, K.E. 2013. Chimpanzee food calls are directed at specific individuals. *Animal Behaviour*, 86, 955–965.

Schelling, T.C. 1967. *Arms and Influence*. New Haven, CT: Yale University Press.

Schink, B. 2002. Synergistic interactions in the microbial world. *Antonie Van Leeuwenhoek*, 81, 257–261.

Schino, G. 2007. Grooming and agonistic support: a meta-analysis of primate reciprocal altruism. *Behavioral Ecology*, 18, 115–120.

Schino, G. & Aureli, F. 2008a. Grooming reciprocation among female primates: a meta-analysis. *Biology Letters*, 4, 9–11.

Schino, G. & Aureli, F. 2008b. Trade-offs in primate grooming reciprocation: testing behavioural flexibility and correlated evolution. *Biological Journal of the Linnean Society*, 95, 439–446.

Schino, G. & Aureli, F. 2009. Reciprocal altruism in primates: partner choice, cognition, and emotions. *Advances in the Study of Behavior*, 39, 45–69.

Schino, G. & Aureli, F. 2010a. The relative roles of kinship and reciprocity in explaining primate altruism. *Ecology Letters*, 13, 45–50.

Schino, G. & Aureli, F. 2010b. A few misunderstandings about reciprocal altruism. *Communicative & Integrative Biology*, 3, 561–563.

Schino, G. & Aureli, F. 2010c. Primate reciprocity and its cognitive requirements. *Evolutionary Anthropology*, 19, 130–135.

Schino, G. & Aureli, F. 2017. Reciprocity in group-living animals: partner control versus partner choice. *Biological Reviews*, 92, 665–672.

Schino, G. & Pellegrini, B. 2009. Grooming in mandrills and the time frame of reciprocal partner choice. *American Journal of Primatology*, 71, 884–888.

Schino, G. & Pellegrini, B. 2011. Grooming and the expectation of reciprocation in mandrills (*Mandrillus sphinx*). *International Journal of Primatology*, 32, 406–414.

Schino, G., Ventura, R. & Troisi, A. 2003. Grooming among female Japanese macaques: distinguishing between reciprocation and interchange. *Behavioral Ecology*, 14, 887–891.

Schino, G., Di Sorrentino, E.P. & Tiddi, B. 2007. Grooming and coalitions in Japanese macaques (*Macaca fuscata*): partner choice and the time frame of reciprocation. *Journal of Comparative Psychology*, 121, 181–188.

Schino, G., Di Giuseppe, F. & Visalberghi, E. 2009. The time frame of partner choice in the grooming reciprocation of *Cebus apella*. *Ethology*, 115, 70–76.

Schjelderup-Ebbe, T. 1935. Social behavior of birds. In Murchison, C.A. & Allee, W.C. (eds), *A Handbook of Social Psychology*, pp. 947–972. Worcester, MA: Clark University Press.

Schluter, D. & Grant, P.R. 1984. Determinants of morphological patterns in communities of Darwin's finches. *The American Naturalist*, 123, 175–196.

Schmelz, M., Grueneisen, S., Kabalak, A., Jost, J. & Tomasello, M. 2017. Chimpanzees return favors at a personal cost. *Proceedings of the National Academy of Sciences of the United States of America*, 114, 7462–7467.

Schmelz, M., Grueneisen, S. & Tomasello, M. 2020. The psychological mechanisms underlying reciprocal prosociality in chimpanzees (*Pan troglodytes*). *Journal of Comparative Psychology*, 134, 149–157.

Schmid, J. 1998. Tree holes used for resting by gray mouse lemurs (*Microcebus murinus*) in Madagascar: insulation capacities and energetic consequences. *International Journal of Primatology*, 19, 797–809.

Schmid, R., Schneeberger, K. & Taborsky, M. 2017. Feel good, do good? Disentangling reciprocity from unconditional prosociality. *Ethology*, 123, 640–647.

Schmidt, K. & Kuijper, D.P. 2015. A 'death trap' in the landscape of fear. *Mammal Research*, 60, 275–284.

Schneeberger, K., Dietz, M. & Taborsky, M. 2012. Reciprocal cooperation between unrelated rats depends on cost to donor and benefit to recipient. *BMC Evolutionary Biology*, 12, 41.

Schneeberger, K., Röder, G. & Taborsky, M. 2020. The smell of hunger: Norway rats provision social partners based on odour cues of need. *PLoS Biology*, 18, e3000628.

Schneider-Orelli, O. 1913. Untersuchungen über den pilzzüchtenden Obstbaumborkenkäfer *Xyleborus* (*Anisandrus*) *dispar* und seinen Nährpilz. *Centralblatt für Bakteriologie und Parasitenkunde*, 38, 25–110.

Schoener, T.W. 1983. Field experiments on interspecific competition. *The American Naturalist*, 122, 240–285.

Schoener, T.W. 1987. Time budgets and territory size: some simultaneous optimization models for energy maximizers. *American Zoologist*, 27, 259–291.

Schonmann, R.H. & Boyd, R. 2016. A simple rule for the evolution of contingent cooperation in large groups. *Philosophical Transactions of the Royal Society of London B: Biological Sciences*, 371, 20150099.

Schonmann, R.H., Vicente, R. & Caticha, N. 2013. Altruism can proliferate through population viscosity despite high random gene flow. *PLoS One*, 8, e72043.

Schrader, E. 1993. Untersuchungen zum Brutparasitismus von Fiederbartwelsen. *DATZ*, 46, 426–434.

Schradin, C. 2019. Alternative reproductive tactics. In *Encyclopedia of Animal Cognition and Behavior*, pp. 1–11. Cham: Springer.

Schradin, C. & Lindholm, A.K. 2011. Relative fitness of alternative male reproductive tactics in a mammal varies between years. *Journal of Animal Ecology*, 80, 908–917.

Schreier, T. 2013. Punishment motivates subordinate helper to pay to stay and to compensate after a period of reduced helping. BSc thesis, University of Bern, Switzerland.

Schuster, R. 2002. Cooperative coordination as a social behavior – experiments with an animal model. *Human Nature – An Interdisciplinary Biosocial Perspective*, 13, 47–83.

Schuster, R. & Perelberg, A. 2004. Why cooperate? An economic perspective is not enough. *Behavioural Processes*, 66, 261–277.

Schusterman, R.J. & Berkson, G. 1962. Reciprocal food sharing of gibbons. *American Zoologist*, 2, 556.

Schürch, R. & Heg, D. 2010a. Life history and behavioral type in the highly social cichlid *Neolamprologus pulcher*. *Behavioral Ecology*, 21, 588–598.

Schürch, R. & Heg, D. 2010b. Variation in helper type affects group stability and reproductive decisions in a cooperative breeder. *Ethology*, 116, 257–269.

Schürch, R. & Taborsky, B. 2005. The functional significance of buccal feeding in the mouthbrooding cichlid *Tropheus moorii*. *Behaviour*, 142, 265–281.

Schürch, R., Rothenberger, S. & Heg, D. 2010. The building-up of social relationships: behavioural types, social networks and cooperative breeding in a cichlid. *Philosophical Transactions of the Royal Society of London B: Biological Sciences*, 365, 4089–4098.

Schütz, D., Parker, G.A., Taborsky, M. & Sato, T. 2006. An optimality approach to male and female body sizes in an extremely size-dimorphic cichlid fish. *Evolutionary Ecology Research*, 8, 1393–1408.

Schweinfurth, M.K. & Call, J. 2019a. Reciprocity: different behavioural strategies, cognitive mechanisms and psychological processes. *Learning & Behavior*, 47, 284–301.

Schweinfurth, M.K. & Call, J. 2019b. Revisiting the possibility of reciprocal help in non-human primates. *Neuroscience and Biobehavioral Reviews*, 104, 73–86.

Schweinfurth, M.K. & Taborsky, M. 2016. No evidence for audience effects in reciprocal cooperation of Norway rats. *Ethology*, 122, 513–521.

Schweinfurth, M.K. & Taborsky, M. 2017. The transfer of alternative tasks in reciprocal cooperation. *Animal Behaviour*, 131, 35–41.

Schweinfurth, M.K. & Taborsky, M. 2018a. Relatedness decreases and reciprocity increases cooperation in Norway rats. *Proceedings of the Royal Society of London B: Biological Sciences*, 285, 20180035.

Schweinfurth, M.K. & Taborsky, M. 2018b. Reciprocal trading of different commodities in Norway rats. *Current Biology*, 28, 594–599.

Schweinfurth, M.K. & Taborsky, M. 2018c. Norway rats (*Rattus norvegicus*) communicate need, which elicits donation of food. *Journal of Comparative Psychology*, 132, 119–129.

Schweinfurth, M.K. & Taborsky, M. 2020. Rats play tit-for-tat instead of integrating social experience over multiple interactions. *Proceedings of the Royal Society of London B: Biological Sciences*, 287, 20192423.

Schweinfurth, M.K., Stieger, B. & Taborsky, M. 2017a. Experimental evidence for reciprocity in allogrooming among wild-type Norway rats. *Scientific Reports*, 7, 4010.

Schweinfurth, M.K., Neuenschwander, J., Engqvist, L., et al. 2017b. Do female Norway rats form social bonds? *Behavioral Ecology and Sociobiology*, 71, 98.

Schweinfurth, M.K., Aeschbacher, J., Santi, M. & Taborsky, M. 2019. Male Norway rats cooperate according to direct but not generalized reciprocity rules. *Animal Behaviour*, 152, 93–101.

Scott, D.K. 1980. Functional aspects of prolonged parental care in Bewick's swans. *Animal Behaviour*, 28, 938–952.

Searcy, W.A. & Nowicki, S. 2005. *The Evolution of Animal Communication: Reliability and Deception in Signaling Systems*. Princeton, NJ: Princeton University Press.

Sefc, K.M. 2011. Mating and parental care in Lake Tanganyika's cichlids. *International Journal of Evolutionary Biology*, 2011, 470875.

Segelbacher, G., Wegge, P., Sivkov, A.V. & Höglund, J. 2007. Kin groups in closely spaced capercaillie leks. *Journal of Ornithology*, 148, 79–84.

Segers, F.H.I.D. & Taborsky, B. 2012. Competition level determines compensatory growth abilities. *Behavioral Ecology*, 23, 665–671.

Seinen, I. & Schram, A. 2006. Social status and group norms: indirect reciprocity in a repeated helping experiment. *European Economic Review*, 50, 581–602.

Sella, G. 1985. Reciprocal egg trading and brood care in a hermaphroditic polychaete worm. *Animal Behaviour*, 33, 938–944.

Sella, G. 1988. Reciprocation, reproductive success, and safeguards against cheating in a hermaphroditic polychaete worm, *Ophryotrocha diadema* Akesson, 1976. *Biological Bulletin*, 175, 212–217.

Sella, G. & Lorenzi, M.C. 2000. Partner fidelity and egg reciprocation in the simultaneously hermaphroditic polychaete worm *Ophryotrocha diadema*. *Behavioral Ecology*, 11, 260–264.

Sella, G., Premoli, M.C. & Turri, F. 1997. Egg trading in the simultaneously hermaphroditic polychaete worm *Ophryotrocha gracilis* (Huth). *Behavioral Ecology*, 8, 83–86.

Semel, B. & Sherman, P.W. 2001. Intraspecific parasitism and nest-site competition in wood ducks. *Animal Behaviour*, 61, 787–803.

Semmann, D., Krambeck, H.J. & Milinski, M. 2005. Reputation is valuable within and outside one's own social group. *Behavioral Ecology and Sociobiology*, 57, 611–616.

Semple, K., Wayne, R.K. & Gibson, R.M. 2001. Microsatellite analysis of female mating behaviour in lek-breeding sage grouse. *Molecular Ecology*, 10, 2043–2048.

Seppä, P., Queller, D.C. & Strassmann, J.E. 2012. Why wasp foundresses change nests: relatedness, dominance, and nest quality. *PLoS One*, 7, e45386.

Sergio, F. & Bogliani, G. 2001. Nest defense as parental care in the northern hobby (*Falco subbuteo*). *The Auk*, 118, 1047–1053.

Seyfarth, R.M. 1976. Social relationships among adult female baboons. *Animal Behaviour*, 24, 917–938.

Seyfarth, R.M. 1977. Model of social grooming among adult female monkeys. *Journal of Theoretical Biology*, 65, 671–698.

Seyfarth, R.M. & Cheney, D.L. 1984. Grooming, alliances and reciprocal altruism in vervet monkeys. *Nature*, 308, 541–543.

Seyfarth, R.M. & Cheney, D.L. 1988. Empirical tests of reciprocity theory – problems in assessment. *Ethology and Sociobiology*, 9, 181–187.

Shapiro, D.Y., Hensley, D.A. & Appeldoorn, R.S. 1988. Pelagic spawning and egg transport in coral-reef fishes – a skeptical overview. *Environmental Biology of Fishes*, 22, 3–14.

Sharp, S.P. & Clutton-Brock, T.H. 2011. Reluctant challengers: why do subordinate female meerkats rarely displace their dominant mothers? *Behavioral Ecology*, 22, 1337–1343.

Sharp, S.P., McGowan, A., Wood, M.J. & Hatchwell, B.J. 2005. Learned kin recognition cues in a social bird. *Nature*, 434, 1127.

Sharp, S.P., Simeoni, M. & Hatchwell, B.J. 2008. Dispersal of sibling coalitions promotes helping among immigrants in a cooperatively breeding bird. *Proceedings of the Royal Society of London B: Biological Sciences*, 275, 2125–2130.

Sharpe, R.V. & Aviles, L. 2016. Prey size and scramble vs. contest competition in a social spider: implications for population dynamics. *Journal of Animal Ecology*, 85, 1401–1410.

Shaw, J.J., Tregenza, T., Parker, G.A. & Harvey, I.F. 1995. Evolutionarily stable foraging speeds in feeding scrambles: a model and an experimental test. *Proceedings of the Royal Society of London B: Biological Sciences*, 260, 273–277.

Sheehan, M.J. & Tibbetts, E.A. 2008. Robust long-term social memories in a paper wasp. *Current Biology*, 18, R851–R852.

Sheehan, M.J. & Tibbetts, E.A. 2010. Selection for individual recognition and the evolution of polymorphic identity signals in *Polistes* paper wasps. *Journal of Evolutionary Biology*, 23, 570–577.

Sheehan, M.J. & Tibbetts, E.A. 2011. Specialized face learning is associated with individual recognition in paper wasps. *Science*, 334, 1272–1275.

Sheehan, M.J., Botero, C.A., Hendry, T.A., et al. 2015. Different axes of environmental variation explain the presence vs. extent of cooperative nest founding associations in *Polistes* paper wasps. *Ecology Letters*, 18, 1057–1067.

Sheldon, B.C. 2002. Relating paternity to paternal care. *Philosophical Transactions of the Royal Society of London B: Biological Sciences*, 357, 341–350.

Shelly, T.E. 2001. Lek size and female visitation in two species of tephritid fruit flies. *Animal Behaviour*, 62, 33–40.

Shen, S.F., Vehrencamp, S.L., Johnstone, R.A., et al. 2012. Unfavourable environment limits social conflict in *Yuhina brunneiceps*. *Nature Communications*, 3, 885.

Shen, S., Emlen, S.T., Koenig, W.D. & Rubenstein, D.R. 2017. The ecology of cooperative breeding behaviour. *Ecology Letters*, 20, 708–720.

Sheppard, C.E., Marshall, H.H., Inger, R., et al. 2018. Decoupling of genetic and cultural inheritance in a wild mammal. *Current Biology*, 28, 1846–1850.

Sherley, G.H. 1990. Co-operative breeding in riflemen (*Acanthissitta chloris*) benefits to parents, offspring and helpers. *Behaviour*, 112, 1–22.

Sherman, C.D.H., Wapstra, E., Uller, T. & Olsson, M. 2008. Males with high genetic similarity to females sire more offspring in sperm competition in Peron's tree frog *Litoria peronii*. *Proceedings of the Royal Society of London B: Biological Sciences*, 275, 971–978.

Sherman, P.W. 1977. Nepotism and the evolution of alarm calls. *Science*, 197, 1246–1253.

Sherman, P.W., Reeve, H. & Pfennig, D. 1997. Recognition systems. In Krebs, J.R. & Davies, N.B. (eds), *Behavioural Ecology* (4th ed.), pp. 69–96. Oxford: Blackwell Scientific.

Shorey, L. 2002. Mating success on white-bearded manakin (*Manacus manacus*) leks: male characteristics and relatedness. *Behavioral Ecology and Sociobiology*, 52, 451–457.

Shorey, L., Piertney, S., Stone, J. & Höglund, J. 2000. Fine-scale genetic structuring on *Manacus manacus* leks. *Nature*, 408, 352.

Shorter, J.R. & Rueppell, O. 2012. A review on self-destructive defense behaviors in social insects. *Insectes Sociaux*, 59(1), 1–10.

Shrader, A.M., Brown, J.S., Kerley, G.I. & Kotler, B.P. 2008. Do free-ranging domestic goats show 'landscapes of fear'? Patch use in response to habitat features and predator cues. *Journal of Arid Environments*, 72, 1811–1819.

Shuster, S.M. & Sassaman, C. 1997. Genetic interaction between male mating strategy and sex ratio in a marine isopod. *Nature*, 388, 373–377.

Shuster, S.M. & Wade, M.J. 1991. Equal mating success among male reproductive strategies in a marine isopod. *Nature*, 350, 608–610.

Shutt, K., MacLarnon, A., Heistermann, M. & Semple, S. 2007. Grooming in Barbary macaques: better to give than to receive? *Biology Letters*, 3, 231–233.

Sibly, R.M. 1983. Optimal group size is unstable. *Animal Behaviour*, 31, 947–948.

Sicardi, E.A., Fort, H., Vainstein, M.H. & Arenzon, J.J. 2009. Random mobility and spatial structure often enhance cooperation. *Journal of Theoretical Biology*, 256, 240–246.

Sigmund, K. 2010. *The Calculus of Selfishness*. Princeton, NJ: Princeton University Press.

Sih, A., Hanser, S.F. & McHugh, K.A. 2009. Social network theory: new insights and issues for behavioral ecologists. *Behavioral Ecology and Sociobiology*, 63, 975–988.

Sikkel, P.C. 1989. Egg presence and developmental stage influence spawning-site choice by female garibaldi. *Animal Behaviour*, 38, 447–456.

Silberberg, A., Allouch, C., Sandfort, S., et al. 2014. Desire for social contact, not empathy, may explain 'rescue' behavior in rats. *Animal Cognition*, 17, 609–618.

Silk, J.B. 1992. The patterning of intervention among male bonnet macaques – reciprocity, revenge, and loyalty. *Current Anthropology*, 33, 318–325.

Silk, J.B. 2007. The strategic dynamics of cooperation in primate groups. *Advances in the Study of Behavior*, 37, 1–41.

Silk, J.B., Seyfarth, R.M. & Cheney, D.L. 1999. The structure of social relationships among female savanna baboons in Moremi Reserve, Botswana. *Behaviour*, 136, 679–703.

Silk, J.B., Rendall, D., Cheney, D.L. & Seyfarth, R.M. 2003. Natal attraction in adult female baboons (*Papio cynocephalus ursinus*) in the Moremi Reserve, Botswana. *Ethology*, 109, 627–644.

Silk, J.B., Brosnan, S.F., Henrich, J., Lambeth, S.P. & Shapiro, S. 2013. Chimpanzees share food for many reasons: the role of kinship, reciprocity, social bonds and harassment on food transfers. *Animal Behaviour*, 85, 941–947.

Simmons, L.W. & Kotiaho, J.S. 2007. The effects of reproduction on courtship, fertility and longevity within and between alternative male mating tactics of the horned beetle, *Onthophagus binodis*. *Journal of Evolutionary Biology*, 20, 488–495.

Sinervo, B. & Clobert, J. 2003. Morphs, dispersal behavior, genetic similarity, and the evolution of cooperation. *Science*, 300, 1949–1951.

Sinervo, B., Chaine, A., Clobert, J., et al. 2006. Self-recognition, color signals, and cycles of greenbeard mutualism and altruism. *Proceedings of the National Academy of Sciences of the United States of America*, 103, 7372–7377.

Singh, M. & Boomsma, J.J. 2015. Policing and punishment across the domains of social evolution. *Oikos*, 124, 971–982.

Skaperdas, S. 1996. Contest success functions. *Economic Theory*, 7, 283–290.

Skjærvø, G.R. & Røskaft, E. 2013. Menopause: no support for an evolutionary explanation among historical Norwegians. *Experimental Gerontology*, 48, 408–413.

Skutch, A.F. 1935. Helpers at the nest. *The Auk*, 52, 257–273.

Skutch, A.F. 1961. Helpers among birds. *Condor*, 63, 198–226.

Slater, K.Y., Schaffner, C.M. & Aureli, F. 2007. Embraces for infant handling in spider monkeys: evidence for a biological market? *Animal Behaviour*, 74, 455–461.

Smiseth, P.T. 2019. Coordination, cooperation and conflict between caring parents in burying beetles. *Frontiers in Ecology and Evolution*, 7, 397.

Smith, B.D. 1998. *The Emergence of Agriculture*. New York, NY: American Library.

Smith, C. & Wootton, R.J. 1994. The cost of parental care in *Haplochromis* 'argens' (Cichlidae). *Environmental Biology of Fishes*, 40, 99–104.

Smith, C. & Wootton, R.J. 1995. The costs of parental care in teleost fishes. *Reviews in Fish Biology and Fisheries*, 5, 7–22.

Smith, J.E. 2014. Hamilton's legacy: kinship, cooperation and social tolerance in mammalian groups. *Animal Behaviour*, 92, 291–304.

Smith, S.M., Kent, D.S., Boomsma, J.J. & Stow, A.J. 2018. Monogamous sperm storage and permanent worker sterility in a long-lived ambrosia beetle. *Nature Ecology & Evolution*, 2, 1009–1018.

Smuts, B.B. 1985. *Sex and Friendship in Baboons*. New York, NY: Aldine Publishing.

Smyers, S.D., Rubbo, M.J., Townsend, V.R. & Swart, C.C. 2002. Intra- and interspecific characterizations of burrow use and defense by juvenile ambystomatid salamanders. *Herpetologica*, 58, 422–429.

Sober, E. & Wilson, D.S. 1998. *Unto Others: The Evolution and Psychology of Unselfish Behavior*. Cambridge, MA: Harvard University Press.

Soler, M. 2014. Long-term coevolution between avian brood parasites and their hosts. *Biological Reviews*, 89, 688–704.

Solomon, N.G. & French, J.A. 1997. *Cooperative Breeding in Mammals*. Cambridge: Cambridge University Press.

Sorato, E., Gullett, P.R., Creasey, M.J.S., Griffith, S.C. & Russell, A.F. 2015. Plastic territoriality in group-living chestnut-crowned babblers: roles of resource value, holding potential and predation risk. *Animal Behaviour*, 101, 155–168.

Spahni, C. 2005. Indirect reciprocity in Norway rats (*Rattus norvegicus*). MSc thesis, University of Bern, Switzerland.

Spottiswoode, C.N., Begg, K.S. & Begg, C.M. 2016. Reciprocal signaling in honeyguide–human mutualism. *Science*, 353, 387–389.

Sridhar, H., Beauchamp, G. & Shanker, K. 2009. Why do birds participate in mixed-species foraging flocks? A large-scale synthesis. *Animal Behaviour*, 78, 337–347.

Sridhar, H., Srinivasan, U., Askins, R.A., et al. 2012. Positive relationships between association strength and phenotypic similarity characterize the assembly of mixed-species bird flocks worldwide. *American Naturalist*, 180, 777–790.

St-Pierre, A., Larose, K. & Dubois, F. 2009. Long-term social bonds promote cooperation in the iterated Prisoner's Dilemma. *Proceedings of the Royal Society of London B: Biological Sciences*, 276, 4223–4228.

Stacey, P.B. & Koenig, W.D. 1990. *Cooperative Breeding in Birds: Long Term Studies of Ecology and Behaviour*. Cambridge: Cambridge University Press.

Stacey, P.B. & Ligon, J.D. 1987. Territory quality and dispersal options in the acorn woodpecker, and a challenge to the habitat-saturation model of cooperative breeding. *The American Naturalist*, 130, 654–676.

Stacey, P.B. & Ligon, J.D. 1991. The benefits-of-philopatry hypothesis for the evolution of cooperative breeding: variation in territory quality and group size effects. *The American Naturalist*, 137, 831–846.

Stadler, B. & Dixon, T. 2008. *Mutualism. Ants and Their Insect Partners*. Cambridge: Cambridge University Press.

Stanca, L. 2009. Measuring indirect reciprocity: whose back do we scratch? *Journal of Economic Psychology*, 30, 190–202.

Stander, P.E. 1992. Cooperative hunting in lions – the role of the individual. *Behavioral Ecology and Sociobiology*, 29, 445–454.

Stein, A.C. & Uy, J.A. 2005. Plumage brightness predicts male mating success in the lekking golden-collared manakin, *Manacus vitellinus*. *Behavioral Ecology*, 17, 41–47.

Steinegger, M. & Taborsky, B. 2007. Asymmetric sexual conflict over parental care in a biparental cichlid. *Behavioral Ecology and Sociobiology*, 61, 933–941.

Steinhart, G.B., Sandrene, M.E., Weaver, S., Stein, R.A. & Marschall, E.A. 2005. Increased parental care cost for nest-guarding fish in a lake with hyperabundant nest predators. *Behavioral Ecology*, 16, 427–434.

Stephens, D.W., McLinn, C.M. & Stevens, J.R. 2002. Discounting and reciprocity in an iterated prisoner's dilemma. *Science*, 298, 2216–2218.

Stevens, J.R. & Gilby, I.C. 2004. A conceptual framework for nonkin food sharing: timing and currency of benefits. *Animal Behaviour*, 67, 603–614.

Stevens, J.R. & Hauser, M.D. 2004. Why be nice? Psychological constraints on the evolution of cooperation. *Trends in Cognitive Sciences*, 8, 60–65.

Stevens, J.R., Cushman, F.A. & Hauser, M.D. 2005. Evolving the psychological mechanisms for cooperation. *Annual Review of Ecology Evolution and Systematics*, 36, 499–518.

Stevens, J.R., Volstorf, J., Schooler, L.J., & Rieskamp, J. 2011. Forgetting constrains the emergence of cooperative decision strategies. *Frontiers in Psychology*, 1, 235.

Stieger, B., Schweinfurth, M.K. & Taborsky, M. 2017. Reciprocal allogrooming among unrelated Norway rats (*Rattus norvegicus*) is affected by previously received cooperative, affiliative and aggressive behaviours. *Behavioral Ecology and Sociobiology*, 71, 182.

Stilwell, A.R., Smith, S.M., Cognato, A.I., Martinez, M. & Flowers, R.W. 2014. *Coptoborus ochromactonus*, n. sp. (Coleoptera: Curculionidae: Scolytinae), an emerging pest of cultivated balsa (Malvales: Malvaceae) in Ecuador. *Journal of Economic Entomology*, 107, 675–683.

Stiver, K.A. & Alonzo, S.H. 2011. Alloparental care increases mating success. *Behavioral Ecology*, 22, 206–211.

Stiver, K.A. & Alonzo, S.H. 2013. Does the risk of sperm competition help explain cooperation between reproductive competitors? A study in the ocellated wrasse (*Symphodus ocellatus*). *American Naturalist*, 181, 357–368.

Stiver, K.A., Dierkes, P., Taborsky, M. & Balshine, S. 2004. Dispersal patterns and status change in a co-operatively breeding cichlid *Neolamprologus pulcher*: evidence from microsatellite analyses and behavioural observations. *Journal of Fish Biology*, 65, 91–105.

Stiver, K.A., Dierkes, P., Taborsky, M., Gibbs, H.L. & Balshine, S. 2005. Relatedness and helping in fish: examining the theoretical predictions. *Proceedings of the Royal Society of London B: Biological Sciences*, 272, 1593–1599.

Stiver, K.A., Fitzpatrick, J., Desjardins, J.K. & Balshine, S. 2006. Sex differences in rates of territory joining and inheritance in a cooperatively breeding cichlid fish. *Animal Behaviour*, 71, 449–456.

Stiver, K., Desjardins, J., Fitzpatrick, J., et al. 2007. Evidence for size and sex-specific dispersal in a cooperatively breeding cichlid fish. *Molecular Ecology*, 16, 2974–2984.

Stiver, K., Fitzpatrick, J., Desjardins, J., et al. 2008. The role of genetic relatedness among social mates in a cooperative breeder. *Behavioral Ecology*, 19, 816–823.

Stiver, K.A., Wolff, S.H. & Alonzo, S.H. 2012. Adoption and cuckoldry lead to alloparental care in the tessellated darter (*Etheostoma olmstedi*), a non-group-living species with no evidence of nest site limitation. *Behavioral Ecology and Sociobiology*, 66, 855–864.

Stockley, P. & Bro-Jørgensen, J. 2011. Female competition and its evolutionary consequences in mammals. *Biological Reviews*, 86, 34–366.

Stojkoski, V., Utkovski, Z., Basnarkov, L. & Kocarev, L. 2018. Cooperation dynamics of generalized reciprocity in state-based social dilemmas. *Physical Review E*, 97, 052305.

Stokes, A.W. 1971. Parental and courtship feeding in red jungle fowl. *The Auk*, 88, 21–29.

Stokkebo, S. & Hardy, I.C. 2000. The importance of being gravid: egg load and contest outcome in a parasitoid wasp. *Animal Behaviour*, 59, 1111–1118.

Stopka, P. & Graciasova, R. 2001. Conditional allogrooming in the herb-field mouse. *Behavioral Ecology*, 12, 584–589.

Storey, A., Wilhelm, S. & Walsh, C. 2020. Negotiation of parental duties in chick-rearing common murres (*Uria aalge*) in different foraging conditions. *Frontiers in Ecology and Evolution*, 7, 506.

Strickland, D. 1991. Juvenile dispersal in gray jays: dominant brood member expels siblings from natal territory. *Canadian Journal of Zoology*, 69, 2935–2945.

Stutt, A.D. & Siva-Jothy, M.T. 2001. Traumatic insemination and sexual conflict in the bed bug *Cimex lectularius*. *Proceedings of the National Academy of Sciences of the United States of America*, 98, 5683–5687.

Suchak, M. & de Waal, F.B.M. 2012. Monkeys benefit from reciprocity without the cognitive burden. *Proceedings of the National Academy of Sciences of the United States of America*, 109, 15191–15196.

Sugiyama, Y. 1971. Characteristics of the social life of bonnet macaques (*Macaca radiata*). *Primates*, 12, 247–266.

Suhonen, J. 1993a. Risk of predation and foraging sites of individuals in mixed-species tit flocks. *Animal Behaviour*, 45, 1193–1198.

Suhonen, J. 1993b. Predation risk influences the use of foraging sites by tits. *Ecology*, 74, 1197–1203.

Suhonen, J., Ilvonen, J.J., Nyman, T. & Sorvari, J. 2019. Brood parasitism in eusocial insects (Hymenoptera): role of host geographical range size and phylogeny. *Philosophical Transactions of the Royal Society of London B: Biological Sciences*, 374, 20180203.

Sulloway, F.J. & Kleindorfer, S. 2013. Adaptive divergence in Darwin's small ground finch (*Geospiza fuliginosa*): divergent selection along a cline. *Biological Journal of the Linnean Society*, 110, 45–59.

Sumana, A. & Starks, P.T. 2004. The function of dart behavior in the paper wasp, *Polistes fuscatus*. *Naturwissenschaften*, 91, 220–223.

Sumpter, D.J.T. 2006. The principles of collective animal behaviour. *Philosophical Transactions of the Royal Society of London B: Biological Sciences*, 361, 5–22.

Surbeck, M. & Hohmann, G. 2015. Social preferences influence the short-term exchange of social grooming among male bonobos. *Animal Cognition*, 18, 573–579.

Surridge, A.K., Bell, D.J. & Hewitt, G.M. 1999. From population structure to individual behaviour: genetic analysis of social structure in the European wild rabbit (*Oryctolagus cuniculus*). *Biological Journal of the Linnean Society*, 68, 57–71.

Sutherland, W.J. 1983. Aggregation and the ideal 'free' distribution. *The Journal of Animal Ecology*, 821–828.

Suzuki, S. 2013. Biparental care in insects: paternal care, life history, and the function of the nest. *Journal of Insect Science*, 13, 131.

Suzuki, S. & Kimura, H. 2011. Oscillatory dynamics in the coevolution of cooperation and mobility. *Journal of Theoretical Biology*, 287, 42–47.

Suzuki, S. & Kimura, H. 2013. Indirect reciprocity is sensitive to costs of information transfer. *Scientific Reports*, 3, 1435.

Svanbäck, R. & Bolnick, D.I. 2005. Intraspecific competition affects the strength of individual specialization: an optimal diet theory method. *Evolutionary Ecology Research*, 7, 993–1012.

Svensson, B.G. & Petersson, E. 1994. Mate choice tactics and swarm size: a model and a test in a dance fly. *Behavioral Ecology and Sociobiology*, 35, 161–168.

Syrop, S. 1974. Three selected aspects of the territorial behavior of a pomacentrid fish, *Pomacentrus jenkinsi*. Master's thesis, University of Hawaii.

Szabo, G. & Fath, G. 2007. Evolutionary games on graphs. *Physics Reports*, 446, 97–216.

Számadó, S. 2008. How threat displays work: species-specific fighting techniques, weaponry and proximity risk. *Animal Behaviour*, 76, 1455–1463.

Számadó, S. 2011. Long-term commitment promotes honest status signalling. *Animal Behaviour*, 82, 295–302.

Szathmáry, E. 2015. Toward major evolutionary transitions theory 2.0. *Proceedings of the National Academy of Sciences of the United States of America*, 112, 10104–10111.

Szekely, T., Weissing, F.J. & Komdeur, J. 2014. Adult sex ratio variation: implications for breeding system evolution. *Journal of Evolutionary Biology*, 27, 1500–1512.

Szolnoki, A., Wang, Z. & Perc, M. 2012. Wisdom of groups promotes cooperation in evolutionary social dilemmas. *Scientific Reports*, 2, 576.

Taborsky, B. 2006. The influence of juvenile and adult environments on life-history trajectories. *Proceedings of the Royal Society of London B: Biological Sciences*, 273, 741–750.

Taborsky, B. & Oliveira, R.F. 2012. Social competence: an evolutionary approach. *Trends in Ecology & Evolution*, 27, 679–688.

Taborsky, B., Skubic, E. & Bruintjes, R. 2007. Mothers adjust egg size to helper number in a cooperatively breeding cichlid. *Behavioral Ecology*, 18, 652–657.

Taborsky, B., Arnold, C., Junker, J. & Tschopp, A. 2012. The early social environment affects social competence in a cooperative breeder. *Animal Behaviour*, 83, 1067–1074.

Taborsky, B., Tschirren, L., Meunier, C. & Aubin-Horth, N. 2013. Stable reprogramming of brain transcription profiles by the early social environment in a cooperatively breeding fish. *Proceedings of the Royal Society of London B: Biological Sciences*, 280, 20122605.

Taborsky, M. 1984. Broodcare helpers in the cichlid fish *Lamprologus brichardi*: their costs and benefits. *Animal Behaviour*, 32, 1236–1252.

Taborsky, M. 1985. Breeder–helper conflict in a cichlid fish with broodcare helpers: an experimental analysis. *Behaviour*, 95, 45–75.

Taborsky, M. 1994. Sneakers, satellites, and helpers: parasitic and cooperative behavior in fish reproduction. *Advances in the Study of Behavior*, 23, 1–100.

Taborsky, M. 1998. Sperm competition in fish: 'bourgeois' males and parasitic spawning. *Trends in Ecology & Evolution*, 13, 222–227.

Taborsky, M. 2001. The evolution of bourgeois, parasitic, and cooperative reproductive behaviors in fishes. *Journal of Heredity*, 92, 100–110.

Taborsky, M. 2007. Cooperation built the Tower of Babel. *Behavioural Processes*, 76, 95–99.

Taborsky, M. 2008. Alternative reproductive tactics in fish. In Oliveira, R.F., Taborsky, M. & Brockmann, H.J. (eds), *Alternative Reproductive Tactics. An Integrative Approach*, pp. 251–299. Cambridge: Cambridge University Press.

Taborsky, M. 2009. Reproductive skew in cooperative fish groups: virtue and limitations of alternative modeling approaches. In Hager, R. & Jones, C. (eds), *Reproductive Skew in Vertebrates: Proximate and Ultimate Causes*, pp. 265–304. Cambridge: Cambridge University Press.

Taborsky, M. 2013. Social evolution: reciprocity there is. *Current Biology*, 23, R486–R488.

Taborsky, M. 2014. Tribute to Tinbergen: the four problems of biology. A critical appraisal. *Ethology*, 120, 224–227.

Taborsky, M. 2016. Cichlid fishes: a model for the integrative study of social behavior. In Koenig, W.D. &

Dickinson, J.L. (eds), *Cooperative Breeding in Vertebrates*, pp. 272–293. Cambridge: Cambridge University Press.

Taborsky, M. & Brockmann, H.J. 2010. Alternative reproductive tactics and life history phenotypes. In Kappeler, P. (ed.), *Animal Behaviour: Evolution and Mechanisms*, pp. 537–586. Heidelberg Springer.

Taborsky, M. & Grantner, A. 1998. Behavioural time-energy budgets of cooperatively breeding *Neolamprologus pulcher* (Pisces: Cichlidae). *Animal Behaviour*, 56, 1375–1382.

Taborsky, M. & Limberger, D. 1981. Helpers in fish. *Behavioral Ecology and Sociobiology*, 8, 143–145.

Taborsky, M. & Riebli, T. 2020. Coaction vs. reciprocal cooperation among unrelated individuals in social cichlids. *Frontiers in Ecology and Evolution*, 7, 515.

Taborsky, M. & Taborsky, B. 2015. Evolution of genetic and physiological mechanisms of cooperative behaviour. *Current Opinion in Behavioral Sciences*, 6, 132–138.

Taborsky, M. & Wong, M. 2017. Sociality in fishes. In Rubenstein, D.R. & Abbot, P. (eds), *Comparative Social Evolution*, pp. 354–389. Cambridge: Cambridge University Press.

Taborsky, M., Hert, E., Siemens, M. & Stoerig, P. 1986. Social behaviour of *Lamprologus* species: functions and mechanisms. *Annales du Musee Royale de l'Afrique Centrale Serie 8: Sciences Zoologique (Tervuren, Belgium)*, 251, 7–11.

Taborsky, M., Hudde, B. & Wirtz, P. 1987. Reproductive behaviour and ecology of *Symphodus* (*Crenilabrus*) *ocellatus*, a European wrasse with four types of male behaviour. *Behaviour*, 102, 82–118.

Taborsky, M., Oliveira, R.F. & Brockmann, H.J. 2008. The evolution of alternative reproductive tactics: concepts and questions. In Oliveira, R.F., Taborsky, M. & Brockmann, H.J. (eds), *Alternative Reproductive Tactics: An Integrative Approach*, pp. 1–21. Cambridge: Cambridge University Press.

Taborsky, M., Hofmann, H.A., Beery, A.K., et al. 2015. Taxon matters: promoting integrative studies of social behavior. *Trends in Neurosciences*, 38, 189–191.

Taborsky, M., Frommen, J.G. & Riehl, C. 2016. Correlated pay-offs are key to cooperation. *Philosophical Transactions of the Royal Society of London B: Biological Sciences*, 371, 20150084.

Taborsky, M., Schütz, D., Goffinet, O. & van Doorn, G.S. 2018. Alternative male morphs solve sperm performance/longevity trade-off in opposite directions. *Science Advances*, 4, eaap8563.

Takahashi, M., Suzuki, N. & Koga, T. 2001. Burrow defense behaviors in a sand-bubbler crab: *Scopimera globosa*, in relation to body size and prior residence. *Journal of Ethology*, 19, 93–96.

Takezawa, M. & Price, M.E. 2010. Revisiting 'the evolution of reciprocity in sizable groups': continuous reciprocity in the repeated n-person prisoner's dilemma. *Journal of Theoretical Biology*, 264, 188–196.

Tallamy, D.W. 1985. 'Egg dumping' in lace bugs (*Gargaphia solani*, Hemiptera; Tingidae). *Behavioral Ecology and Sociobiology*, 17, 357–362.

Tallamy, D.W. 2005. Egg dumping in insects. *Annual Review of Entomology*, 50, 347–370.

Tan, L. & Hackenberg, T.D. 2016. Functional analysis of mutual behavior in laboratory rats (*Rattus norvegicus*). *Journal of Comparative Psychology*, 130, 13–23.

Tanaka, H., Heg, D., Takeshima, H., et al. 2015. Group composition, relatedness, and dispersal in the cooperatively breeding cichlid *Neolamprologus obscurus*. *Behavioral Ecology and Sociobiology*, 69, 169–181.

Tanaka, H., Frommen, J.G., Takahashi, T. & Kohda, M. 2016. Predation risk promotes delayed dispersal in the cooperatively breeding cichlid *Neolamprologus obscurus*. *Animal Behaviour*, 117, 51–58.

Tanaka, H., Frommen, J.G. & Kohda, M. 2018a. Helpers increase food abundance in the territory of a cooperatively breeding fish. *Behavioral Ecology and Sociobiology*, 72, 52.

Tanaka, H., Kohda, M. & Frommen, J.G. 2018b. Helpers increase the reproductive success of breeders in the cooperatively breeding cichlid *Neolamprologus obscurus*. *Behavioral Ecology and Sociobiology*, 72, 152.

Tanaka, H., Frommen, J.G., Engqvist, L. & Kohda, M. 2018c. Task-dependent workload adjustment of female breeders in a cooperatively breeding fish. *Behavioral Ecology*, 29, 221–229.

Tanaka, H., Frommen, J.G., Koblmuller, S., et al. 2018d. Evolutionary transitions to cooperative societies in fishes revisited. *Ethology*, 124, 777–789.

Tang-Martinez, Z. 2001. The mechanisms of kin discrimination and the evolution of kin recognition in vertebrates: a critical re-evaluation. *Behavioural Processes*, 53, 21–40.

Taylor, P.D. 1988. An inclusive fitness model for dispersal of offspring. *Journal of Theoretical Biology*, 130, 363–378.

Taylor, P.D. 1990. Allele-frequency change in a class-structured population. *The American Naturalist*, 135, 95–106.

Taylor, P.D. 1992a. Altruism in viscous populations – an inclusive fitness model. *Evolutionary Ecology*, 6, 352–356.

Taylor, P.D. 1992b. Inclusive fitness in a homogeneous environment. *Proceedings of the Royal Society of London B: Biological Sciences*, 249, 299–302.

Taylor, P.D. & Day, T. 2004. Stability in negotiation games and the emergence of cooperation. *Proceedings of the Royal Society of London B: Biological Sciences*, 271, 669–674.

Taylor, P.D. & Frank, S.A. 1996. How to make a kin selection model. *Journal of Theoretical Biology*, 180, 27–37.

Taylor, P.D. & Jonker, L.B. 1978. Evolutionary stable strategies and game dynamics. *Mathematical Biosciences*, 40, 145–156.

Taylor, P.D., Day, T. & Wild, G. 2007a. Evolution of cooperation in a finite homogeneous graph. *Nature*, 447, 469–472.

Taylor, P.D., Wild, G. & Gardner, A. 2007b. Direct fitness or inclusive fitness: how shall we model kin selection? *Journal of Evolutionary Biology*, 20, 301–309.

Taylor, P.W. & Elwood, R.W. 2003. The mismeasure of animal contests. *Animal Behaviour*, 65, 1195–1202.

Tebbich, S., Taborsky, M. & Winkler, H. 1996. Social manipulation causes cooperation in keas. *Animal Behaviour*, 52, 1–10.

Teichroeb, J.A. & Sicotte, P. 2018. Cascading competition: the seasonal strength of scramble influences between-group contest in a folivorous primate. *Behavioral Ecology and Sociobiology*, 72, 6.

Telle, H.-J. 1965. Beitrag zur Kenntnis der Verhaltensweise von Ratten, vergleichend dargestellt bei *Rattus norvegicus* und *Rattus rattus*. *Zeitschrift für Angewandte Zoologie*, 53, 129–196.

Temple, H.J., Hoffman, J.I. & Amos, W. 2006. Dispersal, philopatry and intergroup relatedness: fine-scale genetic structure in the white-breasted thrasher, *Ramphocinclus brachyurus*. *Molecular Ecology*, 15, 3449–3458.

Temple, H.J., Hoffman, J.I. & Amos, W. 2009. Group structure, mating system and extra-group paternity in the co-operatively breeding white-breasted thrasher *Ramphocinclus brachyurus*. *Ibis*, 151, 99–112.

Templeton, J.J. & Giraldeau, L.A. 1995. Patch assessment in foraging flocks of european starlings – evidence for the use of public information. *Behavioral Ecology*, 6, 65–72.

Terry, R.L. 1970. Primate grooming as a tension reduction mechanism. *Journal of Psychology*, 76, 129–136.

Teunissen, N., Kingma, S.A., Hall, M.L., et al. 2018. More than kin: subordinates foster strong bonds with relatives and potential mates in a social bird. *Behavioral Ecology*, 29, 1316–1324.

Thayer, B.A. 2004. *Darwin and International Relations: On the Evolutionary Origins of War and Ethnic Conflict.* Lexington, KY: University Press of Kentucky.

Theberge, J.B. & Wedeles, C.H.R. 1989. Prey selection and habitat partitioning in sympatric coyote and red fox populations, southwest Yukon. *Canadian Journal of Zoology*, 67, 1285–1290.

Theimer, T.C. 1987. The effect of seed dispersion on the foraging success of dominant and subordinate dark-eyed juncos, *Junco hyemalis*. *Animal Behaviour*, 35, 1883–1890.

Thomas, L.K. & Manica, A. 2003. Filial cannibalism in an assassin bug. *Animal Behaviour*, 66, 205–210.

Thomas, M.L., Makrisâ, C.M., Suarez, A.V., Tsutsui, N.D. & Holway, D.A. 2006. When supercolonies collide: territorial aggression in an invasive and unicolonial social insect. *Molecular Ecology*, 15, 4303–4315.

Thompson, F.J. & Cant, M.A. 2018. Dynamic conflict among heterogeneous groups: a comment on Christensen and Radford. *Behavioral Ecology*, 29, 1016–1017.

Thompson, F.J., Donaldson, L., Johnstone, R.A., Field, J. & Cant, M.A. 2014. Dominant aggression as a deterrent signal in paper wasps. *Behavioral Ecology*, 25, 706–715.

Thompson, F.J., Marshall, H.H., Sanderson, J.L., et al. 2016. Reproductive competition triggers mass eviction in cooperative banded mongooses. *Proceedings of the Royal Society of London B: Biological Sciences*, 283, 20152607.

Thompson, F.J., Cant, M.A., Marshall, H.H., et al. 2017a. Explaining negative kin discrimination in a cooperative mammal society. *Proceedings of the National Academy of Sciences of the United States of America*, 114, 5207–5212.

Thompson, F.J., Marshall, H.H., Vitikainen, E.I. & Cant, M.A. 2017b. Causes and consequences of intergroup conflict in cooperative banded mongooses. *Animal Behaviour*, 126, 31–40.

Thompson, F.J., Marshall, H.H., Vitikainen, E.I.K., Young, A.J. & Cant, M.A. 2017c. Individual and demographic consequences of mass eviction in cooperative banded mongooses. *Animal Behaviour*, 134, 103–112.

Thompson, F.J., Hunt, K.L., Wright, K., et al. 2020. Who goes there? Social surveillance as a response to intergroup conflict in a primitive termite. *Biology Letters*, 16, 20200131.

Thompson, J.N. 1994. *The Coevolutionary Process.* Chicago, IL: University of Chicago Press.

Thorne, B.L. 1997. Evolution of eusociality in termites. *Annual Review of Ecology and Systematics*, 28, 27–54.

Thorne, B.L., Breisch, N.L. & Muscedere, M.L. 2003. Evolution of eusociality and the soldier caste in termites: influence of intraspecific competition and accelerated inheritance. *Proceedings of the National Academy of Sciences of the United States of America*, 100, 12808–12813.

Thorpe, W.H. 1956. *Learning and Instinct in Animals.* Cambridge, MA: Harvard University Press.

Thresher, R.E. 1976. Field analysis of the territoriality of the threespot damselfish, *Eupomacentrus planifrons* (Pomacentridae). *Copeia*, 1976, 266–276.

Thünken, T., Bakker, T.C., Baldauf, S.A. & Kullmann, H. 2007. Active inbreeding in a cichlid fish and its adaptive significance. *Current Biology*, 17, 225–229.

Thünken, T., Meuthen, D., Bakker, T.C. & Baldauf, S.A. 2012. A sex-specific trade-off between mating preferences for genetic compatibility and body size in a cichlid fish with mutual mate choice. *Proceedings of the Royal Society of London B: Biological Sciences*, 279, 20120333.

Thünken, T., Eigster, M. & Frommen, J.G. 2014a. Context-dependent group size preferences in large shoals of three-spined sticklebacks. *Animal Behaviour*, 90, 205–210.

Thünken, T., Bakker, T.C. & Baldauf, S.A. 2014b. Armpit effect in an African cichlid fish: self-referent kin recognition in mating decisions of male *Pelvicachromis taeniatus*. *Behavioral Ecology and Sociobiology*, 68, 99–104.

Tibbetts, E.A. & Dale, J. 2004. A socially enforced signal of quality in a paper wasp. *Nature*, 432, 218–222.

Tibbetts, E.A. & Reeve, H.K. 2000. Aggression and resource sharing among foundresses in the social wasp *Polistes dominulus*: testing transactional theories of conflict. *Behavioral Ecology and Sociobiology*, 48, 344–352.

Tibbetts, E.A. & Sheehan, M.J. 2013. Individual recognition and the evolution of learning and memory in *Polistes* paper wasps. In Menzel, E. & Benjamin, P.R. (eds), *Invertebrate Learning and Memory* (Handbook of Behavioral Neuroscience Volume 22), pp. 561–571. London: Academic Press.

Tibbetts, E.A., Skaldina, O., Zhao, V., et al. 2011. Geographic variation in the status signals of *Polistes* dominulus paper wasps. *PLoS One*, 6, e28173.

Tibbetts, E.A., Agudelo, J., Pandit, S. & Riojas, J. 2019. Transitive inference in *Polistes* paper wasps. *Biology Letters*, 15, 20190015.

Tiddi, B., Aureli, F. & Schino, G. 2010. Grooming for infant handling in tufted capuchin monkeys: a reappraisal of the primate infant market. *Animal Behaviour*, 79, 1115–1123.

Tiddi, B., Aureli, F., di Sorrentino, E.P., Janson, C.H. & Schino, G. 2011. Grooming for tolerance? Two mechanisms of exchange in wild tufted capuchin monkeys. *Behavioral Ecology*, 22, 663–669.

Tiedemann, R. & Noer, H. 1998. Geographic partitioning of mitochondrial DNA patterns in European eider *Somateria mollissima*. *Hereditas*, 128, 159–166.

Timms, S., Ferro, D.N. & Emberson, R.M. 1982. Andropolymorphism and its heritability in *Sancassania berlesei* (Michael) (Acari: Acaridae). *Acarologia*, 22, 391–398.

Tinbergen, N. 1951. *The Study of Instinct*. Oxford: Clarendon Press.

Tinbergen, N. 1963. On aims and methods of ethology. *Zeitschrift für Tierpsychologie – Journal of Comparative Ethology*, 20, 410–433.

Tittle, C.R. & Rowe, A.R. 1974. Certainty of arrest and crime rates: a further test of the deterrence hypothesis. *Social Forces*, 52, 455–462.

Tolker-Nielsen, T. & Molin, S. 2000. Spatial organization of microbial biofilm communities. *Microbial Ecology*, 40, 75–84.

Tomkins, J.L. & Brown, G.S. 2004. Population density drives the local evolution of a threshold dimorphism. *Nature*, 431, 1099.

Tomkins, J.L., LeBas, N.R., Unrug, J. & Radwan, J. 2004. Testing the status-dependent ESS model: population variation in fighter expression in the mite *Sancassania berlesei*. *Journal of Evolutionary Biology*, 17, 1377–1388.

Toobaie, A. & Grant, J.W. 2013. Effect of food abundance on aggressiveness and territory size of juvenile rainbow trout, *Oncorhynchus mykiss*. *Animal Behaviour*, 85, 241–246.

Townsend, A.K., Clark, A.B., McGowan, K.J. & Lovette, I.J. 2009. Reproductive partitioning and the assumptions of reproductive skew models in the cooperatively breeding American crow. *Animal Behaviour*, 77, 503–512.

Travisano, M. & Velicer, G.J. 2004. Strategies of microbial cheater control. *Trends in Microbiology*, 12, 72–78.

Tregenza, T. 1995. Building on the ideal free distribution. *Advances in Ecological Research*, 26, 253–307.

Tregenza, T., Wedell, N. & Chapman, T. 2006. Introduction. Sexual conflict: a new paradigm? *Philosophical Transactions of the Royal Society of London B: Biological Sciences*, 361, 229–234.

Tripet, F., Glaser, M. & Richner, H. 2002. Behavioural responses to ectoparasites: time-budget adjustments and what matters to blue tits *Parus caeruleus* infested by fleas. *Ibis*, 144, 461–469.

Trivers, R.L. 1971. The evolution of reciprocal altruism. *The Quarterly Review of Biology*, 46, 35–57.

Trivers, R.L. 1972. Parental investment and sexual selection. In Campbell, B. (ed.), *Sexual Selection and the Descent of Man*, pp. 136–179. Chicago, IL: Aldine.

Trivers, R.L. 1974. Parent–offspring conflict. *American Zoologist*, 14, 249–264.

Trivers, R.L. 1985. *Social Evolution*. Menlo Park, CA: Benjamin Cummings.

Trivers, R.L. & Hare, H. 1976. Haplodiploidy and the evolution of the social insects. *Science*, 191, 249–263.

Troisi, C.A., Hoppitt, W.J., Ruiz-Miranda, C.R. & Laland, K.N. 2018. Food-offering calls in wild golden lion tamarins (*Leontopithecus rosalia*): evidence for teaching behavior? *International Journal of Primatology*, 39, 1105–1123.

Tsubaki, Y. 2003. The genetic polymorphism linked to mate-securing strategies in the male damselfly *Mnais costalis* Selys (Odonata: Calopterygidae). *Population Ecology*, 45, 263–266.

Tsuji, K. & Tsuji, N. 2005. Why is dominance hierarchy age-related in social insects? The relative longevity hypothesis. *Behavioral Ecology and Sociobiology*, 58, 517–526.

Tsvetkova, M. & Macy, M.W. 2014. The social contagion of generosity. *PLoS One*, 9, e87275.

Tsvetkova, M. & Macy, M.W. 2015. The social contagion of antisocial behavior. *Sociological Science*, 2, 36–49.

Tuljapurkar, S. 1990. Delayed reproduction and fitness in variable environments. *Proceedings of the National Academy of Sciences of the United States of America*, 87, 1139–1143.

Turillazzi, S. & West-Eberhard, M.J. 1996. *Natural History and Evolution of Paper Wasps*. Oxford: Oxford University Press.

Ueno, M., Yamada, K. & Nakamichi, M. 2015. Emotional states after grooming interactions in Japanese macaques (*Macaca fuscata*). *Journal of Comparative Psychology*, 129, 394–401.

Ummenhofer, C.C. & Meehl, G.A. 2017. Extreme weather and climate events with ecological relevance: a review. *Philosophical Transactions of the Royal Society B: Biological Sciences*, 372, 20160135.

Unger, L.M. & Sargent, R.C. 1988. Allopaternal care in the fathead minnow, *Pimephales promelas*: females prefer males with eggs. *Behavioral Ecology and Sociobiology*, 23, 27–32.

Utkovski, Z., Stojkoski, V., Basnarkov, L. & Kocarev, L. 2017. Promoting cooperation by preventing exploitation: the role of network structure. *Physical Review E*, 96, 022315.

Vahl, W.K. & Kingma, S.A. 2007. Food divisibility and interference competition among captive ruddy turnstones, *Arenaria interpres*. *Animal Behaviour*, 74, 1391–1401.

Vahl, W.K., Van Der Meer, J., Meijer, K., Piersma, T. & Weissing, F.J. 2007. Interference competition, the spatial distribution of food and free-living foragers. *Animal Behaviour*, 74, 1493–1503.

Vaidya, N., Walker, S.I. & Lehman, N. 2013. Recycling of informational units leads to selection of replicators in a prebiotic soup. *Chemistry & Biology*, 20, 241–252.

Vail, A.L., Manica, A. & Bshary, R. 2013. Referential gestures in fish collaborative hunting. *Nature Communications*, 4, 1765.

Vail, A.L., Manica, A. & Bshary, R. 2014. Fish choose appropriately when and with whom to collaborate. *Current Biology*, 24, R791–R793.

Valone, T.J. 1989. Group foraging, public information, and patch estimation. *Oikos*, 56, 357–363.

Valone, T.J. 2007. From eavesdropping on performance to copying the behavior of others: a review of public information use. *Behavioral Ecology and Sociobiology*, 62, 1–14.

van Boheemen, L.A., Hammers, M., Kingma, S.A., et al. 2019. Compensatory and additive helper effects in the cooperatively breeding Seychelles warbler (*Acrocephalus sechellensis*). *Ecology and Evolution*, 9, 2986–2995.

Van Cleve, J. & Akcay, E. 2014. Pathways to social evolution: reciprocity, relatedness, and synergy. *Evolution*, 68, 2245–2258.

van de Crommenacker, J., Komdeur, J., Burke, T. & Richardson, D.S. 2011a. Spatio-temporal variation in territory quality and oxidative status: a natural experiment in the Seychelles warbler (*Acrocephalus sechellensis*). *Journal of Animal Ecology*, 80, 668–680.

van de Crommenacker, J., Komdeur, J. & Richardson, D.S. 2011b. Assessing the cost of helping: the roles of body condition and oxidative balance in the Seychelles warbler (*Acrocephalus sechellensis*). *PLoS One*, 6, e26423.

van de Pol, M., Jenouvrier, S.p., Cornelissen, J.H. & Visser, M.E. 2017. Behavioural, ecological and evolutionary responses to extreme climatic events: challenges and directions. *Philosophical Transactions of the Royal Society of London B*, 372, 20160134.

van de Waal, E., Spinelli, M., Bshary, R., Ros, A.F.H. & Noe, R. 2013. Negotiations over grooming in wild vervet monkeys (*Chlorocebus pygerythrus*). *International Journal of Primatology*, 34, 1153–1171.

van der Marel, A., Lopez-Darias, M. & Waterman, J.M. 2019. Group-enhanced predator detection and quality of vigilance in a social ground squirrel. *Animal Behaviour*, 151, 43–52.

van Doorn, G.S. & Taborsky, M. 2012. The evolution of generalized reciprocity on social interaction networks. *Evolution*, 66, 651–664.

van Doorn, G.S., Riebli, T. & Taborsky, M. 2014. Coaction versus reciprocity in continuous-time models of cooperation. *Journal of Theoretical Biology*, 356, 1–10.

van Honk, C. & Hogeweg, P. 1981. The ontogeny of the social structure in a captive *Bombus terrestris* colony. *Behavioral Ecology and Sociobiology*, 9, 111–119.

van Zweden, J.S., Fuerst, M.A., Heinze, J. & D'Ettorre, P. 2007. Specialization in policing behaviour among workers in the ant *Pachycondyla inversae*. *Proceedings of the Royal Society of London B: Biological Sciences*, 274, 1421–1428.

Van Zweden, J.S., Cardoen, D. & Wenseleers, T. 2012. Social evolution: when promiscuity breeds cooperation. *Current Biology*, 22, R922–R924.

Vanderveldt, A., Oliveira, L. & Green, L. 2016. Delay discounting: pigeon, rat, human – does it matter? *Journal of Experimental Psychology. Animal Learning and Cognition*, 42, 141–162.

Vangestel, C., Callens, T., Vandomme, V. & Lens, L. 2013. Sex-biased dispersal at different geographical scales in a cooperative breeder from fragmented rainforest. *PLoS One*, 8, e71624.

Varley, G.C. & Gradwell, G.R. 1960. Key factors in population studies. *Journal of Animal Ecology*, 29, 399–401.

Välimäki, P., Kivelä, S.M. & Mäenpää, M.I. 2011. Mating with a kin decreases female remating interval: a possible example of inbreeding avoidance. *Behavioral Ecology and Sociobiology*, 65, 2037.

Vehrencamp, S.L. 1977. Relative fecundity and parental effort in the communally nesting anis, *Crotophaga sulcirostris*. *Science*, 197, 403–405.

Vehrencamp, S.L. 1978. The adaptive significance of communal nesting in groove-billed anis (*Crotophaga sulcirostris*). *Behavioral Ecology and Sociobiology*, 4, 1–33.

Vehrencamp, S.L. 1983. A model for the evolution of despotic versus egalitarian societies. *Animal Behaviour*, 31, 667–682.

Vehrencamp, S.L. & Quinn, J.S. 2004. Joint laying systems. In Koenig, W.D. & Dickinson, J.L. (eds), *Ecology and Evolution of Cooperative Breeding in*

Birds, pp. 177–196. Cambridge: Cambridge University Press.

Venkataraman, V.V., Kerby, J.T., Nguyen, N., Ashenafi, Z.T. & Fashing, P.J. 2015. Solitary Ethiopian wolves increase predation success on rodents when among grazing gelada monkey herds. *Journal of Mammalogy*, 96, 129–137.

Ventura, R., Majolo, B., Koyama, N.F., Hardie, S. & Schino, G. 2006. Reciprocation and interchange in wild Japanese macaques: grooming, cofeeding, and agonistic support. *American Journal of Primatology: Official Journal of the American Society of Primatologists*, 68, 1138–1149.

Verbeek, N.A. & Butler, R.W. 1981. Cooperative breeding of the northwestern crow *Corvus caurinus* in British Columbia. *Ibis*, 123, 183–189.

Vestergaard, K. & Magnhagen, C. 1993. Brood size and offspring age affect risk-taking and aggression in nest-guarding common gobies. *Behaviour*, 125, 233–243.

Viana, D.S., Gordo, I., Sucena, E. & Moita, M.A. 2010. Cognitive and motivational requirements for the emergence of cooperation in a rat social game. *Plos One*, 5, e8483.

Viblanc, V.A., Arnaud, C.M., Dobson, F.S. & Murie, J.O. 2009. Kin selection in Columbian ground squirrels (*Urocitellus columbianus*): littermate kin provide individual fitness benefits. *Proceedings of the Royal Society of London B: Biological Sciences*, 277, 989–994.

Viblanc, V.A., Mathien, A., Saraux, C., Viera, V.M. & Groscolas, R. 2011. It costs to be clean and fit: energetics of comfort behavior in breeding-fasting penguins. *PLoS One*, 6, e21110.

Vick, L.G. & Pereira, M.E. 1989. Episodic targeting aggression and the histories of *Lemur* social groups. *Behavioral Ecology and Sociobiology*, 25, 3–12.

Vidya, T.N.C., Balmforth, Z., Roux, A.L. & Cherry, M.I. 2009. Genetic structure, relatedness and helping behaviour in the yellow mongoose in a farmland and a natural habitat. *Journal of Zoology*, 278, 57–64.

Villet, M. 1990. Qualitative relations of egg size, egg production and colony size in some ponerine ants (Hymenoptera: Formicidae). *Journal of Natural History*, 24, 1321–1331.

Vitikainen, E.I.K., Marshall, H.H., Thompson, F.J., et al. 2017. Biased escorts: offspring sex, not relatedness explains alloparental care patterns in a cooperative breeder. *Proceedings of the Royal Society of London B: Biological Sciences*, 284, 20162384.

Vitikainen, E.I., Thompson, F.J., Marshall, H.H. & Cant, M.A. 2019. Live long and prosper: durable benefits of early-life care in banded mongooses. *Philosophical Transactions of the Royal Society of London B*, 374, 20180114.

Voelkl, B. 2015. The evolution of generalized reciprocity in social interaction networks. *Theoretical Population Biology*, 104, 17–25.

Voelkl, B., Portugal, S.J., Unsold, M., Usherwood, J.R., Wilson, A.M. & Fritz, J. 2015. Matching times of leading and following suggest cooperation through direct reciprocity during V-formation flight in ibis. *Proceedings of the National Academy of Sciences of the United States of America*, 112, 2115–2120.

Voigt, D.R. & Earle, B.D. 1983. Avoidance of coyotes by red fox families. *The Journal of Wildlife Management*, 47, 852–857.

von Bayern, A.M., de Kort, S.R., Clayton, N.S. & Emery, N.J. 2007. The role of food- and object-sharing in the development of social bonds in juvenile jackdaws (*Corvus monedula*). *Behaviour*, 144, 711–733.

Wade, M.J. 1976. Group selection among laboratory populations of *Tribolium*. *Proceedings of the National Academy of Sciences of the United States of America*, 73, 4604–4607.

Wade, M.J. 1977. Experimental study of group selection. *Evolution*, 31, 134–153.

Waldeck, P., Andersson, M., Kilpi, M. & Öst, M. 2007. Spatial relatedness and brood parasitism in a female-philopatric bird population. *Behavioral Ecology*, 19, 67–73.

Waldman, B. 1988. The ecology of kin recognition. *Annual Review of Ecology and Systematics*, 19, 543–571.

Wallace, J.C., Kolbeinshavn, A.G. & Reinsnes, T.G. 1988. The effects of stocking density on early growth in Arctic charr, *Salvelinus alpinus* (L.). *Aquaculture*, 73, 101–110.

Walter, B., Brunner, E. & Heinze, J. 2011. Policing effectiveness depends on relatedness and group size. *The American Naturalist*, 177, 368–376.

Walters, J.R. 1990. Red-cockaded woodpeckers: a 'primitive' cooperative breeder. In Stacey, P.B. & Koenig, W.D. (eds), *Cooperative Breeding in Birds*, pp. 69–101. Cambridge: Cambridge University Press.

Walters, J.R., Copeyon, C.K. & Carter III, J.H. 1992. Test of the ecological basis of cooperative breeding in red-cockaded woodpeckers. *The Auk*, 109, 90–97.

Wang, C. & Lu, X.IN. 2011. Female ground tits prefer relatives as extra-pair partners: driven by kin-selection? *Molecular Ecology*, 20, 2851–2863.

Ward, P. & Zahavi, A. 1973. The importance of certain assemblages of birds as 'information centres' for food-finding. *Ibis*, 115, 517–534.

Ward, P.I. 2000. Cryptic female choice in the yellow dung fly *Scathophaga stercoraria* (L.). *Evolution*, 54, 1680–1686.

Ward, P.I. & Enders, M.M. 1985. Conflict and cooperation in the group feeding of the social spider *Stegodyphus mimosarum*. *Behaviour*, 94, 167–182.

Warner, R.R. & Hoffman, S.G. 1980. Population density and the economics of territorial defense in a coral reef fish. *Ecology*, 61, 772–780.

Waser, P.M. 1981. Sociality or territorial defense? The influence of resource renewal. *Behavioral Ecology and Sociobiology*, 8, 231–237.

Wasser, S.K. & Barash, D.P. 1983. Reproductive suppression among females – implications for biomedicine and sexual selection theory. *Quarterly Review of Biology*, 58, 513–538.

Watts, D.P. 1998. Coalitionary mate guarding by male chimpanzees at Ngogo, Kibale National Park, Uganda. *Behavioral Ecology and Sociobiology*, 44, 43–55.

Watts, D.P. 2002. Reciprocity and interchange in the social relationships of wild male chimpanzees. *Behaviour*, 139, 343–370.

Weatherhead, P.J. 1983. Two principal strategies in avian communal roosts. *The American Naturalist*, 121, 237–243.

Weatherhead, P.J. 1987. Field tests of information transfer in communally roosting birds. *Animal Behaviour*, 35, 614–615.

Webster, M.S. 1994. Female-defence polygyny in a Neotropical bird, the *Montezuma oropendola*. *Animal Behaviour*, 48, 779–794.

Wedekind, C. & Braithwaite, V.A. 2002. The long-term benefits of human generosity in indirect reciprocity. *Current Biology*, 12, 1012–1015.

Wedekind, C. & Milinski, M. 2000. Cooperation through image scoring in humans. *Science*, 288, 850–852.

Weeks, P. 1999. Interactions between red-billed oxpeckers, *Buphagus erythrorhynchus*, and domesticated cattle, *Bos taurus*, in Zimbabwe. *Animal Behaviour*, 58, 1253–1259.

Weisel, O. 2016. Social motives in intergroup conflict: group identity and perceived target of threat. *European Economic Review*, 90, 122–133.

Weladji, R.B., Gaillard, J.M., Yoccoz, N.G., et al. 2006. Good reindeer mothers live longer and become better in raising offspring. *Proceedings of the Royal Society of London B: Biological Sciences*, 273, 1239–1244.

Wells, D.A., Cant, M.A., Nichols, H.J. & Hoffman, J.I. 2018. A high-quality pedigree and genetic markers both reveal inbreeding depression for quality but not survival in a cooperative mammal. *Molecular Ecology*, 27, 2271–2288.

Wenseleers, T. & Ratnieks, F.L.W. 2006a. Comparative analysis of worker reproduction and policing in eusocial Hymenoptera supports relatedness theory. *American Naturalist*, 168, E163–E179.

Wenseleers, T. & Ratnieks, F.L.W. 2006b. Enforced altruism in insect societies. *Nature*, 444, 50.

Wenseleers, T., Ratnieks, F.L.W. & Billen, J. 2003. Caste fate conflict in swarm-founding social Hymenoptera: an inclusive fitness analysis. *Journal of Evolutionary Biology*, 16, 647–658.

Wenseleers, T., Hart, A.G. & Ratnieks, F.L.W. 2004a. When resistance is useless: policing and the evolution of reproductive acquiescence in insect societies. *American Naturalist*, 164, E154–E167.

Wenseleers, T., Helantera, H., Hart, A. & Ratnieks, F.L.W. 2004b. Worker reproduction and policing in insect societies: an ESS analysis. *Journal of Evolutionary Biology*, 17, 1035–1047.

Werner, G.D.A., Strassmann, J.E., Ivens, A.B.F., et al. 2014. Evolution of microbial markets. *Proceedings of the National Academy of Sciences of the United States of America*, 111, 1237–1244.

Werner, N.Y., Balshine, S., Leach, B. & Lotem, A. 2003. Helping opportunities and space segregation in cooperatively breeding cichlids. *Behavioral Ecology*, 14, 749–756.

West, S. 2009. *Sex Allocation* (48th ed.). Princeton, NJ: Princeton University Press.

West, S.A. & Gardner, A. 2010. Altruism, spite, and greenbeards. *Science*, 327, 1341–1344.

West, S.A. & Gardner, A. 2013. Adaptation and inclusive fitness. *Current Biology*, 23, R577–R584.

West, S.A. & Ghoul, M. 2019. Conflict within cooperation. *Current Biology*, 29, R42–R426.

West, S.A., Murray, M.G., Machado, C.A., Griffin, A.S. & Herre, E.A. 2001. Testing Hamilton's rule with competition between relatives. *Nature*, 409, 510.

West, S.A., Pen, I. & Griffin, A.S. 2002. Conflict and cooperation – cooperation and competition between relatives. *Science*, 296, 72–75.

West, S., Griffin, A. & Gardner, A. 2007a. Social semantics: altruism, cooperation, mutualism, strong reciprocity and group selection. *Journal of Evolutionary Biology*, 20, 415–432.

West, S.A., Diggle, S.P., Buckling, A., Gardner, A. & Griffins, A.S. 2007b. The social lives of microbes. *Annual Review of Ecology Evolution and Systematics*, 38, 53–77.

West, S.A., Griffin, A.S. & Gardner, A. 2007c. Evolutionary explanations for cooperation. *Current Biology*, 17, R661–R672.

West, S.A., Fisher, R.M., Gardner, A. & Kiers, E.T. 2015. Major evolutionary transitions in individuality. *Proceedings of the National Academy of Sciences of the United States of America*, 112, 10112–10119.

West-Eberhard, M.J. 1975. The evolution of social behavior by kin selection. *The Quarterly Review of Biology*, 50, 1–33.

West-Eberhard, M.J. 1978. Polygyny and the evolution of social behavior in wasps. *Journal of the Kansas Entomological Society*, 51, 832–856.

West-Eberhard, M.J. 1979. Sexual selection, social competition, and evolution. *Proceedings of the American Philosophical Society*, 123, 222–234.

Westergaard, G.C. & Suomi, S.J. 1997. Transfer of tools and food between groups of tufted capuchins (*Cebus apella*). *American Journal of Primatology*, 43, 33–41.

Wheller, W.M. 1911. The ant-colony as an organism. *Journal of Morphology*, 22, 307–325.

Whitehouse, M.E.A. & Lubin, Y. 2005. The functions of societies and the evolution of group living: spider societies as a test case. *Biological Reviews*, 80, 347–361.

Whiten, A. & Byrne, R.W. 1988. Tactical deception in primates. *Behavioral and Brain Sciences*, 11, 233–244.

Whittingham, L.A., Dunn, P.O. & Magrath, R.D. 1997. Relatedness, polyandry and extra-group paternity in the cooperatively-breeding white-browed scrubwren (*Sericornis frontalis*). *Behavioral Ecology and Sociobiology*, 40, 261–270.

Wickler, W. & Seibt, U. 1981. Monogamy in Crustacea and Man. *Zeitschrift für Tierpsychologie – Journal of Comparative Ethology*, 57, 215–234.

Wickler, W. & Seibt, U. 1983. Monogamy: an ambiguous concept. In Bateson, P.P.G. (ed.), *Mate Choice*, pp. 33–50. Cambridge: Cambridge University Press.

Wiklund, C.G. 1979. Increased breeding success for merlins *Falco columbarius* nesting among colonies of fieldfares *Turdus pilaris*. *Ibis*, 121, 109–111.

Wiklund, C.G. 1982. Fieldfare (*Turdus pilaris*) breeding success in relation to colony size, nest position and association with merlins (*Falco columbarius*). *Behavioral Ecology and Sociobiology*, 11, 165–172.

Wilcox, R.S. & Ruckdeschel, T. 1982. Food threshold territoriality in a water strider (*Gerris remigis*). *Behavioral Ecology and Sociobiology*, 11, 85–90.

Wild, G., Pizzari, T. & West, S.A. 2011. Sexual conflict in viscous populations: the effect of the timing of dispersal. *Theoretical Population Biology*, 80, 298–316.

Wiley, R.H. & Rabenold, K.N. 1984. The evolution of cooperative breeding by delayed reciprocity and queuing for favorable social positions. *Evolution*, 38, 609–621.

Wilkins, A.S. & Holliday, R. 2009. The evolution of meiosis from mitosis. *Genetics*, 181, 3–12.

Wilkinson, G.S. 1984. Reciprocal food sharing in the vampire bat. *Nature*, 308, 181–184.

Wilkinson, G.S. 1986. Social grooming in the common vampire bat, *Desmodus rotundus*. *Animal Behaviour*, 34, 1880–1889.

Wilkinson, G.S. 1988. Reciprocal altruism in bats and other mammals. *Ethology and Sociobiology*, 9, 85–100.

Wilkinson, G.S. 1992. Communal nursing in the evening bat, *Nycticeius humeralis*. *Behavioral Ecology and Sociobiology*, 31, 225–235.

Wilkinson, G.S. 2019. Vampire bats. *Current Biology*, 29, R1216–R1217.

Wilkinson, G.S., Carter, G.G., Bohn, K.M. & Adams, D.M. 2016. Non-kin cooperation in bats. *Philosophical Transactions of the Royal Society of London B: Biological Sciences*, 371, 20150095.

Wilkinson, G.S., Carter, G., Bohn, K.M., et al. 2019. Kinship, association, and social complexity in bats. *Behavioral Ecology and Sociobiology*, 73, 7.

Williams, D.A. & Rabenold, K.N. 2005. Male-biased dispersal, female philopatry, and routes to fitness in a social corvid. *Journal of Animal Ecology*, 74, 150–159.

Williams, G.C. 1966. *Adaptation and Natural Selection*. Princeton, NJ: Princeton University Press.

Williams, J.M., Lonsdorf, E.V., Wilson, M.L., et al. 2008. Causes of death in the Kasekela chimpanzees of Gombe National Park, Tanzania. *American Journal of Primatology*, 70, 766–777.

Williams, P., Winzer, K., Chan, W.C. & Camara, M. 2007. Look who's talking: communication and quorum sensing in the bacterial world. *Philosophical Transactions of the Royal Society of London B: Biological Sciences*, 362, 1119–1134.

Wilson, A.J. & Nussey, D.H. 2010. What is individual quality? An evolutionary perspective. *Trends in Ecology & Evolution*, 25, 207–214.

Wilson, D.S. 1975. Theory of group selection. *Proceedings of the National Academy of Sciences of the United States of America*, 72, 143–146.

Wilson, D.S., Pollock, G.B. & Dugatkin, L.A. 1992. Can altruism evolve in purely viscous populations? *Evolutionary Ecology*, 6, 331–341.

Wilson, E.O. 1971. *The Insect Societies*. Cambridge, MA: Bellknap Press.

Wilson, E.O. 1975. *Sociobiology*. Cambridge, MA: Belknap Press.

Wilson, E.O. & Hölldobler, B. 2005. Eusociality: origin and consequences. *Proceedings of the National Academy of Sciences of the United States of America*, 102, 13367–13371.

Wilson, M.L., Boesch, C., Fruth, B., et al. 2014. Lethal aggression in *Pan* is better explained by adaptive strategies than human impacts. *Nature*, 513, 414–417.

Wiltermuth, S.S. & Heath, C. 2009. Synchrony and cooperation. *Psychological Science*, 20, 1–5.

Winterhalder, B. 1996. A marginal model of tolerated theft. *Ethology and Sociobiology*, 17, 37–53.

Winterrowd, M.F. & Weigl, P.D. 2006. Mechanisms of cache retrieval in the group nesting southern flying squirrel (*Glaucomys volans*). *Ethology*, 112, 1136–1144.

Wirtz, P. 1999. Mother species–father species: unidirectional hybridization in animals with female choice. *Animal Behaviour*, 58, 1–12.

Wirtz-Ocaña, S., Schütz, D., Pachler, G., & Taborsky, M. 2013. Paternal inheritance of growth in fish pursuing alternative reproductive tactics. *Ecology and Evolution*, 3, 1614–1625.

Wirtz-Ocaña, S., Meidl, P., Bonfils, D. & Taborsky, M. 2014. Y-linked Mendelian inheritance of giant and dwarf male morphs in shell-brooding cichlids. *Proceedings of the Royal Society of London B: Biological Sciences*, 281, 20140253.

Wisenden, B.D. 1999. Alloparental care in fishes. *Reviews in Fish Biology and Fisheries*, 9, 45–70.

Wisenden, B.D. & Keenleyside, M.H.A. 1992. Intraspecific brood adoption in convict cichlids: a mutual benefit. *Behavioral Ecology and Sociobiology*, 31, 263–269.

Wisenden, B.D. & Keenleyside, M.H.A. 1994. The dilution effect and differential predation following brood adoption in free-ranging convict cichlids (*Cichlasoma nigrofasciatum*). *Ethology*, 96, 203–212.

Witsenburg, F., Schuerch, R., Otti, O. & Heg, D. 2010. Behavioural types and ecological effects in a natural population of the cooperative cichlid *Neolamprologus pulcher*. *Animal Behaviour*, 80, 757–767.

Witte, V., Schliessmann, D. & Hashim, R. 2010. Attack or call for help? Rapid individual decisions in a group-hunting ant. *Behavioral Ecology*, 21, 1040–1047.

Wittig, R.M., Crockford, C., Deschner, T., et al. 2014. Food sharing is linked to urinary oxytocin levels and bonding in related and unrelated wild chimpanzees. *Proceedings of the Royal Society of London B: Biological Sciences*, 281, 20133096.

Wogel, H., Abrunhosa, P.A. & Pombal Jr, J.P. 2002. Atividade reprodutiva de *Physalaemus signifer* (Anura, Leptodactylidae) em ambiente temporário. *Iheringia Série Zoologia*, 92, 57–70.

Wolf, J.B.W. & Trillmich, F. 2008. Kin in space: social viscosity in a spatially and genetically substructured network. *Proceedings of the Royal Society of London B: Biological Sciences*, 275, 2063–2069.

Wolf, M. & Weissing, F.J. 2012. Animal personalities: consequences for ecology and evolution. *Trends in Ecology & Evolution*, 27, 452–461.

Wolff, J.O. & Plissner, J.H. 1998. Sex biases in avian natal dispersal: an extension of the mammalian model. *Oikos*, 327–330.

Wong, M.Y.L. & Balshine, S. 2010. Fight for your breeding right: hierarchy re-establishment predicts aggression in a social queue. *Biology Letters*, 7, 190–193.

Wong, M. & Balshine, S. 2011. The evolution of cooperative breeding in the African cichlid fish, *Neolamprologus pulcher*. *Biological Reviews*, 86, 511–530.

Wong, M.Y.L., Buston, P.M., Munday, P.L. & Jones, G.P. 2007. The threat of punishment enforces peaceful cooperation and stable queues in a coral-reef fish. *Proceedings of the Royal Society of London B: Biological Sciences*, 274, 1093–1099.

Wong, M.Y.L., Munday, P.L., Buston, P.M. & Jones, G.R. 2008. Fasting or feasting in a fish social hierarchy. *Current Biology*, 18, R372–R373.

Wood, R.I., Kim, J.Y. & Li, G.R. 2016. Cooperation in rats playing the iterated Prisoner's Dilemma game. *Animal Behaviour*, 114, 27–35.

Woodburn, J. 1982. Egalitarian societies. *Man*, 17, 431–451.

Woolfenden, G.E. & Fitzpatrick, J.W. 1978. The inheritance of territory in group-breeding birds. *Bioscience*, 28, 104–108.

Woolfenden, G.E. & Fitzpatrick, J.W. 1984. *The Florida Scrub Jay: Demography of a Cooperative-Breeding Bird* (20th ed.). Princeton, NJ: Princeton University Press.

Wootton, R.J. 1985. Effects of food and density on the reproductive biology of the threespine stickleback with a hypothesis on population limitation in sticklebacks. *Behaviour*, 93, 101–111.

Woxvold, I.A., Adcock, G.J. & Mulder, R.A. 2006. Fine-scale genetic structure and dispersal in cooperatively breeding apostlebirds. *Molecular Ecology*, 15, 3139–3146.

Wrangham, R.W. 1999. Evolution of coalitionary killing. *American Journal of Physical Anthropology*, 110, 1–30.

Wrangham, R.W. 2018. Two types of aggression in human evolution. *Proceedings of the National Academy of Sciences of the United States of America*, 115, 245–253.

Wrangham, R.W. & Glowacki, L. 2012. Intergroup aggression in chimpanzees and war in nomadic hunter-gatherers. *Human Nature*, 23, 5–29.

Wright, J. 1999. Altruism as a signal: Zahavi's alternative to kin selection and reciprocity. *Journal of Avian Biology*, 108–115.

Wright, J. & Cuthill, I. 1989. Manipulation of sex differences in parental care. *Behavioral Ecology and Sociobiology*, 25, 171–181.

Wright, J., McDonald, P.G., Te Marvelde, L., Kazem, A.J. & Bishop, C.M. 2009. Helping effort increases with relatedness in bell miners, but 'unrelated' helpers of both sexes still provide substantial care. *Proceedings of the Royal Society of London B: Biological Sciences*, 277, 437–445.

Wright, S. 1922. Coefficients of inbreeding and relationship. *The American Naturalist*, 56, 330–338.

Wright, S. 1931. Evolution in Mendelian populations. *Genetics*, 16, 97–159.

Wrighten, S.A. & Hall, C.R. 2016. Support for altruistic behavior in rats. *Open Journal of Social Sciences*, 4, 93–102.

Wyatt, G.A.K., West, S.A. & Gardner, A. 2013. Can natural selection favour altruism between species? *Journal of Evolutionary Biology*, 26, 1854–1865.

Wynne-Edwards, V.C. 1962. *Animal Dispersion in Relation to Social Behaviour*. London: Oliver and Boyd.

Xia, D., Li, J., Garber, P.A., et al. 2012. Grooming reciprocity in female tibetan macaques *Macaca thibetana*. *American Journal of Primatology*, 74, 569–579.

Yaber, M.a.C. & Rabenold, K.N. 2002. Effects of sociality on short-distance, female-biased dispersal in tropical wrens. *Journal of Animal Ecology*, 71, 1042–1055.

Yamamura, N., Higashi, M., Behera, N. & Yuichiro Wakano, J. 2004. Evolution of mutualism through spatial effects. *Journal of Theoretical Biology*, 226, 421–428.

Yamane, S. 1986. The colony cycle of the Sumatran paper wasp *Ropalidia (Icariola) variegata jacobsoni* (Buysson), with reference to the possible occurrence of serial polygyny (Hymenoptera Vespidae). *Monitore Zoologico Italiano – Italian Journal of Zoology*, 20, 135–161.

Yanagisawa, Y. 1983. Reproduction and parental care of the scale-eating fish *Perissodus microlepis* in Lake

Tanganyika. *Physiology and Ecology of Japan*, 20, 23–31.

Yanagisawa, Y. 1985. Parental strategy of the cichlid fish *Perissodus microlepis*, with particular reference to intraspecific brood 'farming out'. *Environmental Biology of Fishes*, 12, 241–249.

Yanagisawa, Y. 1986. Parental care in a monogamous mouthbrooding cichlid *Xenotilapia flavipinnis* in Lake Tanganyika. *Japanese Journal of Ichthyology*, 33, 249–261.

Yanagisawa, Y., Ochi, H. & Rossiter, A. 1996. Intra-buccal feeding of young in an undescribed Tanganyikan cichlid *Microdontochromis* sp. *Environmental Biology of Fishes*, 47, 191–201.

Yee, J.R., Cavigelli, S.A., Delgado, B. & McClintock, M.K. 2008. Reciprocal affiliation among adolescent rats during a mild group stressor predicts mammary tumors and lifespan. *Psychosomatic Medicine*, 70, 1050–1059.

Yom-Tov, Y. 1980. Intraspecific nest parasitism in birds. *Biological Reviews*, 55, 93–108.

Yom-Tov, Y. 2001. An updated list and some comments on the occurrence of intraspecific nest parasitism in birds. *Ibis*, 143, 133–143.

Young, A.J. & Clutton-Brock, T. 2006. Infanticide by subordinates influences reproductive sharing in cooperatively breeding meerkats. *Biology Letters*, 2, 385–387.

Young, A.J., Carlson, A.A., Monfort, S.L., et al. 2006. Stress and the suppression of subordinate reproduction in cooperatively breeding meerkats. *Proceedings of the National Academy of Sciences of the United States of America*, 103, 12005–12010.

Young, A.J., Oosthuizen, M.K., Lutermann, H. & Bennett, N.C. 2010. Physiological suppression eases in Damaraland mole-rat societies when ecological constraints on dispersal are relaxed. *Hormones and Behavior*, 57, 177–183.

Young, K.A., Genner, M.J., Joyce, D.A. & Haesler, M.P. 2009. Hotshots, hot spots, and female preference: exploring lek formation models with a bower-building cichlid fish. *Behavioral Ecology*, 20, 609–615.

Zack, S. 1990. Coupling delayed breeding with short-distance dispersal in cooperatively breeding birds. *Ethology*, 86, 265–286.

Zahavi, A. 1990. Arabian babblers: the quest for social status in a cooperative breeder. In Stacey, P.B. & Koenig, W.D. (eds), *Cooperative Breeding in Birds*, pp. 103–130. Cambridge: Cambridge University Press.

Zamudio, K.R. & Chan, L.M. 2008. Alternative reproductive tactics in amphibians. In Oliveira, R.F., Taborsky, M. & Brockmann, H.J. (eds), *Alternative Reproductive Tactics. An Integrative Approach*, pp. 300–331. Cambridge: Cambridge University Press.

Zanette, L.R. & Field, J. 2008. Genetic relatedness in early associations of *Polistes dominulus*: from related to unrelated helpers. *Molecular Ecology*, 17, 2590–2597.

Zanette, L.R. & Field, J. 2011. Founders versus joiners: group formation in the paper wasp *Polistes dominulus*. *Animal Behaviour*, 82, 699–705.

Zanette, L.R., Miller, S.D., Faria, C., et al. 2012. Reproductive conflict in bumblebees and the evolution of worker policing. *Evolution*, 66, 3765–3777.

Zeyl, E., Aars, J., Ehrich, D. & Wiig, O. 2009. Families in space: relatedness in the Barents Sea population of polar bears (*Ursus maritimus*). *Molecular Ecology*, 18, 735–749.

Zickler, D. & Kleckner, N. 2016 A few of our favorite things: pairing, the bouquet, crossover interference and evolution of meiosis. *Seminars in Cell & Developmental Biology*, 54, 135–148.

Zink, A.G. 2000. The evolution of intraspecific brood parasitism in birds and insects. *American Naturalist*, 155, 395–405.

Zöttl, M., Heg, D., Chervet, N. & Taborsky, M. 2013a. Kinship reduces alloparental care in cooperative cichlids where helpers pay-to-stay. *Nature Communications*, 4, 1341.

Zöttl, M., Frommen, J.G. & Taborsky, M. 2013b. Group size adjustment to ecological demand in a cooperative breeder. *Proceedings of the Royal Society of London B: Biological Sciences*, 280, 20122772.

Zöttl, M., Fischer, S. & Taborsky, M. 2013c. Partial brood care compensation by female breeders in response to experimental manipulation of alloparental care. *Animal Behaviour*, 85, 1471–1478.

Zöttl, M., Chapuis, L., Freiburghaus, M. & Taborsky, M. 2013d. Strategic reduction of help before dispersal in a cooperative breeder. *Biology Letters*, 9, 20120878.

Zupan, M., Štuhec, I., & Jordan, D. 2020. The effect of an irregular feeding schedule on equine behavior. *Journal of Applied Animal Welfare Science*, 23, 156–163.

Subject Index

adaptation xii, 21, 32, 62, 68–71, 87, 89, 117–118, 129, 282, 304, 308, 326
adoption 207, 278, 279, 281
affiliative 50, 126–127, 135, 169, 252
aggregation 1–2, 7, 47, 56, 76, 192–202, 252, 280, 317
aggression 37–42, 54, 77–82, 87, 91–100, 120–135, 178, 224, 228, 242–244, 253, 272–280, 310–311
agonistic support 149–151, 174
alarm call 51, 196–197, 215, 285, 294–295, 316
allogrooming 128, 141, 152, 158, 161, 164, 169, 171, 174–175, 178, 240, 302–306
allonursing 152–153, 161, 241
alloparental care 148–149, 166, 179, 183, 247, 257, 259, 297, 302, 305–307
alternative reproductive tactics 55, 246
altruism 3–4, 16–20, 92, 117, 122, 137, 139, 144, 178, 181–184, 210, 238, 242, 246, 259, 313
  reciprocal altruism 4, 7, 9, 17, 144, 145, 155, 201, 238, 291–292, 314
appeasement 81, 91, 244, 253, 257
arms race 23, 246, 282, 284, 314, 316
assessment model 113–115
associations 110, 131–134, 187, 189, 195–196, 221–222, 249, 274–280, 285, 295
associative learning 190, 209

battleground models 97
benefits
  by-product benefits 138–139, 144, 247, 295, 315, 318
  delayed benefits 141, 290
  fitness benefits 5, 17, 20, 22, 27, 50, 60, 63–64, 77, 130, 132, 179, 187, 189, 201–202, 234, 259, 313
  immediate benefits 140–141, 239, 286
  mutual benefits 201, 288, 293
biparental 15, 71, 88, 177, 226, 229, 315, 320
body condition 158, 169, 179, 237
bonanza resource 8, 306
breeder turnover 189–190, 204
breeding experience 29, 236

brood care 147–148, 179, 184, 227–228, 235–237, 245, 252–261, 279–281, 302, 313–317
  interspecific brood care 276–285
brood parasitism 5, 212, 238, 246, 249, 277, 281, 283, 314, 316
broods
  mixed-species broods 276–280, 317
by-product mutualism 137–139, 146, 176, 247, 288, 295, 316

caste 2, 21, 69, 181, 242–243, 249, 297
character displacement 266–267, 272, 316
cheating 79, 85, 140, 145, 212, 238, 284, 286–289, 294, 316
clumping 35–39
coalitions 59, 119, 123, 151, 163, 195–196, 199, 202, 204–205, 243, 280
co-breeding 61, 183, 225, 324
coercion 17, 23, 91, 107–108, 111, 136, 176–177, 236, 238, 241–242, 247, 251, 263, 314, 316, 318–319
coevolution 97, 99–100, 107, 122, 129, 135, 282, 310, 312, 316
coexistence 141, 210, 266, 268, 270, 294, 316
cognition 135, 155, 157, 174, 177, 212, 248, 314
collective
  collective action 66, 73–74, 119
  collective behaviour 47
  collective movement 46–47, 60, 66, 309
colonies 48, 90–91, 118, 121, 123, 127–128, 182, 192–195, 212, 239, 247, 256, 259, 279, 298–308
colouration 52, 272
commensalism 266, 285–286, 294–295, 316
commodity 19, 147, 163, 174
common descent 20, 137, 139–140, 180, 190, 249, 313
communal
  communal breeding 17
  communal care 63, 224
  communal litter 63–66
  communal thatch 90
communication 14, 17, 50, 290, 292

communities 266, 293
competition
  among-kin competition 187, 234
  destructive competition 106
  interference competition 267, 269, 280
  interspecific competition 266, 273
  intrabuccal competition 278
  local mate competition 299
  non-interference competition 269
  resource competition 6, 21–24, 38, 54, 224, 257,
    273, 316
  scramble competition 35–48, 59–60, 309–310
competitive exclusion 266
conflict
  conflict behaviour 22, 69, 72, 99, 107, 129, 295
  conflict of interest 256, 274, 288, 318
  evolutionary conflict 68–69, 97–105, 107, 117, 128
  interspecific conflict 265, 274
  sexual conflict 20, 55, 87, 216, 221, 226, 314, 321
conflict–cohesion hypothesis 126
contest 2, 18, 35–47, 53–59, 77–80, 99–117, 123,
  134–135, 146, 309–312, 317–318
contest success functions 99–104, 113, 312
cooperation
  (cn)forced cooperation 4, 23, 28, 108, 136,
    236–251, 281, 314, 316
  indiscriminate cooperation 183, 190, 265, 316
  interspecific cooperation 264, 284, 288, 295, 315
  mutual cooperation 264, 285, 295
  nepotistic cooperation 196
  reciprocal cooperation 19, 141, 145–178, 205,
    256, 289, 313–314, 319
cooperative
  cooperative breeders 21, 61, 84, 131, 164,
    180–185, 192–193, 205, 207, 209, 234, 241,
    243, 251–262, 297, 308, 315, 318
  cooperative hunting 8, 136, 140, 172, 247, 291
  cooperative transitions 67–71, 118, 127–129
correlated pay-offs 12, 18, 137–138, 140, 165, 175,
  179, 247–248, 288, 313
cost–benefit analysis 285, 295
courtship 16, 51, 53, 57–58, 197–203, 221, 320
credible threats 5, 92, 98, 108–110
cross-feeding 293
cryptic female choice 85

deceit 212, 263, 316
deception 23, 48, 51–52, 247–249, 310, 313–314
decision rules 4, 19, 147, 154–160, 166–178, 205,
  237, 248, 263, 310, 314, 319
decisions
  adaptive decisions 319
  behavioural decisions 2, 21, 156
  collective decisions 47
  cooperation decisions 262
  foraging decisions 7
  life-history decisions 94, 261

  optimal decisions 22
  social decisions 2, 21
decisiveness 103–104, 106, 117
defection 108, 111, 154, 157, 159, 167, 170, 248,
  256, 289
defence 11, 16, 22, 37–39, 72, 96, 129, 141, 144,
  147–153, 172, 241, 244, 251–261, 273–281, 284
density 37, 43, 53–60, 96, 141, 221, 224–225, 259,
  267, 270, 284, 300, 310
deterrence 108, 112
dictatorship 118, 129
direct fitness benefits 17, 23, 25, 29, 130, 195, 199,
  206, 212, 214, 223, 226, 234
dispersal
  delayed dispersal 26, 73, 189, 193, 195,
    213–214, 216, 297, 302, 306–307
  dispersal in kin coalitions 202
  limited dispersal 122, 192, 194, 221, 224, 313
  natal dispersal 192–193, 195, 202, 213
dispersal constraints 182
divisibility 38, 41
division of labour 4, 78, 131, 243, 260, 297,
  302–308, 315, 318
divorce 54, 190
dominance hierarchy 62, 77, 80, 82, 87, 110–111,
  124, 129–131, 252, 311

eavesdropping 49, 143, 156, 285, 289, 295
ecological constraints 22, 27, 60, 95, 310
economic defendability 36, 55
effort-matching 89
energetic war-of-attrition 114
environmental conditions 33, 56, 159, 171, 268
eusocial 12, 18–20, 21, 68–69, 118, 181, 192,
  242–243, 249, 259, 297–298, 302–308, 318
eviction 63–76, 81, 98, 107–110, 129, 178, 205,
  243, 310, 315
evolutionarily stable strategy (ESS) 45, 100–101,
  109, 113
exploitation 5, 44, 50, 77, 121, 136, 138, 144, 166,
  172–173, 179, 237, 246, 248, 252, 267, 310,
  317
extortion 246

familiarity 159, 166, 209, 211, 313
family groups 97, 141–142, 181, 192, 195, 211,
  214, 324
farming out 277–278
fecundity 34, 82, 92–93, 189, 216, 226–227, 273,
  304, 311
fertility 75, 83, 119–120, 273, 321–322, 325–326
fertilization 10, 144, 147, 174, 230, 275, 286, 300,
  317
fighting 7, 12–13, 22, 35–36, 38, 52, 56, 60, 64, 67,
  77–78, 80, 94, 106, 110, 114–116, 121, 123,
  126, 134–136, 156, 219, 224, 311, 388
filial cannibalism 18, 229–230

fish schools 1, 47, 76
fitness costs 17, 23, 31, 44, 103, 120, 122,
    139–140, 160, 180, 207, 216, 230, 238, 252,
    260, 263, 281, 293, 295, 305, 313, 324, 326
food provisioning 149–150, 152, 161, 169, 194,
    235, 238
food resources 30, 214, 295, 355
foraging
    cooperative foraging 290
    foraging success 33, 50, 285, 291, 294
forced altruism 23

generalists 266, 268, 270, 316
generosity 157, 313, 319
genetic altruism 18–20, 259
Goldilocks principle 48
group
    group composition 1, 181, 259–260
    group size 1, 7, 18, 30–34, 40–41, 44, 71–75,
        127, 133, 139–144, 154, 159, 212, 234, 255,
        259, 261
    group structure 47, 147, 252, 260–261
    group transformation 68, 117, 128–129
    grouping 10, 33, 46, 49, 68, 72–76, 129, 275, 310
group augmentation 18, 140, 142–143, 195, 234
group selection xi, 71, 118, 138, 312

habitat
    habitat quality 25, 30–32, 271
    habitat saturation 25, 27, 32, 213, 224, 244
Hamilton's rule 3, 19, 92, 137–138, 180, 202, 248,
    313
harassment 79, 87, 176, 221
harming 97, 216–221, 311, 324
helpfulness 145, 154, 157, 171
helping
    helping behaviour 25–32, 61, 82, 95, 122,
        130–131, 181, 190, 193, 195, 204, 207, 236,
        244
    helping experience 29, 236
hierarchical information hypothesis of reciprocal
    cooperation 156, 167
hierarchy 41, 67, 77, 79, 128, 132, 134
home ranges 55, 62, 274
hybridization 272–273, 395

ideal despotic distribution 6, 44
ideal free distribution 6, 42, 46, 48, 60
image-scoring 157, 289
imprinting 15, 209
inbreeding 55, 63, 210, 221, 226–229, 300, 304,
    306, 314, 390
    inbreeding depression 63, 226
inclusive fitness 3, 16, 50, 63, 71–74, 79, 89, 91,
    100–101, 103, 117, 120, 134, 139, 141, 196,
    205–208, 226–227, 238, 305, 326
indirect fitness benefits 5, 17–20, 22, 25, 27–28,
    180–184, 187, 192–209, 214, 259, 313

indiscriminate altruism 182
individual quality 190
infant handling 150–151, 176
infanticide 62, 69, 86, 94, 102, 105, 108, 129, 204,
    230, 238, 311
infidelity 190, 204
    mate infidelity 206
infinite island model 93, 123
information centres 48
information parasitism 51
inheritance rank 80, 130, 133–134
insider–outsider conflict 72–74, 310
interactions
    acoustic interactions 294
    agonistic interactions 280
    competitive interactions 135
    cooperative interactions 192, 249, 262, 315, 318
    host–parasite interactions 271
    predator–prey interactions 23
interdependence 49, 72, 178, 315
interference
    interference rivalry 21, 35, 77, 263, 266, 271,
        294, 316
    reproductive interference 272
intergroup conflict 22, 55, 61, 65–66, 72, 88,
    120–129, 239, 312
intergroup cooperation 127–128
interspecific
    interspecific mutualism 69, 105, 144, 175, 276,
        287, 294–295, 315, 318
interspecific interactions 4, 178, 263, 265, 294, 317
interspecific relations 23, 263, 281, 286, 316–317
investment 10, 31, 39, 69, 76, 84, 88–91, 97, 99,
    105, 112, 143–145, 166, 177, 180–183, 186,
    190, 212, 224, 233, 245, 249, 251–252, 258,
    260, 305, 315, 325–326
    parental investment 55, 88, 97, 161, 229, 245,
        247, 259, 315
    reproductive investment 83

kidnapping 11, 142, 212, 232, 235
kin clustering 193, 216
kin discrimination 5, 23, 64, 92, 182, 189–190,
    192–193, 202–207, 234–235, 313
    active kin discrimination 204, 207, 209
    fine-scale kin discrimination 207, 212
kin recognition 19, 186, 189, 202–213
kin selection 4–6, 19, 92–97, 100, 102, 107, 129,
    137–140, 164, 166, 180–184, 196, 198, 201,
    205–208, 218, 233, 242–251, 259, 263, 285,
    294–297, 305, 312–324
kinship viii, 5, 28, 118, 159, 183, 187, 190–193,
    204, 207–212, 221, 233, 311, 314, 319, 321,
    324, 326

landscape of fear 42
learning 155, 171, 190, 209–210, 212
lekking 55, 196–202

life-history segregation 119–120, 312
lifetime reproductive success xii, 88, 125, 206, 218, 220
linkage disequilibrium 210
load lightening 31, 84, 245
local enhancement 49
longevity 79, 171, 187, 189, 192, 216, 219, 274

major transitions 20, 67–71, 117–129, 311, 316, 318
maladaptive 110, 272, 278, 284, 314
manipulation 57, 66, 88, 133, 137, 158, 167, 223, 230, 237–251, 258, 268, 281, 294, 312, 319
mate attraction 196, 200
mate guarding 54, 64, 87, 210, 311
mate sharing 162, 196, 200
mating skew 87, 196
mating system 1, 5, 10–11, 181, 300, 309
memory 71, 111, 116, 134–135, 157, 166, 171, 319
menopause 96, 119, 321–322, 324, 326
monogamy 2, 39, 54, 87–88, 118, 227, 305
monopolization 2, 6–12, 36–41, 55, 62, 77, 84, 87, 119, 129, 164, 243, 271, 310, 322
morphological divergence 242, 249, 271, 295, 297
morphology 14, 20, 243, 266–269
mortality 31, 33, 64, 94, 121–124, 203, 258, 277, 321–326
mortality risk 219, 267, 278, 287
mouthbrooding 277–278, 281
multilevel selection 117, 122, 139
mutualism
    by-product mutualism 17, 137–139, 143, 176, 179, 247, 288, 295, 316
    interspecific mutualism 14, 69, 105, 175, 276, 287, 294–295, 315, 318
mutual benefits 126, 143, 200, 235, 258, 288–289, 294

natural selection xii, 3, 19, 22, 35, 44, 67, 113, 138, 140, 177–178, 210, 249, 262, 283, 294, 310, 312, 322
negotiations 99, 106–107, 112, 129, 147, 176–177, 240, 248–249, 257, 259, 288, 310–311, 315, 318
nepotism 196, 249
nest building 26, 200
networks
    interaction networks 68, 154, 158–161, 258
    social networks 68, 156, 160, 191, 262
niche
    ecological niche 266, 293
    foraging niche 61, 64–65, 267
    social niche 78, 236, 262
    niche differentiation 64, 266
    niche overlap 267
    niche shifts 266

olfactory cues 211, 227, 230
open box models 116

opportunity costs 10, 160, 273, 277, 288, 291
optimal group size 75, 310
organismality 70, 123, 318
outgroup threat 120
outside options 97, 100, 236, 240–241, 243, 246, 249, 251, 288, 315, 318

parasites 5, 9, 160, 222, 264, 271, 280–281, 289, 297, 316–317
parasitism
    nest parasitism 281
    reproductive parasitism 59, 229–230, 280
parentage 26, 29, 66, 69, 83, 190–191, 229
parental
    parental care 31, 87–88, 112, 177, 209, 226–233, 249, 277, 279, 281, 294, 311
    parental facilitation 213–214
partial compensation 88
partner choice 176, 290
partnership 68, 88–89, 178
pay-off 11–12, 18, 41, 43, 50, 52, 55–60, 80, 97, 109, 113, 118, 126, 137–138, 145, 165, 176, 247, 249, 313–314
pay-to-stay 19, 29, 91, 147, 149, 178, 243–259
pedigree
    genetic pedigree 199, 208, 211
    multi-generational pedigree 202
    social pedigree 184
personality 23, 47, 55, 159, 236, 262, 319
phenotype matching 209–210, 313
philopatry 25, 27, 32, 96, 182, 187–189, 192–196, 202, 216, 252, 306, 323
policing 76, 85, 107, 118, 236, 238–239, 242, 249
policing model 100–105
polydomy 127
population demography 129, 223, 326
population viscosity 23, 92, 97, 154, 182, 192, 223–224, 265, 314
post-reproductive lifespan 321
power asymmetry 73, 238–247
power symmetry 238
predation
    predation risk 2, 9, 25, 31–32, 42, 46, 50, 196, 213, 228, 251, 258–261, 267, 275–276, 278–279, 287, 295, 317
    predator deterrence 294
    predator inspection 147–148, 160, 172
predictability 2, 38–40
predictive adaptive response 84
prisoner's dilemma 2, 126, 155, 165, 167, 246
producer 50, 91
promiscuity 11, 189–191
prosocial behaviour 9
protection 41, 144, 166, 195, 213–214, 251, 254, 256, 258, 274–280, 286, 306
provisioning rate 184, 207, 282
proximate mechanisms 14, 19, 145, 160, 166, 186
pseudoreciprocity 140, 143

public goods 6, 19, 90–91, 172, 222, 239, 293, 297, 305
punishment 17, 19, 51, 91, 109, 111, 129, 236, 238–240, 288, 306, 316

ratio form contest success function 100–101, 104–105
reciprocity
  direct reciprocity 4, 20, 149, 152–159, 164–169, 177, 190, 248, 288
  generalized reciprocity 4, 9, 59, 150–159, 163–165, 167, 171–179, 182, 248, 265, 314, 316, 319
  indirect reciprocity 4, 20, 146, 155–158, 163–164, 166, 168, 248, 289, 314, 319
  interspecific reciprocity 289
recognition 71, 134, 166, 186, 190, 192, 202–213, 249, 272, 313, 319
recognition errors 190, 205, 212, 234, 272
recruitment 48, 203, 290
reproductive
  reproductive altruism 16, 18–20, 182
  reproductive competition 61, 63, 75, 84, 94, 96, 99, 103, 129, 225, 257, 260, 305
  reproductive conflict 97–98, 321–326
  reproductive levelling 66, 118–120, 129, 312
  reproductive restraint 76, 94, 238, 252
  reproductive skew 37, 61, 65, 82, 95, 97–99, 107, 239, 243, 260
  reproductive success 27–32, 57–58, 63–66, 75–76, 84–88, 95, 105, 141, 192, 196–200, 206, 212, 216, 218, 220, 231, 279, 283, 305
  reproductive suppression 61–63, 83, 86, 118, 120
reputation 111, 155–156, 166
resolution models 97, 99–100
resources
  resource availability 37–38, 53
  resource defence 32, 37–42, 53, 73–74
  resource holding potential (RHP) 9, 52, 56, 78, 80–81, 98, 113–116, 126, 311, 318
  resource overlap 272, 295
robots 50

safety in numbers 143, 275, 278, 287, 295
satellite males 56, 58, 147, 317
schooling 36, 47, 59, 76
scramble 6, 8, 22, 35–45, 48, 55, 58–60, 77, 97, 105, 266–267, 309–310, 317–318
scrounger 50
sealed-bid models 97, 99, 106, 126, 129
selfish herd 76–77
selfishness 22, 100–105, 111, 126, 137
sequential assessment 113, 115
sequential models 107, 129
sex allocation 182
sex-biased dispersal 187, 193, 228, 323

shared genes 23, 137, 145, 164, 176, 243, 247, 250, 313, 315, 318
shared interests 285, 288, 295
shoals 2, 7, 47, 287
simultaneous hermaphrodites 11, 173
site-fidelity 187
sneaking 53, 55–58, 317
social
  social behaviour 1, 14–17, 21–24, 35, 60, 129–130, 134–135, 139, 193, 221, 233–234, 252, 262, 310, 319
  social conflict 22, 59, 67, 69, 72, 131, 310–311
  social immunity 302
  social interactions 1, 4–6, 23, 36, 59, 95, 100, 102, 129, 138, 159, 167, 184, 252, 280, 309, 318
  social learning 49
  social parasitism 5, 23, 136, 246
  social queue 79, 130, 133
  social rank 77–80, 123, 129–130, 132, 134
  social structure 2, 6, 13, 47, 71, 95, 250, 252, 260, 262
  social support 150–153, 174
solicitation 169
spawning 173, 200, 202, 228, 230–231, 278, 317
specialists 266, 268, 270, 316
spite 94, 281
stable group size 73–74
structured environments 293
structured population models 92, 94–95, 311, 325
submission 16, 80–83, 91, 130, 244, 249, 253
surveillance 126, 163, 289
survival 21, 25–34, 63–65, 75, 133, 141, 163, 180, 195, 214, 218, 220, 233, 244–245, 258, 279, 281, 303, 324
swarming 43, 143
symbiosis 105, 143, 264–265, 307
sympatry 267, 272
synergistic effects 4, 6, 22, 136, 178, 241, 252, 260

territoriality
  interspecific territoriality 271, 295, 316
  serial territoriality 273–274, 295
territory
  territory defence 141, 147, 152, 172, 236, 244, 254, 257, 260
  territory inheritance 29, 142, 152, 235
thermoregulation 9, 141
threats 5, 76, 84, 91, 98, 107–112, 120, 129, 134, 178, 238, 241, 244, 312, 315, 318
Tinbergen's four questions 15
tit-for-tat 146, 169
trade-offs 71, 89–90, 124, 166, 237, 258, 276, 295, 297
trading 20, 147–153, 172–176, 248–251, 254, 288, 295, 315–316, 318
tragedy of the commons 77, 97, 256, 284

tug-of-war model 100–104, 123, 323
turn-taking 129, 148, 161
   unconditional prosociality 168

uncorrelated asymmetry 8, 78
undermatching 43–44
unpredictability 40

veil of ignorance 66, 106, 118
vigilance 42, 121, 141, 147, 160, 185, 197, 267, 280, 285, 287, 294–295
viscous populations 182, 192, 223, 314
vocalizations 203, 206

winner/loser effects 146, 172

Taxonomic Index

Acanthisitta chloris. See rifleman
Accipiter gentilis. See goshawk
Accipiter nisus. See sparrowhawk
Acinetobacter baylyi 293
acorn woodpecker 84, 191, 194, 214, 225, 241
Acrocephalus scirpaceus. See reed warbler
Acrocephalus sechellensis. See Seychelles warbler
Actinia equina. See sea anemone
Aegithalos caudatus. See long-tailed tit
Aepyceros melampus. See impala
Aetobatus narinari. See spotted eagle ray
African grey parrot 148
African honeybee 247
African wild dog 141, 185–186, 188
Agelaius phoeniceus. See red-winged blackbird
Aidablennius sphynx. See sphynx blenny
Alces alces. See moose
Alopex lagopus. See Arctic fox
Alpheus spp. *See* burrowing shrimp
ambrosia beetle 188, 226, 297–308
American white pelican 140
American wood warblers 272
Amphiprion percula. See orange clownfish
Ancistrus spinosus 43
Amphiprion. See clownfish
Antarctic plunder fish 178–179
Apholecoma coerulescens. See Florida scrub jay
Aphelocoma ultramarine. See Mexican jay
Apis cerana 85
Apis florea. See Asian honeybee
Apis mellifera capensis. See Cape bee
Apis mellifera scuttelata. See honeybee
Apis mellifera. See honeybee
Apodemus microps. See herb-field mouse
apostlebird 188
Aptenodytes patagonicus. See king penguin
Arabian babbler 75, 186
Archocentrus nigrofasciatum. See convict cichlids
Arctic fox 276
Arctic ground squirrel 269
Arenaria interpres. See ruddy turnstone
Argya squamiceps. See Arabian babbler
Artibeus jamaicensis. See Jamaican fruit-eating bat
Asemichthys taylori. See spinynose sculpin

Asian honeybee 85
Assamese macaque 151
Ateles geoffroyi. See spider monkey
Atlantic salmon 40, 42
Attini 297
Auchenoglanis occidentalis. See bagrid catfish
Australian magpie 190–191
Australopithecus africanus 322
Austroplatypus incompertus 307

baboon 119, 151
bacteria 69, 95, 172, 222–223, 264, 293, 306
bacterial symbionts 264
bagrid catfish 278, 287
Bagrus meridionalis. See bagrid catfish
banded mongoose 11, 55, 59, 61–66, 75–88, 98, 108, 124, 185, 188, 194, 202, 205, 224, 235
bank vole 280
Barbary macaque 150, 158, 178
barn owl 148
barnacle goose 188
Bechstein's bat 49
bed bug 216–217
Belding's ground squirrel 185, 197–198
bell miner 185, 193
belted sandfish 148
beluga whale 321
Betta splendens. See fighting fish
black grouse 188, 196
black hamlet 148
black skimmer 276
blue chromis 53
blue jay 149
blue monkey 126, 150
bluegill sunfish 47, 230
bluehead wrasse 202
Bombus terrestris. See bumblebee
bonnet macaque 126, 151
bonobo 152, 322
Boulengerochromis microlepis 277
Brachydanio rario. See zebrafish
Branta canadensis. See Canada goose
Branta leucopsis. See barnacle goose
Branta ruficollis. See red-breasted geese

brown hare 39
brown jay 30, 194
brown tree creeper 193
brown-headed nuthatch 149
buffalo sculpin 281
buff-breasted wren 149, 173
Bullock's oriole 275
bumblebee 85
Buphagus spp. *See* oxpecker
burrowing shrimp 286
burying beetle 227–228
Buteo galapagoensis. See Galápagos hawk

Cabanis's greenbuls 188
cactus finch 187, 270
Callithrix jacchus. See common marmoset
Calocitta formosa. See white-throated magpie-jays
Campylorhynchus nuchalis. See stripe-backed wren
Canada goose 188
Canis familiaris. See dog
Canis latrans. See coyote
Canis lupus. See wolf
Canis simensis. See Ethiopian wolf
Cantorchilus leucotis. See buff-breasted wren
Cape bee 246
capercaillie 196
capuchin monkey 155, 158, 161
Carollia perspicillata. See short-tailed fruit bat
carrion crow 84, 185, 213–214
Castor canadensis. See North American beaver
catenulid flatworm 264
Cebus apella. See tufted capuchin
Cebus capucinus. See white-faced capuchin
Cercocebus atys. See sooty mangabey
Cercopithecus mitis. See blue monkey
Cercotrichas coryphaeus. See Karoo scrub-robin
Cervidae. *See* deer
Ceryle rudis. See pied kingfisher
chaffinch 271
Chalinochromis 262
chalk bass 148
chestnut-crowned babblers 241
chimpanzee 50–51, 64, 87, 120, 122, 140, 151, 155, 158, 161, 173–174, 322, 326
Chinese crested tern 280
Chinook salmon 56
Chironomus plumosus 46
Chiroxiphia lanceolata. See lance-tailed manakin
Chiroxiphia linearis. See long-tailed manakin
Chlorocebus pygerythrus. See vervet monkey
Chordeiles rupestris. See sand-coloured nighthawk
Chromis cyanea. See blue chromis
Chrysolophus pictus 288
Cichlasoma dovii 283
Cichlasoma nicaraguense. See Nicaragua cichlid
Cimex lectularius. See bed bug
cleaner wrasse 92, 157, 288–289, 316

Clethrionomys gapperi. See red-backed vole
cliff swallow 49
Climacteris picumnus. See brown tree creeper
clownfish 41, 109–110
coal tit 266
coati 153
cockatiel 148
coho salmon 41
Columba livia. See pigeon
Columba palumbus. See woodpigeon
Columbian ground squirrel 185, 186, 197
common cactus finch 268
common cuckoo 282, 288
common degu 186
common eider 188, 195
common guillemot 148, 163
common marmoset 150, 188
common shiner 276
convict cichlid 38
cooperative cichlid ix, 74, 76, 81, 84, 85, 92, 110, 115, 126, 127, 141, 147, 165, 201, 204, 228, 229, 236, 240, 241, 245, 251–262, 315
Copidosoma floridanum. See polyembryonic wasp
coral trout 292
Corcorax melanorhamphos. See white-winged chough
Corthylus columbianus 308
Corthylus zulmae 308
Corvus corax. See raven
Corvus corone. See carrion crow
Corvus frugilegus. See rook
Corvus macrorhynchos. See large-billed crow
Corvus monedula. See jackdaw
cotton-top tamarin 149
Cottus gobio. See river bullhead
Coturnix japonica. See Japanese quail
coyote 269
crested tit 266
Crotophaga ani. See smooth-billed ani
Crotophaga major. See greater ani
Crotophaga sulcirostris. See groove-billed ani
Ctenochaetus striatus. See striated surgeonfish
Ctenodactylus gundi. See gundi
cuckoo catfish 281, 288
Cuculus canorus. See common cuckoo
Cyanocitta cristata. See blue jay
Cyanocorax morio. See brown jay
Cynictis penicillata. See yellow mongoose
Cyrtocara pleurostigmoides 288

Dactylopus ceylonicus. See mealybug
Damaraland mole-rat 119
damselfish 273
dark-eyed junco 39
Darwin's ground finch 267
Dascyllus aruanus. See humbug damselfish
deer 42, 153

deer mouse 270
Delphinapterus leucas. See beluga whale
Dendroplatypus impar 308
Desmodus rotundus. See common vampire bat
Dicrurus adsimilis. See fork-tailed drongo
Dinotopterus cunningtoni 278
dog 81, 140, 153, 155–159
Doliopygus dubius 308
dolphin 82, 153
Dorylus wilverthi. See driver ant
driver ant 69
Drosophila melanogaster. See fruit fly
dung fly 43
dunnock 75
dusky-footed woodrat 188
dwarf mongoose 61, 141, 153, 185

Egyptian fruit bat 152
El Oro parakeet 241
Elassoma spp. See pygmy sunfish
emerald coral goby 75, 110–111
Enophrys bison. See buffalo sculpin
Equus caballus. See horse
Equus quagga. See zebra
Escherichia coli 293
Etheostoma flabellare. See fantail darter
Etheostoma olmstedi. See tessellated darter
Ethiopian wolf 285, 286
Eulemur fulvus. See common brown lemur
Eulemur rufifrons. See red-fronted lemur
Eurasian hobby 276
European bee-eater 185
European earwig 57
eusocial hymenoptera 181, 298, 303
eusocial insects 68–69, 118, 123, 192, 242–243,
    249, 297, 302, 307, 318
evening bat 49, 222

Falco columbarius. See merlin
Falco naumanni. See lesser kestrel
Falco peregrinus. See peregrine falcon
Falco subbeteo. See Eurasian hobby
fantail darter 233
fathead minnow 233
Ficedula hypoleuca. See pied flycatcher
field vole 280
fieldfare 276
fig wasp 95, 224
fighting fish 156
Florida scrub jay 185–186, 236
Forficula auricularia. See European earwig
fork-tailed drongo 51
Foudia sechellarum. See Seychelles fody
Fregata minor. See great frigatebird
Fringilla coelebs. See chaffinch
fruit fly 189, 218
Fukomys damarensis. See Damaraland mole-rat

Galápagos hawk 186
Galápagos mockingbird 185, 190
garibaldi 233
Gasterosteus aculeatus. See threespine stickleback
gelada monkey 160, 285
Geospiza spp. See Darwin's ground finch
Geospiza fortis. See medium ground finch
Geospiza fuliginosa. See small ground finch
Geospiza scandens. See common cactus finch
Geospiza magnirostris. See large ground finch
Geronticus eremita. See northern bald ibis
giant moray eel 291
Giraffa camelopardalis. See giraffe
giraffe 153
Globicephala macrorhynchus. See short-finned
    pilot whale
Globicephala melas. See pilot whale
goby 111, 286
goldcrest 266
Gorilla gorilla. See western gorilla
goshawk 198
great frigatebird 226
great gerbil 188
great tit 50, 148, 160, 188, 271
greater ani 85
greater crested tern 280
greater honeyguide 289
greater mouse-eared bat 160
green woodhoopoe 141, 148, 186
grey-cheeked mangabey 150
grey-crowned babbler 188
groove-billed ani 82
ground tit 84, 194
ground-hopper 273
grouper 291
Gryllidae 53
Gryllus 53
guira cuckoo 188
Guira guira. See guira cuckoo
gundi 188
guppy 53, 147, 156, 160, 188
Gymnorhina tibicen. See Australian magpie
Gymnorhinus cyamocephalus. See pinyon jay
Gymnothorax javanicus. See giant moray eel

harlequin bass 148
Harpagifer bispinis. See Antarctic plunder fish
Helogale parvula. See dwarf mongoose
herb-field mouse 152
hermit crab 41
Hetaerina damselflies 272
Heterocephalus glaber. See naked mole-rat
Homo neanderthalensis 322
Homo sapiens. See human
honeybee 84–85
hornyhead chub 276
horse 153

house mouse 86, 185, 286
house sparrows 50
hover wasp 78–79, 133
human 20, 59–70, 89, 96, 118–128, 154–158, 168–175, 286–291, 321–326
humbug damselfish 202
hummingbird 37
hyaena 82
Hybopsis biguttata. See hornyhead chub
Hylobates lar. See white-handed gibbon
Hypoplectrus nigricans. See black hamlet
Hypsypops rubicundus. See garibaldi

Icterus galbula bullockii. See Bullock's oriole
impala 153, 160
Indicator indicator. See greater honeyguide

jackdaw 149
Jamaican fruit-eating bat 152, 222
Japanese macaque 120, 151
Japanese quail 221, 276
Julidochromis 262
Junco hyemalis. See dark-eyed junco

Karoo scrub-robin 188, 193
kea 237
killer whale 96, 325
king penguin 160
Kribensis cichlid 147

Labroides dimidiatus. See cleaner wrasse
Lake Tanganyika cichlid 186, 188, 201, 228, 236, 274
Lamprologini 262
Lamprologus brichardi 251, 255
Lamprologus callipterus 230–231
Lamprotornis superbus. See superb starling
lance-tailed manakin 198
large ground finch 268, 270
large-billed crow 149
large-billed tern 276
Lepidiolamprologus attenuates 277
Lepidiolamprologus elongates 253–254
Lepidiolamprologus 262
Lepomis macrochirus. See bluegill sunfish
Lepus americanus. See snowshoe hare, *See* brown hare
lesser kestrel 188
lichen 143
Linepithema humile 127
lion 82, 95, 99, 140, 161, 194–204
Liostenogaster flaveolina 133
Liostenogaster flavolineata. See hover wasp
Litoria peronei. See Peron's tree frog
Lonchura punctulata. See spice finches
long-tailed macaque 87, 150
long-tailed manakin 199

long-tailed tit 185, 192, 194, 202, 205–207, 209
Lophocebus albigena. See grey-cheeked mangabey
Lycaon pictus. See African wild dog
lynx 42
Lynx lynx. See lynx
Lyrurus tetrix. See black grouse

Macaca arctoides. See stump-tailed macaque
Macaca assamensis. See Assamese macaque
Macaca fascicularis. See long-tailed macaque
Macaca fuscata. See Japanese macaque
Macaca mulatta. See rhesus macaque
Macaca radiata. See bonnet macaque
Macaca sylvanus. See barbary macaque
Macaca thibetana. See Tibetan macaque
mackerel 46–47
macrotermites 243
Macrotermitinae 297
Malurus cyaneus. See superb fairy-wren
Malurus splendens. See splendid fairy-wren
Manacus manacus. See white-bearded manakin
mandrill 151
Mandrillus sphinx. See mandrill
Manorina malanophrys. See bell miner
mantis shrimp 115
mealybug 131
medium ground finch 268
meerkat 51–92, 119, 141, 152, 178–186, 205–212, 234–241
Melanerpes formicivorus. See acorn woodpecker
Meleagris gallopavo. See wild turkey
merlin 276
Merops apiaster. See European bee-eater
Merops bullockoides. See white-fronted bee-eater
Mexican jay 186, 236
Microtus agrestis. See field vole
Monodon monocerus. See narwhal
moose 160
mound-building mouse 188
mountain bluebird 95
mourning cuttlefish 51
mouthbrooding cichlids 281
Mungos mungo. See banded mongoose
Mus domestica. See house mouse
Mus spicilegus. See mound-building mouse
Mustela erminea. See stoat
mycophagous beetle 189
mycorrhiza 143
Myodes glareolus. See bank vole
Myotis bechsteinii. See Bechstein's bat
Myotis myotis. See greater mouse-eared bat
Myotis septentrionalis 222

naked mole-rat 119, 244
narwhal 322
Nasua nasua. See coati
Neetroplus nematopus 284

Neogonodactylus bredini. See mantis shrimp
Neolamprologus obscurus 245
Neolamprologus pulcher. See cooperative cichlid
Neolamprologus tetracanthus 274–275
Neotoma fuscipes. See dusky-footed woodrat
Nesomimus parvulus. See Galápagos mockingbird
Nestor notabilis. See kea
Nicaragua cichlid 283
Nicrophorus vespilloides. See burying beetle
North American beaver 188
Northern bald ibis 148
Northern paper wasp 245
Norway rat 146, 152, 155–158, 165–171, 211, 286, 315
Notropis cornutus. See common shiner
Nycticeius humeralis. See evening bat
Nymphicus hollandicus. See cockatiel

ocellated wrasse 86, 147, 317
Octodon degus. See common degu
Oecophylla. See weaver ant
Oncorhynchus tshawytscha. See Chinook salmon
Oncorynchus kisutch. See coho salmon
Ophryotrocha diadema. See polychaete worm
orange clownfish 75, 202
orangutan 120, 151
Orcinus orca. See killer whale
oxpecker 287

Paguroidea. See hermit crab
Pan paniscus. See bonobo
Pan troglodytes. See chimpanzee
Panthera leo. See lion
paper wasp 72, 78, 80–81, 85, 110, 115, 130–135, 186
Papio cynocephalus. See baboon
Paracatenula 264
Paragobiodon xanthosomus. See emerald coral goby
Paranthropus robustus 322
Parulidae. See American wood warblers
Parus ater. See coal tit
Parus cristatus. See crested tit
Parus humilis. See ground tit
Parus major. See great tit
Parus montanus. See willow tit
Passer domesticus 50
Pavo cristatus. See peafowl
peafowl 196
Pelecanus erythrorhynchos. See American white pelican
Pelvicachromis pulcher. See Kribensis cichlid
Pelvicachromis taeniatus 227–228
Pemphigus obesinymphase. See social aphid
peregrine falcon 276
Perisoreus infaustus. See Siberian jay
Perissodus microlepis 277

Peromyscus maniculatus. See deer mouse
Peron's tree frog 226
Petrochelidon pyrrhonota. See cliff swallow
Phaetusa simplex. See large-billed tern
Phalacrus substriatus. See mycophagous beetle
Philetairus socius. See sociable weaver
Philomachus pugnax. See ruff
Phoeniculus purpureus. See green woodhoopoe
Phyllastrephus cabanisis. See Cabanis's greenbuls
Phyllostomus hastatus 222
Pica nuttali. See yellow-billed magpie
Picoides borealis. See red-cockaded woodpecker
pied babbler 11, 50, 51, 90, 294
pied flycatcher 148
pied kingfisher 75, 186–187
pigeon 47
pilot whale 188
Pimephales promelas. See fathead minnow
pinyon jay 185
Pipra filicauda. See wire-tailed manakins
platypodid 298, 307
Platypodinae 297
Plectropomus leopardus. See coral trout
Plectropomus pessuliferus. See grouper
Plectropous arealoatus. See squaretail coral grouper
Poecilia reticulata. See guppy
polar bear 69, 188
Polistes chinensis 85
Polistes dominula. See paper wasp
Polistes fuscatus. See Northern paper wasp
Polistes semenowi 72
Polistes versicolor 240
polistine wasp 79
Polybia occidentalis 240
polychaete worm 173, 179
polyembryonic wasp 185
Polyrhachis 303
Pomacentrus. See damselfish
Pomatostomus ruficeps. See chestnut-crowned babbler
Pomatostomus temporalis. See grey-crowned babbler
Pongo pygmaeus. See orangutan
Porphyrio porphyrio. See pukeko
Princess of Lake Tanganyika 147, 214, 251, 255, 262
Procyon lotor. See raccoon
Prunella modularis. See dunnock
Pseudomonas aeruginosa 222–223, 240
Psittacus erithacus. See African grey parrot
pukeko 82
pygmy sunfish 39
Pyrrhura orcesi. See El Oro parakeet

rabbitfish 147
raccoon 286
Ramphocinclus rachyurus. See white-breasted thrasher

Rangifer tarandus. See reindeer
Rattus norvegicus. See Norway rat
raven 49, 149
red fire ant 210
red flour beetle 189
red fox 269
red squirrel 207
red-backed vole 270
red-breasted geese 276
red-cockaded woodpecker 73, 186, 214
redfronted lemur 75, 149, 194
red-winged blackbird 149
reed warbler 282–283
Regulus regulus. See goldcrest
reindeer 153
rhesus macaque 53, 151
Rhombomys opimus. See great gerbil
Rhynchonycteris naso 222
rifleman 186
river bullhead 233
rook 149
Ropalidia marginata. See social wasp
round-tailed ground squirrel 185, 197
Rousettus aegyptiacus. See Egyptian fruit bat
ruddy turnstone 39
ruff 201
Rynchops niger. See black skimmer

Saccopteryx bilineata 222
Saguinus oedipus. See Saguinus oedipus
Salmo salar. See Atlantic salmon
Sancassania berleisei 57
sand-coloured nighthawk 276
Scarus croicensis. See striped parrotfish
Scathophaga stercoraria. See dung fly
Scolytinae 297
Scombridae. See mackerel
sea anemone 98
Sepia plangon. See mourning cuttlefish
Sericornis frontalis. See white-browed scrubwren
Serranus subligarius. See belted sandfish
Serranus tabacarius. See tobaccofish
Serranus tigrinus. See harlequin bass
Serranus tortugarum. See chalk bass
Seychelles fody 31
Seychelles warbler 25–34, 54, 88, 185, 189–192, 204–216, 235–238
short-finned pilot whale 96
short-tailed fruit bat 49
Sialia currucoides. See mountain bluebird
Sialia mexicana. See western bluebird
Siberian jay 185, 196–197, 215
side-blotched lizards 210
Siganus corallinus. See rabbitfish
Sinosuthora webbiana. See vinous-throated parrotbill
Sitta pusilla. See brown-headed nuthatch

slave-making ant 212
small ground finch 268
smooth-billed ani 84
snowshoe hare 269
sociable weaver 73, 91, 185, 188
social aphid 96
social cichlid *See* cooperative cichlid
social wasp 238
Solenopsis invicta. See red fire ant
Somateria mollissima. See common eider
sooty mangabey 150, 186
spadefoot toad 273
sparrowhawk 198
Spea bombifrons. See spadefoot toad
Spea multiplicata 273
Spermophilus beldingi. See Belding's ground squirrel
Spermophilus parryii. See Arctic ground squirrel
Spermophilus tereticaudus. See round-tailed ground squirrel
sphynx blenny 233
spice finches 50
spider monkey 39
spinynose sculpin 281
splendid fairy wren 84
spotted eagle ray 188
squaretail coral grouper 188
Stenella coeruleoalba. See striped dolphin
Sterna superciliari. See yellow-billed tern
stoat 280
striated surgeonfish 288
stripe-backed wren 30, 149, 186, 188
striped dolphin 188
striped parrotfish 59
Struthidea cinerea. See apostlebird
stump-tailed macaque 150
superb fairy-wren 73, 75, 149, 185, 188, 190–193, 205, 214
superb starling 87
Suricata suricatta. See meerkat
Symphodus ocellatus. See ocellated wrasse
Synodontis multipunctatus. See cuckoo catfish

Taeniopygia guttata. See zebra finch
Tasmanian native hen 75, 194, 199
Tasmiasciurus hudsonicus. See red squirrel
Telmatochromis vittatus 231
tessellated darter 179, 231
Tetrao urogallus. See capercaillie
Tetrix ceperoi 273
Tetrix subulata 273
Thalasseus bernsteini. See Chinese crested tern
Thalassoma bifasciatum. See bluehead wrasse
Thallasseus bergii. See greater crested tern
Theropithecus gelada. See gelada monkey
three-spined stickleback 47, 148, 179, 231, 233

Thyroptera tricolor 222
Tibetan macaque 151
tobaccofish 148
Trachyostus ghanaensis 308
Tribolium castaneum. See red flour beetle
Tribonyx mortierii. See Tasmanian native hen
Trochilidae. See hummingbirds
tufted capuchin 150
Turdoides bicolor 11
Turdus pilar. See fieldfare
Tyto alba. See barn owl

Uria aalge. See common guillemot
Urocitellus columbianus. See Columbian ground
    squirrel
Ursus maritimus. See polar bear
Uta stansburiana. See side-blotched lizard

vampire bat 152, 161, 163, 166, 173–174, 315
vervet monkey 126, 150
Vibrio bacteria 69
vinous-throated parrotbill 188, 194
Vulpes vulpes. See red fox

waterfowl 195
weaver ant 303
western bluebird 95, 186, 190, 214
western gorilla 194
white fronted bee-eater 185
white-bearded manakin 188, 196
white-breasted thrasher 188, 193

white-browed scrubwren 185–186
white-faced capuchin 150
white-fronted bee-eater 190
white-handed gibbon 151
white-throated magpie-jays 188
white-winged chough 11, 149, 186, 188, 194, 212
wild turkey 196, 202
willow tit 266
wire-tailed manakins 226
Wolbachia 300
wolf 42, 121
woodpigeon 276

Xyleborini 298
Xyleborinus saxesenii 298–299. *See* ambrosia
    beetle
Xyleborus affinis 305
Xylosandrus germanus 298. *See* ambrosia beetle

yellow mongoose 188
yellow-billed magpie 275
yellow-billed tern 276
Yuhina 84
Yuhina brunneiceps. See yuhina

zebra 7, 149, 173, 287
zebra finch 7, 149, 173
zebrafish 39, 42
Zenaida aurita. See Zenaida dove
Zenaida dove 39–40
zooxanthellae 69, 143, 178